Handbook of Neuroendocrinology

Handbook of Neuroendocrinology

Editor: Cooper Grant

MURPHY & MOORE
www.murphy-moorepublishing.com

www.murphy-moorepublishing.com

MURPHY & MOORE

Cataloging-in-Publication Data

Handbook of neuroendocrinology / edited by Cooper Grant.
p. cm.
Includes bibliographical references and index.
ISBN 978-1-63987-291-6
1. Neuroendocrinology. 2. Neurohormones. 3. Neurology. 4. Endocrinology. I. Grant, Cooper.
QP356.4 .H36 2022
612.8--dc23

Murphy & Moore Publishing,
1 Rockefeller Plaza,
New York City, NY 10020, USA

ISBN 978-1-63987-291-6 (Hardback)

Contents

Preface

The functional and anatomical interactions between the endocrine system and the nervous system are studied under the field of neuroendocrinology. The neuroendocrine system is responsible for maintaining homeostasis, and managing reproduction, eating and drinking behavior, metabolism, energy utilization, and blood pressure. The advances in neuroendocrinology are essential to the study and management of neurobiological brain disorders. The endocrine system is made up of several glands which are responsible for the production and secretion of different hormones. The hypothalamus is an integral part of the neuroendocrine system. It connects the nervous system to the endocrine system through the pituitary gland. The pituitary gland consists of two portions, the anterior pituitary gland and the posterior pituitary gland. This book unravels the recent studies in the field of neuroendocrinology. It presents researches and studies performed by experts across the globe. Researchers and students in this field will be assisted by this book.

This book unites the global concepts and researches in an organized manner for a comprehensive understanding of the subject. It is a ripe text for all researchers, students, scientists or anyone else who is interested in acquiring a better knowledge of this dynamic field.

I extend my sincere thanks to the contributors for such eloquent research chapters. Finally, I thank my family for being a source of support and help.

Editor

1

Receptor oligomerization: from early evidence to current understanding in class B GPCRs

Stephanie Y. L. Ng, Leo T. O. Lee and Billy K. C. Chow*

Endocrinology, School of Biological Sciences, The University of Hong Kong, Hong Kong, China

Edited by:
Hubert Vaudry, University of Rouen, France

Reviewed by:
Ralf Jockers, University of Paris, France
Pedro A. Jose, Georgetown University, USA

***Correspondence:**
Billy K. C. Chow, Endocrinology, School of Biological Sciences, The University of Hong Kong, Pokfulam Road, Hong Kong, China.
e-mail: bkcc@hku.hk

Dimerization or oligomerization of G protein-coupled receptors (GPCRs) are known to modulate receptor functions in terms of ontogeny, ligand-oriented regulation, pharmacological diversity, signal transduction, and internalization. Class B GPCRs are receptors to a family of hormones including secretin, growth hormone-releasing hormone, vasoactive intestinal polypeptide and parathyroid hormone, among others. The functional implications of receptor dimerization have extensively been studied in class A GPCRs, while less is known regarding its function in class B GPCRs. This article reviews receptor oligomerization in terms of the early evidence and current understanding particularly of class B GPCRs.

Keywords: GPCR, class B, secretin receptor, oligomerization, BRET

INTRODUCTION

G protein-coupled receptors (GPCRs) comprise the largest subset of cell surface receptors which transduce signals via coupling to heterotrimeric G proteins and are extensively involved in the fine-tuning of physiological processes. They constitute at least 3% of the human genome and have great pathophysiological importance with an abundance of information indicating their dysfunction to be associated with diseases such as diabetes, visual disability, and chronic inflammation. As a result, at least 30–40% of pharmaceutical drugs developed are targeted at GPCRs. Traditionally, GPCRs were recognized to elicit physiological responses via coupling as monomeric units to G proteins in a 1:1 stoichiometric ratio. However there is now a growing body of evidence confirming that GPCRs can self-associate or associate with different receptors to form homo-and/or hetero-oligomers. With the wealth of information recently discovered, oligomerization has been implicated to play important roles in maturation, cell surface delivery, signaling, and internalization of GPCRs. The concept of oligomerization is groundbreaking as it not only widens our perspective in understanding the molecular determinants to receptor regulation and function, but also provides new opportunities in the development of personalized drug treatments. In recent years, the small 15-member class B [secretin (SCT) or class II] GPCRs are emerging as oligomerization candidates with efforts contributed predominantly by Laurence Miller's and Dominik Schelshorn's groups. In this article, we will provide an overview of the history of oligomerization and review the available information on class B GPCRs and its functional implications.

EARLY EVIDENCE OF GPCR DIMERIZATION BY PHARMACOLOGICAL AND BIOCHEMICAL APPROACHES

Although GPCR oligomerization is now a widely accepted phenomenon with modern non-radiative techniques such as resonance energy transfer (RET) strategies that are effective in demonstrating homo- and/or hetero-oligomer interactions, early clues to their existence were often indirect and overlooked. In 1975, a binding experiment of a potent antagonist to β_2-adrenergic receptors (ADRB2) in frog erythrocyte membranes led to findings of negative cooperativity among binding sites (Limbird et al., 1975; Limbird and Lefkowitz, 1976). This was pioneering evidence for oligomerization and can be better explained as site–site interactions amongst ADRB2 oligomers based on today's knowledge. Soon after, radiation inactivation, cross-linking and co-immunoprecipitation studies have also provided biochemical evidence complementing earlier observations of oligomerization. For example, immunoaffinity chromatography and sodium dodecyl sulfate-polyacrylamide gel electrophoresis (SDS-PAGE) showed the subunit molecular weight of mammalian lung ADRB2 to be 59 kDa, while radiation inactivation of ADRB2 resulted in a functional subunit molecular weight of 109 kDa (Fraser and Venter, 1982). Taken together, the contrasting molecular sizes indicate that ADRB2s exist in the membrane as dimers of two subunits (Fraser and Venter, 1982). Similar suggestions have also been made for the rat liver membrane α_1-adrenergic receptor (ADRA1; Venter et al., 1984) and human platelet α_2-adrenergic receptor (ADRA2; Venter et al., 1983) which each have molecular masses of 160 kDa. Alternatively, cross-linking experiments, using photoaffinity labeling reagents, cell permeable cross-linkers, agonists, and antagonists (Capponi and Catt, 1980; Paglin and Jamieson, 1982; Guillemette and Escher, 1983; Rogers, 1984; Carson et al., 1987; Rondeau et al., 1990; Siemens et al., 1991) have been used to study the dimeric nature of angiotensin II (ANGII) receptors. Using similar methods, other GPCRs such as the dopamine D_2 (Ng et al., 1996), calcium-sensing (Bai et al., 1998), and chemokine (Rodriguez-Frade et al., 1999) receptors have also been demonstrated to exist as dimeric units. Other experiments such as photoaffinity labeling of MRs from various brain regions and the heart have also provided evidence for the presence of inter convertible dimers and tetramers (Avissar et al., 1983). The idea of higher order oligomerization was further supported by comparable findings of thyrotropin hormone receptor complexes (Gennick et al., 1987).

In the 1990s, another line of evidence demonstrating GPCR oligomerization stemmed from *trans*-complementation, and dominant-negative and -positive effect studies on co-expression of chimeric and mutant receptor constructs. One of the first experiments of these series was performed in 1993 by co-expression of chimeric muscarinic and adrenergic receptors composed of their C-terminal units (Maggio et al., 1993). Although no binding activity was detected when the chimeras were expressed individually, co-expression restored ligand binding to a level comparable to wild-type receptors and allowed agonist-dependent phospholipase C (PLC) activation (Maggio et al., 1993). These observations were explained as molecular interaction of the chimeras restoring functionality in a heteromeric complex (Maggio et al., 1993). Other *trans*-complementation studies for GPCRs such as the ANGII type 1a (AGTR1a; Monnot et al., 1996), somatostatin (SST – SST_1 and SST_5; Rocheville et al., 2000) and dopamine (D_2 and D_3; Scarselli et al., 2001) receptors have also provided useful information in support of GPCR oligomerization. This concept was further explored in experiments showing dominant-negative or -positive effects such those observed with the antidiuretic V2 vasopressin (Zhu and Wess, 1998) and ADRB2 (Hebert et al., 1998), respectively. Although there are reports of different functional effects, the various studies described are useful in offering more clues to molecular interactions amongst GPCRs.

Though earlier experiments provided a large pool of information suggesting GPCR oligomerization, there was still no direct evidence to support this concept. Early western blot studies often showed presence of immuno-reactive bands with molecular masses two or more times greater than a single receptor (Harrison and van der Graaf, 2006). Western blot was later performed in combination with immunoprecipitation using antibodies to endogenous or epitope tagged-receptors, providing for the first time direct evidence of GPCR interaction. Using this technique, homodimerization of ADRB2 (Hebert et al., 1996) was demonstrated. For example, cross-species oligomerization was also detected in select serotonin receptors with lysophosphatidic acid receptors 1 and 3 and γ-aminobutyric acid B_2 receptors (Salim et al., 2002), dopamine D_1 and D_2 receptors (Lee et al., 2004), and α_{1b} and β_2 adrenergic receptors (Uberti et al., 2005).

RET APPROACH IN GPCR OLIGOMERIZATION

Since the days of radioactive inactivation experiments, the concept of GPCR oligomerization has been confirmed with emergence of biophysical data providing more in-depth evidence. In the last decade, RET techniques have gained popularity and are one of the best resolution strategies developed for direct study of GPCR interactions. The basis of these techniques lies in non-radiative energy transfer from an excited "donor" molecule to an "acceptor" (Wu and Brand, 1994). Bioluminescence RET (BRET) and fluorescence RET (FRET) are two of the most widely used RET approaches. BRET relies on a naturally occurring biophysical process in marine species between a luminescent donor and fluorescent acceptor, while only fluorescent molecules are utilized in FRET (Wu and Brand, 1994). These have provided advantages over traditional biochemical methods including high signal to noise ratios, use of intact cells, precise targeting of fusion receptors and actual quantification of the proportion and type of GPCR oligomers formed, and therefore are currently the most commonly used methods. Based on these approaches, a wide range of GPCRs have since been identified to function as oligomers, including the yeast α-factor (Overton and Blumer, 2000), dopamine D_2 (Wurch et al., 2001), thyrotropin (Latif et al., 2001, 2002), opioid (Ramsay et al., 2002), neuropeptide Y (Dinger et al., 2003), melatonin (Ayoub et al., 2004), adrenergic (Mercier et al., 2002; Ramsay et al., 2002; Carrillo et al., 2004), and chemokine (Percherancier et al., 2005) receptors. Despite the successes in identifying various oligomers, there are several drawbacks of the BRET and FRET techniques. With regards to these aforementioned RET techniques, a primary concern is that the signals generated cannot be used to discriminate between non-mature and mature proteins within the various cellular locations (e.g., intracellular complexes and plasma membrane; Gandia et al., 2008; Cottet et al., 2011). Therefore, the information provided is essentially limited and more steps may be needed to address this concern. Moreover, another drawback of BRET and FRET is potential bleed-through artifacts which may be due to spectral overlaps, substrate instability, and auto-luminescence from serum containing medium, which together skew the interpretation of the results (Pfleger et al., 2006; Gandia et al., 2008). Therefore, the careful use of appropriate controls and fluorescent molecules need to be considered when using these RET techniques for the study of oligomerization. More recently, homogeneous time-resolved fluorescence (HTRF) which combines FRET with time-resolved measurements has also been considered. HTRF provides the advantage of increasing assay sensitivity and accuracy via replacing donor molecules with rare-earth lanthanides (e.g., europium cryptate) whose properties include non-auto-fluorescence and long emission half-lives (Degorce et al., 2009). Using HTRF, a number of receptors have been identified to dimerize, e.g., GABA (Maurel et al., 2004) and metabotropic glutamate-like receptors (Rondard et al., 2006; Brock et al., 2007) and oligomerize, e.g., dopamine D_2 (Guo et al., 2008) and histamine H4 (Albizu et al., 2006) receptors. Fluorescence life-time imaging microscopy (FLIM) is also useful in overcoming the drawback of the use of intact cells and bleed-through in BRET and FRET assays. Moreover, FLIM can also provide useful information on the proportion of non-dimerizing and dimerizing partners and also visual images indicating where the signals are localized, for example the dimerization of the transcription factor CCAAT and enhancer binding protein-α in live mouse pituitary cell nuclei (Sun et al., 2011).

OLIGOMERIZATION OF CLASS B GPCRs

Although techniques in studying oligomerization have existed for more than three decades, information with regards to the class B GPCRs is still in its infancy and largely contributed by the newer RET techniques. In class A GPCRs, several important interfaces including the transmembrane (TM) domains have been identified to contribute toward oligomerization. Moreover, oligomerization has also been shown to play a role in modulating function, via altering parameters such as ligand binding, signaling, and trafficking. Though the SCT receptor (SCTR) remains to be the most extensively studied class B GPCR, information regarding other class B

GPCRs continues to grow. Collectively, the SCT superfamily of hormones and receptors represent important drug targets due to their physiological roles in glucose homeostasis, feeding behavior, and vascular contractility. They are characterized by a large N-terminal extracellular domain (ECD) containing six cysteine residues for disulfide bond formation and *N*-glycosylation sites for receptor conformation and ligand binding. The N-terminal ectodomain is linked to seven hydrophobic TM domains arranged in α-helical bundles connected by three exoloops, three endoloops, and a short cytosolic C-terminus (Miller et al., 2007). Currently, there are intense efforts to link the various structural domains to oligomerization in hopes of unraveling the specific molecular determinants that may affect certain pathological conditions. Taken together, information regarding the oligomerization of class B GPCRs will be highly valuable in enhancing the specificity of future drug design.

SECRETIN RECEPTORS

The SCTR was first cloned from the rat in 1991 (Ishihara et al., 1991) and is now recognized as one of the most extensively studied class B GPCRs, and the first that was demonstrated to have the ability to form oligomers. By investigating wild-type and exon-3 splice variants using confocal imaging and BRET, SCTR has been shown to be capable of homo- and heterodimerization (Ding et al., 2002a,b; **Tables 1 and 2**). When expressed alone, the exon-3 splice variant receptors lack SCT binding and signaling activity but are able to traffic normally to the cell surface. However, co-expression of the variant with the wild-type SCT results in a dominant-negative effect, indicating direct physical interaction. Since the variant receptor is predominantly expressed, comprising up to 70% of SCTRs in gastrinoma, over the wild-type receptor, heterodimerization has been suggested to be an underlying factor in facilitating tumor growth through its dominant-negative effects.

Table 1 | Homodimerization of class B GPCRs.

Homodimer	Technique	Key domain	Reference
SCTR/SCTR	Morphological FRET BRET	GxxxG motif independent Lipid-exposed TM4 residues (human: Gly^{243}, Ile^{247})	Ding et al. (2002a), Harikumar et al. (2006, 2007, 2008a), Lisenbee and Miller (2006)
GCGR/GCGR	BRET	n/a	Roed et al. (2012), Schelshorn et al. (2012)
GLP1R/GLP1R	BRET	n/a	Schelshorn et al. (2012), Whitaker et al. (2012)
GLP2R/GLP2R	BRET	n/a	Schelshorn et al. (2012)
GIPR/GIPR	BRET	n/a	Schelshorn et al. (2012), Whitaker et al. (2012)
VIPR1/ VIPR1	Immunohistochemistry Co-immunoprecipitation Morphological FRET BRET	n/a	Harikumar et al. (2006)
VIPR2/VIPR2	Morphological FRET BRET	n/a	Harikumar et al. (2006)
ADCYAP1R1/ADCYAP1R1	Time-resolved FRET	n/a	Maurel et al. (2008)
GHRHR/GHRHR	Co-immunoprecipitation		McElvaine and Mayo (2006)
PTHR1/PTHR1	Crystallography FRET BRET	ECD α-helix (human: Ile^{135}, Arg^{179}, Val^{183}, Leu^{187})	Pioszak et al. (2010)
CALCR/CALCR	Co-immunoprecipitation FRET BRET	Lipid-exposed TM4 residues (human: Arg^{236}, Val^{250}, Thr^{253}) C-terminal tail	Seck et al. (2003), Harikumar et al. (2010)
CALCRL/CALCRL	Co-immunoprecipitation FRET BRET	n/a	Heroux et al. (2007)
CRHR1/CRHR1	FRET BRET	Pseudo signal peptide (based on rat CRHR2a: Asn^{13} prevents oligomerization)	Kraetke et al. (2005), Young et al. (2007), Teichmann et al. (2012)

Techniques used for study and domains indicated to be important are described. SCTR, secretin receptor; GCGR, glucagon receptor; GLP1R, glucagon-like peptide 1 receptor; GLP2R, glucagon-like peptide 2 receptor; GIPR, glucose-dependent insulinotropic polypeptide receptor; VIPR1, vasoactive intestinal peptide (VIP) receptor 1; VIPR2, VIP receptor 2; ADCYAP1R1, PACAP type 1 receptor; GHRHR, growth hormone-releasing hormone receptor; PTHR1, parathyroid hormone receptor type 1; CALCR, calcitonin receptor; CALCRL, CALCR-like receptor; CRHR, corticotropin-releasing hormone receptor; FRET, fluorescence resonance energy transfer; BRET, bioluminescence resonance energy transfer; n/a, information not available.

Table 2 | Heterodimerization of class B GPCRs.

Heterodimer	Technique	Key domain	Reference
SCTR/GLP1R	BRET	n/a	Harikumar et al. (2008b)
SCTR/GLP2R	BRET	n/a	Harikumar et al. (2008b)
SCTR/VIPR1	Morphological FRET BRET	n/a	Harikumar et al. (2006, 2008b)
SCTR/VIPR2	Morphological FRET BRET	n/a	Harikumar et al. (2006, 2008b)
SCTR/GHRHR	BRET	n/a	Harikumar et al. (2008b)
SCTR/PTHR1	BRET	n/a	Harikumar et al. (2008b)
SCTR/PTHR2	BRET	n/a	Harikumar et al. (2008b)
SCTR/CALCRL	BRET	n/a	Harikumar et al. (2008b)
GCGR/GLP1R	BRET	n/a	Roed et al. (2012), Schelshorn et al. (2012)
GCGR/GLP2R	BRET	n/a	Schelshorn et al. (2012)
GCGR/GIPR	BRET	n/a	Schelshorn et al. (2012)
GLP1R/GIPR	BRET	n/a	Schelshorn et al. (2012), Whitaker et al. (2012)
GLP2R/GIPR	BRET	n/a	Schelshorn et al. (2012)
VIPR1/VIPR2	Co-immunoprecipitation BRET	n/a	Harikumar et al. (2006)

Techniques used for study are described.

This study in 2002 was a breakthrough for class B GPCRs, showing the first physiological relevance of class B GPCR oligomerization. Taken together with data from subsequent studies, SCTR homodimerization is now recognized to occur, independent of ligand binding (Ding et al., 2002a; Harikumar et al., 2006).

To decipher the molecular determinants of oligomerization, receptors with mutated N- and C- terminal domains were studied (Lisenbee and Miller, 2006). Mutant receptors, as expected, were unable to bind SCT or sort efficiently to the plasma membrane, but the ability to still produce BRET signals above background suggested that the TM spanning core alone was sufficient for oligomerization (Lisenbee and Miller, 2006). Moreover, SCTR dimerization was also found to be independent of the GxxxG helix–helix motif (Lisenbee and Miller, 2006), which is essential for oligomerization of class A receptors, such as the yeast α-factor (Overton et al., 2003) and β_2 adrenergic (Salahpour et al., 2004) receptors. In addition, FRET signals within organelles of the receptor biosynthetic pathway including the endoplasmic reticulum, Golgi clusters, and plasma membrane were also detected, suggesting the occurrence of oligomerization even during the maturation of nascent molecules (Lisenbee and Miller, 2006). To further explore the domains responsible for homodimerization, TM peptide competition experiments have been performed. Of the seven TM peptides applied, TM4 was the only segment that disrupted BRET signals, suggesting it to be a functionally important interface for oligomerization (Harikumar et al., 2007). Using alanine mutagenesis, the contribution of TM4 in SCTR oligomers was pinpointed to two lipid-facing residues: Gly^{243} and Ile^{247} (Harikumar et al., 2007). Although no direct pathophysiological connection has been made regarding these new data, reduced signaling of monomeric forms suggests that SCTR dimers are necessary in optimizing functionality (Harikumar et al., 2007). Most recently, bimolecular luminescence complementation and BRET experiments have clarified SCTR's existence as homodimers and not higher order oligomers (Harikumar et al., 2008a). Therefore, previous references to oligomerization of SCTRs should be referred to as homodimerization unless otherwise stated. Aside from homodimers, SCTRs have also been implicated to form heterodimers with a wide range of class B GPCRs, including the glucagon-like peptide 1 receptor (GLP1R), glucagon-like peptide 2 receptor (GLP2R), vasoactive intestinal peptide receptor 1 (VIPR1), vasoactive intestinal peptide receptor 2 (VIPR2), growth hormone-releasing hormone receptor (GHRHR), parathyroid hormone 1 receptor (PTHR1), parathyroid hormone 2 receptor (PTHR2), and calcitonin receptor-like (CALCRL; Harikumar et al., 2006, 2008b; **Table 2**).

GCG, GLP1, GLP2, AND GIP RECEPTORS

Receptors for glucagon (GCG), glucagon-like peptide 1 (GLP1), glucagon-like peptide 2 (GLP2), and glucose-independent insulinotropic polypeptide (GIP) are well-known regulators of carbohydrate, fat, and protein metabolism. Oligomerization within the GCG subfamily of receptors was recently identified but with some controversy (Roed et al., 2012; Schelshorn et al., 2012). Homodimerization of each GCG family receptor member has been reported through BRET experiments (Schelshorn et al., 2012), however, these events remained unconfirmed with the lack of appropriate negative controls and the fact that another group was unable to repeat some of these results (Roed et al., 2012). Amongst the receptors, the GCG receptor (GCGR) and GIP receptor (GIPR) exhibited the strongest ability to homodimerize but BRET signals were slightly reduced upon application of GCG or GIP, while the GLP receptors were weakly responsive and unaffected by agonist stimulation (Schelshorn et al., 2012). Further studies with BRET saturation experiments confirmed GLP1R and GIPR homodimerization, with some agonist-induced reduction (Schelshorn et al., 2012). On the basis of these results, it was suggested that ligand binding leads to a decrease in affinity and conformational change of the homodimers (Schelshorn et al., 2012). In a similar study, the same BRET saturation results were obtained for the GLP1R, however no changes were observed when GLP1 was added (Roed et al., 2012). This was similarly the case for GCGRs (Roed et al., 2012). Taken together, it is highly likely that the GCG subfamily receptors are able to form homodimers (**Table 1**), while further studies with appropriate use of controls are necessary to solidify this conclusion.

Despite the controversy, heterodimerization of GLP1R and GIPR has been confirmed by BRET saturation and kinetic experiments (Roed et al., 2012; Schelshorn et al., 2012; Whitaker et al., 2012; **Table 2**). The heterodimerization event between GLP1R and GIPR was found to be dose-dependently induced by GLP1 and inhibited by GIP (Schelshorn et al., 2012). Further application of GLP1 and its antagonists to this system showed heterodimerization to occur independently to GLP1R activation, but was induced by ligand binding, with BRET signals reaching a maximum 10–30 s after addition of GLP1 (Schelshorn et al., 2012). More specifically, the heterodimers were suggested to play a role in allosteric modulation with arrestin recruitment. In basal conditions, GLP1R and GIPR are proposed to exist mainly as monomers or homodimers, GLP1, under low concentrations (<30 nM), acts as a high affinity ligand for functioning of GLP1R but switches to become a low affinity ligand to GIPR with high concentrations (>30 nM). This promotes formation of heterodimers with altered G protein coupling resulting in GIP-like activity that can later be dissociated in the presence of GIP (Schelshorn et al., 2012). Heterodimerization of GLP1R and GIPR was also confirmed by a later study with wild-type GLP1R rescuing mutant GIPR function (Whitaker et al., 2012).

VIP/PACAP RECEPTORS

To elicit physiological response, vasoactive intestinal peptide (VIP) and pituitary adenylate cyclase activating polypeptide (PACAP) bind to three receptors, namely VIPR1, VIPR2, and PACAP receptor type 1 (ADCYAP1R1). Discoveries of VIPR1 and VIPR2 homodimers were made during the study of SCTR oligomerization in 2006 (Harikumar et al., 2006; **Table 1**). These physical interactions were demonstrated by BRET experiments and found to be modulated by agonist but not antagonist binding (Harikumar et al., 2006). In the same study, BRET results also indicated that VIPR1 and VIPR2 to form hetero-oligomers and VIP binding was found to affect this association negatively (Harikumar et al., 2006; **Table 2**). Formation of these oligomeric complexes was also supported by co-immunoprecipitation studies (Langer et al., 2006). Besides formation of hetero-oligomers between the two subtypes, both VIPRs can oligomerize with SCTR. Interestingly, co-expression of SCTR with either VIPR resulted in strong intracellular FRET signals, suggesting the trapping of hetero-oligomers within organelles of the biosynthetic pathway (Harikumar et al., 2006). Since this retention occurred independent to SCT and VIP stimulation, it has been described as a regulatory step, allowing SCTR to have dominant-negative effects by inhibiting VIP's action on cells expressing both receptors (Harikumar et al., 2006). Within a physiological context, the SCT and VIPR are often co-expressed; therefore information regarding their physical interactions may provide some insights toward diseases such as pancreatic carcinoma (Estival et al., 1981; Ding et al., 2002a). Of the receptor trio, information regarding ADCYAP1R1 oligomerization is scarce with only one study indicating its homodimerization by time-resolved FRET studies (Maurel et al., 2008; **Table 1**).

GROWTH HORMONE-RELEASING HORMONE RECEPTORS

Growth hormone-releasing hormone (GHRH) is a hypothalamic peptide responsible for stimulating growth hormone release and disruption of the peptide–receptor pair often results in abnormal growth, such as dwarfism or gigantism. GHRHRs have been suggested to form oligomers, with co-expression of mutant and wild-type receptors having dominant-negative effects (McElvaine and Mayo, 2006). The physical interaction amongst GHRHRs was implied with the reduction of ligand binding ability and cyclic adenosine monophosphate (cAMP) production to 60% in presence of truncated receptors (McElvaine and Mayo, 2006). These observations were further supported by detection of both receptor forms by differentially tagged co-immunoprecipitation studies (McElvaine and Mayo, 2006). The relevance of these findings has been hypothesized in the context of pituitary adenomas for example, with preferential expression of the mutant receptor down-regulating signaling and thus modulating growth hormone release (Matsuno et al., 1999).

PARATHYROID HORMONE RECEPTORS

Parathyroid hormone receptors (PTHRs) play an important role in calcium homeostasis and bone maintenance, mediating the effects of its natural ligands parathyroid hormone (PTH) and PTH-related protein (PTHrP). In 2008 and 2009, the crystal structures of PTH and PTHrP bound human PTHR1 were determined by engineering the receptor as a readily crystallizing maltose binding protein (Pioszak and Xu, 2008; Pioszak et al., 2009). A "hot dog bun" three-layer α-β-βα fold structure was described, forming the central hydrophobic groove within which the ligands in an amphipathic helical fashion docked (Pioszak and Xu, 2008; Pioszak et al., 2009). More importantly, the crystal structures depicted ligand binding to PTHR1 ECD monomers in a 1:1 stoichiometric ratio (Pioszak and Xu, 2008; Pioszak et al., 2009). Interestingly a year later, the crystal structure of ligand-free PTHR1 showed the ECDs as dimers (Pioszak et al., 2010). These ECD dimers were formed in a similar fashion to ligand-bound PTHR1, with the C-terminal of one ECD forming α-helices to occupy the peptide-binding groove of the other (Pioszak et al., 2010). Besides crystallography, BRET and FRET experiments also supported existence of these ECD-mediated PTHR1 homodimers (Pioszak et al., 2010). To confirm the ligand-independent nature of ECD dimerization shown by the crystal structures, PTH was applied to PTHR1s in BRET studies and as predicted, led to agonist-induced dissociation of the PTHR1 homodimers (Pioszak et al., 2010). Furthermore, co-expression of mutant and wild-type ECD PTHR1s showed that monomeric units of the PTHR1 were sufficient for functionality (Pioszak et al., 2010). With the discovery of monomeric and dimeric units of PTHR1, this may be useful in understanding how the two biologically distinct peptides PTH and PTHrP are able to modulate function through binding to the same receptor (Pioszak et al., 2010).

CALCITONIN AND CORTICOTROPIN-RELEASING HORMONE RECEPTORS

Targeting mainly osteoblasts, calcitonin is important in calcium homeostasis and has anorexic and analgesic effects in the central nervous system. In a study focused on rabbit calcitonin receptors (CALCRs), homo- and heterodimers of the alternatively spliced CALCR (Δe13) and CALCR type 1a isoform (CALCR1a) were detected by co-immunoprecipitation and FRET analyses (Seck et al., 2003). Co-expression resulted in a dominant-negative effect of the splice variant Δe13 over CALCR1a, resulting in reduced CALCR1a surface expression, cAMP response, and extracellular signal-regulated kinase (ERK) phosphorylation (Seck et al., 2003). The combined data highlight the importance of CALCR1a homodimers in proper expression and functioning, and also suggest a role of Δe13 in regulating CALCR1a expression (Seck et al., 2003). In contrast, both static and saturation BRET studies on the human CALCR were found unable to form homodimers

(Harikumar et al., 2010). On the basis of SCTR studies where TM4 was identified to be an important interface (Harikumar et al., 2007), the same TM was also considered for CALCR (Harikumar et al., 2010). Comparing human and rabbit TM4 domains, only one single amino acid was found to differ between the two species, namely Arg and His at position 236, respectively (Harikumar et al., 2010). Synthetic TM4 peptides were constructed by exchange of these identified lipid-facing residues to those from respective CALCR species and human SCTR, and their application enhanced human CALCR BRET signals (Harikumar et al., 2010). Similar to the SCTR, lipid-exposed residues in TM4 are also key in facilitating homodimerization events in human CALCR (Harikumar et al., 2010). Though not studied in-depth, the closely related CALCRL has also been demonstrated to exist as homodimers (Heroux and Bouvie, 2005).

Within the class B GPCRs, the corticotropin-releasing hormone receptors (CRHRs) are the least studied. CRHRs are mediators of stress response, modulating the release of adrenocorticotropic hormone from the anterior pituitary. Two subtypes of the receptors exist, but only subtype 1 (CRHR1) has been studied for oligomerization. Data from FRET and co-immunoprecipitation studies show evidence of CRHR1 forming constitutive homodimers independent to ligand binding but their physiological relevance remains unexplored (Kraetke et al., 2005; Young et al., 2007).

FUNCTIONAL CONSEQUENCES OF OLIGOMERIZATION IN CLASS B GPCRs

Within the large superfamily of cell surface proteins, obligatory oligomerization is unique only to class C GPCRs and recognized as a prerequisite for activation and allosteric modulation (Kniazeff et al., 2011; Chun et al., 2012). However, in the case of class A and B GPCRs where oligomerization has also been established as a real event, the implications on their functions remain unresolved. This is further complicated by the fact that monomeric GPCRs are demonstrated to be independently capable of regulating signal transduction via a series of processes including the activation of G proteins (White et al., 2007; Whorton et al., 2007, 2008; Kuszak et al., 2009), kinase phosphorylation and signal "switch-off" by arrestin binding (Xu et al., 1997; Bayburt et al., 2011). To decipher the underlying functional significance, the effect of GPCR oligomerization on various functional properties needs to be examined with emphasis on class B GPCRs, as examples.

LIGAND BINDING

Ligand binding, either with an agonist or antagonist, is fundamental in activating subsequent downstream signaling cascades. Natural ligands for the class B GPCRs share common features, comprising of 25 or more amino acids and have diffuse pharmacophoric domains (Ulrich et al., 1998). Critical residues have been identified throughout the length of the peptides (Dong et al., 2011), with the N-terminus recognized as necessary for receptor binding and signaling, whilst the C-terminus contributes mainly to high affinity binding and receptor specificity. Crystallography (Sasaki et al., 1975; Parthier et al., 2007) and nuclear magnetic resonance (NMR; Grace et al., 2007; Venneti and Hewage, 2011) analyses have also been useful, elucidating the class B ligands to preferentially assume an α-helical conformation particularly in their C-terminal regions. Structure–activity studies have further implicated the specific interaction of ligand–receptor regions, with the C-terminal ligand domain first fitting into the receptor ECD peptide-binding cleft, thus facilitating the N-terminal ligand domain to associate with the receptor core helical bundle domain (Dong et al., 2004, 2008; Mann et al., 2007; Parthier et al., 2009). Though the molecular interactions described are on the basis of monomeric GPCRs, similar associations may be expected from oligomeric forms. Similarly, molecular modeling and crystallization studies have predicted the binding pockets in SCTR and PTHR homodimers, respectively, to be localized in the extracellular N-terminal domains (Gao et al., 2009; Pioszak et al., 2010). Moreover, the SCTR homodimer peptide-binding clefts are demonstrated to reside opposite to the dimerization interfaces that may allow structural freedom for each protomer to bind to its respective ligand in a 1:1 stoichiometric ratio, as expected for monomeric GPCRs (Gao et al., 2009). Though limited, the two models show oligomerization to have minimal structural modifications in terms of adequately exposing the binding pockets, allowing ligand–receptor interactions in class B GPCRs.

In majority of studies for this receptor class, the use of peptide or mutant receptors to inhibit dimerization events have been utilized to explore the contribution of such receptor interactions toward functionality. On the basis of these studies, oligomerization has been demonstrated to have differential effects on the ligand binding affinity of class B GPCRs. Using TM4 peptides that are known to disrupt SCTR homodimerization, both monomeric and dimeric SCTR forms were found to have analogous ligand binding properties (Harikumar et al., 2007). Similarly, oligomerization was also found to have null effects on the ligand binding affinity of PTHR1, with the non-dimerizing R179A/V183A double mutant maintaining wild-type PTH binding activity (Pioszak et al., 2010). In another study, CALCR mutants also bound calcitonin saturably with no statistically significant differences in binding affinity (Harikumar et al., 2010). In contrast, disruption of GLP1R homodimerization by TM4 peptides resulted in elimination of G protein-dependent high affinity binding to GLP1(7–36)NH_2 (Harikumar et al., 2012). Moreover, co-expression of full-length and truncated GHRHRs resulted in a decrease in GHRH ligand binding and has been described to be resultant of the truncated receptor inducing a dominant-negative effect, leading to conformational changes which inhibit proper binding (McElvaine and Mayo, 2006). Nevertheless, these contrasting findings are consistent with recent reports of oligomerization having variable effects on the kinetics and efficiencies amongst receptors (Dorsch et al., 2009; Hern et al., 2010). Therefore, oligomerization may be important in modulating receptor activity via altering ligand binding affinity only in certain class B GPCRs.

ALLOSTERY

In recent studies, a link between oligomerization and allosteric regulation has been established in class B GPCRs. Allostery concerns association of a ligand or molecule to the receptor other than its orthosteric site, modifying its functional properties in either a positive or negative manner (May et al., 2007). Using a classical radio-ligand binding approach, the dissociation of labeled

SCT in the absence or presence of unlabeled SCT was monitored to study the negative binding cooperativity of SCTRs (Gao et al., 2009). The wild-type dimerizing receptors were found to shift from monophasic to biphasic dissociation upon presence of unlabeled SCT peptide, whilst the non-dimerizing mutant receptors maintained monophasic dissociation, regardless of treatment (Gao et al., 2009). On the basis of these results, the homodimeric SCTRs have been speculated to predominantly exist in a G protein-coupled high affinity state and the monomeric forms in a G protein-uncoupled low affinity state (Gao et al., 2009). Though the molecular basis responsible for the allosteric effects are still unknown, steric hindrance by the two large extracellular amino-terminal domain or selective coupling may be underlying factors contributing to the negative cooperativity observed in SCTRs (Miller et al., 2012). Similarly, the homodimerization event amongst the GCGR and GLP1R have also been identified to exhibit negative cooperativity with addition of labeled native peptides to their respective receptors leading to accelerated dissociation of unlabeled ligands (Roed et al., 2012). More recently, the ECD of the GCGR has been demonstrated to act as a negative regulator of receptor activity through interaction with the third extracellular loop (Koth et al., 2012), a region not only recognized to contribute to receptor affinity and efficacy, but may also aid in optimizing the arrangement of the TM bundle for efficient ligand binding (Peeters et al., 2011). As this case, agonist-occupied homodimers may induce negative cooperativity through structural modifications that affect ligand binding. Though the molecular determinants remain to be confirmed, there is a clear relation between dimerization and negative allostery. Aside from the typical ligand-induced allostery, physical coupling of each protomer in a oligomeric complex may also play a role (Haack and McCarty, 2011). Within the class B GPCRs, this has only been demonstrated in heteromers of the GLP1R and GIPR, where GIPR is suggested to act allosterically on the GLP1R to decrease maximal responses in calcium flux and β-arrestin recruitment assays (Schelshorn et al., 2012). In a later study, mutant GIPR function rescue by wild-type GLP1R was observed, with reduction in GLP1 responsiveness (Whitaker et al., 2012). Again GIPR may be exerting an allosteric effect on GLP1R, but the precise molecular basis needs to be explored with further structural and functional studies.

EFFECTS OF AGONIST OCCUPATION

Besides allostery, agonist occupation of class B GPCRs can also promote the association or dissociation of oligomeric complexes. In contrast to SCT homodimers that are unaffected by ligand binding (Ding et al., 2002a; Harikumar et al., 2006), GLP1 binding was found to encourage the dimerization between GLP1R and GIPR (Schelshorn et al., 2012). A model proposed describes GLP1 to act as a high affinity ligand for GLP1R at low concentrations, but also becomes a low affinity ligand for GIPR at higher concentrations to trigger formation of the GLP1 and GIPR dimer (Schelshorn et al., 2012). Interestingly, the presence of the high affinity GIP reverses the GLP1 induced association, dissolving the heteromer to a monomeric state (Schelshorn et al., 2012). As previously discussed, the GIPR has allosteric effects on the GLP1R when heterodimerized. Taken together with the agonist-induced association and/or dissociation of receptors, this may be a mechanism by which the receptors activate their G proteins and subsequent downstream signaling cascades (Gomes et al., 2001). Agonist-induced dissociation has also been reported for the PTHR1 via structural mimicry of PTH/PTHrP binding (Pioszak et al., 2010), however the functional relevance remains unclear. Other examples of agonist-induced disruption of oligomerization include VIPR1 and VIPR2 homodimers and VIPR1/VIPR2 heterodimers (Harikumar et al., 2006).

SIGNALING

Another prominent effect of oligomerization in class B GPCRs is on signaling selectivity and efficiency. In particular, cAMP and PLC are two of the predominant pathways in which physiological responses are elicited through in class B GPCRs. Therefore most oligomerization studies have extended their focus beyond information from ligand binding and BRET studies, but also rely on the cAMP and calcium mobilization responses of receptors. In particular, SCTRs are one of the first class B GPCRs demonstrated to have altered functionality due to homodimerization. By TM4 peptide competition studies, the disruption of SCTR dimerization was found to result in impairment of the generation of cAMP (Harikumar et al., 2007). The dimeric form of SCTR was, therefore, suggested be the optimal conformation for G protein activation (Harikumar et al., 2007). Similarly, disruption of the GLP1R homodimers was found to not only affect cAMP formation and ERK phosphorylation, but also lead to a complete loss of intracellular calcium mobilization response (Harikumar et al., 2012). In the case of GLP1R homodimers, signal transduction involves more than one G protein and/or accessory proteins such as β-arrestins. Nonetheless, dimerization is likely the basis in altering G protein coupling efficiency (Harikumar et al., 2012). This was also evident in the heterodimerization of GLP1 and GIP receptors, with the heteromer having more "GIP-like" (Schelshorn et al., 2012) pharmacological characteristics. Based on most of the studied class B GPCRs, oligomerization seems to exhibit a general trend in affecting G protein activation and signaling efficiency. However, oligomerization should not be a prerequisite for signaling, as monomers such as the PTHRs have been demonstrated to be capable of activating G proteins on their own (Pioszak et al., 2010). Therefore, oligomerization is likely important in providing structural framework to facilitate G protein coupling and thus modulate function.

TRAFFICKING

A number of studies have suggested the importance of oligomerization in cellular trafficking of the receptors and is a process that occurs early in the biosynthetic pathway (Bulenger et al., 2005). Within the class B GPCRs, this aspect of oligomerization has been most thoroughly explored for the SCTRs. Indeed using a combination of fluorescence and morphologic FRET microscopy studies, the SCTR homodimers were localized within organelles of the biosynthetic pathway including the tubular endoplasmic reticulum, Golgi clusters and the plasma membrane (Lisenbee and Miller, 2006). The homodimerization of SCTRs has therefore been suggested to occur as early as newly synthesized receptors and continue throughout their maturation process

(Lisenbee and Miller, 2006). Moreover, non-dimerizing SCTR constructs were not expressed nor yielded a significant morphological FRET signal both intracellularly and on the plasma membrane (Harikumar et al., 2007). Taken together, the SCTR data support the idea that oligomerization may be necessary for receptors to by-pass quality checkpoints before being delivered to their site of action (Bulenger et al., 2005). Consistent with the SCTR data, the VIPRs have also been identified in the biosynthetic pathway and plasma membrane as homo- and heterodimeric complexes (Harikumar et al., 2006). Interestingly, heterodimerization involving the SCTR and VIPR impaired trafficking to the plasma membrane with morphological FRET analyses revealing these heteromers to be trapped within the biosynthetic pathway, lacking cell surface expression (Harikumar et al., 2006). In the case of VIPRs, heterodimerization with SCTR predominates over the homodimerization of VIPRs (Harikumar et al., 2006). This demonstrates dominant-negative inhibition of oligomerization on cellular trafficking, which may be useful for modulating function in cells expressing both the SCTR and VIPR (Harikumar et al., 2006). In a later study, a small amount of mutant GIPR completely lacking *N*-glycosylation and cell surface expression was rescued by coexpression with GLP1R but not GIPR, suggesting the possibility of a heteromer which has a dominant-positive effect in facilitating the trafficking of GIPR (Whitaker et al., 2012).

STRUCTURAL ELEMENTS GOVERNING OLIGOMERIZATION IN CLASS B GPCRs

With the class B GPCRs key in a number of pathophysiological diseases and mounting evidence indicating their oligomerization to have influence in modulating various functional properties, this has fueled research in unraveling the structural determinants. To date, majority of studies have suggested the importance of different domains in GPCR oligomerization. However within the class B GPCRs, a common theme seems to prevail with several lines of evidence indicating the TM domains to be important. More specifically, it is the fourth TM domain, which has been implicated as a key molecular domain in class B receptor homodimerization (**Table 1**). This has been well documented by the disruption of SCTR homodimerization by TM4 peptides, with mutation studies identifying the lipid-facing residues namely Gly^{243} and Ile^{247} as important interfaces (Harikumar et al., 2007). Similarly, TM4 also provides the primary interface for GLP1R homodimerization, as supported by experimental data with TM4 peptide treatment dissociating the complex (Harikumar et al., 2012). Consistent with findings from the SCTR studies, lipid-facing residues within TM4 of the CALCR were also found to be necessary for dimerization (Harikumar et al., 2010). Though TM4 has been indicated to provide basis for dimerization in class B GPCRs, other domains including the ECD in PTHR (Pioszak et al., 2010) and C-terminal tail in CALCR (Harikumar et al., 2010) may also have some role. More recently, a pseudo signal peptide unique to the CRHR2a was identified to inhibit oligomerization (Teichmann et al., 2012). Steric hindrance by the bulky nature of the high mannose glycan protruding from this N-terminal domain has been suggested, thus preserving CRHR2a as monomers (Teichmann et al., 2012). Current prediction programs are unable to differentiate between canonical and pseudo signal peptides, as a result the presence of similar structures may also exist in other class B GPCRs (Rutz et al., 2006; Teichmann et al., 2012). Taken together, dimerization of class B GPCRs may not necessarily be dependent solely on one structural motif but instead is a highly complex interaction amongst several domains to achieve optimal structural basis for the fine-tuning of physiological processes.

FUTURE PERSPECTIVES

Over the last three decades, there has been a rapid development of techniques for studying the molecular interaction between GPCRs. Though early evidence was largely overlooked and limited to the class A GPCRS, establishment of RET techniques, in particular, have led to reinterpretation and strongly supports the concept of GPCR oligomerization. In recent years, class B GPCRs are also gaining merit in their ability to form homo- and hetero- oligomers, with the SCTRs being the most extensively studied. Though still nascent, the information available supports the role of dimerization in modulating function of class B GPCRs. Naturally, ligand binding to a receptor results in conformational changes in G protein arrangement to elicit downstream signaling pathways. When GPCRs associate, conformational arrangements also occur to modulate functionality. For example, SCTR homodimers have greater signaling responses than its monomeric counterparts. Furthermore, GPCR dimerization may also act as a repair mechanism, *trans*-complementing domains to restore binding sites and thus signaling, as observed for spliced SCTRs (Ding et al., 2002a,b). In terms of trafficking, oligomerization may also play a role with evidence of SCTR homodimers present as early as nascent molecules throughout the biosynthetic pathway (Lisenbee and Miller, 2006). Though seemingly simple when considering homodimeric units, evidence of GPCR heterodimerization, for example of SCTRs with a wide range of class B GPCRs, such as VIPR and GCGR, suggests a more complex role. Attempts have also been made to link these physical characteristics to pathophysiological responses in class B GPCRs, for example, association of SCTR homodimers to gastrinoma (Ding et al., 2002b) and GLP1R/GIPR heterodimers to diabetes (Whitaker et al., 2012). GPCR oligomerization is therefore functionally relevant and further research will be useful in providing more insights in understanding the molecular determinants to *in vivo* responses and for drug design.

ACKNOWLEDGMENTS

The present study was supported by the Hong Kong Government RGC grant GRF764510, CRFHKU6/CRF/11G to Billy K. C. Chow and GRF770212 to Leo T. O. Lee.

REFERENCES

Albizu, L., Balestre, M. N., Breton, C., Pin, J. P., Manning, M., Mouillac, B., et al. (2006). Probing the existence of G protein-coupled receptor dimers by positive and negative ligand-dependent cooperative binding. *Mol. Pharmacol.* 70, 1783–1791.

Avissar, S., Amitai, G., and Sokolovsky, M. (1983). Oligomeric structure of muscarinic receptors is shown by photoaffinity labeling: subunit assembly may explain high- and low-affinity agonist states. *Proc. Natl. Acad. Sci. U.S.A.* 80, 156–159.

Ayoub, M. A., Levoye, A., Delagrange, P., and Jockers, R. (2004). Preferential formation of MT1/MT2 melatonin receptor heterodimers with distinct ligand interaction properties compared with MT2 homodimers. *Mol. Pharmacol.* 66, 312–321.

Bai, M., Trivedi, S., and Brown, E. M. (1998). Dimerization of the extracellular calcium-sensing receptor (CaR) on the cell surface of CaR-transfected HEK293 cells. *J. Biol. Chem.* 273, 23605–23610.

Bayburt, T. H., Vishnivetskiy, S. A., Mclean, M. A., Morizumi, T., Huang, C. C., Tesmer, J. J., et al. (2011). Monomeric rhodopsin is sufficient for normal rhodopsin kinase (GRK1) phosphorylation and arrestin-1 binding. *J. Biol. Chem.* 286, 1420–1428.

Brock, C., Oueslati, N., Soler, S., Boudier, L., Rondard, P., and Pin, J. P. (2007). Activation of a dimeric metabotropic glutamate receptor by intersubunit rearrangement. *J. Biol. Chem.* 282, 33000–33008.

Bulenger, S., Marullo, S., and Bouvier, M. (2005). Emerging role of homo- and heterodimerization in G-protein-coupled receptor biosynthesis and maturation. *Trends Pharmacol. Sci.* 26, 131–137.

Capponi, A. M., and Catt, K. J. (1980). Solubilization and characterization of adrenal and uterine angiotensin II receptors after photoaffinity labeling. *J. Biol. Chem.* 255, 12081–12086.

Carrillo, J. J., Lopez-Gimenez, J. F., and Milligan, G. (2004). Multiple interactions between transmembrane helices generate the oligomeric alpha1b-adrenoceptor. *Mol. Pharmacol.* 66, 1123–1137.

Carson, M. C., Harper, C. M., Baukal, A. J., Aguilera, G., and Catt, K. J. (1987). Physicochemical characterization of photoaffinity-labeled angiotensin II receptors. *Mol. Endocrinol.* 1, 147–153.

Chun, L., Zhang, W. H., and Liu, J. F. (2012). Structure and ligand recognition of class C GPCRs. *Acta Pharmacol. Sin.* 33, 312–323.

Cottet, M., Albizu, L., Comps-Agrar, L., Trinquet, E., Pin, J. P., Mouillac, B., et al. (2011). Time resolved FRET strategy with fluorescent ligands to analyze receptor interactions in native tissues: application to GPCR oligomerization. *Methods Mol. Biol.* 746, 373–387.

Degorce, F., Card, A., Soh, S., Trinquet, E., Knapik, G. P., and Xie, B. (2009). HTRF: a technology tailored for drug discovery - a review of theoretical aspects and recent applications. *Curr. Chem. Genomics* 3, 22–32.

Ding, W. Q., Cheng, Z. J., Mcelhiney, J., Kuntz, S. M., and Miller, L. J. (2002a). Silencing of secretin receptor function by dimerization with a misspliced variant secretin receptor in ductal pancreatic adenocarcinoma. *Cancer Res.* 62, 5223–5229.

Ding, W. Q., Kuntz, S., Bohmig, M., Wiedenmann, B., and Miller, L. J. (2002b). Dominant negative action of an abnormal secretin receptor arising from mRNA missplicing in a gastrinoma. *Gastroenterology* 122, 500–511.

Dinger, M. C., Bader, J. E., Kobor, A. D., Kretzschmar, A. K., and Beck-Sickinger, A. G. (2003). Homodimerization of neuropeptide y receptors investigated by fluorescence resonance energy transfer in living cells. *J. Biol. Chem.* 278, 10562–10571.

Dong, M., Lam, P. C., Pinon, D. I., Sexton, P. M., Abagyan, R., and Miller, L. J. (2008). Spatial approximation between secretin residue five and the third extracellular loop of its receptor provides new insight into the molecular basis of natural agonist binding. *Mol. Pharmacol.* 74, 413–422.

Dong, M., Le, A., Te, J. A., Pinon, D. I., Bordner, A. J., and Miller, L. J. (2011). Importance of each residue within secretin for receptor binding and biological activity. *Biochemistry* 50, 2983–2993.

Dong, M., Pinon, D. I., Cox, R. F., and Miller, L. J. (2004). Importance of the amino terminus in secretin family G protein-coupled receptors. Intrinsic photoaffinity labeling establishes initial docking constraints for the calcitonin receptor. *J. Biol. Chem.* 279, 1167–1175.

Dorsch, S., Klotz, K. N., Engelhardt, S., Lohse, M. J., and Bunemann, M. (2009). Analysis of receptor oligomerization by FRAP microscopy. *Nat. Methods* 6, 225–230.

Estival, A., Clemente, F., and Ribet, A. (1981). Adenocarcinoma of the human exocrine pancreas: presence of secretin and caerulein receptors. *Biochem. Biophys. Res. Commun.* 102, 1336–1341.

Fraser, C. M., and Venter, J. C. (1982). The size of the mammalian lung beta 2-adrenergic receptor as determined by target size analysis and immunoaffinity chromatography. *Biochem. Biophys. Res. Commun.* 109, 21–29.

Gandia, J., Lluis, C., Ferré, S., Franco, R., and Ciruela, F. (2008). Light resonance energy transfer-based methods in the study of G protein-coupled receptor oligomerization. *Bioessays* 30, 82–89.

Gao, F., Harikumar, K. G., Dong, M., Lam, P. C., Sexton, P. M., Christopoulos, A., et al. (2009). Functional importance of a structurally distinct homodimeric complex of the family B G protein-coupled secretin receptor. *Mol. Pharmacol.* 76, 264–274.

Gennick, S. E., Thomas, C. G. Jr., and Nayfeh, S. N. (1987). Characterization of the subunit structure of the thyrotropin receptor in the FRTL-5 rat thyroid cell line. *Endocrinology* 121, 2119–2130.

Gomes, I., Jordan, B. A., Gupta, A., Rios, C., Trapaidze, N., and Devi, L. A. (2001). G protein coupled receptor dimerization: implications in modulating receptor function. *J. Mol. Med. (Berl)* 79, 226–242.

Grace, C. R., Perrin, M. H., Cantle, J. P., Vale, W. W., Rivier, J. E., and Riek, R. (2007). Common and divergent structural features of a series of corticotropin releasing factor-related peptides. *J. Am. Chem. Soc.* 129, 16102–16114.

Guillemette, G., and Escher, E. (1983). Analysis of the adrenal angiotensin II receptor with the photoaffinity labeling method. *Biochemistry* 22, 5591–5596.

Guo, W., Urizar, E., Kralikova, M., Mobarec, J. C., Shi, L., Filizola, M., et al. (2008). Dopamine D2 receptors form higher order oligomers at physiological expression levels. *EMBO J.* 27, 2293–2304.

Haack, K. K. V., and McCarty, N. A. (2011). Functional consequences of GPCR heterodimerziation: GPCRs as allosteric modulators. *Pharmaceuticals* 4, 509–523.

Harikumar, K. G., Ball, A. M., Sexton, P. M., and Miller, L. J. (2010). Importance of lipid-exposed residues in transmembrane segment four for family B calcitonin receptor homo-dimerization. *Regul. Pept.* 164, 113–119.

Harikumar, K. G., Happs, R. M., and Miller, L. J. (2008a). Dimerization in the absence of higher-order oligomerization of the G protein-coupled secretin receptor. *Biochim. Biophys. Acta* 1778, 2555–2563.

Harikumar, K. G., Morfis, M. M., Sexton, P. M., and Miller, L. J. (2008b). Pattern of intra-family hetero-oligomerization involving the G-protein-coupled secretin receptor. *J. Mol. Neurosci.* 36, 279–285.

Harikumar, K. G., Morfis, M. M., Lisenbee, C. S., Sexton, P. M., and Miller, L. J. (2006). Constitutive formation of oligomeric complexes between family B G protein-coupled vasoactive intestinal polypeptide and secretin receptors. *Mol. Pharmacol.* 69, 363–373.

Harikumar, K. G., Pinon, D. I., and Miller, L. J. (2007). Transmembrane segment IV contributes a functionally important interface for oligomerization of the class II G protein-coupled secretin receptor. *J. Biol. Chem.* 282, 30363–30372.

Harikumar, K. G., Wootten, D., Pinon, D. I., Koole, C., Ball, A. M., Furness, S. G., et al. (2012). Glucagon-like peptide-1 receptor dimerization differentially regulates agonist signaling but does not affect small molecule allostery. *Proc. Natl. Acad. Sci. U.S.A.* 109, 18607–18612.

Harrison, C., and van der Graaf, P. H. (2006). Current methods used to investigate G protein coupled receptor oligomerisation. *J. Pharmacol. Toxicol. Methods* 54, 26–35.

Hebert, T. E., Loisel, T. P., Adam, L., Ethier, N., Onge, S. S., and Bouvier, M. (1998). Functional rescue of a constitutively desensitized beta2AR through receptor dimerization. *Biochem. J.* 330(Pt 1), 287–293.

Hebert, T. E., Moffett, S., Morello, J. P., Loisel, T. P., Bichet, D. G., Barret, C., et al. (1996). A peptide derived from a beta2-adrenergic receptor transmembrane domain inhibits both receptor dimerization and activation. *J. Biol. Chem.* 271, 16384–16392.

Hern, J. A., Baig, A. H., Mashanov, G. I., Birdsall, B., Corrie, J. E., Lazareno, S., et al. (2010). Formation and dissociation of M1 muscarinic receptor dimers seen by total internal reflection fluorescence imaging of single molecules. *Proc. Natl. Acad. Sci. U.S.A.* 107, 2693–2698.

Heroux, M., Breton, B., Hogue, M., and Bouvier, M. (2007). Assembly and signaling of CRLR and RAMP1 complexes assessed by BRET. *Biochemistry* 46, 7022–7033.

Heroux, M., and Bouvie, M. (2005). Homo- and hetero-dimerization of receptor activity modifying proteins. *FASEB J.* 19, A254.

Ishihara, T., Nakamura, S., Kaziro, Y., Takahashi, T., Takahashi, K., and Nagata, S. (1991). Molecular cloning and expression of a cDNA encoding the secretin receptor. *EMBO J.* 10, 1635–1641.

Kniazeff, J., Prézeau, L., Rondard, P., Pin, J. P., and Goudet, C. (2011). Dimers and beyond: the functional puzzles of class C GPCRs. *Pharmacol. Ther.* 130, 9–25.

Koth, C. M., Murray, J. M., Mukund, S., Madjidi, A., Minn, A., Clarke, H. J., et al. (2012). Molecular basis for negative regulation of the glucagon receptor. *Proc. Natl. Acad. Sci. U.S.A.* 109, 14393–14398.

Kraetke, O., Wiesner, B., Eichhorst, J., Furkert, J., Bienert, M., and Beyermann, M. (2005). Dimerization of corticotropin-releasing factor receptor type 1 is not coupled to ligand binding. *J. Recept. Signal Transduct. Res.* 25, 251–276.

Kuszak, A. J., Pitchiaya, S., Anand, J. P., Mosberg, H. I., Walter, N. G., and Sunahara, R. K. (2009). Purification and functional reconstitution of monomeric mu-opioid receptors: allosteric modulation of agonist binding by Gi2. *J. Biol. Chem.* 284, 26732–26741.

Langer, I., Gaspard, N., and Robberecht, P. (2006). Pharmacological properties of Chinese hamster ovary cells coexpressing two vasoactive intestinal peptide receptors (hVPAC1 and hVPAC2). *Br. J. Pharmacol.* 148, 1051–1059.

Latif, R., Graves, P., and Davies, T. F. (2001). Oligomerization of the human thyrotropin receptor: fluorescent protein-tagged hTSHR reveals post-translational complexes. *J. Biol. Chem.* 276, 45217–45224.

Latif, R., Graves, P., and Davies, T. F. (2002). Ligand-dependent inhibition of oligomerization at the human thyrotropin receptor. *J. Biol. Chem.* 277, 45059–45067.

Lee, S. P., So, C. H., Rashid, A. J., Varghese, G., Cheng, R., Lanca, A. J., et al. (2004). Dopamine D1 and D2 receptor co-activation generates a novel phospholipase C-mediated calcium signal. *J. Biol. Chem.* 279, 35671–35678.

Limbird, L. E., and Lefkowitz, R. J. (1976). Negative cooperativity among beta-adrenergic receptors in frog erythrocyte membranes. *J. Biol. Chem.* 251, 5007–5014.

Limbird, L. E., Meyts, P. D., and Lefkowitz, R. J. (1975). Beta-adrenergic receptors: evidence for negative cooperativity. *Biochem. Biophys. Res. Commun.* 64, 1160–1168.

Lisenbee, C. S., and Miller, L. J. (2006). Secretin receptor oligomers form intracellularly during maturation through receptor core domains. *Biochemistry* 45, 8216–8226.

Maggio, R., Vogel, Z., and Wess, J. (1993). Coexpression studies with mutant muscarinic/adrenergic receptors provide evidence for intermolecular "cross-talk" between G-protein-linked receptors. *Proc. Natl. Acad. Sci. U.S.A.* 90, 3103–3107.

Mann, R., Nasr, N., Hadden, D., Sinfield, J., Abidi, F., Al-Sabah, S., et al. (2007). Peptide binding at the GLP-1 receptor. *Biochem. Soc. Trans.* 35, 713–716.

Matsuno, A., Katakami, H., Sanno, N., Ogino, Y., Osamura, R. Y., Matsukura, S., et al. (1999). Pituitary somatotroph adenoma producing growth hormone (GH)-releasing hormone (GHRH) with an elevated plasma GHRH concentration: a model case for autocrine and paracrine regulation of GH secretion by GHRH. *J. Clin. Endocrinol. Metab.* 84, 3241–3247.

Maurel, D., Comps-Agrar, L., Brock, C., Rives, M. L., Bourrier, E., Ayoub, M. A., et al. (2008). Cell-surface protein–protein interaction analysis with time-resolved FRET and snap-tag technologies: application to GPCR oligomerization. *Nat. Methods* 5, 561–567.

Maurel, D., Kniazeff, J., Mathis, G., Trinquet, E., Pin, J. P., and Ansanay, H. (2004). Cell surface detection of membrane protein interaction with homogeneous time-resolved fluorescence resonance energy transfer technology. *Anal. Biochem.* 329, 253–262.

May, L. T., Leach, K., Sexton, P. M., and Christopoulos, A. (2007). Allosteric modulation of G protein-coupled receptors. *Annu. Rev. Pharmacol. Toxicol.* 47, 1–51.

McElvaine, A. T., and Mayo, K. E. (2006). A dominant-negative human growth hormone-releasing hormone (GHRH) receptor splice variant inhibits GHRH binding. *Endocrinology* 147, 1884–1894.

Mercier, J. F., Salahpour, A., Angers, S., Breit, A., and Bouvier, M. (2002). Quantitative assessment of beta 1- and beta 2-adrenergic receptor homo- and heterodimerization by bioluminescence resonance energy transfer. *J. Biol. Chem.* 277, 44925–44931.

Miller, L. J., Dong, M., and Harikumar, K. G. (2012). Ligand binding and activation of the secretin receptor, a prototypic family B G protein-coupled receptor. *Br. J. Pharmacol.* 166, 18–26.

Miller, L. J., Dong, M., Harikumar, K. G., and Gao, F. (2007). Structural basis of natural ligand binding and activation of the class II G-protein-coupled secretin receptor. *Biochem. Soc. Trans.* 35, 709–712.

Monnot, C., Bihoreau, C., Conchon, S., Curnow, K. M., Corvol, P., and Clauser, E. (1996). Polar residues in the transmembrane domains of the type 1 angiotensin II receptor are required for binding and coupling. Reconstitution of the binding site by co-expression of two deficient mutants. *J. Biol. Chem.* 271, 1507–1513.

Ng, G. Y., O'Dowd, B. F., Lee, S. P., Chung, H. T., Brann, M. R., Seeman, P., et al. (1996). Dopamine D2 receptor dimers and receptor-blocking peptides. *Biochem. Biophys. Res. Commun.* 227, 200–204.

Overton, M. C., and Blumer, K. J. (2000). G-protein-coupled receptors function as oligomers in vivo. *Curr. Biol.* 10, 341–344.

Overton, M. C., Chinault, S. L., and Blumer, K. J. (2003). Oligomerization, biogenesis, and signaling is promoted by a glycophorin A-like dimerization motif in transmembrane domain 1 of a yeast G protein-coupled receptor. *J. Biol. Chem.* 278, 49369–49377.

Paglin, S., and Jamieson, J. D. (1982). Covalent crosslinking of angiotensin II to its binding sites in rat adrenal membranes. *Proc. Natl. Acad. Sci. U.S.A.* 79, 3739–3743.

Parthier, C., Kleinschmidt, M., Neumann, P., Rudolph, R., Manhart, S., Schlenzig, D., et al. (2007). Crystal structure of the incretin-bound extracellular domain of a G protein-coupled receptor. *Proc. Natl. Acad. Sci. U.S.A.* 104, 13942–13947.

Parthier, C., Reedtz-Runge, S., Rudolph, R., and Stubbs, M. T. (2009). Passing the baton in class B GPCRs: peptide hormone activation via helix induction? *Trends Biochem. Sci.* 34, 303–310.

Peeters, M. C., Van Westen, G. J., Li, Q., and Ap, I. J. (2011). Importance of the extracellular loops in G protein-coupled receptors for ligand recognition and receptor activation. *Trends Pharmacol. Sci.* 32, 35–42.

Percherancier, Y., Berchiche, Y. A., Slight, I., Volkmer-Engert, R., Tamamura, H., Fujii, N., et al. (2005). Bioluminescence resonance energy transfer reveals ligand-induced conformational changes in CXCR4 homo- and heterodimers. *J. Biol. Chem.* 280, 9895–9903.

Pfleger, K. D., Dromey, J. R., Dalrymple, M. B., Lim, E. M., Thomas, W. G., and Eidne, K. A. (2006). Extended bioluminescence resonance energy transfer (eBRET) for monitoring prolonged protein–protein interactions in live cells. *Cell. Signal.* 18, 1664–1670.

Pioszak, A. A., Harikumar, K. G., Parker, N. R., Miller, L. J., and Xu, H. E. (2010). Dimeric arrangement of the parathyroid hormone receptor and a structural mechanism for ligand-induced dissociation. *J. Biol. Chem.* 285, 12435–12444.

Pioszak, A. A., and Xu, H. E. (2008). Molecular recognition of parathyroid hormone by its G protein-coupled receptor. *Proc. Natl. Acad. Sci. U.S.A.* 105, 5034–5039.

Pioszak, A. A., Parker, N. R., Gardella, T. J., and Xu, H. E. (2009). Structural basis for parathyroid hormone-related protein binding to the parathyroid hormone receptor and design of conformation-selective peptides. *J. Biol. Chem.* 284, 28382–28391.

Ramsay, D., Kellett, E., Mcvey, M., Rees, S., and Milligan, G. (2002). Homo- and hetero-oligomeric interactions between G-protein-coupled receptors in living cells monitored by two variants of bioluminescence resonance energy transfer (BRET): hetero-oligomers between receptor subtypes form more efficiently than between less closely related sequences. *Biochem. J.* 365, 429–440.

Rocheville, M., Lange, D. C., Kumar, U., Sasi, R., Patel, R. C., and Patel, Y. C. (2000). Subtypes of the somatostatin receptor assemble as functional homo- and heterodimers. *J. Biol. Chem.* 275, 7862–7869.

Rodriguez-Frade, J. M., Vila-Coro, A. J., De Ana, A. M., Albar, J. P., Martinez, A. C., and Mellado, M. (1999). The chemokine monocyte chemoattractant protein-1 induces functional responses through dimerization of its receptor CCR2. *Proc. Natl. Acad. Sci. U.S.A.* 96, 3628–3633.

Roed, S. N., Orgaard, A., Jorgensen, R., and De Meyts, P. (2012). Receptor oligomerization in family B1 of G-protein-coupled receptors: focus on BRET investigations and the link between GPCR oligomerization and binding cooperativity. *Front. Endocrinol. (Lausanne)* 3, 62.

Rogers, T. B. (1984). High affinity angiotensin II receptors in myocardial sarcolemmal membranes. Characterization of receptors and covalent linkage of 125I-angiotensin II to a membrane component of 116,000 daltons. *J. Biol. Chem.* 259, 8106–8114.

Rondard, P., Liu, J., Huang, S., Malhaire, F., Vol, C., Pinault, A., et al. (2006). Coupling of agonist binding to effector domain activation in metabotropic glutamate-like receptors. *J. Biol. Chem.* 281, 24653–24661.

Rondeau, J. J., Mcnicoll, N., Escher, E., Meloche, S., Ong, H., and De Lean, A. (1990). Hydrodynamic properties of the angiotensin II receptor from bovine adrenal zona glomerulosa. *Biochem. J.* 268, 443–448.

Rutz, C., Renner, A., Alken, M., Schulz, K., Beyermann, M., Wiesner, B., et al. (2006). The corticotropin-releasing factor receptor type 2a contains an N-terminal pseudo signal peptide. *J. Biol. Chem.* 281, 24910–24921.

Salahpour, A., Angers, S., Mercier, J. F., Lagace, M., Marullo, S., and Bouvier, M. (2004). Homodimerization of the beta2-adrenergic receptor as a prerequisite for cell surface targeting. *J. Biol. Chem.* 279, 33390–33397.

Salim, K., Fenton, T., Bacha, J., Urien-Rodriguez, H., Bonnert, T., Skynner, H. A., et al. (2002). Oligomerization of G-protein-coupled receptors shown by selective co-immunoprecipitation. *J. Biol. Chem.* 277, 15482–15485.

Sasaki, K., Dockerill, S., Adamiak, D. A., Tickle, I. J., and Blundell, T. (1975). X-ray analysis of glucagon and its relationship to receptor binding. *Nature* 257, 751–757.

Scarselli, M., Novi, F., Schallmach, E., Lin, R., Baragli, A., Colzi, A., et al. (2001). D2/D3 dopamine receptor heterodimers exhibit unique functional properties. *J. Biol. Chem.* 276, 30308–30314.

Schelshorn, D., Joly, F., Mutel, S., Hampe, C., Breton, B., Mutel, V., et al. (2012). Lateral allosterism in the glucagon receptor family: glucagon-like peptide 1 induces G-protein-coupled receptor heteromer formation. *Mol. Pharmacol.* 81, 309–318.

Seck, T., Baron, R., and Horne, W. C. (2003). The alternatively spliced deltae13 transcript of the rabbit calcitonin receptor dimerizes with the C1a isoform and inhibits its surface expression. *J. Biol. Chem.* 278, 23085–23093.

Siemens, I. R., Swanson, G. N., Fluharty, S. J., and Harding, J. W. (1991). Solubilization and partial characterization of angiotensin II receptors from rat brain. *J. Neurochem.* 57, 690–700.

Sun, Y., Day, R. N., and Periasamy, A. (2011). Investigating protein-protein interactions in living cells using fluorescence lifetime imaging microscopy. *Nat. Protoc.* 6, 1324–1340.

Teichmann, A., Rutz, C., Kreuchwig, A., Krause, G., Wiesner, B., and Schulein, R. (2012). The Pseudo signal peptide of the corticotropin-releasing factor receptor type 2A prevents receptor oligomerization. *J. Biol. Chem.* 287, 27265–27274.

Uberti, M. A., Hague, C., Oller, H., Minneman, K. P., and Hall, R. A. (2005). Heterodimerization with beta2-adrenergic receptors promotes surface expression and functional activity of alpha1D-adrenergic receptors. *J. Pharmacol. Exp. Ther.* 313, 16–23.

Ulrich, C. D. II, Holtmann, M., and Miller, L. J. (1998). Secretin and vasoactive intestinal peptide receptors: members of a unique family of G protein-coupled receptors. *Gastroenterology* 114, 382–397.

Venneti, K. C., and Hewage, C. M. (2011). Conformational and molecular interaction studies of glucagon-like peptide-2 with its N-terminal extracellular receptor domain. *FEBS Lett.* 585, 346–352.

Venter, J. C., Horne, P., Eddy, B., Greguski, R., and Fraser, C. M. (1984). Alpha 1-adrenergic receptor structure. *Mol. Pharmacol.* 26, 196–205.

Venter, J. C., Schaber, J. S., U'Prichard, D. C., and Fraser, C. M. (1983). Molecular size of the human platelet alpha 2-adrenergic receptor as determined by radiation inactivation. *Biochem. Biophys. Res. Commun.* 116, 1070–1075.

Whitaker, G. M., Lynn, F. C., McIntosh, C. H., and Accili, E. A. (2012). Regulation of GIP and GLP1 receptor cell surface expression by *N*-glycosylation and receptor heteromerization. *PLoS ONE* 7:e32675. doi: 10.1371/journal.pone.0032675

White, J. F., Grodnitzky, J., Louis, J. M., Trinh, L. B., Shiloach, J., Gutierrez, J., et al. (2007). Dimerization of the class A G protein-coupled neurotensin receptor NTS1 alters G protein interaction. *Proc. Natl. Acad. Sci. U.S.A.* 104, 12199–12204.

Whorton, M. R., Bokoch, M. P., Rasmussen, S. G., Huang, B., Zare, R. N., Kobilka, B., et al. (2007). A monomeric G protein-coupled receptor isolated in a high-density lipoprotein particle efficiently activates its G protein. *Proc. Natl. Acad. Sci. U.S.A.* 104, 7682–7687.

Whorton, M. R., Jastrzebska, B., Park, P. S., Fotiadis, D., Engel, A., Palczewski, K., et al. (2008). Efficient coupling of transducin to monomeric rhodopsin in a phospholipid bilayer. *J. Biol. Chem.* 283, 4387–4394.

Wu, P., and Brand, L. (1994). Resonance energy transfer: methods and applications. *Anal. Biochem.* 218, 1–13.

Wurch, T., Matsumoto, A., and Pauwels, P. J. (2001). Agonist-independent and -dependent oligomerization of dopamine D(2) receptors by fusion to fluorescent proteins. *FEBS Lett.* 507, 109–113.

Xu, J., Dodd, R. L., Makino, C. L., Simon, M. I., Baylor, D. A., and Chen, J. (1997). Prolonged photoresponses in transgenic mouse rods lacking arrestin. *Nature* 389, 505–509.

Young, S. F., Griffante C., and Aguilera, G. (2007). Dimerization between vasopressin V1b and corticotropin releasing hormone type 1 receptors. *Cell. Mol. Neurobiol.* 27, 439–461.

Zhu, X., and Wess, J. (1998). Truncated V2 vasopressin receptors as negative regulators of wild-type V2 receptor function. *Biochemistry* 37, 15773–15784.

2

The VPAC1 receptor: structure and function of a class B GPCR prototype

A. Couvineau*, E. Ceraudo, Y.-V. Tan, P. Nicole and M. Laburthe*

Faculté de Médecine Xavier Bichat, INSERM 773/Centre de Recherche Biomédicale Bichat Beaujon (CRB3), Université Paris 7, Paris Cedex 18, France

Edited by:
Hubert Vaudry, University of Rouen, France

Reviewed by:
James Waschek, University of California at Los Angeles, USA
Daniel Fourmy, University of Toulouse 3, France

***Correspondence:**
A. Couvineau and M. Laburthe, Faculté de Médecine X. Bichat, INSERM U773/CRB3, 16 Rue Henri Huchard, 75018 Paris, France.
e-mail: alain.couvineau@inserm.fr; marc.laburthe@inserm.fr

The class B G protein-coupled receptors (GPCRs) represents a small sub-family encompassing 15 members, and are very promising targets for the development of drugs to treat many diseases such as chronic inflammation, neurodegeneration, diabetes, stress, and osteoporosis. The VPAC1 receptor which is an archetype of the class B GPCRs binds Vasoactive Intestinal Peptide (VIP), a neuropeptide widely distributed in central and peripheral nervous system modulating many physiological processes including regulation of exocrine secretions, hormone release, foetal development, immune response ... VIP appears to exert beneficial effect in neurodegenerative and inflammatory diseases. This article reviews the current knowledge regarding the structure and molecular pharmacology of VPAC1 receptors. Over the past decade, structure–function relationship studies have demonstrated that the N-terminal ectodomain (N-ted) of VPAC1 plays a pivotal role in VIP recognition. The use of different approaches such as directed mutagenesis, photoaffinity labeling, Nuclear Magnetic Resonance (NMR), molecular modeling, and molecular dynamic simulation has led to demonstrate that: (1) the central and C-terminal part of the VIP molecule interacts with the N-ted of VPAC1 receptor which is itself structured as a ≪ Sushi ≫ domain; (2) the N-terminal end of the VIP molecule interacts with the first transmembrane domain of the receptor where three residues (K^{143}, T^{144}, and T^{147}) play an important role in VPAC1 interaction with the first histidine residue of VIP.

Keywords: GPCR, photolabeling, VPAC1, VIP, mutagenesis, inflammation, neuroprotection, molecular modeling

INTRODUCTION

Vasoactive Intestinal Peptide (VIP) discovered by Said and Mutt (1970) is an ubiquitous 28-aminoacid neuropeptide that is widely distributed in central and peripheral nervous system. During the past 10 years, VIP was also identified in the immune system where it plays the role of a "cytokine-like peptide" (Delgado et al., 2004). VIP plays an important role in human physiology (**Table 1**) such as in development, growth, immune responses, circadian rhythms, neuronal and endocrine control, neuroprotective actions, and in the functions of the digestive, respiratory, reproductive, and cardiovascular systems (Laburthe et al., 2007). Associated to its large distribution and biological functions, VIP may also play a role in various pathologies (**Table 1**). It has been identified as a very promising agent in the treatment of inflammatory and neurodegenerative diseases (Gozes et al., 2003; Delgado et al., 2004). Indeed, VIP appears to be a very potent anti-inflammatory peptide in animal models of Crohn disease (Abad et al., 2003), rheumatoid polyarthritis (Delgado et al., 2001), or septic shock. This neuropeptide belongs to the structural-related peptide named secretin/VIP family (**Table 2**) encompassing VIP, pituitary adenylate cyclase activating peptide (PACAP), secretin, growth hormone releasing factor (GRF), peptide having an histidine residue in N-terminal position and an isoleucine residue in C-terminal position (PHI and its human homolog PHM), helodermin, glucagon, gastric inhibitory polypeptide (GIP), glucagon-like peptide 1 and 2 (GLP-1 and GLP-2).

List of non-standard abbreviations: VIP, Vasoactive Intestinal Peptide; PACAP, Pituitary Adenylate Cyclase Activating Peptide; VPAC, VIP and PACAP receptor; Bpa, Benzophenone; N-ted, N-terminal ectodomain; ITF, Intrinsic Tryptophan Fluorescence.

VIP A POTENTIAL THERAPEUTICAL AGENTS

Few years ago, VIP emerged as a potential therapeutic agent for various diseases including asthma (Groneberg et al., 2006), sexual impotence (Fahrenkrug, 2001), brain strokes (Dogrukol-Ak et al., 2004), chronic inflammation (Delgado et al., 2004), neurodegenerative disorders (Dejda et al., 2005), and cancers (Moody et al., 2011). Recently, a lot of reports have focused on the role of VIP and its receptors in chronic inflammation and neurodegenerative diseases.

VIP has been identified as a very promising agent in treatment of inflammatory diseases (Delgado et al., 2004). Indeed, VIP appeared to be a very potent anti-inflammatory peptide in animal models of various chronic inflammatory diseases (Couvineau and Laburthe, 2012a,b). The VIP anti-inflammatory effect has been widely studied (Delgado et al., 2004). These studies showed, in homeostasis condition, innate and adaptive immunity, that VIP can help to preserve the equilibrium between pro-inflammatory and anti-inflammatory response. In chronic

Table 1 | Major physiological and pathophysiological actions of VIP[a].

Short-term	Neurotransmition, exocrine secretions (water, ions), hormone release (prolactin, luteinizing hormone, growth hormone, insulin...), muscle relaxation (vasodilator, bronchodilator, gastro–intestinal motility), metabolism
Long-term	Circadian rhythms, learning and behavior, growth regulator of whole fetuses and embryonic brain
Other effects	Neuroprotection, suppression of inflammation, immunomodulation, effects on cell proliferation in cancer

[a]Reviewed in Gozes et al. (2003); Dickson and Finlayson (2009); Delgado and Ganea (2011); Moody et al. (2011); Harmar et al. (2012).

Table 2 | Sequence alignments of class B GPCR ligands[b].

VIP[a]	HSDAVFTDNYTRLRKQMAVKKYLNSILN----------------	28[b]
PACAP27	HSDGIFTDSYSRYRKQMAVKKYLAAVL-----------------	27
PACAP38	HSDGIFTDSYSRYRKQMAVKKYLAAVLGKRYKQRVKNK------	38
Helodermin	HSDAIFTEEYSKLLAKLALQKYLASILGSRTSPPP---------	35
PHM	HADGVFTSDFSKLLGQLSAKKYLESLM-----------------	27
Secretin	HSDGTFTSELSRLREGARLQRLLQGLV-----------------	27
GRF	YADAIFTNSYRKVLGQLSARKLLQDIMSRQQGESNQERGARARL	44
Glucagon	HSQGTFTSDYSKYLDSRRAQDFVQWLMNT---------------	29
GLP-1	HAEGTFTSDVSSYLEGQAAKEFIAWLVKGR-------------	30
GLP-2	HADGSFSDEMNTILDNLAARDFINWLIQTKITD-----------	33
GIP	YAEGTFISDYSIAMDKIHQQDFVNWLLAQKGKKNDWKHNITQ--	42
PTH	---SVSEIQLMHNLGKHLNSMERVEWLRKKLQDVHNF	34
PTHrP	---AVSEHQLLHDKGKSIQDLRRRFFLHHLIAEIHTA----	34
Calcitonin	----CGNLSTCMLGTYTQDFNKFHTFPQTAIGVGAP-----	32
CRF	SEEPPISLDLTFHLLREVLEMARAEQLAQQAHSNRKLMEII	41

[a]Black boxes represent sequence identity and light gray boxes represent sequence homology.

[b]Numbers indicate the length of the peptides.

inflammatory diseases (Crohn disease, rheumatoid polyarthritis, hepatitis, encephalomyelitis...) a modification of this equilibrium can be induce by various stimuli such as pathogenic agents, auto-immunity, environment, genetic background...which lead to the stimulation of production of pro-inflammatory cytokines (IL-17, IL-1, IFNγ, TNFα...) by macrophages and lymphocytes T (Th1 and Th17). Conversely, the anti-inflammatory response mediated by anti-inflammatory cytokines (IL-10, IL-4, IL-13, TGFβ...) secreted by lymphocytes T (Th2 and Treg), was strongly inhibited. The VIP anti-inflammatory effect involves a "rebalancing" of immune system (Firestein, 2001) by inhibition of pro-inflammatory response (Th1 and Th17) and stimulation of anti-inflammatory response mediated by Th2 and Tregs. In parallel, VIP induces an inhibitory effect on innate immunity by inhibition of production of pro-inflammatory cytokines and chemokines secreted by macrophage. Moreover, VIP is able to strongly inhibit the production of reactive oxygen species (ROS) induced by fMLP in monocytes (personnal data). Moreover, various reports clearly demonstrate that VIP promotes tolerance by inducing expansion of Treg cells (Leceta et al., 2007). Whereas, some reports reveal that VIP-deficient mice are resistant to the development of induced-encephalomyelitis or induced-endotoxemia indicating that in these conditions VIP plays unexpected permissive and/or pro-inflammatory actions (Abad et al., 2010, 2012). Despite this effect, VIP represents a potential anti-inflammatory agent that could be used in human therapeutic treatment, although the VIP anti-inflammatory effects have been mainly described in animal models (Couvineau and Laburthe, 2012a,b). Whereas, the major obstacle to the use of VIP in clinic therapies is its high sensitivity to protease degradation. Indeed, removing of the first residues by peptidases, such as dipeptidyl peptidase IV (DPPIV), induces a drastic loss of affinity of VIP peptide family (Lambeir et al., 2001). To circumvent these labile properties, VIP can be modified to increase its resistance to degradation by N-acylation of the peptide N-terminal end or by substitution of residues involved in proteolytic consensus sequences (dibasic doublets). Recent data indicate that PACAP N-terminal modifications confer resistance to DPPIV (Bourgault et al., 2008). In the same way acetylation of the VIP N-terminal end increase its stability in the presence of human serum (personal data). Other strategies consist to protect peptide against degradation by insertion of VIP into micelles or nanoparticles (Fernandez-Montesinos et al., 2009; Onyüksel et al., 2009). Despite these limitations, VIP has been tested in a phase I clinical trial for the treatment of acute respiratory distress syndrome and sepsis (id: NCT00004494, http://www.clinicaltrials.gov).

In the mid-1980s, the first report of VIP neuroprotection, demonstrated that this peptide is able to prevent neuronal death associated with electrical blockade induced by tetrodotoxin (TTX) addition to primary spinal cord cultures (Brenneman and Eiden, 1986). Further studies have demonstrated that VIP plays a neuroprotective effects in various neurodegenerative diseases developed in animal models including Alzheimer's disease (Gozes et al., 1996), Parkinson's disease or encephalomyelitis (Gonzalez-Rey et al., 2005; Tan and Waschek, 2011). Some of these VIP neuroprotective actions were associated with glial cells possessing VPAC receptors. Clearly, VIP induced, on glial cells, a secretion of various trophic molecules having neuroprotective properties such as IL-1, IL-6, protease nexin-1, the chemokine RANTES and MIP (Dejda et al., 2005). Moreover, VIP inhibits the production of pro-inflammatory cytokines as TNFα and/or IL-1β secreted by activated microglia which is involved in neuroinflammation observed in Parkinson's disease or brain trauma models (Delgado et al., 2004). VIP also induces neuroprotective effect by increasing the secretion of activity-dependent neurotrophic factor (ADNF) and/or activity-dependent neurotrophic protein (ADNP) (Gozes et al., 2003). These two protective proteins, which belong to the heat shock protein family, are able to prevent the neuronal death (Dejda et al., 2005) and represent one of the most potent neuroprotective agents secreted by astroglia in response to VIP. Recently, it was suggested that the VPAC2 receptor, which binds VIP and/or PACAP with the same affinity, could be a potential target for the development of anti-psychotic drugs. Effectively, the VPAC2 receptor gene has been found to be duplicated in schizophrenia (Vacic et al., 2011). Although VIP is able to cross the brain blood barrier (Dogrukol-Ak et al., 2004), no clinical trials in humans were developed to evaluate its neuroprotective role in brain diseases. However, some human clinical trials based on VIP vasoactive properties on cerebral arteries and hemodynamics have been performed (id: NCT00272896 and NCT00255320 http://www.clinicaltrials.gov) to evaluate its role in development of headache/migraine.

VPAC RECEPTORS, A REPRESENTATIVE MEMBERS OF CLASS B GPCR

Biological responses induced by VIP are triggered by interaction with two receptors, VPAC1 and VPAC2, which are mainly coupled to the G-protein, Gs, resulting in the stimulation of cell adenylyl cyclase (Couvineau et al., 2010). Furthermore, some groups have reported the ability of VIP to increase calcium levels in different cells (Dickson and Finlayson, 2009). Moreover, VPAC1 receptor is able to interact with RAMP (Receptor Activity-Modifying Proteins) proteins, in particular RAMP2, inducing a significant enhancement of agonist-mediated inositol triphosphate production but do not modify the coupling to adenylate cyclase (Christopoulos et al., 2002). VPAC1 and VPAC2 receptors bind, with the same affinity, VIP and another neuropeptide named PACAP. It should be noted that VIP interacts also with the specific PACAP receptor (PAC1) but with a lower affinity (Couvineau and Laburthe, 2012a). Previous report indicate that VPAC1 receptor is able to homo-dimerize and hetero-dimerize with VPAC2 or secretin receptors (Harikumar et al., 2006). However, the relation between receptor oligomerization and the ability to VPAC1 receptor to interact with RAMPs remains unclear.

In the nineties secretin and VPAC receptors have been cloned (Ishihara et al., 1991, 1992; Lutz et al., 1993; Sreedharan et al., 1993; Couvineau et al., 1994) revealing a new G protein-coupled receptor (GPCR) sub-family termed class B GPCR. This GPCR sub-family shares with the other GPCR classes (A, C, D, E, F) the same general structural scheme characterized by the presence of seven-transmembrane helices denoted as TM I through TM VII which are interconnected by extracellular and intracellular loops (Fredrikson and Schiöth, 2006). The class B receptors family is composed of 15 members including receptors for VIP, PACAP, secretin, glucagon, glucagon-like peptide-1, glucagon-like peptide-2, GRF, GIP, and also include receptors for parathyroid hormone, calcitonin, calcitonin gene-related peptide, and corticotropin-releasing factor (CRF) (Couvineau and Laburthe, 2012b). Class B receptors display very low sequence homologies with others GPCRs (Laburthe et al., 2007) and share several specific characteristics: the presence of a large (>120 residues) and structured N-terminal ectodomain (N-ted) which is usually small in most class A GPCRs. The N-teds contain six highly conserved cysteine residues connected by three disulfide bridges, this sequence is the signature of class B GPCRs. The N-ted of class B receptor which represents the major binding site for its cognate natural peptide ligand, is characterized by; (1) the presence of a signal peptide probably involved in insertion of receptor in plasma membrane; (2) the absence of archetypical class A GPCR motifs such as E/D-R-Y or NP-xx(x)-Y; (3) a complex gene organization with many introns (Laburthe et al., 2002).

Currently, no data are available regarding the full-length structure of class B receptors as compare to class A receptors (Shoichet and Kobilka, 2012), although the structural properties of the class B GPCR N-ted, have recently been described, representing the first step toward better understanding of the binding receptor site at the atomic level. Recently, six N-ted structures, including those of the human PACAP receptor (PAC1), human PTH receptor (PTH1R), human GLP-1 receptor (GLP-1R), human GIP receptor (GIPR), and human type-1 and type-2 CRF receptor (CRFR1 and CRFR2) have been elucidated by Nuclear Magnetic Resonance (NMR) spectroscopy and X-ray crystallography in the presence of bound antagonist or agonists (Couvineau et al., 2010). These studies reveal the presence in the N-ted of a common core (**Figure 1**) formed by a Sushi domain (Parthier et al., 2009; Pal et al., 2012). This shared structure is composed of two anti-parallel β sheets (**Figure 1**) stabilized by (1) three disulfide bonds involving the typical six highly conserved cysteine residues (**Figure 1**); (2) a putative salt bridge involving acidic and basic residues, sandwiched between hydrophobic aromatic rings (**Figure 1**). The high conservation of the Sushi domain in the N-ted of class B GPCRs supports the idea that this structure plays a crucial role for peptide recognition (Grace et al., 2004). A "two-site" model for the binding of native ligands to class B GPCRs has been postulated (Hoare, 2005). In short, the central and the C-terminal portions of the peptide ligand are captured by the N-ted of the class B GPCRs. This step is essential for the peptide structuration, allowing the ligand N-terminus to interact with the transmembrane region of the receptor (Hoare, 2005).

As mentioned above VIP belongs to the secretin/VIP/PACAP family. The emergence of the class B GPCR has enlarged this peptide family (**Table 2**) by including parathyroid hormone (PTH), calcitonin, and CRF. All these natural ligands share some common properties: (1) they are all peptides with 27–44 amino acid residues; (2) they are synthesized and released by endocrine cells, neurons, and/or immune cells; (3) all these peptides exhibit a marked propensity to form α-helices; (4) all these peptides contain a N-Cap structure in the N-terminal part (Neumann et al.,

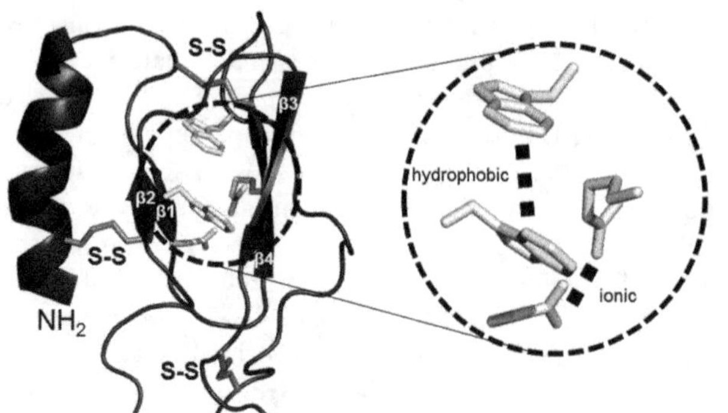

FIGURE 1 | Representation of generic Sushi domain core of Class B GPCR N-ted. Common structural elements of class B GPCR N-ted are represented by the presence of (1) a N-terminal α-helix (*black* ribbon); (2) two anti-parallel β-sheets (β1-β2 and β3-β4, *black* ribbon). The Sushi domain structural core is stabilized by the presence of three conserved disulfide bonds (*middle gray* sticks) and represented in magnified inset an ionic and hydrophobic interactions (*light gray* sticks). All figures were obtained by using PyMOL software (http://www.pymol.org).

2008). The presence of this structural signature which includes a hydrophobic cluster between N-terminal hydrophobic residues and a hydrogen bond between two polar residues (**Figure 2**) have been recently confirmed (Watkins et al., 2012). All these peptides play an important role in physiological processes and strongly impact human physiopathology including chronic inflammation diseases, neurodegenerative disorders, schizophrenia, diabetes, osteoporosis, stress (Couvineau and Laburthe, 2012a).

Cloning of the human VPAC1 receptor (Couvineau et al., 1994) allowed its extensive studied for many years by site-directed mutagenesis and molecular chimerism (Laburthe et al., 2007) laying its molecular basis in terms of: (1) affinity (Couvineau et al., 1995); (2) specificity (Couvineau et al., 1996a); (3) cellular addressing (Couvineau et al., 2004); (4) desensitization (Marie et al., 2003); (5) association with RAMP proteins (Christopoulos et al., 2002); (6) adenylyl cyclase coupling (Couvineau et al., 2003). These studies have revealed that the receptor N-ted plays a crucial role in peptide agonist binding (Couvineau et al., 2010). In parallel, structure–function relationships analysis of VIP by a complete alanine scanning (Nicole et al., 2000) showed that the peptide has a diffuse pharmacophoric domain. In this study we have demonstrated that the N-terminal 1–5 segment plays a crucial role in receptor activation e.g., mainly adenylyl cyclase activation.

THE VPAC1 BINDING SITE, CONTRIBUTION OF PHOTOLABELING APPROACH

The physical interaction sites between VIP and the VPAC1 receptor had remained elusive until the development of a photoaffinity labeling strategy, which allowed the demonstration that VIP side chains are physically in contact with the N-ted of VPAC1 (Couvineau et al., 2010). This strategy has two advantages over structural studies of purified recombinant receptors or receptor fragments: (1) the labeled ligand has an affinity for its receptor in the nanomolar range, which is similar to the high affinity measured under physiological conditions; and (2) the labeled ligand can interact with the glycosylated native receptor expressed in plasma membranes of eukaryotic cells. This is particularly important, given to the critical role of glycosylation in VPAC1 expression and function (Couvineau et al., 1996b). Addition of a benzophenone group (Bpa) to the VIP peptide has extensively contributed to the elucidation VIP biochemistry and of its receptor (Couvineau and Laburthe, 2012b). The use of photolabeling probes has clearly demonstrated that VIP residues in position 0, 6, 22, 24, or 28 were in physical contact with different amino acids in N-ted of the VPAC1 e.g., Gln^{135}, Asp^{107}, Gly^{116}, Cys^{122}, and Lys^{127} (**Figure 3**), respectively (Tan et al., 2003, 2004, 2006; Ceraudo et al., 2008, 2012). To dock VIP within the receptor N-ted, we determined the structure of VIP by NMR (**Figure 2**) and also developed a structural model of the VPAC1 receptor N-ted (Tan et al., 2006). Determination of VIP structure by NMR revealed that most of the 28 amino acids sequence has an α-helice structure (sequence 7–28) with the exception of the N-terminal 1–5 sequence, which has no defined structure in solution (**Figure 2**). In parallel, the structural model development of the VPAC1 receptor N-ted, by homology with the NMR structure of the CRF 2β receptor N-ted, allowed us to localize the VIP binding site in the N-ted. As expected, the structure contains two anti-parallel β sheets that are stabilized by three disulfide bonds between residues Cys^{50} and Cys^{72}, Cys^{63} and Cys^{105}, and Cys^{86} and Cys^{122}, and by a putative salt bridge involving Asp^{68}-Arg^{103}, sandwiched between the aromatic rings of Trp^{73} and Trp^{110} (**Figure 3**). The NMR structure of VIP has been docked in the VPAC1 receptor N-ted giving rise to a valid model in which, the N-ted C-terminal part, nicely accommodates the VIP molecule at least for the 6-28 sequence (**Figure 3**). This model has

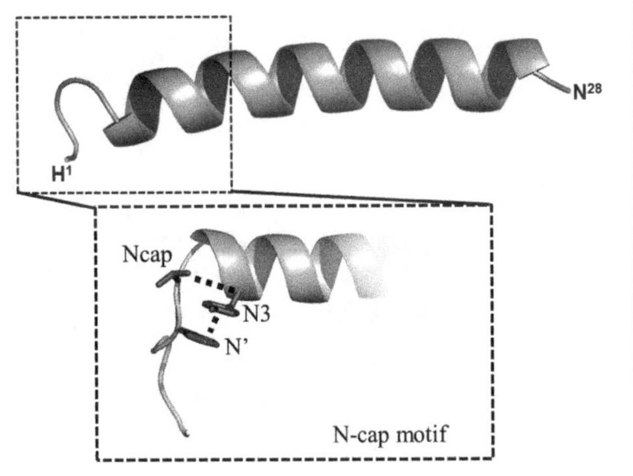

FIGURE 2 | NMR structure of VIP and representation of N-capping motif. *Middle gray* ribbon represents the average conformation of VIP structure. In magnified inset the N-capping motif is represented as (1) the hydrophobic interactions between side-chain groups of N' and N3 residues (dashed lines); (2) the hydrogen bond between side chain of N-cap residue and backbone atom of N3 residue. See ref. Neumann et al. (2008) for details.

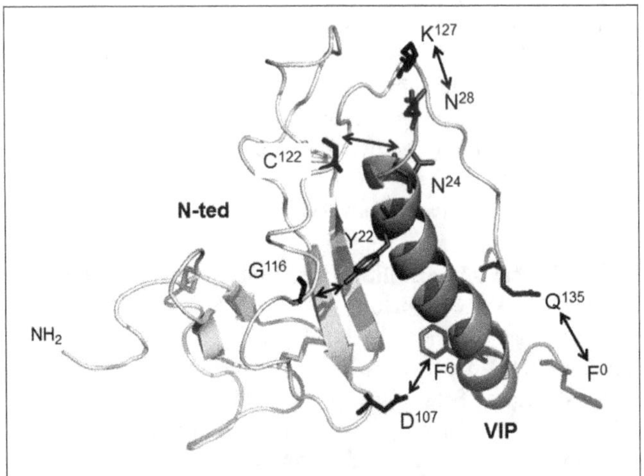

FIGURE 3 | The 3D-structural model of VPAC1 receptor N-ted and docking of VIP. Ribbon representation of the VPAC1 N-ted: *light gray ribbon*, main chain; *white ribbon*, VIP. Docking calculations showed that Q^{135}, D^{107}, G^{116}, C^{122}, and K^{127} residues (*middle gray sticks*) present in the N-ted were in contact (*white arrows*) with the side chains of F^0, F^6, Y^{22}, N^{24}, and N^{28} (*black sticks*) of VIP residues, respectively. Figure was obtained by using PyMOL software (http://www.pymol.org).

been submitted to molecular dynamic simulations over 14 ns in a water box and appears to be highly stable (Ceraudo et al., 2008).

Recently, using similar strategy, we have characterized the interaction site of the VPAC1 receptor-specific VIP antagonist, [Ac-His^{1}, D-Phe^{2}, K^{15}, R^{16}, L^{27}] VIP(3-7)/GRF(8-27) or PG 97-269 (Gourlet et al., 1997). This antagonist is a chimeric peptide between VIP (sequence 1–7) and GRF (sequence 8–27) having a D-phenylalanine residue in position 2. The use of Bpa^{0}-PG97-269 affinity labeling probe revealed that the N-terminal part of antagonist physically interacted with Gly^{62} residue of VPAC1 N-ted (Ceraudo et al., 2012). These observations clearly support that the N-terminal part of VIP (agonist) or PG97-269 (antagonist) were recognized by two different domains present in N-ted of VPAC1 receptor.

As mentioned above, the N-ted structure of different class B GPCRs has been obtained recently by X-ray crystallography or NMR spectroscopy (Parthier et al., 2009). These studies seem to indicate the existence of two different binding sites for ligands in class B receptor N-teds (Couvineau et al., 2010). Analysis of these structure and/or molecular models revealed that N-teds of GIPR, PTHR, CRF1R, CRF2R, and GLP-1R interact with ligands in regions encompassing the loop located between β1 and β2 sheets and the loop located between β3 and β4 sheets (Parthier et al., 2009). In contrast, the N-teds of PAC1R and VPAC1R bind peptides along β3 and β4 sheets of the sushi domain (Couvineau et al., 2010). However, a recent report based on the X-ray crystallography analysis of PAC1 receptor N-ted and the docking of PACAP indicates that PACAP could interact with its receptor as GIPR, PTHR, CRF1R, CRF2R, and GLP-1R (Kumar et al., 2011). The real significance of these differences were unclear but may be tentatively related to the following interpretations: (1) some structural determinations were carried-out in presence of ligands which have a low affinity (micromolar range) for the recombinant N-ted whereas in other studies ligand affinity was higher; it also could be hypothesized that low and high affinity binding occur at different sites in the N-ted structure; (2) the determination of interaction between N-teds and ligands was mainly obtained in the presence of antagonist but it some cases in the presence of an agonist; (3) moreover it could be hypothesized that agonists and antagonists bind to different domains in the N-teds. Finally, we cannot exclude the possibility that ligands can bind by two different ways to N-ted of class B GPCR.

THE KEY ROLE OF THE FIRST TRANSMEMBRANE DOMAIN OF VPAC1 IN VIP BINDING

VPAC1 domain interacting with the N-terminus of VIP (1–5) is still unknown. Up to now, no data are available regarding the full-length structure of class B receptors. To circumvent this unavailability, a 3D-model of the receptor encompassing VIP/N-ted complex and the transmembrane core of the receptor (**Figure 4**) was developed (Ceraudo et al., 2012). The 3D-model of the transmembrane core was constructed by homology modeling based on the recent determination of the X-ray structure of the adenosine A2A receptor (Jaakola et al., 2008). The resulting 3D-model of VPAC1 revealed that the central and C-terminal residues of VIP are in contact with N-ted whereas the N-terminus of VIP lies in a pocket formed by the extracellular side of the first, second and seventh transmembrane domains and the second extracellular loop of VPAC1 (**Figure 4A**). Based on distance calculation (<6Å) between residues of VPAC1 and VIP, substitutions by alanine of residues revealed that many residues are involved in the binding affinity of VIP to VPAC1. Three of them (H^{112}, L^{131}, and Q^{134}) are present in the N-ted, and their substitution to alanine induced an affinity modification of about 100 times as compared to native receptor, indicating that these residues are probably involved in the interaction between the N-ted and the central and C-terminal parts of VIP (Ceraudo et al., 2012). Substitution to alanine of four other residues (K^{143}, T^{144}, T^{147}, and L^{375}) located in the extracellular side of TMI and VII, also induced a strong modification of receptor affinity for VIP (Ceraudo et al., 2012). Moreover site-directed mutagenesis experiments and reciprocal exchange between K^{143}, T^{144}, and T^{147} residues of VPAC1 and H^{1} of VIP, shown that this interaction with (**Figure 4B**) the first histidine residue of VIP play a crucial role (Ceraudo et al., 2012). This step is important for the adenylyl cyclase activation (Couvineau et al., 1984). These observations were in good agreement with previous results indicating that D^{196} present in the second extracellular loop (Du et al., 1997), K^{195} and R^{188} in TMII (Solano et al., 2001), N^{229} in TMIII and Q^{380} in TMVII of VPAC1 play an important role in VIP binding and probably could interact with the D^{3} residue of VIP (Chugunov et al., 2010). Thus, these results along with our data clearly indicate that the N-terminus of VIP interacts with the extracellular side of the VPAC1 core.

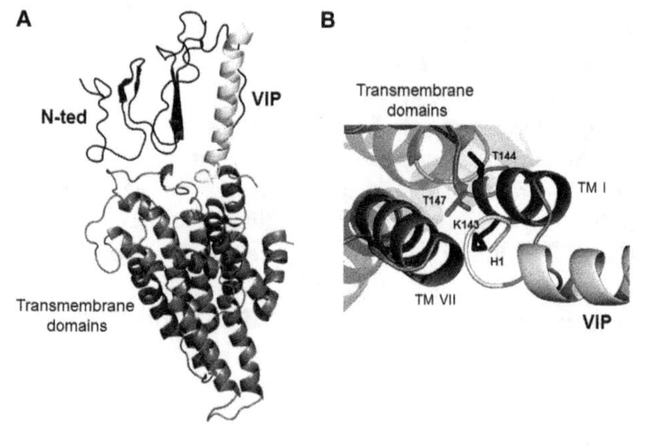

FIGURE 4 | Representation of global 3D-model of VPAC1 docked to VIP. **(A)** 3D-global model of human VPAC1 based on X-ray structure of the A2A receptor. **(B)** Upside view of 3D-global model of human VPAC1 displaying side-chains of residues of the 3D-global model of the receptor (*black sticks*) in close contact (distance <6Å) with the N-terminal end of VIP (*white*). *middle gray ribbon*, transmembrane domains; *black ribbon*, main chain of N-ted; *white ribbon*, main chain of VIP.

THE N-TED DETERMINES THE SPECIFICITY OF THE VPAC1 RECEPTOR

As mentioned above, VPAC1 and VPAC2 receptors do not discriminate between the two neuropeptides, VIP and PACAP. Moreover, some others VIP related-peptides are able to bind to human VPAC1 receptor with low affinity, including peptide histidine methionineamide (PHM), secretin, helodermin and GRF (Laburthe et al., 2007). Potency order being VIP = PACAP>helodermin>PHM>GRF>>secretin. In this context, the development of specific ligands for VPAC1 and VPAC2 receptors represents a major goal. To develop a specific VPAC1 agonist, structure-function relationships analysis of VIP by a complete alanine scanning (Nicole et al., 2000) was used to rationally design the most potent and specific peptide for VPAC1 receptor currently available e.g., $[Ala^{11,22,28}]$-VIP (Nicole et al., 2000). Indeed, this VIP derivative has an affinity 1000 times higher for the VPAC1 receptor, which is mainly involved in VIP anti-inflammatory action, than VPAC2 receptor (Delgado et al., 2004). As mentioned above a high selective antagonist of VPAC1 receptor (PG97-269) has been developed (Gourlet et al., 1997). Regarding VPAC2 receptor, the cyclic peptide analog of VIP $[Ac\text{-}Glu^8$, $OCH3\text{-}Tyr^{10}$, Lys^{12}, Nle^{17}, Ala^{19}, Asp^{25}, Leu^{26}, $\text{-}Lys^{27,28}$ -VIP(cyclo 21–25)] or Ro 25–1392 is a potent and selective agonist (Xia et al., 1997). In our opinion, there is still no satisfactory VPAC2 receptor antagonist since PG 99–465, a VIP analog that antagonizes VIP action on VPAC2 receptor, which also has a significant agonist activity on human VPAC1 receptor (Moreno et al., 2000). Since recently, two non-peptide antagonists specific of VPAC1 (Harikrishnan et al., 2012) or VPAC2 (Chu et al., 2010) have been developed but they display a very low affinity for receptors.

The use of VIP photoaffinity probes associated to receptor mapping and Edman degradation demonstrated that VIP physically interacts with the N-ted of VPAC1 receptor (Couvineau et al., 2010). In order to get a high resolution structure of the VPAC1 receptor N-ted, the production of large quantities of recombinant N-ted protein in bacteria was performed (Couvineau et al., 2008). The 31–144 sequence of human VPAC1 receptor corresponding to the N-ted sequence in which the signal peptide (Couvineau et al., 2004) has been deleted was subcloned in front of 6xHis (His-tag) and behind the thioredoxin sequence containing a thrombin cleavage site (Couvineau et al., 2008). The construction of the thioredoxin-N-ted-6xHis (Trx-N-ted-6xHis) fusion protein was chosen in order to increase the solubility of recombinant proteins as previously described for production of recombinant N-ted of mouse CRF2β receptor (Grace et al., 2004). The soluble recombinant N-ted was purified onto Ni-NTA column and tested for its ability to bind VIP by using the influence of VIP binding on the intrinsic tryptophan fluorescence (ITF) of W^{67}, W^{73}, and W^{110} residues which are present in the N-ted sequence. Indeed, the presence of three tryptophan residues in the N-ted Sushi domain (Couvineau et al., 2008) represents a good fluorescent tag which can be used to measure the interaction between VIP and recombinant N-ted. Based to the ITF parameters, the estimation of dissociation constants revealed a Kd of 0.54 μM for VIP, 0.57 μM for PACAP, and 1 μM for PG96-269 (Couvineau et al., 2008). It should be noted that those Kd values were close to Kd values observed for others purified N-ted such as PAC1 receptor (Sun et al., 2007) and GIP receptor (Parthier et al., 2007). Moreover, the Kd of truncated VIP6–28 is very similar to Kd of native VIP (0.54 μM vs. 0.85 μM) demonstrating that the 6–28 VIP sequence is sufficient to interact with a low affinity to recombinant N-ted (**Table 3**). In contrast, the deletion of large C-terminal (VIP1-12), central (VIP1-9/21-28) and N-terminal (VIP18-28) part of VIP abolishes totally the ability of truncated peptides to bind to recombinant N-ted (**Table 3**). These data clearly indicate that recombinant N-ted is able to recognize with a low affinity the central and C-terminal part of VIP molecule. Using the same approach, the ability of VPAC1 recombinant N-ted to discriminate VIP related-peptides was investigated (**Table 3**). As shown in **Table 2**, the estimation of Kd was of 0.54 μM, 0.57 μM, 2.54 μM, 8 μM, 10.12 μM, and 16 μM for VIP, PACAP, helodermin, PHM, GRF, and secretin respectively, indicating that the order of potency is similar to native receptor i.e., VIP = PACAP>helodermin>PHM>GRF>secretin (Laburthe et al., 2007). Taken altogether these results reveal that: (1) the recombinant N-ted is able to bind with a low affinity and to discriminate VIP related-peptides suggesting that the VPAC1 N-ted contains residues involved in the VPAC1 specificity; (2) the first transmembrane domain of VPAC1 contains three residues (see above) which interact with the first residue of VIP and these three residues are probably involved in the high affinity and the activation of the receptor (**Figure 4B**).

Table 3 | Binding of VIP related-peptides to recombinant N-ted.

Peptides	Kd (μM)[a]
VIP	0.54 ± 0.09
PG97–269	1.05 ± 0.50
PACAP27	0.57 ± 0.06
Helodermine	2.54 ± 0.71
PHM	8.00 ± 2.00
GRF	10.12 ± 0.98
Secretin	16.00 ± 1.00
VIP2–28	0.85 ± 0.36
VIP1–12	ND[b]
VIP18–28	ND
VIP1–9/21–28	ND

[a] *The ITF of W^{67}, W^{73}, and W^{110} residues from the purified N-ted was measured in 2 ml of HEPES buffer pH 7.5 containing 1 μM purified N-ted, in absence or presence of increasing concentration of peptides. Dissociation constants were determined from titration curves using analytical procedure developed by Bechet et al. (Bechet et al., 1986).*

[b] *Not detectable.*

CONCLUSION

The VPAC receptors, in particular VPAC1, are very promising targets for the development of therapeutic molecules in various pathologies including asthma, chronic inflammation diseases (Crohn's disease, rhumatoid arthritis, septic shock, multiple sclerosis...) neurodegenerative disorders, schizophrenia. While new peptide derivatives specifically targeting VPAC receptor sub-types are now available, however, their very short half-life and the inconvenient related to their administration routes make them difficult to use in human therapy. The recent advance in the structural knowledge of the VPAC1 binding site should lead to the design of non-peptide receptor agonists and/or antagonists. The development of such molecules will represent an important overhang in the treatment of many human diseases.

ACKNOWLEDGMENTS

This work was supported by the Institut National de la Santé et de la Recherche Médicale, Centre National de la Recherche Scientifique, Université Paris 7 and by a grant from the Association de Recherche sur la Polyarthrite. E. Ceraudo is supported by grant FDT20070910820 from the Fondation pour la Recherche Médicale and by an ≪ Inter-university Poles of Attraction Program ≫ (PAI) from the Université Libre de Bruxelles (ULB), Belgium.

REFERENCES

Abad, C., Martinez, C., Juarranz, M. G., Arranz, A., Leceta, J., Delgado, M., et al. (2003). Therapeutic effects of vasoactive intestinal peptide in the trinitrobenzene sulfonic acid mice model of Crohn's disease. *Gastroenterology* 124, 961–971.

Abad, C., Tan, Y. V., Cheung-Lau, G., Nobuta, H., and Waschek, J. A. (2012). VIP deficient mice exhibit resistance to lipopolysaccharide induced endotoxemia with an intrinsic defect in proinflammatory cellular responses. *PLoS ONE* 7:e36922. doi: 10.1371/journal.pone.0036922

Abad, C., Tan, Y. V., Lopez, R., Nobuta, H., Dong, H., Phan, P., et al. (2010). Vasoactive intestinal peptide loss leads to impaired CNS parenchymal T-cell infiltration and resistance to experimental autoimmune encephalomyelitis. *Proc. Natl. Acad. Sci. U.S.A.* 107, 19555–19560.

Bechet, J.-J., Houadjeto, M., and D'Albis, A. (1986). Active-site titration of enzymes at high concentration. *Eur. J. Biochem.* 161, 343–349.

Bourgault, S., Vaudry, D., Botia, B., Couvineau, A., Laburthe, M., Vaudry, H., et al. (2008). Novel stable PACAP analogs with potent activity towards the PAC1 receptor. *Peptides* 29, 919–932.

Brenneman, D. E., and Eiden, L. E. (1986). Vasoactive intestinal peptide and electrical activity influence neuronal survival. *Proc. Natl. Acad. Sci. U.S.A.* 83, 1159–1162.

Ceraudo, E., Hierso, R., Tan, Y. V., Murail, S., Rouyer-Fessard, C., Nicole, P., et al. (2012). Spatial proximity between the VPAC1 receptor and the amino terminus of agonist and antagonist peptides reveals distinct sites of interaction. *FASEB J.* 26, 2060–2071.

Ceraudo, E., Murail, S., Tan, Y. V., Lacapère, J. J., Neumann, J. M., Couvineau, A., et al. (2008). The vasoactive intestinal peptide (VIP) alpha-Helix up to C terminus interacts with the N-terminal ectodomain of the human VIP/Pituitary adenylate cyclase-activating peptide 1 receptor: photoaffinity, molecular modeling, and dynamics. *Mol. Endocrinol.* 22, 147–155.

Christopoulos, A., Christopoulos, G., Morfis, M., Adawela, M., Laburthe, M., Couvineau, A., et al. (2002). Novel receptor partners and function of receptor activity-modifying proteins. *J. Biol. Chem.* 278, 3293–3297.

Chu, A., Caldwell, J. S., and Chen, Y. A. (2010). Identification and characterization of a small molecule antagonist of human VPAC2 receptor. *Mol. Pharmacol.* 77, 95–101.

Chugunov, A. O., Simms, J., Poyner, D. R., Dehouck, Y., Rooman, M., Gilis, D., et al. (2010). Evidence that interaction between conserved residues in transmembrane helices 2 3, and 7 are crucial for human VPAC1 receptor activation. *Mol. Pharmacol.* 78, 394–401.

Couvineau, A., Ceraudo, E., Tan, Y. V., and Laburthe, M. (2010). VPAC1 receptor binding site: contribution of photoaffinity labeling approach. *Neuropeptides* 44, 127–132.

Couvineau, A., Gaudin, P., Maoret, J. J., Rouyer-Fessard, C., Nicole, P., and Laburthe, M. (1995). Highly conserved aspartate 68, tryptophane 73 and glycine 109 in the N-terminal extracellular domain of the human VIP receptor are essential for its ability to bind VIP. *Biochem. Biophys. Res. Commun.* 206, 246–252.

Couvineau, A., and Laburthe, M. (2012a). The family B1 GPCR: structural aspects and interaction with accessory proteins. *Curr. Drug Targets* 13, 103–115.

Couvineau, A., and Laburthe, M. (2012b). VPAC receptors: structure, molecular pharmacology and interaction with accessory proteins. *Br. J. Pharmacol.* 166, 42–50.

Couvineau, A., Lacapère, J. J., Tan, Y. V., Rouyer-Fessard, C., Nicole, P., and Laburthe, M. (2003). Identification of cytoplasmic domains of hVPAC1 receptor required for activation of adenylyl cyclase. *J. Biol. Chem.* 278, 24759–24766.

Couvineau, A., Robert, J. C., Ramdani, T., Lacapère, J. J., Rouyer-Fessard, C., and Laburthe, M. (2008). Production and purification of large quantities of the functional N-terminal ectodomain of human VPAC1 receptor. *J. Mol. Neurosci.* 36, 249–253.

Couvineau, A., Rouyer-Fessard, C., Darmoul, D., Maoret, J. J., Carrero, I., Ogier-Denis, E., et al. (1994). Human intestinal VIP receptor: cloning and functional expression of two cDNA encoding proteins with different N-terminal domains. *Biochem. Biophys. Res. Commun.* 200, 769–776.

Couvineau, A., Rouyer-Fessard, C., Fournier, A., St Pierre, S., Pipkorn, R., and Laburthe, M. (1984). Structural requirements for VIP interaction with specific receptors in human and rat intestinal membranes: effect of nine partial sequences. *Biochem. Biophys. Res. Commun.* 121, 493–498.

Couvineau, A., Rouyer-Fessard, C., and Laburthe, M. (2004). Presence of a N-terminal signal peptide in class II G protein-coupled receptors: crucial role for expression of the human VPAC1 receptor. *Regul. Pept.* 123, 181–185.

Couvineau, A., Rouyer-Fessard, C., Maoret, J. J., Gaudin, P., Nicole, P., and Laburthe, M. (1996a). Vasoactive intestinal peptide (VIP) 1 receptor. Three nonadjacent amino acids are responsible for species selectivity with respect to recognition of peptide histidine isoleucineamide. *J. Biol. Chem.* 271, 12795–12800.

Couvineau, A., Fabre, C., Gaudin, P., Maoret, J. J., and Laburthe, M. (1996b). Mutagenesis of N-glycosylation sites in the human vasoactive intestinal peptide 1 receptor. Evidence that asparagine 58 or 69 is crucial for correct delivery of the receptor to plasma membrane. *Biochemistry* 35, 1745–1752.

Dejda, A., Sokołowska, P., and Nowak, J. Z. (2005). Neuroprotective potential of three neuropeptides PACAP, VIP and PHI. *Pharmacol. Rep.* 57, 307–320.

Delgado, M., Abad, C., Martinez, C., Leceta, J., and Gomariz, R. P. (2001). Vasoactive intestinal peptide prevents experimental arthritis by downregulating both autoimmune and inflammatory components of the disease. *Nat. Med.* 7, 563–568.

Delgado, M., and Ganea, D. (2011). Vasoactive intestinal peptide: a neuropeptide with pleiotropic immune functions. *Amino Acids* 11, 1184–1188.

Delgado, M., Pozo, D., and Ganea, D. (2004). The significance of vasoactive intestinal peptide in immunomodulation. *Pharmacol. Rev.* 56, 249–290.

Dickson, L., and Finlayson, K. (2009). VPAC and PAC receptors: from ligands to function. *Pharmacol. Ther.* 121, 294–316.

Dogrukol-Ak, D., Tore, F., and Tuncel, N. (2004). Passage of VIP/PACAP/secretin family across the blood-brain barrier: therapeutic effects. *Curr. Pharm. Des.* 10, 1325–1340.

Du, K., Nicole, P., Couvineau, A., and Laburthe, M. (1997). Aspartate 196 in the first extracellular loop of the human VIP1 receptor is essential for VIP binding and VIP-stimulated cAMP production. *Biochem. Biophys. Res. Commun.* 230, 289–292.

Fahrenkrug, J. (2001). Gut/brain peptides in the genital tract: VIP and PACAP. *Scand. J. Clin. Lab. Invest.* 234, 35–39.

Fernandez-Montesinos, R., Castillo, P. M., Klippstein, R., Gonzalez-Rey, E., Mejias, J. A., Zaderenko, A. P., et al. (2009). Chemical synthesis and characterization of silver-protected vasoactive intestinal peptide nanoparticles. *Nanomedicine (Lond.)* 4, 919–930.

Firestein, G. S. (2001). VIP: a very important protein in arthritis. *Nat. Med.* 7, 537–538.

Fredrikson, R., and Schiöth, B. (2006). "G Protein-coupled receptors in human genome," in *Ligand Design for G Protein-Coupled Receptors, vol. 30*, ed D. Rognan (Weinheim: Wiley-VCH), 1–27.

Gonzalez-Rey, E., Chorny, A., Fernandez-Martin, A., Varela, N., and Delgado, M. (2005). Vasoactive intestinal peptide family as a therapeutic target for Parkinson's disease. *Expert Opin. Ther. Targets* 9, 923–929.

Gourlet, P., De Neef, P., Cnudde, J., Waelbroeck, M., and Robberecht, P. (1997). *In vitro* properties of a high affinity selective antagonist of the VIP1 receptor. *Peptides* 18, 1555–1560.

Gozes, I., Bardea, A., Reshef, A., Zamostiano, R., Zhukovsky, S., Rubinraut, S., et al. (1996). Neuroprotective strategy for Alzheimer disease: intranasal administration of a fatty neuropeptide. *Proc. Natl. Acad. Sci. U.S.A.* 93, 427–432.

Gozes, I., Divinsky, I., Pilzer, I., Fridkin, M., Brenneman, D. E., and Spier, A. D. (2003). From vasoactive intestinal peptide (VIP) through activity-dependent neuroprotective protein (ADNP) to NAP: a view of neuroprotection and cell division. *J. Mol. Neurosci.* 20, 315–322.

Grace, C. R., Perrin, M. H., DiGruccio, M. R., Miller, C. L., Rivier, J. E., Vale, W. W., et al. (2004). NMR structure and peptide hormone binding site of the first extracellular domain of a type B1 G protein-coupled receptor. *Proc. Natl. Acad. Sci. U.S.A.* 101, 12836–12841.

Groneberg, D. A., Rabe, K. F., and Fischer, A. (2006). Novel concepts of neuropeptide-based drug therapy: vasoactive intestinal polypeptide and its receptors. *Eur. J. Pharmacol.* 533, 182–194.

Harikrishnan, L. S., Srivastava, N., Kayser, L. E., Nirschl, D. S., Kumaragurubaran, K., Roy, A., et al. (2012). Identification and optimization of small molecule antagonists of vasoactive intestinal peptide receptor-1 (VIPR1). *Bioorg. Med. Chem. Lett.* 22, 2287–2290.

Harikumar, K. G., Morfis, M. M., Lisenbee, C. S., Sexton, P. M., and Miller, L. J. (2006). Constitutive formation of oligomeric complexes between family B G protein-coupled vasoactive intestinal polypeptide and secretin receptors. *Mol. Pharmacol.* 69, 363–373.

Harmar, A. J., Fahrenkrug, J., Gozes, I., Laburthe, M., May, V., Pisegna, J. R., et al. (2012). Pharmacology and functions of receptors for vasoactive intestinal peptide and pituitary adenylate cyclase-activating polypeptide: IUPHAR review 1. *Br. J. Pharmacol.* 166, 4–17.

Hoare, S. R. J. (2005). Mechanism of peptide and nonpeptide ligand binding to class B G-protein-coupled receptors. *Drug Discov. Today* 10, 417–427.

Ishihara, T., Nakamura, S., Kaziro, Y., Takahashi, T., Takahashi, K., and Nagata, S. (1991). Molecular cloning and expression of a cDNA encoding the secretin receptor. *EMBO J.* 10, 1635–1641.

Ishihara, T., Shigemoto, R., Mori, K., Takahashi, K., and Nagata, S. (1992). Functional expression, and tissue distribution of a novel receptor for vasoactive intestinalpolypeptide. *Neuron* 8, 811–819.

Jaakola, V. P., Griffith, M. T., Hanson, M. A., Cherezov, V., Chien, E. Y., Lane, J. R., et al. (2008). The 2.6 angstrom crystal structure of a human A2A adenosine receptor bound to an antagonist. *Science* 322, 1211–1217.

Kumar, S., Pioszak, A., Zhang, C., Swaminathan, K., and Xu, H. E. (2011). Crystal structure of the PAC1R extracellular domain unifies a consensus fold for hormone recognition by class B G-protein coupled receptors. *PLoS ONE* 6:e19682. doi: 10.1371/journal.pone.0019682

Laburthe, M., Couvineau, A., and Marie, J. C. (2002). VPAC receptors for VIP and PACAP. *Receptors Channels* 8, 137–153.

Laburthe, M., Couvineau, A., and Tan, V. (2007). Class II G protein-coupled receptors for VIP and PACAP: structure, models of activation and pharmacology. *Peptides* 28, 1631–1639.

Lambeir, A. M., Durinx, C., Proost, P., Van Damme, J., Scharpé, S., and De Meester, I. (2001). Kinetic study of the processing by dipeptidyl-peptidase IV/CD26 of neuropeptides involved in pancreatic insulin secretion. *FEBS Lett.* 507, 327–330.

Leceta, J., Gomariz, R. P., Martinez, C., Carrión, M., Arranz, A., and Juarranz, Y. (2007). Vasoactive intestinal peptide regulates Th17 function in autoimmune inflammation. *Neuroimmunomodulation* 14, 134–138.

Lutz, E. M., Sheward, W. J., West, K. M., Morrow, J. A., Fink, G., and Harmar, A. J. (1993). The VIP2 receptor: molecular characterisation of a cDNA encoding a novel receptor for vasoactive intestinal peptide. *FEBS Lett.* 334, 3–8.

Marie, J. C., Rouyer-Fessard, C., Couvineau, A., Nicole, P., Devaud, H., El Benna, J., et al. (2003). Serine 447 in the carboxyl tail of human VPAC1 receptor is crucial for agonist-induced desensitization but not internalization of the receptor. *Mol. Pharmacol.* 64, 1565–1574.

Moody, T. W., Ito, T., Osefo, N., and Jensen, R. T. (2011). VIP and PACAP: recent insights into their functions/roles in physiology and disease from molecular and genetic studies. *Curr. Opin. Endocrinol. Diabetes Obes.* 18, 61–67.

Moreno, D., Gourlet, P., De Neef, P., Cnudde, J., Waelbroeck, M., and Robberecht, P. (2000). Development of selective agonists and antagonists for the human vasoactive intestinal peptide VPAC2 receptor. *Peptides* 21, 1543–1549.

Neumann, J. M., Couvineau, A., Murail, S., Lacapère, J. J., Jamin, N., and Laburthe, M. (2008). Class-B GPCR activation: is ligand helix-capping the key? *Trends Biochem. Sci.* 33, 314–319.

Nicole, P., Lins, L., Rouyer-Fessard, C., Drouot, C., Fulcrand, P., Thomas, A., et al. (2000). Identification of key residues for interaction of vasoactive intestinal peptide with human VPAC1 and VPAC2 receptors and development of a highly selective VPAC1 receptor agonist. *J. Biol. Chem.* 275, 24003–24012.

Onyüksel, H., Mohanty, P. S., and Rubinstein, I. (2009). VIP-grafted sterically stabilized phospholipid nanomicellar 17-allylamino-17-demethoxy geldanamycin: a novel targeted nanomedicine for breast cancer. *Int. J. Pharm.* 365, 157–161.

Pal, K., Melcher, K., and Xu, H. E. (2012). Structure and mechanism for recognition of peptide hormones by Class B G-protein-coupled receptors. *Acta Pharmacol. Sin.* 33, 300–311.

Parthier, C., Kleinschmidt, M., Neumann, P., Rudolph, R., Manhart, S., Schlenzig, D., et al. (2007). Crystal structure of the incretin-bound extracellular domain of a G protein-coupled receptor. *Proc. Natl. Acad. Sci. U.S.A.* 104, 13942–13947.

Parthier, C., Reedtz-Runge, S., Rudolph, R., and Stubbs, M. T. (2009). Passing the baton in class B GPCRs: peptide hormone activation via helix induction? *Trends Biochem. Sci.* 34, 303–310.

Said, S. I., and Mutt, V. (1970). Polypeptide with broad biological activity: isolation from small intestine. *Science* 169, 1217–1228.

Shoichet, B. K., and Kobilka, B. K. (2012). Structure-based drug screening for G-protein-coupled receptors. *Trends Pharmacol. Sci.* 33, 268–272.

Solano, R. M., Langer, I., Perret, J., Vertongen, P., Juarranz, M. G., Robberecht, P., et al. (2001). Two basic residues of the h-VPAC1 receptor second transmembrane helix are essential for ligand binding and signal transduction. *J. Biol. Chem.* 276, 1084–1088.

Sreedharan, S. P., Patel, D. R., Huang, J. X., and Goetzl, E. J. (1993). Cloning and functional expression of a human neuroendocrine vasoactive intestinal peptide receptor. *Biochem. Biophys. Res. Commun.* 193, 546–553.

Sun, C., Song, D., Davis-Taber, R. A., Barrett, L. W., Scott, V. E., Richardson, P. L., et al. (2007). Solution structure and mutational analysis of pituitary adenylate cyclase-activating polypeptide binding to the extracellular domain of PAC1-RS. *Proc. Natl. Acad. Sci. U.S.A.* 104, 7875–7880.

Tan, Y. V., Couvineau, A., and Laburthe, M. (2004). Diffuse pharmacophoric domains of vasoactive intestinal peptide (VIP) and further insights into the interaction of VIP with the N-terminal ectodomain of human VPAC1 receptor by photoaffinity labeling with [Bpa6]-VIP. *J. Biol. Chem.* 279, 38889–38894.

Tan, Y. V., Couvineau, A., Murail, S., Ceraudo, E., Neumann, J. M., Lacapère, J. J., et al. (2006). Peptide agonist docking in the N-terminal ectodomain of a class II G protein-coupled receptor, the VPAC1 receptor. Photoaffinity, NMR, and molecular modeling. *J. Biol. Chem.* 281, 12792–12798.

Tan, Y. V., Couvineau, A., Van Rampelbergh, J., and Laburthe, M. (2003). Photoaffinity labeling demonstrates physical contact between vasoactive intestinal peptide and the N-terminal ectodomain of the human VPAC1 receptor. *J. Biol. Chem.* 278, 36531–36536.

Tan, Y. V., and Waschek, J. A. (2011). Targeting VIP and PACAP receptor signalling: new therapeutic strategies in multiple sclerosis. *ASN Neuro* 3, e00065.

Vacic, V., McCarthy, S., Malhotra, D., Murray, F., Chou, H. H., Peoples, A., et al. (2011). Duplications of the neuropeptide receptor gene VIPR2 confer significant risk for schizophrenia. *Nature* 471, 499–503.

Watkins, H. A., Au, M., and Hay, D. L. (2012). The structure of secretin family GPCR peptide ligands: implications for receptor pharmacology and drug development. *Drug Discov. Today* 17, 1006–1014.

Xia, M., Sreedharan, S. P., Bolin, D. R., Gaufo, G. O., and Goetzl, E. J. (1997). Novel cyclic peptide agonist of high potency and selectivity for the type II vasoactive intestinal peptide receptor. *J. Pharmacol. Exp. Ther.* 281, 629–633.

3

Mechanisms involved in VPAC receptors activation and regulation: lessons from pharmacological and mutagenesis studies

Ingrid Langer*

Institut de Recherche Interdisciplinaire en Biologie Humaine et Moléculaire, Faculté de Médecine, Université Libre de Bruxelles, Brussels, Belgium

Edited by:
Hubert Vaudry, University of Rouen, France

Reviewed by:
Nicholas D. Holliday, University of Nottingham, UK
Alain Couvineau, Institut National de la Santé et de la Recherche Médicale, France

Correspondence:
Ingrid Langer, Institut de Recherche Interdisciplinaire en Biologie Humaine et Moléculaire, Faculté de Médecine, Université Libre de Bruxelles, 808 route de Lennik CP602, B-1070 Brussels, Belgium.
e-mail: ilanger@ulb.ac.be

Vasoactive intestinal peptide (VIP) plays diverse and important role in human physiology and physiopathology and their receptors constitute potential targets for the treatment of several diseases such as neurodegenerative disorder, asthma, diabetes, and inflammatory diseases. This article reviews the current knowledge regarding the two VIP receptors, $VPAC_1$ and $VPAC_2$, with respect to mechanisms involved in receptor activation, G protein coupling, signaling, regulation, and oligomerization.

Keywords: VIP, $VPAC_1$, $VPAC_2$, mutagenesis, activation, signaling, regulation, oligomerization

VASOACTIVE INTESTINAL PEPTIDE

Vasoactive intestinal peptide (VIP) is a 28 amino acids peptide isolated from porcine intestine (Said and Mutt, 1970) and that belongs to a family of structurally related peptide hormones that includes secretin, pituitary adenylate cyclase-activating polypeptide (PACAP), glucagon, glucagon-like peptides (GLP), gastric inhibitory peptide (GIP), and growth hormone-releasing hormone (GHRH). It has initially been shown that VIP has a diverse range of effects such as vasodilation, relaxation of smooth muscle in intestinal and pulmonary tissues, and stimulation of electrolyte secretion in the gut (Dickson and Finlayson, 2009; Harmar et al., 2012). As a consequence, VIP was first classified as a gut hormone. Later studies demonstrated that VIP has a more expanded distribution including peripheral (PNS) and central (CNS) nervous system (Larsson et al., 1976a,b) as well as cells and tissues of the immune system (Delgado et al., 2004), suggesting that VIP may also behave as a neuroendocrine hormone, a neurotransmitter and a cytokine-like peptide. Many studies supported this hypothesis and it is now well accepted that VIP plays important role in the CNS such as control of circadian rhythms, anxiety, response to stress, schizophrenia, learning, and memory (King et al., 2003; Dickson and Finlayson, 2009; Moody et al., 2011; Harmar et al., 2012). In the periphery, it is involved in the control of insulin secretion from the pancreas and the release of catecholamines from the adrenal medulla (Dickson and Finlayson, 2009; Moody et al., 2011; Harmar et al., 2012). VIP also acts as a co-transmitter of non-adrenergic non-cholinergic relaxation of vascular and non-vascular smooth muscles (Said and Rattan, 2004). Finally, in the immune system VIP has potent effects on T cell differentiation and migration and modulates cytokine production by T helper cells (Delgado et al., 2004).

VPAC RECEPTORS

The biological effects of VIP are mediated by two receptors named $VPAC_1$ and $VPAC_2$ that belong to the family B of G protein-coupled receptors (GPCRs) which also includes PAC_1-, secretin-, glucagon-, GLP 1 and 2-, calcitonin-, GIP-, corticotropin-releasing factor (CRF) 1 and 2-, and parathyroid hormone receptors. Besides VIP, $VPAC_1$ and $VPAC_2$ receptors also bind with the same high affinity PACAP. The $VPAC_1$ receptor was initially cloned from rat lung (Sreedharan et al., 1993) and the $VPAC_2$ receptor from rat pituitary (Lutz et al., 1993). Like VIP, VPAC receptors are widely distributed throughout the body. In the CNS, $VPAC_1$ receptors are abundantly localized in piriform cortex, cerebral cortex, suprachiasmatic nucleus, hippocampus, and pineal gland (Usdin et al., 1994) while $VPAC_2$ receptors are mainly found in cerebral cortex, suprachiasmatic nucleus, thalamus, hypothalamus, and amygdala (Sheward et al., 1995). Although both receptors may be co-expressed in the same areas of the CNS, studies suggest that the two receptor subtypes have complementary distribution. In peripheral tissues, $VPAC_1$ receptors have been found in breast, kidney, liver, lung, prostate, spleen, and mucosa of the gastrointestinal tract (Reubi, 2000). Similarly, $VPAC_2$ receptors have a large distribution and have been localized in adrenal medulla, blood vessels, lung, pancreatic acinar cells, smooth muscle, and thyroid follicular cells (Harmar et al., 2004). In the immune system, $VPAC_1$ receptors are constitutively expressed in T cells, monocytes, and macrophages while expression of $VPAC_2$ receptors is induced upon activation of T cells and macrophages (Delgado et al., 2004).

Like all members of the GPCR-B family, VPAC receptors are heptahelical membrane proteins and are characterized by the presence of a large N-terminal extracellular domain. The recent solving of the NMR or X-ray structure of the N-terminus of several family B receptors [CRF, PTH, PAC_1, GIP, GLP-1, CLR/RAMP1, and $VPAC_2$(PDB ID: 2X57)] clarified their role in ligand binding. The structure comprises a crucial sushi domain characterized by two antiparallel β sheets and stabilized by three disulfide bonds and a salt bridge sandwiched between aromatic rings of two tryptophan residues (Harmar et al., 2012). The data support the two-site model for peptide binding to family B GPCR, in which the N-terminal domain of the receptor is the principal binding site for the central and the C-terminal regions of the natural ligand and ensures correct ligand positioning, whereas binding of residues 1–6 of the ligand to the extracellular loops and transmembrane helices drives the receptor activation (Hoare, 2005). More recently, it has also been proposed that a helix N-capping motif, identified in the N-terminus of all GPCR-B family ligands and stabilizing their helical conformation, was probably formed upon receptor binding and could also constitute a key element in receptor activation (Neumann et al., 2008). Although the experimental structure of the $VPAC_1$ has not been solved, a three-dimensional model obtained by homology modeling associated with photoaffinity experiments supports that $VPAC_1$ shares the same features (Couvineau and Laburthe, 2012).

SIGNALING PATHWAYS ACTIVATED BY VPAC RECEPTORS

Like all GPCRs, upon agonist binding VPAC receptors undergo physical/conformational changes that allow interaction of cytoplasmic domains with heterotrimeric G proteins and promote exchange of GDP for GTP on the Gα subunit. This initiates the dissociation of GTP-bound Gα subunit from Gβγ dimer and activation of downstream effector pathways. Signals are terminated following hydrolysis of Gα-bound GTP and reformation of inactive trimeric complex (Pierce et al., 2002). VPAC receptors are preferentially coupled to Gαs leading to activation of adenylate cyclase and subsequent cAMP production. Accumulation of intracellular cAMP also leads to activation of protein kinase A (PKA) that may activate the ERK signaling pathway to promote proliferation (Pechon-Vallee et al., 2000) and neuroendocrine cell differentiation (Gutierrez-Canas et al., 2005) as seen in pituitary cells and prostate cancer cell line, respectively. VIP-induced PKA activation is also responsible for most of the anti-inflammatory activity of VIP by regulating several signaling pathways and transcription factors thus increasing anti-inflammatory cytokines and reducing pro-inflammatory cytokines production (Gonzalez-Rey et al., 2007). Several studies also reported that VPAC receptors were able to activate phospholipase C (PLC) pathway and stimulate calcium levels, either in cells endogenously expressing VPAC receptors or in transfected cell lines. However, the precise mechanisms which contribute to VIP-induced $[Ca^{2+}]_i$ increase remain unclear due to divergent results. Indeed, in transfected cell lines some studies observed that activation of PLC was partly sensitive to pertussis toxin (PTx; MacKenzie et al., 1996; Langer et al., 2002), thus involving both Gαi and Gαq coupling, while others did not observe coupling to Gαi (Sreedharan et al., 1994). Moreover, PTx sensitive mechanisms leading to PLC activation seems different for $VPAC_1$ and $VPAC_2$ receptors. Cross-linking studies demonstrated that physical interaction between $VPAC_1$ and Gαi and $VPAC_1$-induced $[Ca^{2+}]_i$ increase are not affected by chelating of extracellular calcium (Langer et al., 2002), while PTx sensitive activation of PLC by $VPAC_2$ relies on the availability of free Gβγ and on Ca^{2+} entry through receptor-operated Ca^{2+} channels (MacKenzie et al., 2001). Finally, it was also observed that both $VPAC_1$ and $VPAC_2$ are able to couple to Gα16, a G protein of the Gαq family, that enables the coupling of a wide variety of receptors to PLC and whose expression is restricted to hematopoietic cells (with the exception of the mature B cells; Langer et al., 2001). These findings indicate that the specific G protein/second messenger complement of the cell line/type being examined could alter the transduction pathways/pharmacology observed for VPAC receptors (**Figure 1**).

Additional coupling events that are not G protein-mediated may also elicit auxiliary signals. Both $VPAC_1$ and $VPAC_2$ are able to activate phospholipase D (PLD). PLD responses induced by $VPAC_2$ are not affected by PLC inhibitors, PTx or PKA inhibitors but are sensitive to brefeldin A an inhibitor of ADP-ribosylation factor (ARF) known to act as a direct activator of PLD (McCulloch et al., 2000). In pancreatic β cells, VIP induced sustained stimulation of insulin secretion is mediated by phosphatidylinositol 3 kinase activation by $VPAC_2$ receptors (Dickinson et al., 1999). In the rat pineal gland, VIP stimulates cGMP formation through activation of nitric oxide synthase, NO production and activation of cytosolic guanylate cyclase (Spessert, 1993).

MOLECULAR MECHANISMS INVOLVED IN VPAC RECEPTORS ACTIVATION

The recent solving of the X-ray crystal structures of several GPCR-A family members in complex with agonist, antagonist, and G proteins provides clues to the transmembrane helix (TM) rearrangements that result from agonist binding and subsequent receptor activation. These include the disruption of an ionic interaction involving the E/DRY motif located at the cytoplasmic face of TM3 and maintaining the receptor preferentially in a ground inactive conformation in absence of agonist (ionic lock), a "rotamer toggle switch" (modulation of the helix conformation around a proline kink) in TM6 causing key sequences to be exposed to cytoplasmic binding partners and a conformational change of Y residue of the NPXXY motif located in TM7 stabilizing the active conformation (Rosenbaum et al., 2009, 2011; Rasmussen et al., 2011). Surprisingly, the predicted interaction between E/DRY motif located in TM3 and a glutamate residue located in TM6 ("ionic lock") was solely observed in rhodopsin inactive state crystals but not in other GPCR crystals available to date. Instead, as seen for the β2-adrenergic receptor (β2-AR), Arg of the E/DRY motif interacts primarily with the adjacent Asp residue in crystals of β2-AR stabilized with the inverse agonist carazolol (inactive conformation; Rasmussen et al., 2007; Rosenbaum et al., 2007) while in crystals of β2-AR/Gs protein complex (active conformation) this interaction is broken and Arg of the E/DRY motif packs against a Tyr residue of Gs (Rasmussen et al., 2011). In absence of X-ray crystal structure of the VPAC receptors, only model structures of $VPAC_1$ have been reported which used as template the structures of the N-terminal domain of the CRF 2β receptor (Ceraudo et al., 2012) or structures of family A GPCRs for the transmembrane domains (Conner et al., 2005; Chugunov et al., 2010). However, the low sequence identity between the sequence

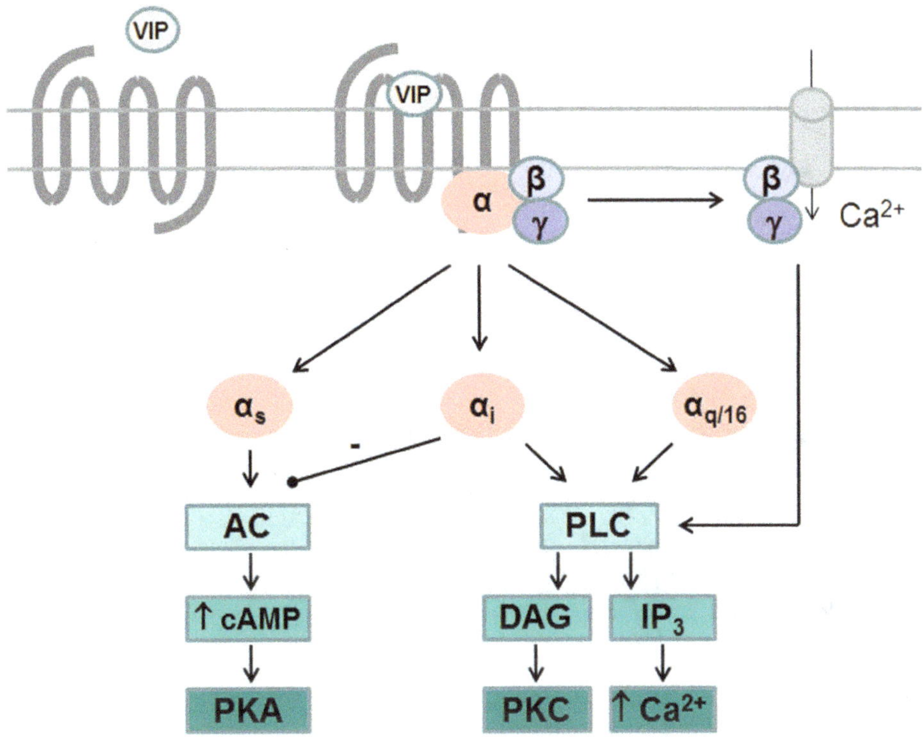

FIGURE 1 | G protein-dependent signaling pathways activated by VPAC receptors. VPAC receptors are preferentially coupled to Gαs leading to activation of adenylate cyclase (AC) and subsequent cAMP production and activation of protein kinase A (PKA). VPAC receptors are able to activate phospholipase C (PLC) pathway after coupling to Gαi, Gαq, or $G\alpha_{16}$ and stimulate calcium levels and protein kinase C (PKC). Gαi-dependent activation of PLC by $VPAC_2$ relies on the availability of free Gβγ and on Ca^{2+} entry through receptor-operated Ca^{2+} channels while Gαi-dependent activation of PLC by $VPAC_1$ is not affected by chelating of extracellular calcium.

of the VPAC receptors and the templates used for homology modeling prevents direct transposition of molecular switches that drive GPCR-A members activation.

As all members of GPCR-B family, VPAC receptors lack the E/DRY sequence. On the basis of subtle changes observed when Y^{239} and L^{240}, located in TM3 of $VPAC_1$, were substituted with alanine it was proposed that this YL sequence was equivalent to the E/DRY motif of GPCR-A family (Tams et al., 2001). Another model based on a three-dimensional analysis of the GLP-1 receptor proposed that a E/DRY motif could be formed by three non-adjacent residues consisting in R^{174} in the cytoplasmic end of TM2, E^{236}, and Y^{239} in the distal part of TM3 of $VPAC_1$ (Frimurer and Bywater, 1999). However, another study showed that $Y^{239}A$, $L^{240}A$, $E^{236}A$, $Y^{239}A$, and $R^{174}A$ mutants were undistinguishable from the wild type receptor (Nachtergael et al., 2006). One possible explanation for the discrepancy can be the fact that Tams et al. (2001) studied cyclic AMP measurements in intact cells a more sensitive model than the adenylate cyclase assay on membrane used in the other study. Nevertheless, even if the YL motif of GPCR-B family and E/DRY motif of GPCR-A family have the same location, they certainly do not have the same importance for receptor activation (**Figure 2**).

As mentioned before structural data confirmed that GPCR activation is accompanied by modification of helix conformation. For the β2-AR, the largest difference between the inactive and active structures is a large outward movement of TM6 and an inward movement of TM7 such as Tyr of the conserved NPxxY sequence (located in TM7) moves into the space occupied by TM6 in the inactive state. In GPCR-A family conserved prolines located in TM6 and laying near the ligand binding pocket and in TM7 (NPxxY sequence) play crucial role in these rearrangements due to their cyclic pyrrolidine ring side chain that introduce kink into the α-helical structure of TM and allow TM flexibility important for G protein coupling and signaling. In this line, a study of Knudsen et al. (2001) investigated the role of prolines located in TM of $VPAC_1$ (**Figure 2**). They found that mutation of P266 (TM4), P300 (TM5), and P348 (TM6) into alanine significantly decrease $VPAC_1$ expression levels but preserve VIP binding. P266A showed decreased ability to stimulate cAMP, while P300A and P348A displayed an increased potency in cAMP production combined with a high sensitivity toward GTP compared to the wild type receptor, thus demonstrating that these prolines are important for overall structure of $VPAC_1$ and receptor activation (Knudsen et al., 2001).

A more recent study, that combined pharmacological and *in silico* approaches, identified a network of interactions between residues located in helices 2, 3, and 7 of the $VPAC_1$ receptor, which could be involved in the stabilization of the receptor in absence of agonist and in early steps of receptor activation. It was proposed that, in absence of ligand, interaction between R^{188}, N^{229}, and Q^{380} ties helices 2, 3, and 7 together (**Figure 3**). Upon VIP

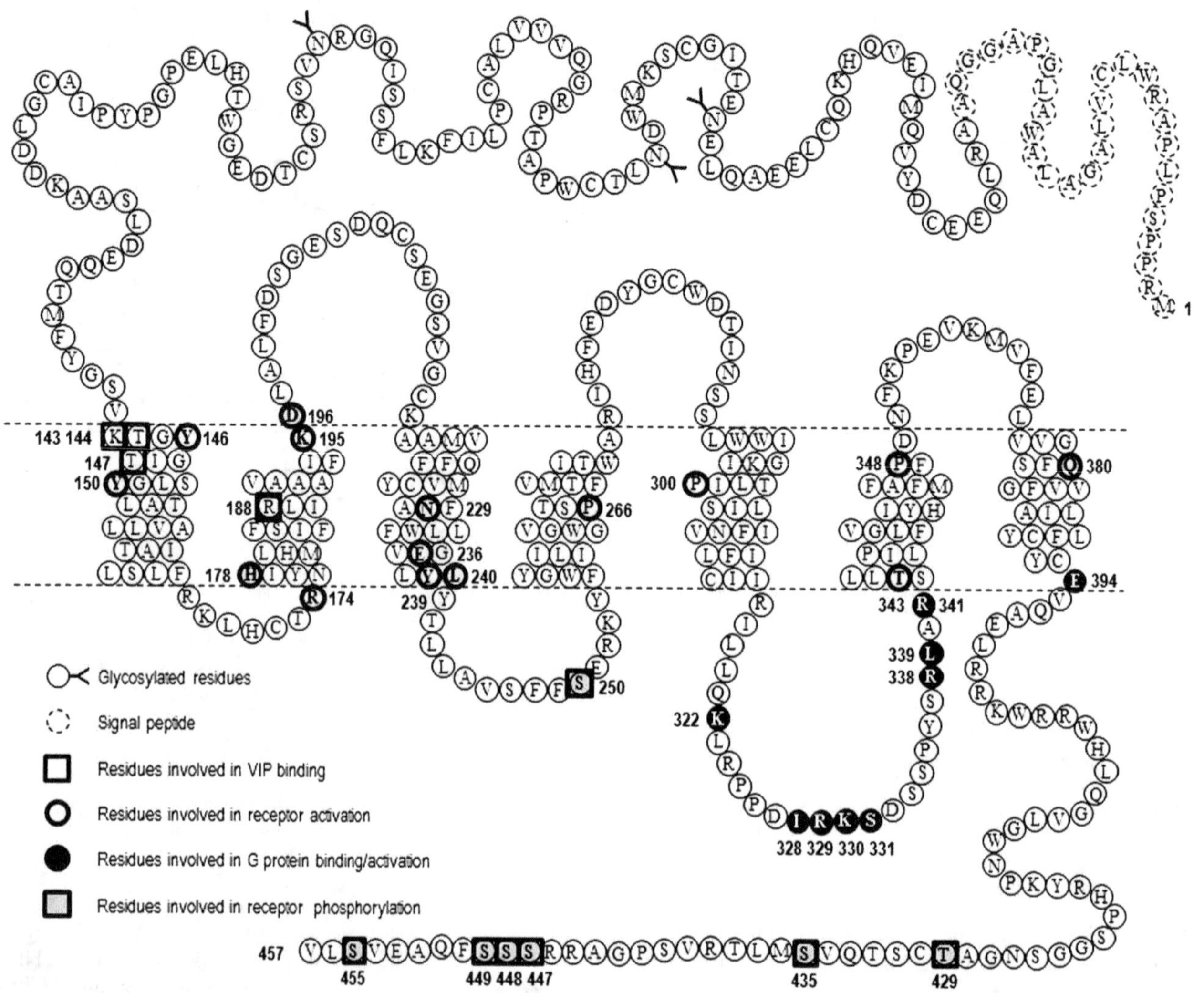

FIGURE 2 | Snake-plot representation of VPAC$_1$ receptor. Amino acid sequence of human VPAC$_1$ receptor, the position of signal peptide, glycosylated residues, and amino acids important for VIP binding, receptor activation, and G protein coupling are also labeled.

binding, the interaction between R^{188} and N^{380} is broken and a stronger interaction (salt bridge) is established between R^{188} and the D^{3} side chain of VIP. TM2 and probably other helices undergo conformational changes causing key sequences located in intracellular loops to be exposed and to interact with the G proteins. In the meantime, the interaction network involving N^{229} and Q^{380} maintains TM7 in a conformation necessary for proper activation of G proteins. The three-dimensional model also suggested that Q^{380} could function as a floating "ferry-boat", switching between R^{188} and N^{229} residues' side-chains hence contributing to signal transduction propagation and activation of G proteins (Chugunov et al., 2010).

When considering other site-directed mutagenesis studies, it is likely that a complex and larger network of interaction between TM helices must be considered for stabilization of VPAC$_1$ inactive and active conformations (**Figure 2**). Indeed, the mutation into arginine of H^{178} located at the bottom of TM2 led to a constitutively activated VPAC$_1$ receptor (Gaudin et al., 1998). Similarly, mutation of T^{343}, located at junction of the third intracellular loop and TM6 of VPAC$_1$, into lysine, proline, or alanine also led to a constitutively activated receptor (Gaudin et al., 1999). Another study showed that Y^{146} and Y^{150}, located in TM1 of VPAC$_1$, do not interact directly with VIP but stabilize the correct active receptor conformation (Perret et al., 2002). It was also observed that K^{195} and D^{196} located at junction of TM2 and the first extracellular loop were essential for VPAC$_1$ activation but were not directly involved in VIP recognition (Langer et al., 2003). How all these residues cooperate to propagate signal transduction after VIP binding remains to be elucidated and would require a model or a structure of the activated receptor in complex with VIP. Particularly the two N-terminal residues of VIP, H^{1} and S^{2}, are likely to affect, directly or indirectly, the interaction network involved in receptor activation. In this line, a very recent study suggested that K^{143}, T^{144}, and T^{147}, located in TM1 of VPAC$_1$ could interact with H^{1} residue of VIP and play an important role in receptor activation (Ceraudo et al., 2012). Mutagenesis studies of VPAC$_2$ are less

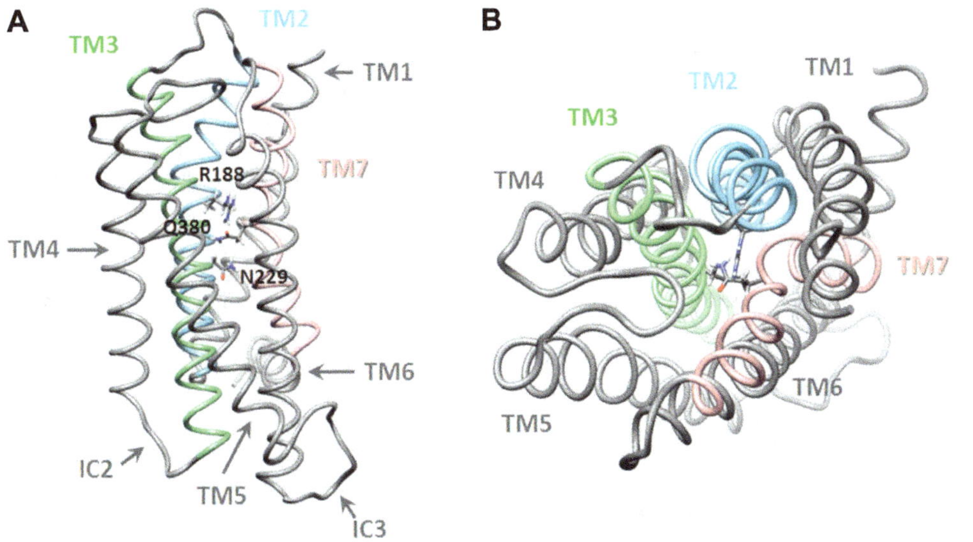

FIGURE 3 | Three-dimensional model of the transmembrane domains of the VPAC$_1$ receptor. Lateral **(A)** and top **(B)** view of a working model of human VPAC$_1$ receptor, TM, and residues identified as important for receptor stabilization are also labeled. Details regarding modeling procedure are described in Chugunov et al. (2010).

exhaustive, however, some studies identified key residues involved in receptor activation such as Y^{130} and Y^{134} located in TM1 (Perret et al., 2002), K^{179} in TM2 (Vertongen et al., 2001), and N^{216} in TM3 (Nachtergael et al., 2006), suggesting that VPAC$_1$ and VPAC$_2$ share a similar pattern of activation. Moreover, so far as all residues that were identified as important for VPAC receptors activation are highly conserved among GPCR-B family members, they may therefore be involved in binding and activation mechanisms that are common to the whole family.

MOLECULAR MECHANISMS INVOLVED IN VPAC/G PROTEIN BINDING AND ACTIVATION

The α subunit of heterotrimeric G proteins has a central role in interaction with both the receptor and the effectors. Several studies have shown that the C-terminal part of Gα subunit can directly bind to the receptor and is involved in the coupling specificity (Conklin et al., 1996). The current model of GPCR activation, based on the study of family A GPCRs, proposes that when the receptor switches to its active conformation, TM movements are accompanied by intracellular loops switches leading to exposure of the G protein binding pocket to cytosol and efficient binding to G protein. However, the diversity of sequences and loop sizes as well as their flexibility has made difficult the identification of a specific set of residues defining the coupling profile.

For the VPAC$_1$ receptor, Gα binding domains are mainly located in the third intracellular loop (IC3) that contains subdomains dedicated to the recognition of the different Gα subunits. K^{322} located in proximal part of IC3 and E^{394} located at the junction of TM7 and the C-terminal tail are required for adenylate cyclase activation but not for the coupling to the inositol trisphosphate/calcium pathway. The former being involved in direct interaction with Gαs (G protein binding), as demonstrated by a reduced sensitivity to GTP, while E^{394} triggering switch of Gαs from inactive to active state (G protein activation; Couvineau et al., 2003; Langer and Robberecht, 2005). Similarly, two other sequences located in IC3 have been identified as important for VIP-induced intracellular calcium increase but not cAMP production. A small sequence, I^{328}-R^{329}-K^{330}-S^{331}, located in the central part of IC3 is involved in efficient binding of VPAC$_1$ to Gαi/o and Gαq (Langer et al., 2002), while R^{338} and L^{339}, located at the distal part of IC3, mediate interaction of VPAC$_1$ with Gαi/o (Langer and Robberecht, 2005). Combining mutations in the proximal and distal part of IC3 together with mutation of E^{394} gave rise to a completely inactive VPAC$_1$ receptor with respect adenylate cyclase activation and intracellular calcium increase (**Figure 2**). In VPAC$_2$ receptors, L^{310} located in the proximal part of IC3 contributes to Gαs activation and the proximal part of IC3 (R^{325} and K^{328}) is involved in both Gαs and Gα16 coupling. The combined mutations of these three amino acids generates an inactive VPAC$_2$ receptor with respect to $[Ca^{2+}]_i$ increase and adenylate cyclase activation (Langer et al., 2005).

Among the different members of the GPCR-B family, proximal and distal domains of IC3 share conserved sequences that could therefore represent common G protein binding motifs. In line with this hypothesis, studies performed on other members of the GPCR-B family identified the proximal domain of IC3 as essential for adenylate cyclase activation but the amino acids involved may differ and additional conserved sequences located in other intracellular regions of the receptor may also be necessary as seen for glucagon (IC2; Cypess et al., 1999) and CGRP receptors (R^{151} located in IC1; Conner et al., 2006). The junctions of IC3 loop are predicted to be α-helical and it is assumed that the correct positioning of charged amino acids plays an important role in G protein interaction. However, other data suggest that lipophilic and aromatic residues are also important for G protein interaction. It is possible that IC3 loop junctions activate G protein directly or that they may serve as regions that control the loop conformation. As mutations may change both direct interaction site and secondary structure, it is difficult to define more precisely the mechanisms involved in IC3 loop/G protein interaction.

REGULATION OF VPAC RECEPTORS ACTIVITY

Besides coupling to the effectors, GPCR activation by agonists also initiates the process of receptor desensitization, an adaptive response contributing to rapidly fade the G protein signaling. This process starts with phosphorylation of the receptors in intracellular loops and carboxyl terminus by activity dependent kinases (PKA and PKC) and/or by receptor activated dependent kinases (GPCR kinases or GRK). GRK mediated phosphorylation of the receptor promotes the high affinity binding of β-arrestins to the receptor, which both sterically interdicts further coupling of G protein and may act as a signal transducer to activate for instance MAPKs, AKT, and PI3 kinases. β-arrestins are also able to bind proteins of the endocytic machinery including clathrin and adaptor protein AP2 and promotes receptor internalization (Shenoy and Lefkowitz, 2011).

Like most GPCRs, $VPAC_1$ and $VPAC_2$ receptors are rapidly phosphorylated after agonist exposure. Absence of inhibitory effect of PKA and PKC inhibitors (Langer et al., 2005; Langlet et al., 2005), use of dominant negative GRK and GRK over-expression experiments (Shetzline et al., 2002; Huang et al., 2007), suggest that GRK are the main kinases involved in VIP receptors phosphorylation. $VPAC_1$ receptor phosphorylation induces β-arrestin translocation to cell membrane, however, over-expression of β-arrestin in HEK 293 cells only causes a minor decrease in cAMP, suggesting $VPAC_1$ desensitization may occur through an arrestin-independent mechanism (Shetzline et al., 2002). By using site-directed mutagenesis studies, T^{429}, S^{435}, S^{447}, S^{448}, S^{449}, S^{455} located in the C-terminus and S^{250} located in IC2 were identified as potential candidates for VIP-induced $VPAC_1$ receptor phosphorylation (Marie et al., 2003; Langlet et al., 2005; **Figure 2**). Combining the mutations of these identified residues indicated that the effect on phosphorylation was not additive and the mutants tested maintained a phosphorylation level of about 30% of that observed for the wild type receptor except when all the Ser/Thr residues of the C-terminus were mutated (Langlet et al., 2005). Although it was shown that $VPAC_1$ forms a complex with β-arrestin and this complex is transported into the cell during endocytosis (Shetzline et al., 2002), direct correlation between the $VPAC_1$ phosphorylation level and internalization was not obvious as in some mutated receptors a significant reduction in phosphorylation has no or little effect on receptor internalization. For instance, some $VPAC_1$ truncated receptors were still internalized while VIP-induced phosphorylation was undetectable thus suggesting an arrestin-independent mechanism of internalization and only mutation of all the Ser/Thr residues of the C-terminus and S250 completely abolished $VPAC_1$ phosphorylation and internalization (Langlet et al., 2005). $VPAC_1$ and $VPAC_2$ receptors are both rapidly internalized following agonist exposure but differ in their trafficking pattern. After internalization, $VPAC_1$ receptors are not re-expressed at the cell surface within 2 h after agonist washing (suggesting that $VPAC_1$ binds with high affinity β-arrestin) while $VPAC_2$ receptors are recycled back to the cell surface (suggesting that $VPAC_2$ binds β-arrestin with low affinity; Langlet et al., 2004, 2005). In $VPAC_2$ receptors, it was found that inactivating mutations that alter G protein coupling reduced both receptor phosphorylation and internalization in a manner that appeared directly linked to the alteration of the Gαs and Gα16 coupling (Langer et al., 2005). As mutants studied do not affect phosphorylatable residues, this suggests that impaired receptor phosphorylation and internalization directly reflect the reduced ability of the mutants to adopt active receptor conformation. However, another study showed that VIP stimulated phosphorylation of $N^{229}Q$ $VPAC_1$ and $N^{216}Q$ $VPAC_2$ (two mutants characterized by a decrease in potency and efficacy of VIP stimulated adenylate cyclase activity, by the absence of agonist stimulated $[Ca^{2+}]_i$ increase, by a preserved receptor recognition of agonists and antagonist and by a preserved sensitivity to GTP) was only slightly decreased, that receptor internalization was comparable to that of the wild type receptors but unlike wild type $VPAC_1$ the $N^{229}Q$ mutant was rapidly re-expressed at the cell surface upon VIP washing (Nachtergael et al., 2006). As $N^{229}$and N^{216} residues are located in the middle of TM3, it seems unlikely that they could be in direct interaction with β-arrestin but probably contribute to receptor conformation necessary for high affinity binding with β-arrestin. This later study thus suggests that receptor conformation necessary for activation and regulatory mechanisms could be different (**Figure 4**). As mentioned before, β-arrestins are also able to act as a signal transducer and activate G protein-independent signaling pathways but to date such a mechanism has not been described for the VIP receptors.

VPAC RECEPTORS OLIGOMERIZATION

It is now well accepted that, like for single transmembrane receptors, GPCRs are also able to form oligomeric complexes either with themselves (homo-oligomerization) or with other receptors (hetero-oligomerization) that may affect the properties of the receptor. When considering the large repertoire of GPCRs, and thus the multitude of potential oligomers that can be formed, a challenging task consists in identifying the specificity and the physiological relevance of the partners, and the functional consequences of these associations. By far, the GPCR-A/rhodopsin family has been the most extensively studied, and data collected indicate that the consequences of oligomerization may be detected at the level of both physiological and pharmacological ligand recognition, in signaling properties as well as at desensitization and internalization levels. Besides pharmacological and functional regulation, it was also demonstrated that GPCR oligomerization plays a role in receptor maturation and in expression at the cell surface (Milligan, 2009; Maurice et al., 2011).

Regarding VPAC receptors, two studies performed on the prostate cancer cell line LNCaP (Juarranz et al., 2001) and adipocytes (Akesson et al., 2005) demonstrated that those cells expressed both $VPAC_1$ and $VPAC_2$ receptors but differed in their pharmacological response with respect to the selective $VPAC_1$ and $VPAC_2$ agonists. LNCaP cells displayed a $VPAC_1$-like phenotype (the $VPAC_2$ selective agonist being inactive) while adipocytes displayed a $VPAC_2$-like phenotype (the $VPAC_1$ selective agonist being inactive). One possible explanation of these results might be the

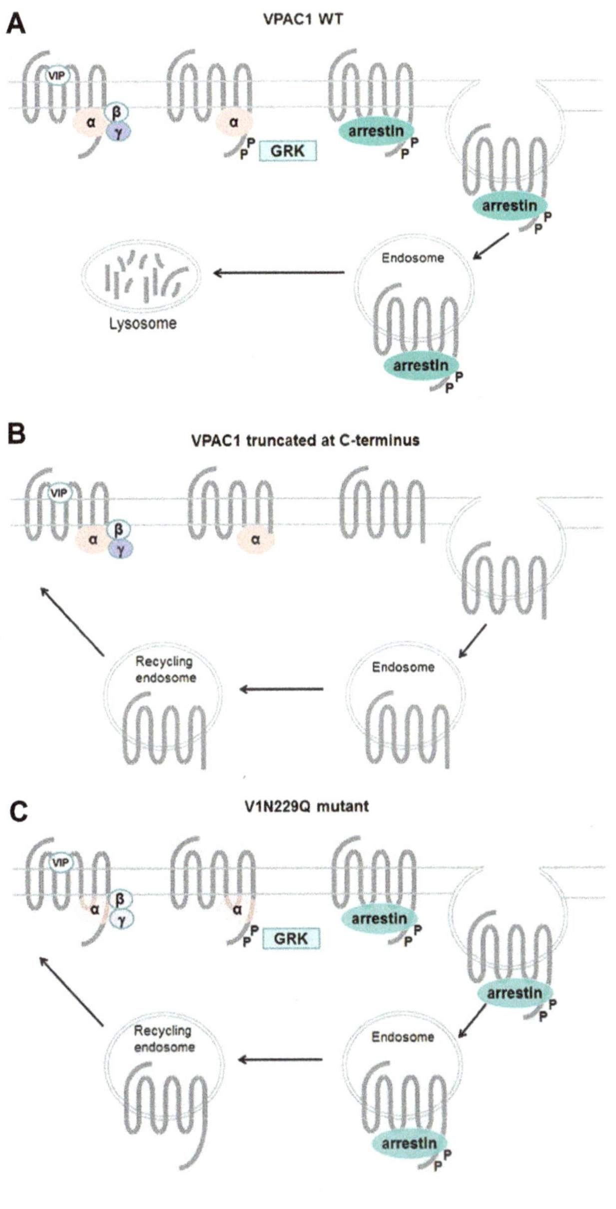

FIGURE 4 | Mechanisms involved in regulation of VPAC$_1$ activity. Upon VIP binding wt VPAC$_1$ **(A)** is rapidly phosphorylated through a GRK-dependent mechanism and desensitized, phosphorylation promotes high affinity binding of β-arrestin to VPAC$_1$ and internalization into endosome through an arrestin- and dynamin-dependent mechanism. After internalization VPAC$_1$ is not re-expressed at the cell surface. In some truncated VPAC$_1$ receptors **(B)**, VIP fails to induce GRK-mediated receptor phosphorylation but the receptor is still able to internalize through an arrestin-independent mechanism and is re-expressed at the cell surface. Some VPAC$_1$ receptor mutants **(C)**, with decrease in potency and efficacy of VIP-stimulated adenylate cyclase activity, preserved receptor recognition of agonists and antagonist and a preserved sensitivity to GTP, are still phosphorylated and internalized and recycle back to cell surface.

formation of inactive receptors dimers neutralizing the receptor expressed at the lowest concentration and letting only one receptor active. First evidence that VPAC receptors form oligomers came from a study of Harikumar et al. (2006) who demonstrated by using biophysical methods that VPAC$_1$ and VPAC$_2$ receptors formed constitutive homo- and hetero-oligomers but also heterodimers with secretin receptors that remained trapped into the cells (Harikumar et al., 2006). In an attempt to evaluate the functional consequences of hetero-oligomerization of VPAC receptors, another study investigated the effect of coexpressing VPAC$_1$ and VPAC$_2$ receptors in Chinese hamster ovary (CHO) cells on ligand binding, adenylate cyclase activation, receptor internalization, and trafficking. Three agonists were used, the natural ligand VIP, and selective VPAC$_1$ [K^{15},R^{16},L^{27}]VIP(1-7)/GRF(8-27)] and VPAC$_2$[Ro 25-1553] agonists. They found that pharmacological properties of cells expressing both receptors were not different from those obtained when mixing cells expressing each receptor individually. Similarly, VIP receptors co-expression did not modify receptor internalization and trafficking patterns following exposure to VIP or selective agonists (Langer et al., 2006). Although this study did not point out any pharmacological consequences of constitutive heterodimerization of VPAC$_1$–VPAC$_2$ receptors, it suggests that the pharmacological profile of the selective VPAC$_1$ and VPAC$_2$ receptors ligands that was established in cells expressing one receptor subtype is also applicable to cells that could express both receptors endogenously. Thus making possible the activation, antagonism, or downregulation of one receptor subtype without affecting the other. Additional experiments are now needed to demonstrate that these oligomers do exist in more physiological conditions and identify physiological consequences, if any, of VIP receptors oligomerization.

Some GPCRs are also able to form hetero-oligomers with receptor activity-modifying proteins (RAMPs), a family of single transmembrane accessory proteins (RAMP1, 2, and 3). More particularly, hetero-oligomerization of RAMPs with two GPCR-B family members, the calcitonin receptor and the calcitonin receptor-like receptor, generates multiple receptor phenotypes with different specificities for endogenous ligands. It has first been shown that VPAC$_1$ receptors, but not VPAC$_2$ receptors, were also able to interact with RAMP1, 2, and 3. VPAC$_1$–RAMP complexes did not display altered ligand specificity compared with VPAC$_1$ alone. However, specific interaction with RAMP2 led to a significant enhancement of VIP- and PACAP-induced inositol phosphate hydrolysis with unaltered cAMP production (Christopoulos et al., 2003). A more recent study, however, observed that VPAC$_2$increases cell surface expression of all three RAMPs. As seen for VPAC$_1$, VPAC$_2$, and RAMP co-expression had no or little effect on agonist-stimulated cAMP production but RAMP1 and RAMP2 significantly enhanced basal coupling to Gαi (Wootten et al., 2012). The RAMPs being largely distributed throughout the nervous system and peripheral tissues, it would be interesting to investigate more deeply the properties of VPAC–RAMP complexes such as for example selective agonists and antagonists specificity, receptor signaling through other pathways, receptor desensitization and internalization.

CONCLUSION AND PERSPECTIVES

Vasoactive intestinal peptide plays diverse and important role in the CNS, PNS, gastrointestinal tract, and immune functions and VPAC receptors constitute potential targets for the treatment of several diseases such as neurodegenerative disorder, schizophrenia, asthma, diabetes, gastrointestinal motility disorder, Crohn's disease, and rheumatoid arthritis. A key limiting factor in this field is that all the currently useful pharmacological tools are peptides, and thus limit their use in human therapy. The first small molecule antagonists of $VPAC_1$ (Harikrishnan et al., 2012) and $VPAC_2$ (Chu et al., 2010) have been described recently and emerge from high throughput screening of compound collection. However, all are low affinity, micro molar range, antagonists and need further improvement to expect to obtain druggable modulators of VPAC receptors activity. Better understand of structure, ligand binding site, and molecular pharmacology of VPAC receptors constitute thus a key information for the rationale design of VPAC receptors modulators and potential druggable compounds.

REFERENCES

Akesson, L., Ahren, B., Edgren, G., and Degerman, E. (2005). VPAC2-R mediates the lipolytic effects of pituitary adenylate cyclase-activating polypeptide/vasoactive intestinal polypeptide in primary rat adipocytes. *Endocrinology* 146, 744–750.

Ceraudo, E., Hierso, R., Tan, Y. V., Murail, S., Rouyer-Fessard, C., Nicole, P., et al. (2012). Spatial proximity between the VPAC1 receptor and the amino terminus of agonist and antagonist peptides reveals distinct sites of interaction. *FASEB J.* 26, 2060–2071.

Christopoulos, A., Christopoulos, G., Morfis, M., Udawela, M., Laburthe, M., Couvineau, A., et al. (2003). Novel receptor partners and function of receptor activity-modifying proteins. *J. Biol. Chem.* 278, 3293–3297.

Chu, A., Caldwell, J. S., and Chen, Y. A. (2010). Identification and characterization of a small molecule antagonist of human VPAC(2) receptor. *Mol. Pharmacol.* 77, 95–101.

Chugunov, A. O., Simms, J., Poyner, D. R., Dehouck, Y., Rooman, M., Gilis, D., et al. (2010). Evidence that interaction between conserved residues in transmembrane helices 2, 3, and 7 are crucial for human VPAC1 receptor activation. *Mol. Pharmacol.* 78, 394–401.

Conklin, B. R., Herzmark, P., Ishida, S., Voyno-Yasenetskaya, T. A., Sun, Y., Farfel, Z., et al. (1996). Carboxyl-terminal mutations of Gq alpha and Gs alpha that alter the fidelity of receptor activation. *Mol. Pharmacol.* 50, 885–890.

Conner, A. C., Hay, D. L., Simms, J., Howitt, S. G., Schindler, M., Smith, D. M., et al. (2005). A key role for transmembrane prolines in calcitonin receptor-like receptor agonist binding and signalling: implications for family B G-protein-coupled receptors. *Mol. Pharmacol.* 67, 20–31.

Conner, A. C., Simms, J., Conner, M. T., Wootten, D. L., Wheatley, M., and Poyner, D. R. (2006). Diverse functional motifs within the three intracellular loops of the CGRP1 receptor. *Biochemistry* 45, 12976–12985.

Couvineau, A., and Laburthe, M. (2012). VPAC receptors: structure, molecular pharmacology and interaction with accessory proteins. *Br. J. Pharmacol.* 166, 42–50.

Couvineau, A., Lacapere, J. J., Tan, Y. V., Rouyer-Fessard, C., Nicole, P., and Laburthe, M. (2003). Identification of cytoplasmic domains of hVPAC1 receptor required for activation of adenylyl cyclase. Crucial role of two charged amino acids strictly conserved in class II G protein-coupled receptors. *J. Biol. Chem.* 278, 24759–24766.

Cypess, A. M., Unson, C. G., Wu, C. R., and Sakmar, T. P. (1999). Two cytoplasmic loops of the glucagon receptor are required to elevate cAMP or intracellular calcium. *J. Biol. Chem.* 274, 19455–19464.

Delgado, M., Pozo, D., and Ganea, D. (2004). The significance of vasoactive intestinal peptide in immunomodulation. *Pharmacol. Rev.* 56, 249–290.

Dickinson, T., Mitchell, R., Robberecht, P., and Fleetwood-Walker, S. M. (1999). The role of VIP/PACAP receptor subtypes in spinal somatosensory processing in rats with an experimental peripheral mononeuropathy. *Neuropharmacology* 38, 167–180.

Dickson, L., and Finlayson, K. (2009). VPAC and PAC receptors: from ligands to function. *Pharmacol. Ther.* 121, 294–316.

Frimurer, T. M., and Bywater, R. P. (1999). Structure of the integral membrane domain of the GLP1 receptor. *Proteins* 35, 375–386.

Gaudin, P., Couvineau, A., Rouyer-Fessard, C., Maoret, J. J., and Laburthe, M. (1999). The human vasoactive intestinal Peptide/Pituitary adenylate cyclase activating peptide receptor 1 (VPAC1): constitutive activation by mutations at threonine 343. *Biochem. Biophys. Res. Commun.* 254, 15–20.

Gaudin, P., Maoret, J. J., Couvineau, A., Rouyer-Fessard, C., and Laburthe, M. (1998). Constitutive activation of the human vasoactive intestinal peptide 1 receptor, a member of the new class II family of G protein-coupled receptors. *J. Biol. Chem.* 273, 4990–4996.

Gonzalez-Rey, E., Chorny, A., and Delgado, M. (2007). Regulation of immune tolerance by anti-inflammatory neuropeptides. *Nat. Rev. Immunol.* 7, 52–63.

Gutierrez-Canas, I., Juarranz, M. G., Collado, B., Rodriguez-Henche, N., Chiloeches, A., Prieto, J. C., et al. (2005). Vasoactive intestinal peptide induces neuroendocrine differentiation in the LNCaP prostate cancer cell line through PKA, ERK, and PI3K. *Prostate* 63, 44–55.

Harikrishnan, L. S., Srivastava, N., Kayser, L. E., Nirschl, D. S., Kumaragurubaran, K., Roy, A., et al. (2012). Identification and optimization of small molecule antagonists of vasoactive intestinal peptide receptor-1 (VIPR1). *Bioorg. Med. Chem. Lett.* 22, 2287–2290.

Harikumar, K. G., Morfis, M. M., Lisenbee, C. S., Sexton, P. M., and Miller, L. J. (2006). Constitutive formation of oligomeric complexes between family B G protein-coupled vasoactive intestinal polypeptide and secretin receptors. *Mol. Pharmacol.* 69, 363–373.

Harmar, A. J., Fahrenkrug, J., Gozes, I., Laburthe, M., May, V., Pisegna, J. R., et al. (2012). Pharmacology and functions of receptors for vasoactive intestinal peptide and pituitary adenylate cyclase-activating polypeptide: IUPHAR review 1. *Br. J. Pharmacol.* 166, 4–17.

Harmar, A. J., Sheward, W. J., Morrison, C. F., Waser, B., Gugger, M., and Reubi, J. C. (2004). Distribution of the VPAC2 receptor in peripheral tissues of the mouse. *Endocrinology* 145, 1203–1210.

Hoare, S. R. (2005). Mechanisms of peptide and nonpeptide ligand binding to Class B G-protein-coupled receptors. *Drug Discov. Today* 10, 417–427.

Huang, J., Mahavadi, S., Sriwai, W., Grider, J. R., and Murthy, K. S. (2007). Cross-regulation of VPAC(2) receptor desensitization by M(3) receptors via PKC-mediated phosphorylation of RKIP and inhibition of GRK2. *Am. J. Physiol. Gastrointest. Liver Physiol.* 292, G867–G874.

Juarranz, M. G., Bolanos, O., Gutierrez-Canas, I., Lerner, E. A., Robberecht, P., Carmena, M. J., et al. (2001). Neuroendocrine differentiation of the LNCaP prostate cancer cell line maintains the expression and function of VIP and PACAP receptors. *Cell. Signal.* 13, 887–894.

King, V. M., Chahad-Ehlers, S., Shen, S., Harmar, A. J., Maywood, E. S., and Hastings, M. H. (2003). A hVIPR transgene as a novel tool for the analysis of circadian function in the mouse suprachiasmatic nucleus. *Eur. J. Neurosci.* 17, 822–832.

Knudsen, S. M., Tams, J. W., and Fahrenkrug, J. (2001). Functional roles of conserved transmembrane prolines in the human VPAC(1) receptor. *FEBS Lett.* 503, 126–130.

Langer, I., Gaspard, N., and Robberecht, P. (2006). Pharmacological properties of Chinese hamster ovary cells coexpressing two vasoactive intestinal peptide receptors (hVPAC1 and hVPAC2). *Br. J. Pharmacol.* 148, 1051–1059.

Langer, I., Langlet, C., and Robberecht, P. (2005). Effect of inactivating mutations on phosphorylation and internalization of the human VPAC2 receptor. *J. Mol. Endocrinol.* 34, 405–414.

Langer, I., Perret, J., Vertongen, P., Waelbroeck, M., and Robberecht, P. (2001). Vasoactive intestinal peptide (VIP) stimulates [Ca2+]i and cyclic AMPin CHO cells expressing Galpha16. *Cell Calcium* 30, 229–234.

Langer, I., and Robberecht, P. (2005). Mutations in the carboxy-terminus of the third intracellular loop of the human recombinant VPAC1 receptor impair VIP-stimulated [Ca2+]i increase but not adenylate cyclase stimulation. *Cell. Signal.* 17, 17–24.

Langer, I., Vertongen, P., Perret, J., Waelbroeck, M., and Robberecht, P. (2002). A small sequence in the third intracellular loop of the VPAC(1) receptor is responsible for its efficient coupling to the calcium effector. *Mol. Endocrinol.* 16, 1089–1096.

Langer, I., Vertongen, P., Perret, J., Waelbroeck, M., and Robberecht, P. (2003). Lysine 195 and aspartate 196 in the first extracellular loop of the VPAC1 receptor are essential for high affinity binding of agonists but not of antagonists. *Neuropharmacology* 44, 125–131.

Langlet, C., Gaspard, N., Nachtergael, I., Robberecht, P., and Langer, I. (2004). Comparative efficacy of VIP and analogs on activation and internalization of the recombinant VPAC2 receptor expressed in CHO cells. *Peptides* 25, 2079–2086.

Langlet, C., Langer, I., Vertongen, P., Gaspard, N., Vanderwinden, J. M., and Robberecht, P. (2005). Contribution of the carboxyl terminus of the VPAC1 receptor to agonist-induced receptor phosphorylation, internalization, and recycling. *J. Biol. Chem.* 280, 28034–28043.

Larsson, L. I., Edvinsson, L., Fahrenkrug, J., Hakanson, R., Owman, C., Schaffalitzky de, M. O., et al. (1976a). Immunohistochemical localization of a vasodilatory polypeptide (VIP) in cerebrovascular nerves. *Brain Res.* 113, 400–404.

Larsson, L. I., Fahrenkrug, J., Schaffalitzky de, M. O., Sundler, F., Hakanson, R., and Rehfeld, J. R. (1976b). Localization of vasoactive intestinal polypeptide (VIP) to central and peripheral neurons. *Proc. Natl. Acad. Sci. U.S.A.* 73, 3197–3200.

Lutz, E. M., Sheward, W. J., West, K. M., Morrow, J. A., Fink, G., and Harmar, A. J. (1993). The VIP2 receptor: molecular characterisation of a cDNA encoding a novel receptor for vasoactive intestinal peptide. *FEBS Lett.* 334, 3–8.

MacKenzie, C. J., Lutz, E. M., Johnson, M. S., Robertson, D. N., Holland, P. J., and Mitchell, R. (2001). Mechanisms of phospholipase C activation by the vasoactive intestinal polypeptide/pituitary adenylate cyclase-activating polypeptide type 2 receptor. *Endocrinology* 142, 1209–1217.

MacKenzie, C. J., Lutz, E. M., McCulloch, D. A., Mitchell, R., and Harmar, A. J. (1996). Phospholipase C activation by VIP1 and VIP2 receptors expressed in COS 7 cells involves a pertussis toxin-sensitive mechanism. *Ann. N. Y. Acad. Sci.* 805, 579–584.

Marie, J. C., Rouyer-Fessard, C., Couvineau, A., Nicole, P., Devaud, H., El Benna, J., et al. (2003). Serine 447 in the carboxyl tail of human VPAC1 receptor is crucial for agonist-induced desensitization but not internalization of the receptor. *Mol. Pharmacol.* 64, 1565–1574.

Maurice, P., Kamal, M., and Jockers, R. (2011). Asymmetry of GPCR oligomers supports their functional relevance. *Trends Pharmacol. Sci.* 32, 514–520.

McCulloch, D. A., Lutz, E. M., Johnson, M. S., MacKenzie, C. J., and Mitchell, R. (2000). Differential activation of phospholipase D by VPAC and PAC1 receptors. *Ann. N. Y. Acad. Sci.* 921, 175–185.

Milligan, G. (2009). G protein-coupled receptor hetero-dimerization: contribution to pharmacology and function. *Br. J. Pharmacol.* 158, 5–14.

Moody, T. W., Ito, T., Osefo, N., and Jensen, R. T. (2011). VIP and PACAP: recent insights into their functions/roles in physiology and disease from molecular and genetic studies. *Curr. Opin. Endocrinol. Diabetes Obes.* 18, 61–67.

Nachtergael, I., Gaspard, N., Langlet, C., Robberecht, P., and Langer, I. (2006). Asn229 in the third helix of VPAC1 receptor is essential for receptor activation but not for receptor phosphorylation and internalization: comparison with Asn216 in VPAC2 receptor. *Cell. Signal.* 18, 2121–2130.

Neumann, J. M., Couvineau, A., Murail, S., Lacapere, J. J., Jamin, N., and Laburthe, M. (2008). Class-B GPCR activation: is ligand helix-capping the key? *Trends Biochem. Sci.* 33, 314–319.

Pechon-Vallee, C., Magalon, K., Rasolonjanahary, R., Enjalbert, A., and Gerard, C. (2000). Vasoactive intestinal polypeptide and pituitary adenylate cyclase-activating polypeptides stimulate mitogen-activated protein kinase in the pituitary cell line GH4C1 by a 3′,5′-cyclic adenosine monophosphate pathway. *Neuroendocrinology* 72, 46–56.

Perret, J., Vertongen, P., Solano, R. M., Langer, I., Cnudde, J., Robberecht, P., et al. (2002). Two tyrosine residues in the first transmembrane helix of the human vasoactive intestinal peptide receptors play a role in supporting the active conformation. *Br. J. Pharmacol.* 136, 1042–1048.

Pierce, K. L., Premont, R. T., and Lefkowitz, R. J. (2002). Seven-transmembrane receptors. *Nat. Rev. Mol. Cell Biol.* 3, 639–650.

Rasmussen, S. G., Choi, H. J., Rosenbaum, D. M., Kobilka, T. S., Thian, F. S., Edwards, P. C., et al. (2007). Crystal structure of the human beta2 adrenergic G-protein-coupled receptor. *Nature* 450, 383–387.

Rasmussen, S. G., Devree, B. T., Zou, Y., Kruse, A. C., Chung, K. Y., Kobilka, T. S., et al. (2011). Crystal structure of the beta2 adrenergic receptor-Gs protein complex. *Nature* 477, 549–555.

Reubi, J. C. (2000). In vitro evaluation of VIP/PACAP receptors in healthy and diseased human tissues. Clinical implications. *Ann. N. Y. Acad. Sci.* 921, 1–25.

Rosenbaum, D. M., Cherezov, V., Hanson, M. A., Rasmussen, S. G., Thian, F. S., Kobilka, T. S., et al. (2007). GPCR engineering yields high-resolution structural insights into beta2-adrenergic receptor function. *Science* 318, 1266–1273.

Rosenbaum, D. M., Rasmussen, S. G., and Kobilka, B. K. (2009). The structure and function of G-protein-coupled receptors. *Nature* 459, 356–363.

Rosenbaum, D. M., Zhang, C., Lyons, J. A., Holl, R., Aragao, D., Arlow, D. H., et al. (2011). Structure and function of an irreversible agonist-beta(2) adrenoceptor complex. *Nature* 469, 236–240.

Said, S. I., and Mutt, V. (1970). Polypeptide with broad biological activity: isolation from small intestine. *Science* 169, 1217–1218.

Said, S. I., and Rattan, S. (2004). The multiple mediators of neurogenic smooth muscle relaxation. *Trends Endocrinol. Metab.* 15, 189–191.

Shenoy, S. K., and Lefkowitz, R. J. (2011). beta-Arrestin-mediated receptor trafficking and signal transduction. *Trends Pharmacol. Sci.* 32, 521–533.

Shetzline, M. A., Walker, J. K., Valenzano, K. J., and Premont, R. T. (2002). Vasoactive intestinal polypeptide type-1 receptor regulation. Desensitization, phosphorylation, and sequestration. *J. Biol. Chem.* 277, 25519–25526.

Sheward, W. J., Lutz, E. M., and Harmar, A. J. (1995). The distribution of vasoactive intestinal peptide2 receptor messenger RNA in the rat brain and pituitary gland as assessed by in situ hybridization. *Neuroscience* 67, 409–418.

Spessert, R. (1993). Vasoactive intestinal peptide stimulation of cyclic guanosine monophosphate formation: further evidence for a role of nitric oxide synthase and cytosolic guanylate cyclase in rat pinealocytes. *Endocrinology* 132, 2513–2517.

Sreedharan, S. P., Patel, D. R., Huang, J. X., and Goetzl, E. J. (1993). Cloning and functional expression of a human neuroendocrine vasoactive intestinal peptide receptor. *Biochem. Biophys. Res. Commun.* 193, 546–553.

Sreedharan, S. P., Patel, D. R., Xia, M., Ichikawa, S., and Goetzl, E. J. (1994). Human vasoactive intestinal peptide1 receptors expressed by stable transfectants couple to two distinct signaling pathways. *Biochem. Biophys. Res. Commun.* 203, 141–148.

Tams, J. W., Knudsen, S. M., and Fahrenkrug, J. (2001). Characterization of a G protein coupling "YL" motif of the human VPAC1 receptor, equivalent to the first two amino acids in the "DRY" motif of the rhodopsin family. *J. Mol. Neurosci.* 17, 325–330.

Usdin, T. B., Bonner, T. I., and Mezey, E. (1994). Two receptors for vasoactive intestinal polypeptide with similar specificity and complementary distributions. *Endocrinology* 135, 2662–2680.

Vertongen, P., Solano, R. M., Perret, J., Langer, I., Robberecht, P., and Waelbroeck, M. (2001). Mutational analysis of the human vasoactive intestinal peptide receptor subtype VPAC(2): role of basic residues in the second transmembrane helix. *Br. J. Pharmacol.* 133, 1249–1254.

Wootten, D., Lindmark, H., Kadmiel, M., Willcockson, H., Caron, K. M., Barwell, J., et al. (2012). Receptor Activity Modifying Proteins (RAMPs) Interact with the VPAC(2) Receptor and CRF(1) Receptors and modulate their function. *Br. J. Pharmacol.* doi: 10.1111/j.1476-5381.2012.02202.x [Epub ahead of print].

4

Alternative splicing of the pituitary adenylate cyclase-activating polypeptide receptor PAC1: mechanisms of fine tuning of brain activity

Janna Blechman and Gil Levkowitz*

Department of Molecular Cell Biology, Weizmann Institute of Science, Rehovot, Israel

Edited by:
Hubert Vaudry, University of Rouen, France

Reviewed by:
Hubert Vaudry, University of Rouen, France
Atsuro Miyata, Kagoshima University, Japan

****Correspondence:***
Gil Levkowitz, Department of Molecular Cell Biology, Weizmann Institute of Science, P. O. Box 26, Rehovot 76100, Israel.
e-mail: gil.levkowitz@weizmann.ac.il

Alternative splicing of the precursor mRNA encoding for the neuropeptide receptor PAC1/ADCYAP1R1 generates multiple protein products that exhibit pleiotropic activities. Recent studies in mammals and zebrafish have implicated some of these splice isoforms in control of both cellular and body homeostasis. Here, we review the regulation of PAC1 splice variants and their underlying signal transduction and physiological processes in the nervous system.

Keywords: ADCYAP1R1, activity-dependent gene regulation, zebrafish model system, PACAP receptor, stress disorders, post-traumatic, hypothalamic hormones, homeostasis

INTRODUCTION

G-protein-coupled receptors (GPCRs) represent the largest family of membrane-associated proteins mediating physiological responses in vertebrates by means of controlling metabolic, neural, and developmental functions (Lefkowitz, 2007; Frooninckx et al., 2012; Zhang and Eggert, 2013). These proteins are expressed in almost all types of tissues and are represented by over 1,000 membrane receptors for extracellular (EC) ligands including hormones, neurotransmitters, pheromones, lipids, and other proteins (Xue et al., 2008; Markovic and Grammatopoulos, 2009; Nordstrom et al., 2009; Hoyer and Bartfai, 2012; Jafurulla and Chattopadhyay, 2013). The basic structure of GPCR proteins consists of a seven-transmembrane (TM) domain with a complex EC structure composed of an N-terminal region and three EC loops involved in the diverse ligand recognition process. Three intracellular (IC) loops and a C-terminal domain transduce a signal into the cell's cytoplasm and nucleus. Typically, ligand binding to the EC loops induces conformational changes in the TM and IC domains of the receptor resulting in specific coupling to a set of cytoplasmic molecules, termed G-proteins, each composed of different isoforms of alpha, beta, and gamma subunits. G-proteins in turn regulate the activity of IC effector molecules, including adenylate cyclase (AC), phospholipase Cβ (PLC), and RhoGEF causing the activation of secondary messengers such as cyclic AMP (cAMP), inositol-1,4,5-triphosphate (InP3), and diacylglycerol leading to the initiation of distinct IC signaling pathways (Simon et al., 1991; Sah et al., 2000; Pierce et al., 2002; Oldham and Hamm, 2008; Mizuno and Itoh, 2009; Mahata et al., 2011; Maurice et al., 2011).

The diversity of the GPCR-initiated signal transduction pathways is determined by the multiplicity of cognate ligands with different receptor binding properties and by the receptors' membrane-interacting partners that form homo- and hetero-dimerized GPCR complexes. These receptor dimers have unique binding properties to both EC ligands and a set of IC G-proteins (Milligan and Kostenis, 2006; Harikumar et al., 2008; Furness et al., 2012). Thus, ligand binding, along with receptor heterodimerization, can generate diversity in G-proteins coupling that can generate varied IC signaling functions.

Beyond the complexity of the aforementioned EC and IC GPCRs interacting effectors, the genetic diversity of the GPCR family can be generated by means of alternative precursor mRNAs (pre-mRNA) splicing of exons encoding specific protein moieties and causing considerable functional differences of the resulting splicing products (Black, 2003; Jaillon et al., 2008; Furness et al., 2012). Alternative splicing mechanisms allow the generation of multiple mRNA transcript variants from a single gene by utilizing different combinations of exons by means of skipping or insertion of alternatively spliced exons. In particular, neuronal cells are known to exhibit high levels of alternative splicing, generating the basis for molecular and cellular diversity important for the patterning and maintenance of the central and peripheral nervous systems (Yeo et al., 2007; Betke et al., 2012; Norris and Calarco, 2012; Sun et al., 2012). In the case of GPCRs, this combinatorial exon assembly can lead to changes in the protein domains responsible for ligand binding, IC effector coupling, as well as receptor stability, and endocytosis.

In this review we focus on one GPCR, the pituitary AC-activating polypeptide (PACAP) receptor (ADCAYP1R1), also known as PAC1. This receptor represents a fascinating example of how alternative splicing of a single GPCR gene leads to different physiological outcomes. We will describe the current knowledge regarding the role and mechanism of action of PAC1 splice variants in development, physiology, and diseases focusing on PAC1's role in the nervous system.

THE PAC1 RECEPTOR

PAC1 belongs to the glucagon/secretin receptor family of GPCRs that consists of hormone and neuropeptide receptors. These receptors signal through coupling to the G-protein alpha subunits Gs and Gq that typically activate AC and phospholipase Cβ enzymes, respectively (McCulloch et al., 2002; Ahren, 2008; Dickson and Finlayson, 2009; Vallejo, 2009; Vaudry et al., 2009). Coupling of PAC1 to Gs may also lead to cAMP-dependent accumulation of IC calcium (Braas and May, 1996; Mustafa et al., 2010). The PAC1 gene contains multiple exons that undergo extensive alternative splicing. The peptide PACAP is the high-affinity ligand for PAC1. Post-translational proteolytic processing of the PACAP precursor protein generates several polypeptides with varying sizes, including PACAP38 and PACAP27 (Miyata et al., 1989; Vaudry et al., 2009; Harmar et al., 2012; Watkins et al., 2012). PAC1 was found to play a pivotal role in the spatio-temporal regulation of proliferation, differentiation, or cell survival during development as well as in the regulation of synthesis and release of neuroendocrine hormones.

Phylogenetic analysis of the vertebrate PAC1 receptor family indicates their origin from a common ancestral gene and demonstrates a tree topology with species-specific paralogs belonging to different separated sub-groups (**Figure 1**). Bony fishes (*teleosts*) genomes typically contain more than one gene due to teleost-specific gene duplication event of both ligand and receptor molecules during the evolution of these species (Wei et al., 1998; Fradinger et al., 2005; Bjarnadottir et al., 2006; Cardoso et al., 2007; Machluf et al., 2011).

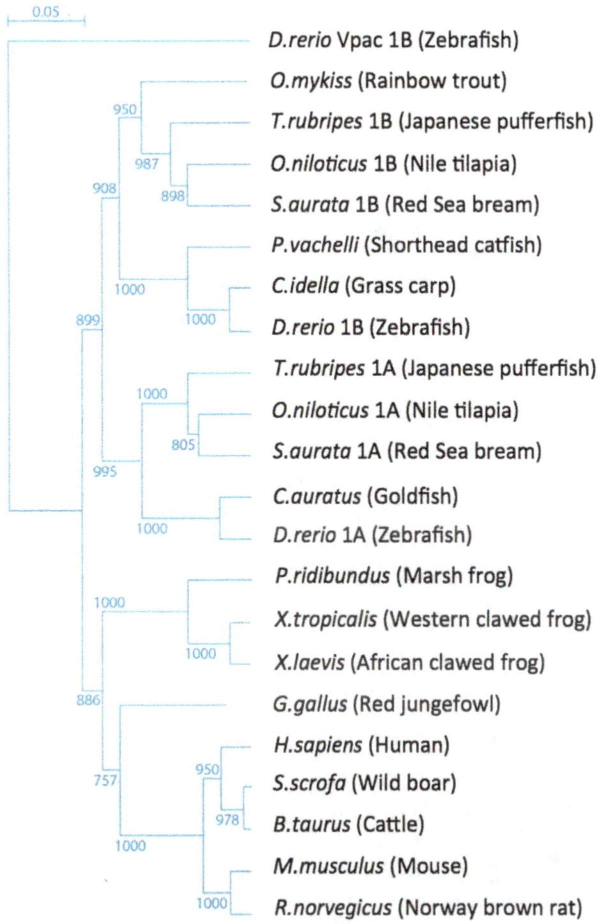

FIGURE 1 | Tree topology of the vertebrate PAC1 receptor family. Phylogenetic relationships of PAC1 receptors analyzed using the zebrafish (*Danio rerio*) Vpac1b gene as an out-group.

ALTERNATIVELY SPLICED PAC1 GENE PRODUCTS

The alternative splicing of PAC1 has been extensively studied. In this review we use the exon numbers designation of the human *PAC1* and otherwise indicate cases where the exons numbers do not match. The human gene was shown to contain 18 exons with the open reading frame encoded by exons 2–18 (Chatterjee et al., 1997; Lutz et al., 2006). Ten of these exons are constitutively expressed (exons 2, 3, 7–13, 18), whereas the rest (exons 4–6, 14, 15, and possibly 16, 17) are regulated by the alternative splicing (**Figure 2**). The N-terminal part of PAC1's EC domain is encoded by six exons. Exons 7–17 encode the seven-TM domains including EC and IC loops and exon 18 encodes the C-terminal cytoplasmic tail including the 3′-untranslated region (**Figures 2** and **3**). PAC1 splicing variants were identified in other vertebrate species including rat, mouse, frog, and fish. In **Table 1** we assembled all known PAC1 splice isoforms from different vertebrate species. The functional outcome of these splicing events will be discussed later. By and large, PAC1 alternative splicing can be divided into four types of splicing events that impact receptor functions (**Figure 3**; **Table 1**): (1) Variations in the EC N-terminal domain altering the ligand-binding specificity and affinity. (2) Variations in exons encoding to part of the third IC loop (IC3) thereby affecting G-protein coupling and/or interaction with other IC signaling proteins. (3) Variations in the TM domains TM2 and TM4 contributing to the receptors heteromerization and IC transport. (4) Variations in the 5′ UTR that may affect mRNA expression dynamics. Notably, splicing products containing different combinations of N-terminal and IC3 splice variants were identified in mammalian species.

The terminology used in independent studies can be somewhat perplexing as different names were designated to PAC1 isoforms corresponding to the same splicing events identified in various species. In the following section we describe the various splice variants and indicate when a different (i.e., specie-specific) name was designated to the same isoform. A splice isoform that includes all N-terminal encoding exons but does not contain IC (IC3) insertion(s) is referred to as "PAC1-null" (**Table 1**). The ligand binding and signaling properties of PAC1-null are often used as a reference when assessing the activities of other splice variants.

N-TERMINAL VARIATIONS

The N-terminal variants were identified in rodents and humans but not in fishes to date. They are generated by alternative splicing of exon 5 (PAC1-δ5), exons 5–6 (PAC1-short or PAC1-δ5,6), or exons 4–6 (PAC1-very short or PAC1-δ4,5,6) leading to deletions of 7, 21, or 57 amino acids, respectively (Journot et al., 1994;

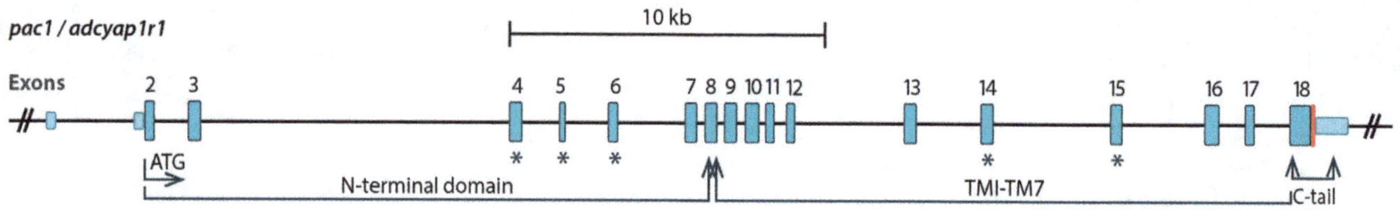

FIGURE 2 | A diagram showing genomic organization of the *PAC1* (*ADCYAP1R1*) gene. Exons 2–18 encode the open reading frame. Exons undergoing the alternative splicing discussed in this review are marked with blue asterisks. Exon 4, 5, and 6 encode parts of the N-terminal domain, whereas exons 14 and 15 encode the third intracellular loop. TM, transmembrane.

Pantaloni et al., 1996; Chatterjee et al., 1997; Dautzenberg et al., 1999; Lutz et al., 2006; Ushiyama et al., 2007, 2010). In the rat, an insertion of 24 amino acids is caused by splicing of a novel exon 3a located between exons 3 and 4 (PAC1-3a) (**Figure 3**) (Daniel et al., 2001; Ajpru et al., 2002; Pilzer and Gozes, 2006a). N-terminal splicing isoforms of PAC1 display alterations both in ligand-binding selectivity and coupling to second messengers compared to PAC1-null.

INTRACELLULAR LOOP VARIATIONS

PAC1 splice variants in the third IC loop (IC3) have been identified in human, amphibian, fishes, and rodents. These splice isoforms are characterized by the presence of one or two cassettes of 84 nucleotides (hip or hop1 variants) or 81 nucleotides (hop2 variant), or a combination of alternative spliced "cassettes" (hip-hop1 or hip-hop2) (Spengler et al., 1993; Journot et al., 1995; Grimaldi and Cavallaro, 1999; McCulloch et al., 2001; Ronaldson et al., 2002; Fradinger et al., 2005; Ushiyama et al., 2007; May et al., 2010; Holighaus et al., 2011). In human, hip and hop variants are also referred to as SV1 and SV2 or SV3 for hip-hop1 (Pisegna and Wank, 1996; Pisegna et al., 1996). In addition, a splice variant formed by a C-terminal deletion of 193 nucleotides (denoted "*hop1 novel*") including two amino acids that are essential for G-protein recognition was identified in rat cochlea samples (Abu-Hamdan et al., 2006). Similar alternative splicing variants of PAC1 are also found in non-mammalian vertebrates such as the frog and bony fishes. Three alternative splice variants were identified in the frog IC3 loop (Alexandre et al., 2002). PAC1-R25, with an insertion of 25 amino acids, corresponds to the mammalian hop cassette. PAC1-R41 contains a cassette with no homology to any other variant. PAC1-RMc with a unique cytoplasmic insertion of 13 amino acid into the TM7 domain is missing a canonical Gs recognition motif. PAC1 genes were also identified in zebrafish, goldfish, stickleback, fugu, sea bream, and several others bony fish species. Three zebrafish PAC1 alternative splice variants with insertions in the IC3 loop were identified. Two of them were found to be homologous to the hop1 (84 nucleotides) and hop2 (81 nucleotides) mammalian isoforms (Fradinger et al., 2005). A unique 107 nucleotides inclusion with a premature stop codon (PAC1-skip) resulting in a truncated PAC1 protein did not correspond to any previously detected PAC1 isoform (Fradinger et al., 2005). This isoform resembles an alternative splicing event in a human gene encoding another secretin family receptor, *VPAC1*. Interestingly, the hip cassette variant was not identified in the mouse and zebrafish genomes. Moreover, teleosts genomes contain two (duplicated) PAC1 paralogs, *pac1a* and *pac1b*, however, only *pac1a* encodes for the hop splicing cassette.

TRANSMEMBRANAL DOMAIN VARIATIONS

A PAC1 variant, cloned from the rat cerebellum, has amino acids deletion/substitution in the TM4 domain along with two amino acid substitutions in the N-terminal (D136N) and TM2 (N190D) domains (Chatterjee et al., 1996; Ajpru et al., 2002). The exact molecular mechanism underlying these variations remains unclear. Notably, the TM4 domain of the secretin family receptors are involved in homo- and hetero-oligomerization of these receptors, associations with receptor activity-modifying proteins (RAMPs), and with GPCR kinases (GRKs) thereby suggesting that splice alterations in the PAC1-TM4 domain may affect receptor function (Morfis et al., 2003; Ritter and Hall, 2009; Magalhaes et al., 2012).

5′ UTR VARIATIONS

Alternative splicing events in exons located at the 5′ UTR were identified for rat *PAC1* gene (Chatterjee et al., 1997). These include different alternative usage of exons located upstream to the ATG translation start codon. Such variations in the 5′ UTR organization and sequences may play a role in the regulation of mRNA expression.

ALTERNATIVE PAC1 SPLICING ALTERS LIGAND-BINDING PROPERTIES

PAC1 is considered as being the high-affinity receptor for PACAP, while it displays low binding affinity to the vasoactive intestinal polypeptide (VIP) (Apostolakis et al., 2005; Vaudry et al., 2009; Harmar et al., 2012). Alternative splicing of PAC1 results in different protein products displaying different ligand-binding properties that may result in changes in affinity and selectivity (**Table 1**). Most studies use the PAC1-null (McCulloch et al., 2001; Holighaus et al., 2011) isoform as a reference for PACAP and VIP binding properties.

Modeling of ligand-receptor binding proposes that the C-terminal part of the ligand PACAP binds to the N-terminus of the PAC1 receptor and that the N-terminal part of PACAP binds to the receptor's EC loops and TM domains (Furness et al., 2012). Consequently, alterations in the EC domain of PAC1 are predicted to affect these ligand-receptor binding properties (**Table 1**). Thus, PAC1-very short (a.k.a. PAC1-δ4,5,6), which lacks 57 amino acids in the EC1 domain displays decreased affinity to PACAP27 and PACAP38 but its affinity toward VIP remains the same (Journot

Table 1 | Biochemical properties of PAC1 splice variants.

PAC1 isoforms	Specie	Sequence alterations	Binding properties	Signaling consequences			Reference
				AC activation (Gs) cAMP production	PLC stimulation (Gq) IP3 turnover	Ca^{2+} mobilization from intracellular and extracellular stores	
null	rat, human mouse* zebrafish	PAC1 containing exons 2–13, 16–18	Pacap38 ≈ Pacap27 ≫ VIP Pacap38 ≫ Pacap27 ≫ VIP*	Pacap38 ≤ Pacap27 ≫ VIP Pacap38 ≤ Pacap27 ≫ VIP*	Pacap38 ≫ Pacap27 > VIP	Pacap38 > Pacap27 ≫ VIP Pacap38 > Pacap27 ≫ VIP* Pacap ≈ VIP (ES cells)	Spengler et al. (1993), Wei et al. (1998), Grumolato et al. (2003), Fradinger et al. (2005), Lutz et al. (2006), Ushiyama et al. (2007, 2010), Chafai et al. (2011), Holighaus et al. (2011)
hop1 SV2*	rat, mouse human*	Insertion of exon 15 into IC3 loop	Pacap38 ≈ Pacap27 ≫ VIP	Pacap38 ≤ Pacap27 ≫ VIP Pacap38 ≤ Pacap27*	Pacap38 ≫ Pacap27 ≈ VIP Pacap38 ≥ Pacap27* Pacap38 ≈ Pacap27 ≫ VIP (SCG)	Pacap38 > Pacap27 ≫ VIP ND*	Spengler et al. (1993), Pisegna and Wank, 1996, Pisegna et al. (1996), McCulloch et al. (2002), Ronaldson et al. (2002), Mustafa et al. (2007), May et al. (2010), Holighaus et al. (2011)
hop1 novel	rat	193 bp deletion: TM6, EC3 loop, TM7, and part of C-terminal tail	Pacap38 ≈ Pacap2 ≫ VIP	No activation – Arg416 and Ser417 are essential for G-protein coupling	No activation	ND	Abu-Hamdan et al. (2006)
hop2	rat zebrafish*	Insertion of exon 15 into IC3 loop	Pacap38 ≈ Pacap27 ≈ VIP Pacap38 > Pacap27 ≫ VIP*	Pacap38 ≤ Pacap27 Pacap38 ≈ VIP Pacap38 < Pacap27 ≫ VIP*	Pacap38 ≫ Pacap27 ND*	Pacap38 ≫ VIP ND*	Spengler et al. (1993), Cavallaro et al. (1995), Wei et al. (1998), Grimaldi and Cavallaro (1999), Pilzer and Gozes (2006b)
hip SV1*	rat human*	Insertion of exon 14 into IC3 loop	Low affinity Pacap38 ≥ VIP Pacap38 ≈ Pacap27 ≫ VIP*	Low potency Pacap38 < Pacap27 ≈ VIP Pacap38 ≤ Pacap27*	No activation Pacap38 > Pacap27 ≈ VIP*	No Ca^{2+} influx ND*	Spengler et al. (1993), Journot et al. (1995), Pisegna and Wank, 1996, Pisegna et al. (1996), Ronaldson et al. (2002), Germano et al. (2004), Lutz et al. (2006)

(Continued)

Table 1 | Continued

PAC1 isoforms	Specie	Sequence alterations	Binding properties	Signaling consequences			Reference
				AC activation (Gs) cAMP production	PLC stimulation (Gq) IP3 turnover	Ca^{2+} mobilization from intracellular and extracellular stores	
hip-hop SV3*	rat, human*	Insertion of exons 14, 15 into IC3 loop	Pacap38 ≈ Pacap27 ≫ VIP	Low potency Pacap38 < Pacap27 ≈ VIP Pacap38 ≤ Pacap27*	Pacap38 ≫ Pacap27 Pacap38 ≥ Pacap27*	No Ca^{2+} influx ND*	Spengler et al. (1993), Pisegna and Wank, 1996, Pisegna et al. (1996), Lu et al. (1998), Abu-Hamdan et al. (2006)
short δ5,6*	rat, mouse, human*	Deletions of exons 5,6	Pacap38 ≈ Pacap27 ≥ VIP Pacap38 ≈ Pacap27 > VIP*	Pacap38 ≈ Pacap27 ≥ VIP Pacap38 ≈ Pacap27 > VIP*	Pacap38 ≈ Pacap27 > VIP	Pacap38 > Pacap27 ≫ VIP	Pantaloni et al. (1996), Dautzenberg et al. (1999), Lutz et al. (2006), Ushiyama et al. (2007, 2010)
short hop1 δ5,6 hop1*	rat, mouse, human*	Deletions of exons 5,6, insertion of exon 15	Pacap38 ≈ Pacap27 ≫ VIP ND*	Pacap38 > Pacap27 ≫ VIP Pacap38 ≥ VIP*	Pacap38 > Pacap27 ≫ VIP Pacap38 > VIP*	ND Pacap38 > Pacap27 ≫ VIP*	Dautzenberg et al. (1999), Lutz et al. (2006), Ushiyama et al. (2007, 2010)
δ5,6-hip	human	Deletions of exons 5,6, insertion of exon 14	Pacap38 ≈ VIP	Low potency Pacap38 ≈ VIP	Low potency Pacap38 ≥ VIP	ND	Lutz et al. (2006)
very short δ4,5,6*	rat, human*	Deletions of exons 4,5,6	Low affinity Pacap38 ≈ Pacap27 > VIP	Low potency Pacap38 ≈ Pacap27 > VIP Pacap38 ≈ Pacap27 ≫ VIP*	No activation	ND Pacap38 > Pacap27 ≫ VIP*	Pantaloni et al. (1996), Dautzenberg et al. (1999), Lutz et al. (2006)
3a	rat	N-terminal insertion of exon 3a (72 bp)	Sixfold increased affinity to Pacap38	Reduced sensitivity to Pacap38; Pacap27 like null	Reduced sensitivity to Pacap38 and Pacap27	Pacap38 and Pacap27 stimulate Ca^{2+} like v null	Daniel et al. (2001), Ajpru et al. (2002), Pilzer and Gozes (2006b)
Pac-TM4	rat	TM4-deletion/insertion (12 to 6 bp), TM2 –D136N in EC1, N190D	Pacap38 ≈ Pacap27	Low potency (BNK cells) Pacap27 ≫ VIP; no activation (CHO cells)	Low potency (BNK) Pacap27 ≫ VIP; no activation (CHO)	Pacap27 via activation of dihydropyridine-sensitive L-type Ca^{2+} channels	Chatterjee et al. (1996), Ajpru et al. (2002)

(Continued)

Table 1 | Continued

PAC1 isoforms	Specie	Sequence alterations	Binding properties	Signaling consequences			Reference
				AC activation (Gs) cAMP production	PLC stimulation (Gq) IP3 turnover	Ca^{2+} mobilization from intracellular and extracellular stores	
δ5	human	Deletion of exon 5	Pacap38 ≈ Pacap27 > VIP	Pacap38 ≈ Pacap27 ≫ VIP	Pacap38 ≫ Pacap27 ≈ VIP	ND	Lutz et al. (2006)
δ5hop1	human	Deletion of exon 5, insertion of exon 15	ND	Pacap38 ≈ Pacap27 ≫ VIP	Pacap38 ≫ Pacap27 ≈ VIP	ND	Lutz et al. (2006)
δ5hip	human	Deletion of exon 5, insertion of exon 14	Pacap38 ≥ VIP	Low potency Pacap38 > VIP	No activation	ND	Lutz et al. (2006)
δ5,6,14–17	human	Deletion of exons 5,6, deletion/ insertion in TM6, EC3 & TM7	Pacap38 ≈ Pacap27 > VIP	No activation	No activation	ND	Lutz et al. (2006)
skip	zebrafish	Insertion into the IC3 loop with premature stop codon	ND	ND	No activation, loss of G-protein coupling epitope	ND	Fradinger et al. (2005)
R25	frog	Insertion of a hop-like cassette into the IC3 loop	Pacap38 > VIP	Pacap38 > VIP (Pac25 > Pac41 > Pac1-null)	ND	ND	Alexandre et al. (2002)
R41	frog	Insertion into the IC3 loop	Pacap38 > VIP	Pacap38 > VIP	ND	ND	Alexandre et al. (2002)
Rmc	frog	Insertion into TM7 C-term.	Pacap38 > VIP	Prevents cAMP formation	Loss of a putative PKC phosphorylation site	ND	Alexandre et al. (2002)

**Information relating to biochemical properties obtained in specific vertebrate species are marked by the asterisk symbol.*

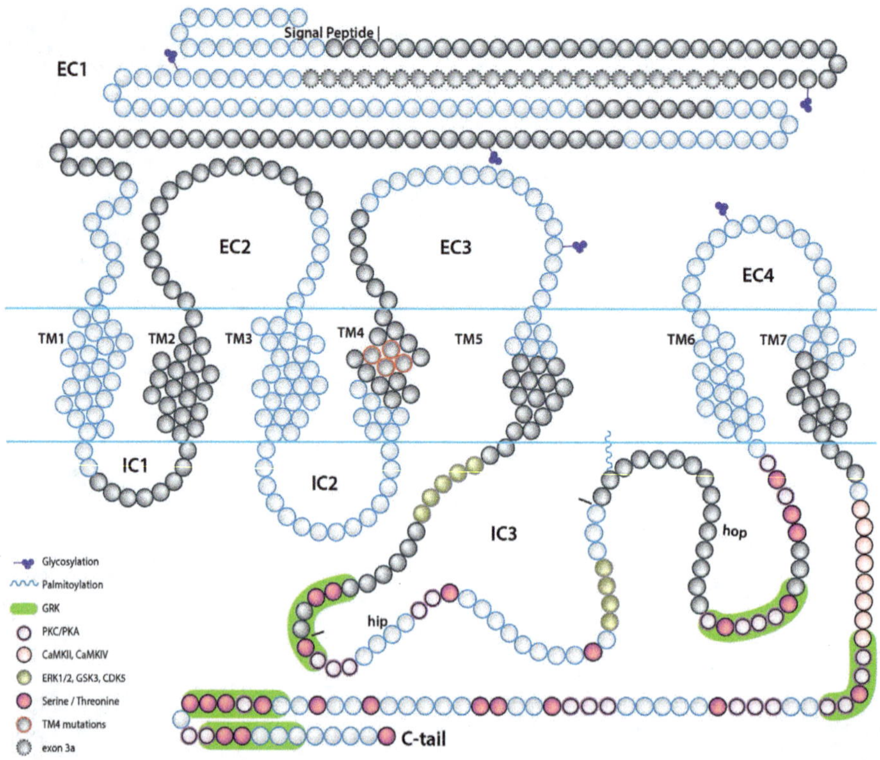

FIGURE 3 | A scheme depicting the topology of the PAC1 receptor. The relative location of amino acids encoded by PAC1 exons are depicted by the blue and gray beads. Predicted PAC1 structural motifs known to be involved in protein-protein interactions determining G-protein mediated PAC1 signaling are marked on the protein diagram with regard to putative motifs formed due to insertions of hop and hip cassettes into the IC3 loop sequence. EC, extracellular loop; IC, intracellular loop; TM, transmembrane domain.

et al., 1995; Pantaloni et al., 1996; Dautzenberg et al., 1999; Lutz et al., 2006). The binding affinities for PACAP38 of the δ5, δ5,6 (a.k.a. short) splice isoforms appeared to be very similar to that of PAC1-null, while δ5,6 isoform has increased affinity toward VIP. The rat-specific PAC1-3a isoform containing a 24 residue N-terminal insertion displays increased affinity to PACAP38 but not to PACAP27 (Daniel et al., 2001; Pilzer and Gozes, 2006a). It should be noted that in all of these examples, PACAP is still the better ligand for PAC1 when compared with VIP (**Table 1**).

The hop1 and hip-hop1 splice isoforms retain similar binding properties to those of PAC1-null. In contrast, insertions into the IC3 loop, namely hip- and hop2-cassettes lead to the elevation of VIP (Spengler et al., 1993; Pisegna et al., 1996; Pilzer and Gozes, 2006b) and the diminution of PACAP binding affinities, thereby suggesting that the alteration in IC3 causes an inside-out conformational change.

Notably, binding analysis of alternative spliced isoforms, which result from combined changes in the EC and IC protein domains yields interesting results. Thus, a splice variant composed of PAC1-short with the inclusion of hop1-cassette, displays similar PACAP and VIP binding properties to that of PAC1-null and different VIP binding properties than PAC1-short alone (Lutz et al., 2006; Ushiyama et al., 2007, 2010). Another combined splice variant composed of PAC1-δ5 or PAC1-δ5,6 together with the hip cassette had different ligand-binding properties to that of PAC1, PAC1-δ5, or PAC1-hip alone (Lutz et al., 2006) (**Table 1**). This imply that the IC3 domain contributes to the association of PAC1 with its cognate ligands.

These results may be explained by a model for agonist binding to the corticotropin-releasing hormone (CRH) receptor, which belongs to the same GPCR sub-family of PAC1 (Dong et al., 2005). According to this model the TM6 protein domain plays a structural role in ligand binding. Thus, insertions into IC3 loop, which is located between TM5 and TM6 region may cause a conformational change in TM6 and possibility affect binding of PACAP and VIP to the EC part of the receptor. A proof for this model awaits a solved three-dimensional protein structural of the different PAC1 isoforms.

ALTERNATIVE PAC1 SPLICING ALTERS INTRACELLULAR SIGNAL TRANSDUCTION

Ligand binding to PAC1 results in allosteric changes in the IC docking sites for effector coupling. A variety of IC signal transduction cascades can be differentially transduced by multiple PAC1 splice variants with altered EC or IC protein domains (**Figure 4**) (Arimura, 1998; Dickson and Finlayson, 2009; Vaudry et al., 2009; Furness et al., 2012). The most studied pathways include coupling of PAC1 to Gs and Gq proteins and activation of AC and phospholipase Cβ PLCβ) which result in the respective stimulation of production of cAMP and/or IP3 (Milligan and Kostenis, 2006;

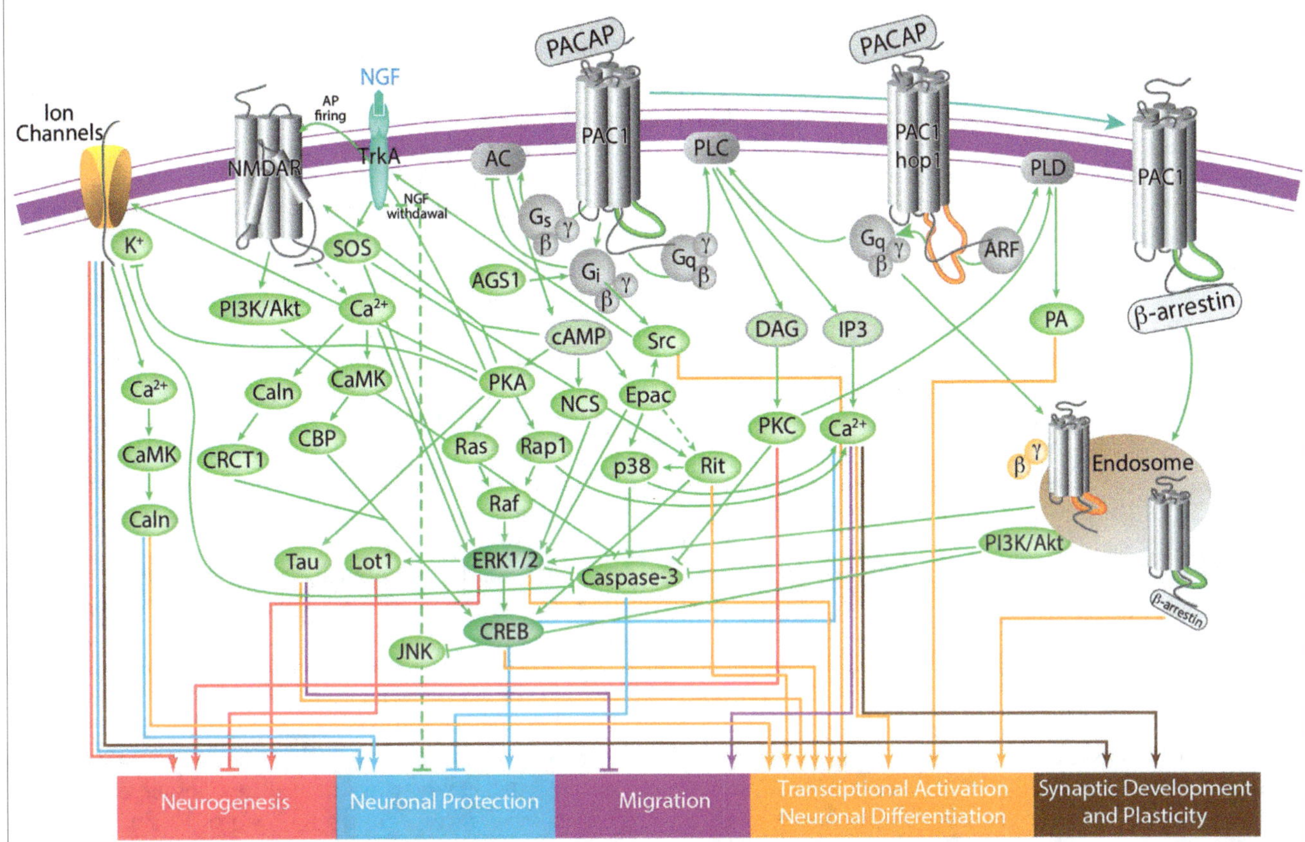

FIGURE 4 | A scheme depicting the current knowledge on PAC1-mediated signaling cascades resulting in a variety of neuronal outcomes. PKA was shown to induce ERK1/2 thereby contributing to PACAP neuroprotective (Villalba et al., 1997; Vaudry et al., 2003; Falluel-Morel et al., 2006; Stumm et al., 2007) and neurotrophic (Ravni et al., 2006; Botia et al., 2007; Monaghan et al., 2008) functions. Action potential (AP) firing induces a CRCT1/CREB mediated neuroprotective effect, presumably through NMDA receptor activation and was shown to be initiated by PKA activation (Baxter et al., 2011). NMDA receptor was also shown to be indirectly activated by PACAP (Llansola et al., 2004) or cAMP/PKA signaling (Costa et al., 2009). PAC1/PKA signaling controls cellular apoptosis through inhibition of potassium channels (Mei et al., 2004; Castel et al., 2006; Pugh and Margiotta, 2006) or induction of calcium channels (Pugh and Margiotta, 2006). PAC1/PKA-mediated activation of ion channels leads to activity-dependent neuronal differentiation and synaptic plasticity (Lee et al., 1999; Maturana et al., 2002; Grumolato et al., 2003; Nishimoto et al., 2007). The tumor suppressor gene Lot1 known as a negative regulator of neuronal precursor proliferation was shown to be controlled by PAC1/cAMP/ERK signaling pathway (Fila et al., 2009). PAC1/PKA-dependent phosphorylation of Tau is involved in the control of granule cell migration during cerebellar development (Falluel-Morel et al., 2006). PAC1-mediated cAMP/ERK-dependent neurite outgrowth was shown to be regulated via a novel neuritogenic factor NCS (Emery and Eiden, 2012) or Epac/ERK (Gerdin and Eiden, 2007) pathways. PAC1/Epac was shown to regulate neuronal differentiation via activation of p38 kinase along with mobilization of Ca^{2+} from intracellular stores (Ster et al., 2007) as well as Epac/Rit-dependent pathway involving CREB signaling (Shi et al., 2006). PAC1 was demonstrated to induce Rit through TrkA/Shc/SOS signaling initiated by Src activation via dual Gs/Epac and Gi stimulation (Shi et al., 2010). PACAP also signals through Gq-linked PLC > IP3 > Ca^{2+}/DAG > PKC, and PLD > phosphatidic acid (PA) pathways (Journot et al., 1994; Makhlouf and Murthy, 1997; Dejda et al., 2006). PAC1 is a mediator of gene transcription, neuronal differentiation, and synaptic development (Masmoudi-Kouki et al., 2006; Vaudry et al., 2007; Andero and Ressler, 2012). As an example of functional diversity caused by PAC1 alternative splicing two additional PAC1-hop1 signaling pathways are presented on the scheme. They depict PAC1-hop1/ARF dependent PLD activation (McCulloch et al., 2001) and internalization-dependent engagement of PI3Kγ/Akt activation (May et al., 2010). AC, adenylate cyclase; AGS, activator of G protein signaling; Akt, serine-threonine protein kinase PKB; cAMP, cyclic adenosine monophosphate; ARF, ADP(adenosine diphosphate) ribosylation factor; Caln, calcineurin; CaMK, calcium calmodulin kinase; CBP, creb binding protein; CRCT1, cysteine-rich C-terminal 1; CREB, cAMP responsive element-binding protein; DAG, diacyl glycerol; Epac, exchange factor directly activated by cAMP; ERK, extracellular signal-regulate kinase; G, guanine nucleotide-binding regulatory protein; IP3, inositol-1,4,5-triphosphate; JNK, c-Jun oncogene N-terminal kinase 1; Lot1, lost on transformation 1; NCS, neuritogenic cAMP sensor; NGF, nerve growth factor; NMDAR, *N*-methyl-d-aspartate receptor; p38, p38 mitogen-activated protein kinase; PA, phosphatidic acid; PI3K, phosphatidylinositol 3′ OH kinase; PKA, protein kinase A; PKC, protein kinase C;PLC, phospholipase; Raf, B-Raf proto-oncogene serine/threonine kinase;Ras, retrovirus-associated DNA sequences; Rap1, Rit, small GTPases of the RAS oncogene family; Sos, son of sevenless homolog 1; Src, sarcoma viral oncogen homolog; Tau, neuron-specific microtubule-associated protein; TrkA, tropomyosin-related kinase.

Couvineau and Laburthe, 2012) (**Figures 3** and **4**). In addition, PAC1 was shown to regulate the level of IC Ca^{2+} in either G-protein dependent or independent manners. The following section reviews the role of PAC1 splice variants in the activation of the above pathways as well as other non-canonical signaling cascades (see also **Table 1**).

AC AND PLCβ

When compared to the PAC1-null isoform, some alternative spliced variants display altered mode of signaling. For example, PAC1 isoform 3a, δ4,5,6 (a.k.a. very short), hip, hip-hop, δ5-hip, and δ5,6-hip show reduction in the potency of agonists-mediated cAMP and IP3 production (Spengler et al., 1993; Dautzenberg et al., 1999; Parsons et al., 2000; Daniel et al., 2001; Germano et al., 2004; Lutz et al., 2006; Pilzer and Gozes, 2006a; Holighaus et al., 2011). Similarly, PAC-TM4, hop1 novel, δ5,6,14–17, skip, and Rmc have lost their ability to stimulate cAMP and IP3 production (Chatterjee et al., 1996; Daniel et al., 2001; Ajpru et al., 2002; Alexandre et al., 2002; Fradinger et al., 2005; Abu-Hamdan et al., 2006; Pilzer and Gozes, 2006a). Notably, all of the above splice variants have modified or deleted IC3, TM, and C-terminal protein domains that are known to be important for G-protein binding (Chatterjee et al., 1996).

In some studies, PAC1-null displays very low or no activation of PLCβ while PAC1-hop1 switches its mode of signaling from AC to PLCβ (Spengler et al., 1993; DiCicco-Bloom et al., 2000; Nicot and DiCicco-Bloom, 2001; Ronaldson et al., 2002; May et al., 2010). For example, PAC1-hop1 was reported to mediate the activation of both AC and phospholipase C signaling in cortical sympathetic neuroblasts, while PAC1-null merely signals via AC stimulated pathway (Braas and May, 1996; DiCicco-Bloom et al., 2000). Other studies report that both isoforms display dual activation of AC and PLCβ pathways, however the hop1 isoform has higher activation of these pathways. Thus, analyses of SV1/hip and SV2/hop1 show that these isoforms display increased coupling to cAMP and PLCβ, respectively (Spengler et al., 1993; Pisegna and Wank, 1996; Lu et al., 1998; Braas and May, 1999; Parsons et al., 2000; Nicot and DiCicco-Bloom, 2001; Germano et al., 2004; Lutz et al., 2006; May et al., 2010; Holighaus et al., 2011). The frog R25 and R41 isoforms containing amino acid insertions into IC3 have higher activation of cAMP compared to PAC1-null (Alexandre et al., 2002).

Consistent with the effect of IC3 loop insertions on ligand-binding properties, hip- and hop2-cassettes conferred comparable potency to induction of cAMP and IP3 accumulation by PACAP and VIP but at the same time characterized by much lower efficacy of this response (Spengler et al., 1993; Pisegna and Wank, 1996; Pisegna et al., 1996; Ronaldson et al., 2002; Lutz et al., 2006). On the other hand, PAC1-hip variant was shown to retain AC mediated signaling but demonstrated impaired coupling to the PLCβ pathway (May et al., 2010).

CA^{2+} SIGNALING

The concentration of calcium ions (Ca^{2+}) in the cytoplasm is controlled by its uptake and release by specific transporter proteins residing in the plasma membrane, the inner mitochondria membrane, and the endoplasmic reticulum (ER) (Clapham, 2007). PAC1-mediated Ca^{2+} signaling was shown to play important roles in regulating neurotransmitter release, and neurotransmitter receptors (Shioda et al., 1997; Taupenot et al., 1999; Germano et al., 2009; Mustafa et al., 2010; Pugh et al., 2010; Amir-Zilberstein et al., 2012; Smith and Eiden, 2012). The effects of PAC1 splice isoforms on the levels of cytoplasmic Ca^{2+} were reported in the cases of PAC1-null hop1/2, δ5,6/short, 3a, and PAC1-TM4 (**Table 1**) (Dautzenberg et al., 1999; Lutz et al., 2006; Mustafa et al., 2007, 2010; Nishimoto et al., 2007; Germano et al., 2009; Hansson et al., 2009; Vallejo, 2009; Ushiyama et al., 2010; Holighaus et al., 2011). PACAP is known to modulate both EC Ca^{2+} influx via voltage-gated calcium channels (VGCC) and Ca^{2+} release from IC ER stores through both IP3/PLCβ and AC pathways but also through other signaling cascades (Tanaka et al., 1997; Shioda et al., 1998; Grimaldi and Cavallaro, 1999).

PAC1-null was reported to modulate cytosolic Ca^{2+} mobilization from both EC and IC stores (Shioda et al., 1997; Masmoudi et al., 2003; Payet et al., 2003; Nishimoto et al., 2007). In acutely dissociated rat melanotrophs, the increase of cytosolic Ca^{2+} was dependent on the activation of non-selective cation channels and the facilitation of voltage-dependent Ca^{2+} channels by PKC- and PKA-dependent phosphorylation, respectively (Tanaka et al., 1997). cAMP-dependent entry of EC calcium was also reported in astrocyte cells (Vallejo, 2009). It was also suggested that PAC1-null-mediated elevation of cytoplasmic Ca^{2+} levels in NG108-15 cells is due to IP_3 receptor-mediated Ca^{2+} release from IC stores (Holighaus et al., 2011).

The PAC1-hop1 variant is responsible for both Ca^{2+} mobilization from IC stores and influx through voltage-gated Ca^{2+} channels in bovine chromaffin cells (Mustafa et al., 2007). Transfection of PAC1-hop to the adrenomedullary pheochromocytoma (PC12) cell line showed sustained IP_3-mediated Ca^{2+} release from IC stores and from store-operated Ca^{2+} entry (SOCE) (Taupenot et al., 1999; Mustafa et al., 2007, 2010). In bovine adrenal chromaffin cells, PAC1-hop was shown to mediate cytosolic Ca^{2+} release from ryanodine/caffeine-sensitive Ca^{2+} stores that was not dependent on either cAMP or IP3 generation (Tanaka et al., 1998; Payet et al., 2003). Heterologous expression of the rat PAC1-hop1 but not PAC1-hip variant in NG108-15 and PC12 cells leads to an increase in IC Ca^{2+} concentration (Mustafa et al., 2007; Holighaus et al., 2011). In both cell lines the response consisted of a rapid and transient rise of Ca^{2+} reminiscent of IP_3 receptor-mediated Ca^{2+} release from IC stores followed by a prolonged Ca^{2+} accumulated from EC source.

When compared with PAC1-null, PAC1-hop1 was more potent in Ca^{2+} elevation (Holighaus et al., 2011). However, following overexpression in Chinese Hamster Ovarian cells, activation of PAC1-null induced higher Ca^{2+} levels when compared with activation of PAC1-hop1 (Ushiyama et al., 2010). PAC1-hop1 also mediated PACAP-induced Ca^{2+} release from ER and PKCγ translocation to the nucleus and plasma membrane resulting in the astrocytic differentiation (Nicot and DiCicco-Bloom, 2001). Finally, stimulation of voltage-gated L-type or non L-type Ca^{2+} channels following initiation of PAC1-hop1 signaling was also reported (Mustafa et al., 2010).

Somewhat limited data was reported with regards to Ca^{2+} signaling via other PAC1 splice variants. Thus, δ5,6/short as well as the PAC1 isoform containing combined "short" deletion in the N-terminal EC1 domain along with hop1-cassette in the IC3 loop exhibit PACAP-induced cytoplasmic calcium elevation (Ushiyama et al., 2010). PAC1-3a was shown to induce Ca^{2+} accumulation through coupling to Gs/cAMP rather than Gq/PLCβ pathway (Pilzer and Gozes, 2006a). PAC1-TM4 that was found to be inactive when assayed for both cAMP and PLCβ activation but it displayed elevation of Ca^{2+} in response to PACAP27. It was demonstrated that this effect involved the modulation of voltage-gated L-type Ca^{2+} channels (Chatterjee et al., 1996).

Taken together, the apparent inconsistent results concerning the mechanisms underlying the aforementioned Ca^{2+} signaling events are most likely due to the different cellular systems (e.g., cell types) employed by the above studies to analyze PAC1-mediated IC Ca^{2+} changes.

OTHER TRANSDUCTION PATHWAYS

Signaling of PAC1 through interaction with cytoplasmic protein partners, other than the canonical Gs and Gq, was reported mainly in the case of the PAC1-hop1 isoform (McCulloch et al., 2001; Ronaldson et al., 2002). Both PAC1-null and -hop1 proteins were reported to activate phospholipase D (PLD). Although PAC1-null-mediated PLD stimulation involved Gq/11 > PLC > PLD pathway, PAC1-hop1 was capable of activating PLD through direct binding to ADP-ribosylation factor (ARF) (McCulloch et al., 2002; Dejda et al., 2006).

EXPRESSION OF PAC1 SPLICE ISOFORMS IN THE NERVOUS SYSTEM

Information on time- and region-specific distribution of PAC1 splice isoforms may shed light on how PAC1 gene products regulate a plethora of biological functions in developmental and physiological processes (D'Agata et al., 1996; Waschek et al., 2000; Waschek, 2003; Vaudry et al., 2009). The distribution of PAC1 has been examined in many species using different techniques that revealed widespread expression in different tissues, including the nervous, cardiovascular, endocrine, immune, and respiratory systems (Aino et al., 1995; Abu-Hamdan et al., 2006; Gomariz et al., 2006; Molnar et al., 2008; Jolivel et al., 2009; Shneider et al., 2010; Lugo et al., 2011; Buljan et al., 2012). However, knowledge concerning the expression of PAC1 splice variants is somewhat limited at it is mainly based on analyses of isolated brain areas and/or primary cell cultures. The reported changes in PAC1 receptor variant expression appear to be most evident during development. We have summarized the existing data concerning the expression of these variants by focusing on expression in the nervous system of different mammalian species.

The major mRNA isoform of PAC1 in the brain is PAC1-null, which contains no splice deletions or insertions. PAC1-null is predominantly expressed in neurons residing in different brain areas although it is also detected in glial cells of the cerebella cortex and in activated astrocytes (Pilzer and Gozes, 2006b; Dickson and Finlayson, 2009; Vaudry et al., 2009).

PAC1 variants with N-terminal deletions are well represented in human fetal brain tissues and in five human neuroblastoma lines (Lutz et al., 2006; Falktoft et al., 2009), thereby suggesting their role in immature nervous tissue. N-terminal splice variants were detected in different brain areas. The PAC1-short variant with 21 amino acids N-terminal deletion was predominantly found in the thalamus, hypothalamus, and the hypophysis, and more moderately in the amygdala and retina (Dautzenberg et al., 1999; Grimaldi and Cavallaro, 1999; Jamen et al., 2002; Girard et al., 2004; Lutz et al., 2006; Ushiyama et al., 2007, 2010; Hammack et al., 2010a). It was shown to be expressed in cochlea subfractions along with the PAC1-δ5 isoform with a seven amino acid deletion (Abu-Hamdan et al., 2006). The PAC1-very short variant (57 amino acid deletion) was also detected at low levels in the mouse amygdala and cortex though not in the retina. All three N-terminal variants (null, short, and very short) were abundantly expressed in neuronal tissues (Dickson and Finlayson, 2009; Vaudry et al., 2009). The PAC1-3a variant containing N-terminal insertion of 24 amino acids was detected in rat cerebral cortex. This splice isoform is also highly expressed in distinct cell populations of the testis, including Sertoli cells, pachytene spermatocytes, and round spermatids (Daniel et al., 2001; Ajpru et al., 2002; Pilzer and Gozes, 2006a).

Contrary to the aforementioned N-terminal splice variants that were only reported in mammals, IC loops (i.e., IC3) splice products are found in all studied vertebrate species. In the postnatal cerebral cortex of rats, the expression of PAC1-null, hop1, hip, and hip-hop1 dramatically decreases during the first neonatal month suggesting a major role for these isoforms in embryonic development (Shneider et al., 2010). Interestingly, the expression of these isoforms was shown to be gender dependent displaying higher levels in female postnatal brain at least during the first 3 months of development. In the developing retina, the proportion of IC3 PAC1 isoforms changes as development proceeds: PAC1-hip-hop1 transcript demonstrated transient elevation at day P10, while a decrease in PAC1-null and hip along with elevation of PAC1-hop1 level was observed by P20 (Lakk et al., 2012). PAC1-hop1 expression was found in the olfactory bulb, hippocampus, cerebral cortex, cerebellum, and striatum of newborn rats. PAC1-hop2 was present in rat cerebral astrocytes from newborn brains, in neuronal enriched cultures, and in PC12 cells that undergo neuronal differentiation following NGF treatment (Jamen et al., 2002; Onoue et al., 2002; Hashimoto et al., 2003; Ravni et al., 2006; Mustafa et al., 2010).

PAC1-hip was detected at much lower levels in adult tissues and it was therefore speculated to be important for the embryonic development (Shneider et al., 2010; Holighaus et al., 2011). The relative expression of human and rat PAC1 splice variants in the frontal cortex was reported to have the following expression level hierarchy: null > SV1/hip > SV2/hop = SV3/hip-hop (Pisegna and Wank, 1996; Pisegna et al., 1996; Germano et al., 2004; Lutz et al., 2006). PAC1-hop1 was found to be expressed in all neuroendocrine cells, suggesting a fine tuning of PAC1-mediated signaling in the neuroendocrine cells (Mustafa et al., 2010). PAC1-hop1 splice isoform was the major form expressed in the superior cervical ganglia (SCG) sympathetic neurons, which also express PAC1-short (Braas and May, 1999). Zebrafish IC3 splice isoforms are widely expressed in the adult tissues with PAC1-hop1 detected in brain and testis, PAC1-hop2 in the ovary and PAC1-skip variant in the gills (Fradinger et al., 2005). Lastly, although PAC1-TM4 isoform is mainly found in pancreatic β-cells it is also expressed in the cerebral cortex, cerebellum, and brain stem (Chatterjee et al., 1996; Ajpru et al., 2002).

In summary, changes in PAC1 receptor variant expression appear to be most evident during development. The fact that PAC1 splice variants display differential expression patterns in the nervous system suggests that alternative splicing of this gene product plays a role in fine tuning of PAC1 activity in these areas.

REGULATION OF PAC1 SPLICING BY NEURONAL-SPECIFIC RNA-BINDING PROTEINS

The regulation of PAC1 splicing is not well understood. Alternative splicing of pre-mRNA is often regulated by conserved cis-regulatory RNA sequence elements that serve as recognition sites for different splicing factors. These RNA-binding splicing factors differ from the general spliceosome machinery proteins due to the formers' ability to either activate or repress the inclusion of alternatively spliced exons, depending on whether the factors' binding site is located upstream, downstream, or inside the exon. Neuronal-specific splicing factors include nova-1/2, Rbfox-1/2, and ELKV2 splicing factors, the neuronal-specific polypyrimidine tract-binding protein (nPTB) as well as a set of heterogeneous nuclear ribonucleoproteins (hnRNP A1,L,F,H1). As the consensus cis-acting binding sequences for the aforementioned splicing factors have been identified, their involvement in regulating the alternative splicing of a given gene by sequence analysis can be predicted. We analyzed the presence of known consensus binding sites for the following RNA-binding proteins: Rbfox-1/2, Nova-1/2 (single and repeatedly organized elements), SC-35, nPTB enhancers and silencers, and CaRRE for Ca^{2+}/CaM kinase IV recognition sequences. Putative binding sites for neuronal-specific splicing factors in the respective PAC1 genes of human, mouse, and zebrafish are shown in **Figure 5**.

A

Trans-acting Splicing factor	Cis elements	Exons of ADCYAP1R1 genes: Rat	Mouse	Human	Zebrafish
Rbfox1/2	(U)GCAUG ■	4,8,17 (upst) 4,11,15,16 (dnst) 3,4,13,18 (inside)	4,8 (upst) 4,11,15,16(dnst) 3,4,18 (inside)	4,8 (upst) 11,15 (dnst) 18 (inside)	4,18 (upst) 4,15,16,17 (dnst) 98 (inside)
CARRE	CACY(N)4A ■	17 (upst) 4 (dnst)	4,15 (upst)	15,17 (upst) 11,15 (dnst)	17,18 (upst) 4,11,15,16 (dnst)
Nova1/2	YCAY ■	7 (dnst) 8,9,10 (inside)	7,8,9,17 (upst) 17,18 (dnst) 8,9,10 (inside)	4,9,13,17 (upst) 6,13 (dnst) 8 (inside)	9 (upst) 4 (dnst) 9,10,13 (inside)
SC-35	UGCUGUU ■		13 (upst) 12 (dnst)		18 (upst) 11 (dnst) 13 (inside)
hnRNPA1	UAGG *	5,6,10,13,17 (upst) 4,6,9,10,17 (dnst) 10 (inside)	6,8,9,10,13 (upst) 8,9,16 (dnst) 10 (inside)	7,8,9,10,13 (upst) 6,9,10,13,16 (dnst) 3 (inside)	9,11,17 (upst) 8,10 (dnst) 4 (inside)
nPTB	CUCUCU ■ UUUUUUUU □ UTGUUU ■	6,13,14 (upst) 9 (inside)	5,13,16 (upst) 4 (dnst)	4,5,10,13,16 (upst) 3 (inside)	10,15,17 (upst) 9 (dnst)

B

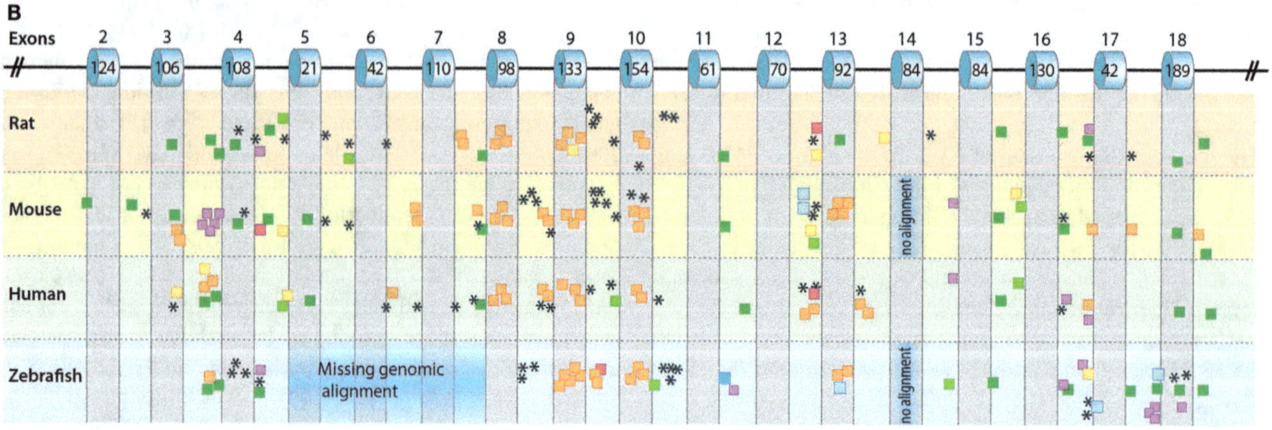

FIGURE 5 | Regulation of PAC1 splicing. (A) A chart depicting the predicted binding sites for neuronal-specific RNA-binding proteins that potentially regulate PAC1 gene splicing by binding in proximity to PAC1 exons. Consensus cis-acting binding DNA elements for the respective RNA-binding protein are depicted with respect to their position in the PAC1 genes of rat, mouse, human, and zebrafish PAC1. We analyzed the presence of putative consensus binding sites located within 300 base-pairs upstream (upst) or downstream (dnst) and inside the exons. **(B)** Schematic representation of the PAC1 gene in which the location of the analyzed cis-acting elements is color-coded as above. Corresponding exons numbers and sizes (bp) are indicated.

Rbfox-1/2 can act either as a splicing enhancer or as an inducer of exon skipping (Zhang et al., 2008). Putative Rbfox-1/2 binding sites located within a short distance downstream of target exons are predicted to induce exon inclusion whereas upstream binding sites are predicted to cause exon skipping. Such Rbfox-1/2 recognition element located within a short distance downstream of hop1 encoding exon has been experimentally validated as a genuine Rbfox-1 binding site (Lee et al., 2009). Our own PAC1 bioinformatic analysis identified a putative Rbfox-1/2 binding element within −30 nucleotides downstream from conserved exon spanning zebrafish TM7 suggesting that this domain might be regulated by alternative splicing (**Figure 5**). Rbfox-1/2 motifs are also present in the sequences of all examined species downstream of exon 16 encoding parts of the TM7 domain. Another recognition site is located upstream of exon 4 consistent with a deletion of the exon resulting in the generation of PAC1-very short splice variant (**Figure 5**). Rbfox-1/2 recognition motif predicts potential deletion of exon 8 that may result in a generation of a soluble PAC1 receptor as in the case of the CRH receptor (Zmijewski and Slominski, 2009, 2010). Rbfox-1/2 binding site is also detected downstream of exon 11, which is known to encode the most hypervariable amino acid sequence among Secretin family GPCRs, as well as part of TM4 domain which undergoes alternative splicing in PAC1-TM4 isoform (Markovic and Grammatopoulos, 2009).

Calcium signaling plays an important role in neuronal development and is involved in the regulation of immediate and long-term neuronal responses to various stimuli such as stressors and hormones (Ghosh et al., 1994; West et al., 2001). Depolarization is known to be critical for modulating the neuronal activity that induces Ca^{2+}-dependent gene regulation, including alternative splicing. Ca^{2+}-dependent splicing is mediated by L-type calcium channels and by Ca^{2+}/calmodulin-dependent protein kinases IV (CaMK IV) (Lee et al., 2007, 2009). The latter was shown to repress splicing of target genes containing specific recognition elements (CaRRE) located within the 3′ splice site or inside the exon. Our own analysis detected additional putative CaRREs that can be responsive to CaMK IV. We predicted single, multiple, and tandemly organized CaRRE repeats upstream of exon 15 and 17 of the zebrafish, human, and mouse PAC1 receptors, suggesting the involvement of CaMK IV in regulating the alternative splicing of these exons. Putative CaRREs are also present proximal to mouse, rat, and zebrafish exon 4 (**Figure 5**).

Exonic and intronic hnRNPA1 and nPTB cis-elements that are important for activity-dependent splicing in neuronal cells were shown to repress the inclusion of target exons (Allemand et al., 2005; An and Grabowski, 2007; Donev et al., 2007; Resnick et al., 2008; Zheng et al., 2012). Putative hnRNPA1 and nPTB recognition sites are located proximal to exons 4, 5, and 6 consistent with the known deletions of these exons that result in the generation of PAC1-short and very short splice variants. Putative hnRNPA1 recognition motifs are also found near exons 8–10 encoding to IC1, IC2, and EC2 domains (**Figure 5**).

Nova-1/2 regulates target exon inclusion or skipping with broad distribution of binding sites across the gene sequence (Ule et al., 2005; Yano et al., 2010; Norris and Calarco, 2012). Predicted Nova-1/2 recognition elements are found in human and mouse PAC1 and in both paralogs of zebrafish PAC1 gene (1a and 1b). Interestingly, higher frequency of putative splicing-inducing AU-rich and Nova-specific sequences are found in intronic regions upstream of alternative spliced exons characteristic of the Secretin family splicing patterns, e.g., around exon 4, 8, 9, 10 (Zmijewski and Slominski, 2009) as well as exon 17. Exons 4–6 encode sequences covering known N-terminal PAC1 deletion regions (deletions of 7, 21, and 57 amino acids). Exon 17 encodes the last amino acids of the seventh TM domain and the beginning of the IC tail shown to represent the highly conserved exon within the secretin family (Markovic and Grammatopoulos, 2009). Skipping of this exon was not detected in the PAC1 receptor gene, but it has been proposed that such exon skipping in the human CRF1 and PTH1 receptors results in a six TM receptor displaying impaired trafficking (Shyu et al., 1996; Grammatopoulos et al., 1999; Markovic et al., 2008). The rabbit calcitonin receptor is also formed as a result of the skipping of the TM7 domain and displays slightly diminished cAMP activation along with deficiency in IP3 induction (Shyu et al., 1996). Taken together the above analysis of potential cis-elements spanning TM7 exons predicts that a PAC1 splice variant containing TM7 skipping may exist in neuronal tissues.

An important question raised in this chapter is whether the aforementioned RNA-binding factors regulate PAC1 splicing *in vivo*. It has been demonstrated that alternative splicing of the PAC1 receptor is regulated by the Rbfox-1 splicing factor in depolarized neurons. In this case, neuronal depolarization induced CaM-kinase dependent self-splicing of Rbfox-1, leading to the translocation of Rbfox-1/2 from the cytoplasm to the nucleus where Rbfox-1 could mediate the alternative splicing of neuronal-specific target genes, including PAC1. Interestingly, Rbfox-1 mRNA levels were shown to be regulated by the Orthopedia (Otp) homedomain-containing protein. The latter is a hypothalamic-specific transcriptional factor, which plays a role in hypothalamic neuronal-specification during development and in regulation of body homeostasis in the mature zebrafish brain (Acampora et al., 1999; Wang and Lufkin, 2000; Blechman et al., 2007; Ryu et al., 2007; Amir-Zilberstein et al., 2012; Fernandes et al., 2012). The involvement and regulation of other neuronal-specific RNA-binding factors in PAC1 splicing remains to be determined.

PLEIOTROPIC ROLES OF PAC1 SPLICE ISOFORMS IN THE NERVOUS SYSTEM

The distribution of PAC1 and its ligands PACAP and VIP in a variety of cell types is reminiscent of the pleiotropic functions of PAC1 in development and physiology. PACAP is described in the literature as a hormone, neuropeptide, endocrine peptide, neurotransmitter, and neurotrophic factor. It affects the central nervous system (CNS), cardiovascular system, pituitary, thyroid, and adrenal glands and provides functional activities in the gonads, gastrointestinal tract, and pancreas (Waschek et al., 2000; Dickson and Finlayson, 2009; Vaudry et al., 2009). In the nervous system, PAC1 was shown to affect a variety of hormones and neuropeptides, including stimulation of oxytocin (Jamen et al., 2003) and melatonin (Nakahara et al., 2002) release and *de novo* mRNA synthesis of CRH (Nakahara et al., 2002; Amir-Zilberstein et al., 2012), arginine-vasopressin (Murase et al., 1995; Gillard et al., 2006), GnRH (Kanasaki et al., 2009; Winters and Moore, 2011), somatostatin (Kageyama et al., 2007), and MSH (Mounien et al., 2006). This overabundance of PAC1-mediated physiological activities can be made possible through the signaling diversity of its alternatively spliced gene products. Moreover, different expression of PAC1 isoforms is common in neuronal ontogeny. Such differences in the expression of PAC1 splice variants might modulate final outputs of VIP and PACAP activities as neurotransmitters, neurotrophic, or differentiation factors. Examples for the involvement of PAC1 splice isoforms in mediating these activities are described below.

NEUROGENESIS, NEUROPROTECTION, AND DIFFERENTIATION

Neural progenitor cells (NPC) and astroglial cells express PAC1-null and PAC1-hop1 variants that mediate both cAMP- and Ca^{2+}-dependent signaling pathways and induce production of a subset of neurotrophic factors resulting in neuronal proliferation and/or differentiation. PAC1-hop2 variant, detected in astrogenic and neuronal populations, promote neuroprotective function induced by VIP. In another study, VIP was also demonstrated to induce PAC1-hop2-mediated astrocytes neuroprotection against oxidative stress. Astrocytic expression of PAC1-hop2 isoform may therefore play a critical role in the NPC shift toward neuronal or astrocytes differentiation (Ashur-Fabian et al., 1997; Pilzer and Gozes, 2006b).

Expression of PAC1-null and PAC1-hop1 define region-specific neurogenesis in the CNS and peripheral nervous systems (Lu et al., 1998). Both variants are differently expressed in proliferating sympathetic (PAC1-hop1) and cortical precursors (PAC1-null) revealing opposing PACAP-mediated mitogenic regulation – either by stimulating sympathetic neuroblast proliferation or by inhibiting cortical precursor mitosis. Ectopic expression of PAC1-hop1 in cortical neuroblasts may transform the anti-mitotic effect of PACAP into promitotic. This promitotic signaling was shown to involve PLC signaling pathway (Nicot and DiCicco-Bloom, 2001). PAC1-hop1 was also shown to promote sympathetic neurons survival following growth factor withdrawal (May et al., 2010).

In conjunction with the abovementioned, PACAP may possess therapeutic potential for neurodegenerative pathologies, such as Parkinson's and Alzheimer's disease (AD). PACAP is enriched in rat mesencephalic dopaminergic neurons and protects them from neurotoxin-induced death (Reglodi et al., 2004). PACAP was shown to be downregulated in several mouse models for AD as well as in the human temporal cortex of AD patients (Kojro et al., 2006; Rat et al., 2011; Postina, 2012). Amyloidogenic processing of the amyloid precursor protein (APP) to $\alpha\beta$-peptides is responsible for the development of AD. However, non-amyloidogenic APP processing pathway results in the α-secretase-dependent cleavage within the $\alpha\beta$-peptide region, preventing AD pathology. Continual PACAP and PAC1 activation resulted also in a feed-forward autocrine elevation of both PACAP and PAC1 in mice that may further facilitate non-amyloidogenic APP cleavage. α-secretase activation was shown to be regulated by ERK1 and ERK 2 and PI-3 kinase, suggesting that PAC1-hop1 is the most efficient isoform with regard to the activation of these downstream PLC effectors (Kojro et al., 2006; Rat et al., 2011; Postina, 2012). It remains to be determined whether specific PAC1 splice variants are involved in these neuroprotective activities.

NEUROSECRETION AND NEUROTRANSMISSION

Pituitary AC-activating polypeptide was shown to elicit catecholamine synthesis and release. Expression of PAC1-hop1 in bovine chromaffin NG108-15 cell line, which lacks endogenous PAC1 receptors, induces the release of norepinephrine via a Ca^{2+} influx-dependent mechanism (Mustafa et al., 2007). Transfected PAC1-hop1 triggers sustained catecholamine secretion by regulating Ca^{2+} levels through both ER and EC Ca^{2+} channels (Mustafa et al., 2010; Smith and Eiden, 2012). Moreover, acute and long-term met-enkephalin secretion and enkephalin biosynthesis were attributed to bovine chromaffin cells upon PAC1-hop1-mediated activation of L-type Ca^{2+} channels. This implies a role of hop1 splice cassette in regulating neuroendocrine secretion. SCG sympathetic neurons were shown to predominantly express the PAC1-hop1 splice isoform and PACAP stimulates neuropeptide Y release in these neurons via a mechanism involving both AC and PLCβ (Braas and May, 1999).

ROLE OF PAC1 SPLICE ISOFORMS IN BODY HOMEOSTASIS

PAC1 is implicated in the regulation of homeostatic processes, including food and liquid consumption (Nomura et al., 1997; Mounien et al., 2006, 2009), sleep (Hannibal and Fahrenkrug, 2004), stress (Pilzer and Gozes, 2006b; Amir-Zilberstein et al., 2012), locomotion (Vaudry et al., 2000), memory and learning activities (Dong et al., 2010; Andero and Ressler, 2012; Holighaus et al., 2012), and circadian functions (Ajpru et al., 2002; Hannibal and Fahrenkrug, 2004). Recent studies have indicated that at least some of these activities are modulated by alternative splicing of PAC1 (Ajpru et al., 2002; Hannibal and Fahrenkrug, 2004; Pilzer and Gozes, 2006b; Holighaus et al., 2011, 2012; Amir-Zilberstein et al., 2012).

Pituitary AC-activating polypeptide/PAC1 signaling was recently implicated in abnormal stress responses underlying post-traumatic stress disorder (PTSD) pathology (Ressler et al., 2011; Andero and Ressler, 2012; Hauger et al., 2012). PACAP38 levels in females were strongly associated with PTSD symptoms. Ressler et al. and May et al. (2010) found that a single nucleotide polymorphism (SNP), rs2267735 in the PAC1 gene is correlated with PTSD in a gender-specific estrogen-dependent manner. This SNP, which resides in the putative estrogen response element within PAC1's promoter/enhancer is associated with sex-dependent PTSD, fear discrimination, PAC1 mRNA expression, and methylation of PAC1. Using mouse models, these authors showed that PAC1 mRNA was induced by fear conditioning or estrogen hormone replacement in the bed nucleus of stria terminalis (BNST), which is a component of the extended amygdala involved in fear- and anxiety-like responses.

In connection to the above, steroid-induced changes in PAC1 splice isoforms were demonstrated in the case of PAC1-hop2 (Apostolakis et al., 2005). PAC1-hop2 and the N-terminal PAC1-short splice variants were detected in the hypothalamic ventromedial nucleus (VMN) upon estradiol or dual estradiol/progesterone treatment. The ratio of PAC1-hop2 mRNA to other PAC1 variants in VMN depends on steroid application, implying its importance for cumulative PAC1 isoforms expression and hence signaling properties. PACAP-induced sexual/mating behavior in female rats was dependent on progesterone receptor in the VMN. Estradiol stimulates synthesis of progesterone, which in turn facilitates PACAP synthesis and activation of PAC1-short and -hop2 signaling critical for the induction of animal sexual receptivity.

PAC1 signaling is known to be required for physiological stress response as activation of PAC1 by PACAP is required for stress-induced CRH transcription *in vivo* and *in vitro* (Agarwal et al., 2005; Kageyama et al., 2007; Hammack et al., 2010b; Stroth and Eiden, 2010; Tsukiyama et al., 2011). The above studies suggest that PAC1 splice variants and their relative expression ratio might be involved in the regulation of body homeostasis including physiological responses to stressor challenges. A recent study performed in our lab, employed various stress paradigms in mouse and zebrafish to demonstrate that activation and termination of CRH transcription caused by stressful stimuli is regulated by an interrelationship of PAC1-null and hop1 isoforms (Amir-Zilberstein et al., 2012). Thus, the generation of PAC1-hop1 by alternative splicing leads to the termination of CRH transcription, normal activation of the hypothalamic-pituitary-adrenal axis, and adaptive anxiety-like behavior (Amir-Zilberstein et al., 2012). We therefore suggested that alternative splicing of the hop1-cassette serves as an ON/OFF stress switch (**Figure 6**).

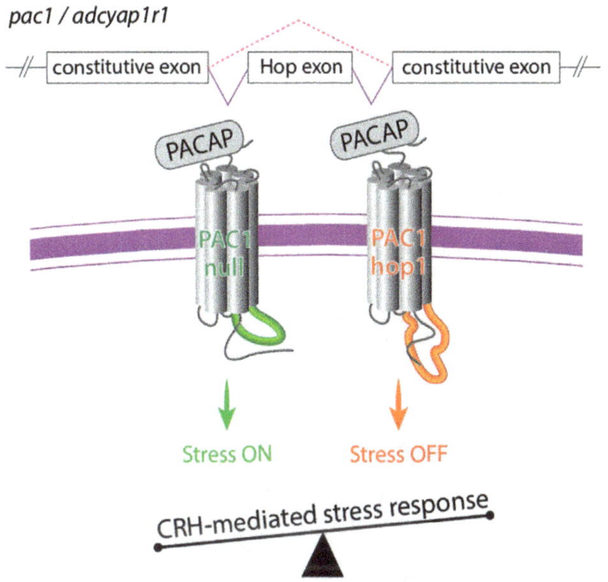

FIGURE 6 | A model illustrating the role of alternative splicing of PAC1 hop cassette that serves as an ON/OFF stress switch. In response to various stressors, the so called PAC1-null splice variant (i.e., no deletion in the N-terminal domain and no addition to the intracellular loops) modulate transcriptional activation of CRH and stress behaviors to adapt to the changes in homeostasis. Termination of CRH-mediated stress response is mediated by means of regulation of PAC1 gene splicing and inclusion of an altered exon (hop1) encoding to 28 amino acids of the third intracellular loop leading to the formation of the PAC1-hop1 splice variant. Generation of the PAC1-hop isoform terminates stress response by means yet to be uncovered (see text and Amir-Zilberstein et al., 2012).

PAC1 rs2267735 gene polymorphism is also associated with increased dark-enhanced startle (DES) in adult females but not males with PTSD (Ressler et al., 2011). Moreover, children of abused mothers show elevated DES and the same PAC1 gene polymorphism associated with PTSD risk in adult females is also associated with increased DES in these children (Jovanovic et al., 2011, 2012). Notably, zebrafish larvae show a strong aversion to the dark side of a two-compartment light/dark arena and this place preference can be mitigated by anxiolytic drugs, such as Diazepam, indicating that this assay measures an anxiety-like behavior (Steenbergen et al., 2011; Schnorr et al., 2012). We found that during the recovery phase that follows a stressful challenge (osmotic shock), wild type larvae decrease their dark-avoidance time, a phenotype indicative of decreased stress-related anxiety, while larvae with depleted PAC1a-hop1 display delayed dark-avoidance recovery (Amir-Zilberstein et al., 2012). Thus, the delayed behavioral response of PAC1a-hop1-depleted embryos correlates with their respective failure to terminate *crh* and cortisol levels following stressors.

CONCLUSION

Alternative splicing is a major gene regulatory process involving cis- and trans-acting factors. PAC1 signaling controls a variety of cellular and physiological responses, such as differentiation, proliferation, cell cycle regulation, neurotransmitter, and hormone release and adaptation to stressful challenges. The PAC1 gene encompasses a relatively long genomic region, which consists of up to 18 exons and contains many putative splicing factors recognition sites that might be activated during different phases of neuronal activation. PAC1 receptor signaling can be fine-tuned by the generation of a set of alternatively spliced variants produced in a spatio-temporal manner. Splicing-dependent alterations in PAC1 protein domains modify its ligand binding and signaling properties leading to a range of cellular activities. Although the physiological function(s) of the vast majority of the alternatively spliced PAC1 gene products is still unknown, recent studies have implicated certain PAC1 splice variants in the regulation of homeostatic processes such as adaptation to stressful challenges. In view of the recent association of PAC1 with PTSD risk, the regulation of PAC1 splicing and its underlying physiological outcomes might prove to be relevant to the etiology of some neurological and psychiatric disorders.

ACKNOWLEDGMENTS

We thank Shifra Ben-Or for PAC1 gene structure and phylogenetic analyses and Danielle Sabah-Israel, Jacob Biran, and Michael Gliksberg for comments on the manuscript. The research in the Levkowitz lab is supported by the Simons Foundation Autism Research Initiative (SFARI); Israel Science Foundation; Kirk Center for Childhood Cancer and Immunological Disorders; The Krenter Institute and Estate of Lore Lennon.

REFERENCES

Abu-Hamdan, M. D., Drescher, M. J., Ramakrishnan, N. A., Khan, K. M., Toma, V. S., Hatfield, J. S., et al. (2006). Pituitary adenylyl cyclase-activating polypeptide (PACAP) and its receptor (PAC1-R) in the cochlea: evidence for specific transcript expression of PAC1-R splice variants in rat microdissected cochlear subfractions. *Neuroscience* 140, 147–161.

Acampora, D., Postiglione, M. P., Avantaggiato, V., Di Bonito, M., Vaccarino, F. M., Michaud, J., et al. (1999). Progressive impairment of developing neuroendocrine cell lineages in the hypothalamus of mice lacking the Orthopedia gene. *Genes Dev.* 13, 2787–2800.

Agarwal, A., Halvorson, L. M., and Legradi, G. (2005). Pituitary adenylate cyclase-activating polypeptide (PACAP) mimics neuroendocrine and behavioral manifestations of stress: evidence for PKA-mediated expression of the corticotropin-releasing hormone (CRH) gene. *Brain Res. Mol. Brain Res.* 138, 45–57.

Ahren, B. (2008). Role of pituitary adenylate cyclase-activating polypeptide in the pancreatic endocrine system. *Ann. N. Y. Acad. Sci.* 1144, 28–35.

Aino, H., Hashimoto, H., Ogawa, N., Nishino, A., Yamamoto, K., Nogi, H., et al. (1995). Structure of the gene encoding the mouse pituitary adenylate cyclase-activating polypeptide receptor. *Gene* 164, 301–304.

Ajpru, S., McArthur, A. J., Piggins, H. D., and Sugden, D. (2002). Identification of PAC1 receptor isoform mRNAs by real-time PCR in rat suprachiasmatic nucleus. *Brain Res. Mol. Brain Res.* 105, 29–37.

Alexandre, D., Vaudry, H., Grumolato, L., Turquier, V., Fournier, A., Jegou, S., et al. (2002). Novel splice variants of type I pituitary adenylate cyclase-activating polypeptide receptor in frog exhibit altered adenylate cyclase stimulation and differential relative abundance. *Endocrinology* 143, 2680–2692.

Allemand, E., Guil, S., Myers, M., Moscat, J., Caceres, J. F., and Krainer, A. R. (2005). Regulation of heterogenous nuclear ribonucleoprotein A1 transport by phosphorylation in cells stressed by osmotic shock. *Proc. Natl. Acad. Sci. U.S.A.* 102, 3605–3610.

Amir-Zilberstein, L., Blechman, J., Sztainberg, Y., Norton, W. H., Reuveny, A., Borodovsky, N., et al. (2012). Homeodomain protein otp and activity-dependent splicing modulate neuronal adaptation to stress. *Neuron* 73, 279–291.

An, P., and Grabowski, P. J. (2007). Exon silencing by UAGG motifs in response to neuronal excitation. *PLoS Biol.* 5:e36. doi:10.1371/journal.pbio.0050036

Andero, R., and Ressler, K. J. (2012). Fear extinction and BDNF: translating animal models of PTSD to the clinic. *Genes Brain Behav.* 11, 503–512.

Apostolakis, E. M., Riherd, D. N., and O'Malley, B. W. (2005). PAC1 receptors mediate pituitary adenylate cyclase-activating polypeptide- and progesterone-facilitated receptivity in female rats. *Mol. Endocrinol.* 19, 2798–2811.

Arimura, A. (1998). Perspectives on pituitary adenylate cyclase activating polypeptide (PACAP) in the neuroendocrine, endocrine, and nervous systems. *Jpn. J. Physiol.* 48, 301–331.

Ashur-Fabian, O., Giladi, E., Brenneman, D. E., and Gozes, I. (1997). Identification of VIP/PACAP receptors on rat astrocytes using antisense oligodeoxynucleotides. *J. Mol. Neurosci.* 9, 211–222.

Baxter, P. S., Martel, M. A., McMahon, A., Kind, P. C., and Hardingham, G. E. (2011). Pituitary adenylate cyclase-activating peptide induces long-lasting neuroprotection through the induction of activity-dependent signaling via the cyclic AMP response element-binding protein-regulated transcription co-activator 1. *J. Neurochem.* 118, 365–378.

Betke, K. M., Wells, C. A., and Hamm, H. E. (2012). GPCR mediated regulation of synaptic transmission. *Prog. Neurobiol.* 96, 304–321.

Bjarnadottir, T. K., Gloriam, D. E., Hellstrand, S. H., Kristiansson, H., Fredriksson, R., and Schioth, H. B. (2006). Comprehensive repertoire and phylogenetic analysis of the G protein-coupled receptors in human and mouse. *Genomics* 88, 263–273.

Black, D. L. (2003). Mechanisms of alternative pre-messenger RNA splicing. *Annu. Rev. Biochem.* 72, 291–336.

Blechman, J., Borodovsky, N., Eisenberg, M., Nabel-Rosen, H., Grimm, J., and Levkowitz, G. (2007). Specification of hypothalamic neurons by dual regulation of the homeodomain protein Orthopedia. *Development* 134, 4417–4426.

Botia, B., Basille, M., Allais, A., Raoult, E., Falluel-Morel, A., Galas, L., et al. (2007). Neurotrophic effects of PACAP in the cerebellar cortex. *Peptides* 28, 1746–1752.

Braas, K. M., and May, V. (1996). Pituitary adenylate cyclase-activating polypeptides, PACAP-38 and PACAP-27, regulation of sympathetic neuron catecholamine, and neuropeptide Y expression through activation of type I PACAP/VIP receptor isoforms. *Ann. N. Y. Acad. Sci.* 805, 204–216; discussion 217–208.

Braas, K. M., and May, V. (1999). Pituitary adenylate cyclase-activating polypeptides directly stimulate sympathetic neuron neuropeptide Y release through PAC(1) receptor isoform activation of specific intracellular signaling pathways. *J. Biol. Chem.* 274, 27702–27710.

Buljan, M., Chalancon, G., Eustermann, S., Wagner, G. P., Fuxreiter, M., Bateman, A., et al. (2012). Tissue-specific splicing of disordered segments that embed binding motifs rewires protein interaction networks. *Mol. Cell* 46, 871–883.

Cardoso, J. C., De Vet, E. C., Louro, B., Elgar, G., Clark, M. S., and Power, D. M. (2007). Persistence of duplicated PAC1 receptors in the teleost, *Sparus auratus*. *BMC Evol. Biol.* 7:221. doi:10.1186/1471-2148-7-221

Castel, H., Vaudry, D., Mei, Y. A., Lefebvre, T., Basille, M., Desrues, L., et al. (2006). The delayed rectifier channel current IK plays a key role in the control of programmed cell death by PACAP and ethanol in cerebellar granule neurons. *Ann. N. Y. Acad. Sci.* 1070, 173–179.

Cavallaro, S., D'Agata, V., Guardabasso, V., Travali, S., Stivala, F., and Canonico, P. L. (1995). Differentiation induces pituitary adenylate cyclase-activating polypeptide receptor expression in PC-12 cells. *Mol. Pharmacol.* 48, 56–62.

Chafai, M., Basille, M., Galas, L., Rostene, W., Gressens, P., Vaudry, H., Gonzalez, B. J., et al. (2011). Pituitary adenylate cyclase-activating polypeptide and vasoactive intestinal polypeptide promote the genesis of calcium currents in differentiating mouse embryonic stem cells. *Neuroscience* 199, 103–115.

Chatterjee, T. K., Liu, X., Davisson, R. L., and Fisher, R. A. (1997). Genomic organization of the rat pituitary adenylate cyclase-activating polypeptide receptor gene. Alternative splicing within the 5'-untranslated region. *J. Biol. Chem.* 272, 12122–12131.

Chatterjee, T. K., Sharma, R. V., and Fisher, R. A. (1996). Molecular cloning of a novel variant of the pituitary adenylate cyclase-activating polypeptide (PACAP) receptor that stimulates calcium influx by activation of L-type calcium channels. *J. Biol. Chem.* 271, 32226–32232.

Clapham, D. E. (2007). Calcium signaling. *Cell* 131, 1047–1058.

Costa, L., Santangelo, F., Volsi, G. L., and Ciranna, L. (2009). Modulation of AMPA receptor-mediated ion current by pituitary adenylate cyclase-activating polypeptide (PACAP) in CA1 pyramidal neurons from rat hippocampus. *Hippocampus* 19, 99–109.

Couvineau, A., and Laburthe, M. (2012). The family B1 GPCR: structural aspects and interaction with accessory proteins. *Curr. Drug Targets* 13, 103–115.

D'Agata, V., Cavallaro, S., Stivala, F., Travali, S., and Canonico, P. L. (1996). Tissue-specific and developmental expression of pituitary adenylate cyclase-activating polypeptide (PACAP) receptors in rat brain. *Eur. J. Neurosci.* 8, 310–318.

Daniel, P. B., Kieffer, T. J., Leech, C. A., and Habener, J. F. (2001). Novel alternatively spliced exon in the extracellular ligand-binding domain of the pituitary adenylate cyclase-activating polypeptide (PACAP) type 1 receptor (PAC1R) selectively increases ligand affinity and alters signal transduction coupling during spermatogenesis. *J. Biol. Chem.* 276, 12938–12944.

Dautzenberg, F. M., Mevenkamp, G., Wille, S., and Hauger, R. L. (1999). N-terminal splice variants of the type I PACAP receptor: isolation, characterization and ligand binding/selectivity determinants. *J. Neuroendocrinol.* 11, 941–949.

Dejda, A., Jozwiak-Bebenista, M., and Nowak, J. Z. (2006). PACAP, VIP, and PHI: effects on AC-, PLC-, and PLD-driven signaling systems in the primary glial cell cultures. *Ann. N. Y. Acad. Sci.* 1070, 220–225.

DiCicco-Bloom, E., Deutsch, P. J., Maltzman, J., Zhang, J., Pintar, J. E., Zheng, J., et al. (2000). Autocrine expression and ontogenetic functions of the PACAP ligand/receptor system during sympathetic development. *Dev. Biol.* 219, 197–213.

Dickson, L., and Finlayson, K. (2009). VPAC and PAC receptors: from ligands to function. *Pharmacol. Ther.* 121, 294–316.

Donev, R., Newall, A., Thome, J., and Sheer, D. (2007). A role for SC35 and hnRNPA1 in the determination of amyloid precursor protein isoforms. *Mol. Psychiatry* 12, 681–690.

Dong, M. Q., Pinon, D. I., and Miller, L. J. (2005). Insights into the structure and molecular basis of ligand docking to the G protein-coupled secretin receptor using charge-modified amino-terminal agonist probes. *Mol. Endocrinol.* 19, 1821–1836.

Dong, Y. X., Fukuchi, M., Inoue, M., Takasaki, I., Tabuchi, A., Wu, C. F., et al. (2010). Pituitary adenylate cyclase-activating polypeptide (PACAP) is an upstream regulator of prodynorphin mRNA expression in neurons. *Neurosci. Lett.* 484, 174–177.

Emery, A. C., and Eiden, L. E. (2012). Signaling through the neuropeptide GPCR PAC1 induces neuritogenesis via a single linear cAMP- and ERK-dependent pathway using a novel cAMP sensor. *FASEB J.* 26, 3199–3211.

Falktoft, B., Georg, B., and Fahrenkrug, J. (2009). Signaling pathways in PACAP regulation of VIP gene expression in human neuroblastoma cells. *Neuropeptides* 43, 387–396.

Falluel-Morel, A., Vaudry, D., Aubert, N., Galas, L., Benard, M., Basille, M., et al. (2006). PACAP and ceramides exert opposite effects on migration, neurite outgrowth, and cytoskeleton remodeling. *Ann. N. Y. Acad. Sci.* 1070, 265–270.

Fernandes, A. M., Fero, K., Arrenberg, A. B., Bergeron, S. A., Driever, W., and Burgess, H. A. (2012). Deep Brain photoreceptors control light-seeking behavior in zebrafish larvae. *Curr. Biol.* 22, 2042–2047.

Fila, T., Trazzi, S., Crochemore, C., Bartesaghi, R., and Ciani, E. (2009). Lot1 is a key element of the pituitary adenylate cyclase-activating polypeptide (PACAP)/cyclic AMP pathway that negatively regulates neuronal precursor proliferation. *J. Biol. Chem.* 284, 15325–15338.

Fradinger, E. A., Tello, J. A., Rivier, J. E., and Sherwood, N. M. (2005). Characterization of four receptor cDNAs: PAC1, VPAC1, a novel PAC1 and a partial GHRH in zebrafish. *Mol. Cell. Endocrinol.* 231, 49–63.

Frooninckx, L., Van Rompay, L., Temmerman, L., Van Sinay, E., Beets, I., Janssen, T., et al. (2012). Neuropeptide GPCRs in *C. elegans*. *Front. Endocrinol.* 3:167. doi:10.3389/fendo.2012.00167

Furness, S. G., Wootten, D., Christopoulos, A., and Sexton, P. M. (2012). Consequences of splice variation on Secretin family G protein-coupled receptor function. *Br. J. Pharmacol.* 166, 98–109.

Gerdin, M. J., and Eiden, L. E. (2007). Regulation of PC12 cell differentiation by cAMP signaling to ERK independent of PKA: do all the connections add up? *Sci. STKE* 2007, e15.

Germano, P. M., Le, S. V., Oh, D. S., Fan, R., Lieu, S., Siu, A., et al. (2004). Differential coupling of the PAC1 SV1 splice variant on human colonic tumors to the activation of intracellular cAMP but not intracellular Ca2+ does not activate tumor proliferation. *J. Mol. Neurosci.* 22, 83–92.

Germano, P. M., Lieu, S. N., Xue, J., Cooke, H. J., Christofi, F. L., Lu, Y., et al. (2009). PACAP induces signaling and stimulation of 5-hydroxytryptamine release and growth in neuroendocrine tumor cells. *J. Mol. Neurosci.* 39, 391–401.

Ghosh, A., Ginty, D. D., Bading, H., and Greenberg, M. E. (1994). Calcium regulation of gene-expression in neuronal cells. *J. Neurobiol.* 25, 294–303.

Gillard, E. R., Leon-Olea, M., Mucio-Ramirez, S., Coburn, C. G., Sanchez-Islas, E., De Leon, A., et al. (2006). A novel role for endogenous pituitary adenylate cyclase activating polypeptide in the magnocellular neuroendocrine system. *Endocrinology* 147, 791–803.

Girard, B. M., Keller, E. T., Schutz, K. C., May, V., and Braas, K. M. (2004). Pituitary adenylate cyclase activating polypeptide and PAC1 receptor signaling increase Homer 1a expression in central and peripheral neurons. *Regul. Pept.* 123, 107–116.

Gomariz, R. P., Juarranz, Y., Abad, C., Arranz, A., Leceta, J., and Martinez, C. (2006). VIP-PACAP system in immunity – new insights for multitarget therapy. *Ann. N. Y. Acad. Sci.* 1070, 51–74.

Grammatopoulos, D. K., Dai, Y., Randeva, H. S., Levine, M. A., Karteris, E., Easton, A. J., et al. (1999). A novel spliced variant of the type 1 corticotropin-releasing hormone receptor with a deletion in the seventh transmembrane domain present in the human pregnant term myometrium and fetal membranes. *Mol. Endocrinol.* 13, 2189–2202.

Grimaldi, M., and Cavallaro, S. (1999). Functional and molecular diversity of PACAP/VIP receptors in cortical neurons and type I astrocytes. *Eur. J. Neurosci.* 11, 2767–2772.

Grumolato, L., Louiset, E., Alexandre, D., Ait-Ali, D., Turquier, V., Fournier, A., et al. (2003). PACAP and NGF regulate common and distinct traits of the sympathoadrenal lineage: effects on electrical properties, gene markers and transcription factors in differentiating PC12 cells. *Eur. J. Neurosci.* 17, 71–82.

Hammack, S. E., Roman, C. W., Lezak, K. R., Kocho-Shellenberg, M., Grimmig, B., Falls, W. A., et al. (2010a). Roles for pituitary adenylate cyclase-activating peptide (PACAP) expression and signaling in the bed nucleus of the stria terminalis (BNST) in mediating the behavioral consequences of chronic stress. *J. Mol. Neurosci.* 42, 327–340.

Hammack, S. E., Roman, C. W., Lezak, K. R., Kocho-Shellenberg, M., Grimmig, B., Falls, W. A., et al. (2010b). Roles for pituitary adenylate cyclase-activating peptide (PACAP) expression and signaling in the bed nucleus of the stria terminalis (BNST) in mediating the behavioral consequences of chronic stress. *J. Mol. Neurosci.* 34, 833–843.

Hannibal, J., and Fahrenkrug, J. (2004). Target areas innervated by PACAP-immunoreactive retinal ganglion cells. *Cell Tissue Res.* 316, 99–113.

Hansson, E., Westerlund, A., Bjorklund, U., and Ronnback, L. (2009). PACAP attenuates 5-HT, histamine, and ATP-evoked Ca2+ transients in astrocytes. *Neuroreport* 20, 957–962.

Harikumar, K. G., Morfis, M. M., Sexton, P. M., and Miller, L. J. (2008). Pattern of intra-family hetero-oligomerization involving the G-protein-coupled secretin receptor. *J. Mol. Neurosci.* 36, 279–285.

Harmar, A. J., Fahrenkrug, J., Gozes, I., Laburthe, M., May, V., Pisegna, J. R., et al. (2012). Pharmacology and functions of receptors for vasoactive intestinal peptide and pituitary adenylate cyclase-activating polypeptide: IUPHAR review 1. *Br. J. Pharmacol.* 166, 4–17.

Hashimoto, H., Kunugi, A., Arakawa, N., Shintani, N., Fujita, T., Kasai, A., et al. (2003). Possible involvement of a cyclic AMP-dependent mechanism in PACAP-induced proliferation and ERK activation in astrocytes. *Biochem. Biophys. Res. Commun.* 311, 337–343.

Hauger, R. L., Olivares-Reyes, J. A., Dautzenberg, F. M., Lohr, J. B., Braun, S., and Oakley, R. H. (2012). Molecular and cell signaling targets for PTSD pathophysiology and pharmacotherapy. *Neuropharmacology* 62, 705–714.

Holighaus, Y., Mustafa, T., and Eiden, L. E. (2011). PAC1hop, null and hip receptors mediate differential signaling through cyclic AMP and calcium leading to splice variant-specific gene induction in neural cells. *Peptides* 32, 1647–1655.

Holighaus, Y., Weihe, E., and Eiden, L. E. (2012). STC1 induction by PACAP is mediated through cAMP and ERK1/2 but not PKA in cultured cortical neurons. *J. Mol. Neurosci.* 46, 75–87.

Hoyer, D., and Bartfai, T. (2012). Neuropeptides and neuropeptide receptors: drug targets, and peptide and non-peptide ligands: a tribute to Prof. Dieter Seebach. *Chem. Biodivers.* 9, 2367–2387.

Jafurulla, M., and Chattopadhyay, A. (2013). Membrane lipids in the function of serotonin and adrenergic receptors. *Curr. Med. Chem.* 20, 47–55.

Jaillon, O., Bouhouche, K., Gout, J. F., Aury, J. M., Noel, B., Saudemont, B., et al. (2008). Translational control of intron splicing in eukaryotes. *Nature* 451, 359–362.

Jamen, F., Alonso, G., Shibuya, I., Widmer, H., Vacher, C. M., Calas, A., et al. (2003). Impaired somatodendritic responses to pituitary adenylate cyclase-activating polypeptide (PACAP) of supraoptic neurones in PACAP type I-receptor deficient mice. *J. Neuroendocrinol.* 15, 871–881.

Jamen, F., Puech, R., Bockaert, J., Brabet, P., and Bertrand, G. (2002). Pituitary adenylate cyclase-activating polypeptide receptors mediating insulin secretion in rodent pancreatic islets are coupled to adenylate cyclase but not to PLC. *Endocrinology* 143, 1253–1259.

Jolivel, V., Basille, M., Aubert, N., De Jouffrey, S., Ancian, P., Le Bigot, J. F., et al. (2009). Distribution and functional characterization of pituitary adenylate cyclase-activating polypeptide receptors in the brain of non-human primates. *Neuroscience* 160, 434–451.

Journot, L., Spengler, D., Pantaloni, C., Dumuis, A., Sebben, M., and Bockaert, J. (1994). The PACAP receptor: generation by alternative splicing of functional diversity among G protein-coupled receptors in nerve cells. *Semin. Cell Biol.* 5, 263–272.

Journot, L., Waeber, C., Pantaloni, C., Holsboer, F., Seeburg, P. H., Bockaert, J., et al. (1995). Differential signal transduction by six splice variants of the pituitary adenylate cyclase-activating peptide (PACAP) receptor. *Biochem. Soc. Trans.* 23, 133–137.

Jovanovic, T., Norrholm, S. D., Davis, J., Mercer, K. B., Almli, L., Nelson, A., et al. (2012). PAC1 receptor (ADCYAP1R1) genotype is associated with dark-enhanced startle in children. *Mol. Psychiatry.* doi:10.1038/mp.2012.98. [Epub ahead of print].

Jovanovic, T., Smith, A., Kamkwalala, A., Poole, J., Samples, T., Norrholm, S. D., et al. (2011). Physiological markers of anxiety are increased in children of abused mothers. *J. Child. Psychol. Psychiatry* 52, 844–852.

Kageyama, K., Hanada, K., Iwasaki, Y., Sakihara, S., Nigawara, T., Kasckow, J., et al. (2007). Pituitary adenylate cyclase-activating polypeptide stimulates corticotropin-releasing factor, vasopressin and interleukin-6 gene transcription in hypothalamic 4B cells. *J. Endocrinol.* 195, 199–211.

Kanasaki, H., Mutiara, S., Oride, A., Purwana, I. N., and Miyazaki, K. (2009). Pulse frequency-dependent gonadotropin gene expression by adenylate cyclase-activating polypeptide 1 in perifused mouse pituitary gonadotroph LbetaT2 cells. *Biol. Reprod.* 81, 465–472.

Kojro, E., Postina, R., Buro, C., Meiringer, C., Gehrig-Burger, K., and Fahrenholz, F. (2006). The neuropeptide PACAP promotes the alpha-secretase pathway for processing the Alzheimer amyloid precursor protein. *FASEB J.* 20, 512–514.

Lakk, M., Szabo, B., Volgyi, B., Gabriel, R., and Denes, V. (2012). Development-related splicing regulates pituitary adenylate cyclase-activating polypeptide (PACAP) receptors in the retina. *Invest. Ophthalmol. Vis. Sci.* 53, 7825–7832.

Lee, H. W., Hahm, S. H., Hsu, C. M., and Eiden, L. E. (1999). Pituitary adenylate cyclase-activating polypeptide regulation of vasoactive intestinal polypeptide transcription requires Ca2+ influx and activation of the serine/threonine phosphatase calcineurin. *J. Neurochem.* 73, 1769–1772.

Lee, J. A., Tang, Z. Z., and Black, D. L. (2009). An inducible change in Fox-1/A2BP1 splicing modulates the alternative splicing of downstream neuronal target exons. *Genes Dev.* 23, 2284–2293.

Lee, J. A., Xing, Y., Nguyen, D., Xie, J., Lee, C. J., and Black, D. L. (2007). Depolarization and CaM kinase IV modulate NMDA receptor splicing through two essential RNA elements. *PLoS Biol.* 5:e40. doi:10.1371/journal.pbio.0050040

Lefkowitz, R. J. (2007). Seven transmembrane receptors: something old, something new. *Acta Physiol. (Oxf.)* 190, 9–19.

Llansola, M., Sanchez-Perez, A. M., Montoliu, C., and Felipo, V. (2004). Modulation of NMDA receptor function by cyclic AMP in cerebellar neurones in culture. *J. Neurochem.* 91, 591–599.

Lu, N., Zhou, R., and DiCicco-Bloom, E. (1998). Opposing mitogenic regulation by PACAP in sympathetic and cerebral cortical precursors correlates with differential expression of PACAP receptor (PAC1-R) isoforms. *J. Neurosci. Res.* 53, 651–662.

Lugo, J. M., Tafalla, C., Leceta, J., Gomariz, R. P., and Estrada, M. P. (2011). Differential expression pattern of pituitary adenylate cyclase-activating polypeptide (PACAP) alternative splicing variants and its receptors in the immune system of rainbow trout (*Oncorhynchus mykiss*). *Fish Shellfish Immunol.* 30, 734–738.

Lutz, E. M., Ronaldson, E., Shaw, P., Johnson, M. S., Holland, P. J., and Mitchell, R. (2006). Characterization of novel splice variants of the PAC1 receptor in human neuroblastoma cells: consequences for signaling by VIP and PACAP. *Mol. Cell. Neurosci.* 31, 193–209.

Machluf, Y., Gutnick, A., and Levkowitz, G. (2011). Development of the zebrafish hypothalamus. *Ann. N. Y. Acad. Sci.* 1220, 93–105.

Magalhaes, A. C., Dunn, H., and Ferguson, S. S. (2012). Regulation of GPCR activity, trafficking and localization by GPCR-interacting proteins. *Br. J. Pharmacol.* 165, 1717–1736.

Mahata, M., Zhang, K., Gayen, J. R., Nandi, S., Brar, B. K., Ghosh, S., et al. (2011). Catecholamine biosynthesis and secretion: physiological and pharmacological effects of secretin. *Cell Tissue Res.* 345, 87–102.

Makhlouf, G. M., and Murthy, K. S. (1997). Signal transduction in gastrointestinal smooth muscle. *Cell. Signal.* 9, 269–276.

Markovic, D., and Grammatopoulos, D. K. (2009). Focus on the splicing of secretin GPCRs transmembrane-domain 7. *Trends Biochem. Sci.* 34, 443–452.

Markovic, D., Lehnert, H., Levine, M. A., and Grammatopoulos, D. K. (2008). Structural determinants critical for localization and signaling within the seventh transmembrane domain of the type 1 corticotropin releasing hormone receptor: lessons from the receptor variant R1d. *Mol. Endocrinol.* 22, 2505–2519.

Masmoudi, O., Gandolfo, P., Leprince, J., Vaudry, D., Fournier, A., Patte-Mensah, C., et al. (2003). Pituitary adenylate cyclase-activating polypeptide (PACAP) stimulates endozepine release from cultured rat astrocytes via a PKA-dependent mechanism. *FASEB J.* 17, 17–27.

Masmoudi-Kouki, O., Gandolfo, P., Leprince, J., Vaudry, D., Pelletier, G., Fournier, A., et al. (2006). PACAP stimulates biosynthesis and release of endozepines from rat astrocytes. *Ann. N. Y. Acad. Sci.* 1070, 411–416.

Maturana, A., Van Haasteren, G., Piuz, I., Castelbou, C., Demaurex, N., and Schlegel, W. (2002). Spontaneous calcium oscillations control c-fos transcription via the serum response element in neuroendocrine cells. *J. Biol. Chem.* 277, 39713–39721.

Maurice, P., Guillaume, J. L., Benleulmi-Chaachoua, A., Daulat, A. M., Kamal, M., and Jockers, R. (2011). GPCR-interacting proteins, major players of GPCR function. *Adv. Pharmacol.* 62, 349–380.

May, V., Lutz, E., MacKenzie, C., Schutz, K. C., Dozark, K., and Braas, K. M. (2010). Pituitary adenylate cyclase-activating polypeptide (PACAP)/PAC1HOP1 receptor activation coordinates multiple neurotrophic signaling pathways: Akt activation through phosphatidylinositol 3-kinase gamma and vesicle endocytosis for neuronal survival. *J. Biol. Chem.* 285, 9749–9761.

McCulloch, D. A., Lutz, E. M., Johnson, M. S., Robertson, D. N., MacKenzie, C. J., Holland, P. J., et al. (2001). ADP-ribosylation factor-dependent phospholipase D activation by VPAC receptors and a PAC(1) receptor splice variant. *Mol. Pharmacol.* 59, 1523–1532.

McCulloch, D. A., MacKenzie, C. J., Johnson, M. S., Robertson, D. N., Holland, P. J., Ronaldson, E., et al. (2002). Additional signals from VPAC/PAC family receptors. *Biochem. Soc. Trans.* 30, 441–446.

Mei, Y. A., Vaudry, D., Basille, M., Castel, H., Fournier, A., Vaudry, H., et al. (2004). PACAP inhibits delayed rectifier potassium current via a cAMP/PKA transduction pathway: evidence for the involvement of I-K in the anti-apoptotic action of PACAP. *Eur. J. Neurosci.* 19, 1446–1458.

Milligan, G., and Kostenis, E. (2006). Heterotrimeric G-proteins: a short history. *Br. J. Pharmacol.* 147(Suppl. 1), S46–S55.

Miyata, A., Arimura, A., Dahl, R. R., Minamino, N., Uehara, A., Jiang, L., et al. (1989). Isolation of a novel 38 residue-hypothalamic polypeptide which stimulates adenylate cyclase in pituitary cells. *Biochem. Biophys. Res. Commun.* 164, 567–574.

Mizuno, N., and Itoh, H. (2009). Functions and regulatory mechanisms of Gq-signaling pathways. *Neurosignals* 17, 42–54.

Molnar, L., Pollak, E., Boros, A., Shioda, S., Nakajo, S., Tamas, A., et al. (2008). PAC1 receptor localization in a model nervous system: light and electron microscopic immunocytochemistry on the earthworm ventral nerve cord ganglia. *Regul. Pept.* 145, 96–104.

Monaghan, T. K., Pou, C., MacKenzie, C. J., Plevin, R., and Lutz, E. M. (2008). Neurotrophic actions of PACAP-38 and LIF on human neuroblastoma SH-SY5Y cells. *J. Mol. Neurosci.* 36, 45–56.

Morfis, M., Christopoulos, A., and Sexton, P. M. (2003). RAMPs: 5 years on, where to now? *Trends Pharmacol. Sci.* 24, 596–601.

Mounien, L., Bizet, P., Boutelet, I., Gourcerol, G., Fournier, A., Vaudry, H., et al. (2006). Pituitary adenylate cyclase-activating polypeptide directly modulates the activity of proopiomelanocortin neurons in the rat arcuate nucleus. *Neuroscience* 143, 155–163.

Mounien, L., Do Rego, J. C., Bizet, P., Boutelet, I., Gourcerol, G., Fournier, A., et al. (2009). Pituitary adenylate cyclase-activating polypeptide inhibits food intake in mice through activation of the hypothalamic melanocortin system. *Neuropsychopharmacology* 34, 424–435.

Murase, T., Kondo, K., Arima, H., Iwasaki, Y., Ito, M., Miura, Y., et al. (1995). The expression of pituitary adenylate cyclase-activating polypeptide (PACAP) mRNA in rat brain: possible role of endogenous PACAP in vasopressin release. *Neurosci. Lett.* 185, 103–106.

Mustafa, T., Grimaldi, M., and Eiden, L. E. (2007). The hop cassette of the PAC1 receptor confers coupling to Ca2+ elevation required for pituitary adenylate cyclase-activating polypeptide-evoked neurosecretion. *J. Biol. Chem.* 282, 8079–8091.

Mustafa, T., Walsh, J., Grimaldi, M., and Eiden, L. E. (2010). PAC1hop receptor activation facilitates catecholamine secretion selectively through 2-APB-sensitive Ca(2+) channels in PC12 cells. *Cell. Signal.* 22, 1420–1426.

Nakahara, K., Abe, Y., Murakami, T., Shiota, K., and Murakami, N. (2002). Pituitary adenylate cyclase-activating polypeptide (PACAP) is involved in melatonin release via the specific receptor PACAP-r1, but not in the circadian oscillator, in chick pineal cells. *Brain Res.* 939, 19–25.

Nicot, A., and DiCicco-Bloom, E. (2001). Regulation of neuroblast mitosis is determined by PACAP receptor isoform expression. *Proc. Natl. Acad. Sci. U.S.A.* 98, 4758–4763.

Nishimoto, M., Furuta, A., Aoki, S., Kudo, Y., Miyakawa, H., and Wada, K. (2007). PACAP/PAC1 autocrine system promotes proliferation and astrogenesis in neural progenitor cells. *Glia* 55, 317–327.

Nomura, M., Ueta, Y., Larsen, P. J., Hannibal, J., Serino, R., Kabashima, N., et al. (1997). Water deprivation increases the expression of pituitary adenylate cyclase-activating polypeptide gene in the rat subfornical organ. *Endocrinology* 138, 4096–4100.

Nordstrom, K. J., Lagerstrom, M. C., Waller, L. M., Fredriksson, R., and Schioth, H. B. (2009). The Secretin GPCRs descended from the family of Adhesion GPCRs. *Mol. Biol. Evol.* 26, 71–84.

Norris, A. D., and Calarco, J. A. (2012). Emerging roles of alternative pre-mRNA splicing regulation in neuronal development and function. *Front. Neurosci.* 6:122. doi:10.3389/fnins.2012.00122

Oldham, W. M., and Hamm, H. E. (2008). Heterotrimeric G protein activation by G-protein-coupled receptors. *Nat. Rev. Mol. Cell Biol.* 9, 60–71.

Onoue, S., Endo, K., Yajima, T., and Kashimoto, K. (2002). Pituitary adenylate cyclase activating polypeptide regulates the basal production of nitric oxide in PC12 cells. *Life Sci.* 71, 205–214.

Pantaloni, C., Brabet, P., Bilanges, B., Dumuis, A., Houssami, S., Spengler, D., et al. (1996). Alternative splicing in the N-terminal extracellular domain of the pituitary adenylate cyclase-activating polypeptide (PACAP) receptor modulates receptor selectivity and relative potencies of PACAP-27 and PACAP-38 in phospholipase C activation. *J. Biol. Chem.* 271, 22146–22151.

Parsons, R. L., Rossignol, T. M., Calupca, M. A., Hardwick, J. C., and Brass, K. M. (2000). PACAP peptides modulate guinea pig cardiac neuron membrane excitability and neuropeptide expression. *Ann. N. Y. Acad. Sci.* 921, 202–210.

Payet, M. D., Bilodeau, L., Breault, L., Fournier, A., Yon, L., Vaudry, H., et al. (2003). PAC1 receptor activation by PACAP-38 mediates Ca2+ release from a cAMP-dependent pool in human fetal adrenal gland chromaffin cells. *J. Biol. Chem.* 278, 1663–1670.

Pierce, K. L., Premont, R. T., and Lefkowitz, R. J. (2002). Seven-transmembrane receptors. *Nat. Rev. Mol. Cell Biol.* 3, 639–650.

Pilzer, I., and Gozes, I. (2006a). A splice variant to PACAP receptor that is involved in spermatogenesis is expressed in astrocytes. *Ann. N. Y. Acad. Sci.* 1070, 484–490.

Pilzer, I., and Gozes, I. (2006b). VIP provides cellular protection through a specific splice variant of the PACAP receptor: a new neuroprotection target. *Peptides* 27, 2867–2876.

Pisegna, J. R., Moody, T. W., and Wank, S. A. (1996). Differential signaling and immediate-early gene activation by four splice variants of the human pituitary adenylate cyclase-activating polypeptide receptor (hPACAP-R). *Ann. N. Y. Acad. Sci.* 805, 54–64; discussion 64–66.

Pisegna, J. R., and Wank, S. A. (1996). Cloning and characterization of the signal transduction of four splice variants of the human pituitary adenylate cyclase activating polypeptide receptor. Evidence for dual coupling to adenylate cyclase and phospholipase C. *J. Biol. Chem.* 271, 17267–17274.

Postina, R. (2012). Activation of alpha-secretase cleavage. *J. Neurochem.* 120(Suppl. 1), 46–54.

Pugh, P. C., Jayakar, S. S., and Margiotta, J. F. (2010). PACAP/PAC(1)R signaling modulates acetylcholine release at neuronal nicotinic synapses. *Mol. Cell. Neurosci.* 43, 244–257.

Pugh, P. C., and Margiotta, J. F. (2006). PACAP support of neuronal survival requires MAPK- and activity-generated signals. *Mol. Cell. Neurosci.* 31, 586–595.

Rat, D., Schmitt, U., Tippmann, F., Dewachter, I., Theunis, C., Wieczerzak, E., et al. (2011). Neuropeptide pituitary adenylate cyclase-activating polypeptide (PACAP) slows down Alzheimer's disease-like pathology in amyloid precursor protein-transgenic mice. *FASEB J.* 25, 3208–3218.

Ravni, A., Bourgault, S., Lebon, A., Chan, P., Galas, L., Fournier, A., et al. (2006). The neurotrophic effects of PACAP in PC12 cells: control by multiple transduction pathways. *J. Neurochem.* 98, 321–329.

Reglodi, D., Lubics, A., Tamas, A., Szalontay, L., and Lengvari, I. (2004). Pituitary adenylate cyclase activating polypeptide protects dopaminergic neurons and improves behavioral deficits in a rat model of Parkinson's disease. *Behav. Brain Res.* 151, 303–312.

Resnick, M., Segall, A., Rozic-Kotliroff, G., Lupowitz, Z., and Zisapel, N. (2008). Alternative splicing of neurexins: a role for neuronal polypyrimidine tract binding protein. *Neurosci. Lett.* 439, 235–240.

Ressler, K. J., Mercer, K. B., Bradley, B., Jovanovic, T., Mahan, A., Kerley, K., et al. (2011). Post-traumatic stress disorder is associated with PACAP and the PAC1 receptor. *Nature* 470, 492–497.

Ritter, S. L., and Hall, R. A. (2009). Fine-tuning of GPCR activity by receptor-interacting proteins. *Nat. Rev. Mol. Cell Biol.* 10, 819–830.

Ronaldson, E., Robertson, D. N., Johnson, M. S., Holland, P. J., Mitchell, R., and Lutz, E. M. (2002). Specific interaction between the hop1 intracellular loop 3 domain of the human PAC(1) receptor and ARF. *Regul. Pept.* 109, 193–198.

Ryu, S., Mahler, J., Acampora, D., Holzschuh, J., Erhardt, S., Omodei, D., et al. (2007). Orthopedia homeodomain protein is essential for diencephalic dopaminergic neuron development. *Curr. Biol.* 17, 873–880.

Sah, V. P., Seasholtz, T. M., Sagi, S. A., and Brown, J. H. (2000). The role of Rho in G protein-coupled receptor signal transduction. *Annu. Rev. Pharmacol. Toxicol.* 40, 459–489.

Schnorr, S. J., Steenbergen, P. J., Richardson, M. K., and Champagne, D. L. (2012). Measuring thigmotaxis in larval zebrafish. *Behav. Brain Res.* 228, 367–374.

Shi, G. X., Jin, L., and Andres, D. A. (2010). Src-dependent TrkA transactivation is required for pituitary adenylate cyclase-activating polypeptide 38-mediated Rit activation and neuronal differentiation. *Mol. Biol. Cell* 21, 1597–1608.

Shi, G. X., Rehmann, H., and Andres, D. A. (2006). A novel cyclic AMP-dependent Epac-Rit signaling pathway contributes to PACAP38-mediated neuronal differentiation. *Mol. Cell. Biol.* 26, 9136–9147.

Shioda, S., Yada, T., and Nakajo, S. (1998). PACAP increases cytosolic calcium in vasopressin neurons: synergism with noradrenaline. *Ann. N. Y. Acad. Sci.* 865, 427–430.

Shioda, S., Yada, T., Nakajo, S., Nakaya, K., Nakai, Y., and Arimura, A. (1997). Pituitary adenylate cyclase-activating polypeptide (PACAP): a novel regulator of vasopressin-containing neurons. *Brain Res.* 765, 81–90.

Shneider, Y., Shtrauss, Y., Yadid, G., and Pinhasov, A. (2010). Differential expression of PACAP receptors in postnatal rat brain. *Neuropeptides* 44, 509–514.

Shyu, J. F., Inoue, D., Baron, R., and Horne, W. C. (1996). The deletion of 14 amino acids in the seventh transmembrane domain of a naturally occurring calcitonin receptor isoform alters ligand binding and selectively abolishes coupling to phospholipase C. *J. Biol. Chem.* 271, 31127–31134.

Simon, M. I., Strathmann, M. P., and Gautam, N. (1991). Diversity of G proteins in signal transduction. *Science* 252, 802–808.

Smith, C. B., and Eiden, L. E. (2012). Is PACAP the major neurotransmitter for stress transduction at the adrenomedullary synapse? *J. Mol. Neurosci.* 48, 403–412.

Spengler, D., Waeber, C., Pantaloni, C., Holsboer, F., Bockaert, J., Seeburg, P. H., et al. (1993). Differential signal transduction by five splice variants of the PACAP receptor. *Nature* 365, 170–175.

Steenbergen, P. J., Richardson, M. K., and Champagne, D. L. (2011). Patterns of avoidance behaviours in the light/dark preference test in young juvenile zebrafish: a pharmacological study. *Behav. Brain Res.* 222, 15–25.

Ster, J., De Bock, F., Guerineau, N. C., Janossy, A., Barrere-Lemaire, S., Bos, J. L., et al. (2007). Exchange protein activated by cAMP (Epac) mediates cAMP activation of p38 MAPK and modulation of Ca2+-dependent K+ channels in cerebellar neurons. *Proc. Natl. Acad. Sci. U.S.A.* 104, 2519–2524.

Stroth, N., and Eiden, L. E. (2010). Stress hormone synthesis in mouse hypothalamus and adrenal gland triggered by restraint is dependent on pituitary adenylate cyclase-activating polypeptide signaling. *Neuroscience* 165, 1025–1030.

Stumm, R., Kolodziej, A., Prinz, V., Endres, M., Wu, D. F., and Hollt, V. (2007). Pituitary adenylate cyclase-activating polypeptide is up-regulated in cortical pyramidal cells after focal ischemia and protects neurons from mild hypoxic/ischemic damage. *J. Neurochem.* 103, 1666–1681.

Sun, S., Zhang, Z., Fregoso, O., and Krainer, A. R. (2012). Mechanisms of activation and repression by the alternative splicing factors RBFOX1/2. *RNA* 18, 274–283.

Tanaka, K., Shibuya, I., Harayama, N., Nomura, M., Kabashima, N., Ueta, Y., et al. (1997). Pituitary adenylate cyclase-activating polypeptide potentiation of Ca2+ entry via protein kinase C and A pathways in melanotrophs of the pituitary pars intermedia of rats. *Endocrinology* 138, 4086–4095.

Tanaka, K., Shibuya, I., Uezono, Y., Ueta, Y., Toyohira, Y., Yanagihara, N., et al. (1998). Pituitary adenylate cyclase-activating polypeptide causes Ca2+ release from ryanodine/caffeine stores through a novel pathway independent of both inositol trisphosphates and cyclic AMP in bovine adrenal medullary cells. *J. Neurochem.* 70, 1652–1661.

Taupenot, L., Mahata, M., Mahata, S. K., and O'Connor, D. T. (1999). Time-dependent effects of the neuropeptide PACAP on catecholamine secretion: stimulation and desensitization. *Hypertension* 34, 1152–1162.

Tsukiyama, N., Saida, Y., Kakuda, M., Shintani, N., Hayata, A., Morita, Y., et al. (2011). PACAP centrally mediates emotional stress-induced corticosterone responses in mice. *Stress* 14, 368–375.

Ule, J., Ule, A., Spencer, J., Williams, A., Hu, J. S., Cline, M., et al. (2005). Nova regulates brain-specific splicing to shape the synapse. *Nat. Genet.* 37, 844–852.

Ushiyama, M., Ikeda, R., Sugawara, H., Yoshida, M., Mori, K., Kangawa, K., et al. (2007). Differential intracellular signaling through PAC1 isoforms as a result of alternative splicing in the first extracellular domain and the third intracellular loop. *Mol. Pharmacol.* 72, 103–111.

Ushiyama, M., Ikeda, R., Yoshida, M., Mori, K., Kangawa, K., Sugawara, H., et al. (2010). Alternative splicing of the pituitary adenylate cyclase-activating polypeptide (PACAP) receptor contributes to function of PACAP-27. *J. Mol. Neurosci.* 42, 341–348.

Vallejo, M. (2009). PACAP signaling to DREAM: a cAMP-dependent pathway that regulates cortical astrogliogenesis. *Mol. Neurobiol.* 39, 90–100.

Vaudry, D., Basille, M., Morel, A. F., Aubert, N., Botia, B., Allais, A., et al. (2007). Neurotrophic effects of PACAP in the cerebellar cortex. *J. Mol. Neurosci.* 33, 312–312.

Vaudry, D., Falluel-Morel, A., Bourgault, S., Basille, M., Burel, D., Wurtz, O., et al. (2009). Pituitary adenylate cyclase-activating polypeptide and its receptors: 20 years after the discovery. *Pharmacol. Rev.* 61, 283–357.

Vaudry, D., Falluel-Morel, A., Leuillet, S., Vaudry, H., and Gonzalez, B. J. (2003). Regulators of cerebellar granule cell development act through specific signaling pathways. *Science* 300, 1532–1534.

Vaudry, D., Gonzalez, B. J., Basille, M., Pamantung, T. F., Fournier, A., and Vaudry, H. (2000). PACAP acts as a neurotrophic factor during histogenesis of the rat cerebellar cortex. *Ann. N. Y. Acad. Sci.* 921, 293–299.

Villalba, M., Bockaert, J., and Journot, L. (1997). Pituitary adenylate cyclase-activating polypeptide (PACAP-38) protects cerebellar granule neurons from apoptosis by activating the mitogen-activated protein kinase (MAP kinase) pathway. *J. Neurosci.* 17, 83–90.

Wang, W., and Lufkin, T. (2000). The murine Otp homeobox gene plays an essential role in the specification of neuronal cell lineages in the developing hypothalamus. *Dev. Biol.* 227, 432–449.

Waschek, J. A. (2003). Multiple actions of pituitary adenylyl cyclase activating peptide in nervous system development and regeneration (vol 24, pg 14, 2002). *Dev. Neurosci.* 25, 393–393.

Waschek, J. A., DiCicco-Bloom, E. M., Lelievre, V., Zhou, X., and Hu, Z. (2000). PACAP action in nervous system development, regeneration, and neuroblastoma cell proliferation. *Ann. N. Y. Acad. Sci.* 921, 129–136.

Watkins, H. A., Au, M., and Hay, D. L. (2012). The structure of secretin family GPCR peptide ligands: implications for receptor pharmacology and drug development. *Drug Discov. Today* 17, 1006–1014.

Wei, Y., Martin, S. C., Heinrich, G., and Mojsov, S. (1998). Cloning and functional characterization of PACAP-specific receptors in zebrafish. *Ann. N. Y. Acad. Sci.* 865, 45–48.

West, A. E., Chen, W. G., Dalva, M. B., Dolmetsch, R. E., Kornhauser, J. M., Shaywitz, A. J., et al. (2001). Calcium regulation of neuronal gene expression. *Proc. Natl. Acad. Sci. U.S.A.* 98, 11024–11031.

Winters, S. J., and Moore, J. P. (2011). PACAP, an autocrine/paracrine regulator of gonadotrophs. *Biol. Reprod.* 84, 844–850.

Xue, C., Hsueh, Y. P., and Heitman, J. (2008). Magnificent seven: roles of G protein-coupled receptors in extracellular sensing in fungi. *FEMS Microbiol. Rev.* 32, 1010–1032.

Yano, M., Hayakawa-Yano, Y., Mele, A., and Darnell, R. B. (2010). Nova2 regulates neuronal migration through an RNA switch in disabled-1 signaling. *Neuron* 66, 848–858.

Yeo, G. W., Xu, X., Liang, T. Y., Muotri, A. R., Carson, C. T., Coufal, N. G., et al. (2007). Alternative splicing events identified in human embryonic stem cells and neural progenitors. *PLoS Comput. Biol.* 3:e196. doi:10.1371/journal.pcbi.0030196

Zhang, C., Zhang, Z., Castle, J., Sun, S., Johnson, J., Krainer, A. R., et al. (2008). Defining the regulatory network of the tissue-specific splicing factors Fox-1 and Fox-2. *Genes Dev.* 22, 2550–2563.

Zhang, X., and Eggert, U. S. (2013). Non-traditional roles of G protein-coupled receptors in basic cell biology. *Mol. Biosyst.* 9, 586–595.

Zheng, S., Gray, E. E., Chawla, G., Porse, B. T., O'Dell, T. J., and Black, D. L. (2012). PSD-95 is post-transcriptionally repressed during early neural development by PTBP1 and PTBP2. *Nat. Neurosci.* 15, 381–388.

Zmijewski, M. A., and Slominski, A. T. (2009). CRF1 receptor splicing in epidermal keratinocytes: potential biological role and environmental regulations. *J. Cell. Physiol.* 218, 593–602.

Zmijewski, M. A., and Slominski, A. T. (2010). Emerging role of alternative splicing of CRF1 receptor in CRF signaling. *Acta Biochim. Pol.* 57, 1–13.

5

Role of PACAP in female fertility and reproduction at gonadal level

Dora Reglodi[1]*, Andrea Tamas[1], Miklos Koppan[2], Donat Szogyi[2] and Laura Welke[3]

[1] Department of Anatomy, Lendulet PACAP-Research Team of the University of Pécs and Hungarian Academy of Sciences, Pécs, Hungary
[2] Department of Obstetrics and Gynaecology, University of Pécs, Pécs, Hungary
[3] Department of Anatomy, Ross University School of Medicine, Roseau, Commonwealth of Dominica

Edited by:
Hubert Vaudry, University of Rouen, France

Reviewed by:
Rita Canipari, University of Rome – La Sapienza, Italy
Khampoun Sayasith, University of Montreal, Canada

***Correspondence:**
Dora Reglodi, Department of Anatomy, University of Pécs, Szigeti u 12, 7624 Pécs, Hungary.
e-mail: dora.reglodi@aok.pte.hu

Pituitary adenylate cyclase activating polypeptide (PACAP) is a pleiotropic neuropeptide, first isolated from hypothalamic extracts, but later shown in peripheral organs, such as endocrine glands, gastrointestinal system, cardiovascular system, and reproductive organs. PACAP plays a role in fertility and reproduction. Numerous studies report on the gonadal regulatory effects of PACAP at hypothalamo-hypophyseal levels. However, the local effects of PACAP at gonadal levels are also important. The present review summarizes the effects of PACAP in the ovary. PACAP and its receptors are present in the ovary, and PACAP plays a role in germ cell migration, meiotic division, follicular development, and atresia. The autocrine-paracrine hormonal effects seem to play a regulatory role in ovulation, luteinization, and follicular atrophy. Altogether, PACAP belongs to the ovarian regulatory peptides.

Keywords: PACAP, ovary, oocyte, ovulation, luteinization

INTRODUCTION

Pituitary adenylate cyclase activating polypeptide (PACAP) was originally isolated from the hypothalamus, and named after its cAMP increasing effect in pituitary cells (Miyata et al., 1989; Arimura, 2007). PACAP belongs to the vasoactive intestinal peptide (VIP)/secretin/glucagon peptide family. It occurs in two amino acid forms: PACAP38 and PACAP27, the longer form is the predominant peptide in mammals. The receptors of PACAP are the VPAC1 and VPAC2 receptors, which bind VIP and PACAP with equal affinity and the specific PAC1 receptor, which binds PACAP selectively (Miyata et al., 1989; Sherwood et al., 2000; Arimura, 2007; Vaudry et al., 2009; Brubel et al., 2010). After the discovery of PACAP, numerous studies described the regulatory effects of PACAP at hypothalamo-pituitary levels, affecting the synthesis and release of several releasing and pituitary hormones. However, soon after its discovery, it was found that PACAP is, and its receptors are, expressed in the peripheral organs, and high levels of the peptide were found in the gonads (Arimura et al., 1991). This immediately drew attention to the peptide playing a central role in fertility and reproduction, not only at central hormonal, but also at local levels.

The last two decades in PACAP research have revealed that PACAP influences fertility and reproduction at several levels. The present mini-review aims to summarize findings on the effects of PACAP in the ovary and how PACAP influences female gonadal functions at the ovarian level.

PACAP IN MAMMALIAN FOLLICULAR DEVELOPMENT

Primordial germ cells (oogonia) migrate from the wall of the yolk sac to the ovaries during early mammalian development. Ovarian germ cells then undergo mitosis and develop further into primary oocytes. Developing oocytes are surrounded by epithelial cells, which build the ovarian follicles. At first, follicular epithelial cells are flattened and surround the primary oocytes entering the first meiotic division. They subsequently are arrested during fetal development until the female reaches sexual maturity. The first meiotic division is only completed during the follicular development before ovulation in each cycle, and the second meiotic division is completed only at the time of fertilization, resulting in the haploid gamete (Sadler, 2012).

A cohort of primordial follicles is activated at the beginning of the maturation process in cyclic manner. Follicular maturation involves changes in the oocyte, the follicular epithelial cells, and the surrounding ovarian stroma. Although significant inter-species differences exist in the follicular growth and its regulation, the major steps show basic similarities in mammalian species, and in most mammals, the vast majority of follicles undergo apoptosis similarly to humans (Matsuda et al., 2012). Therefore, we will focus on mammalian findings and only briefly mention other species. Early follicular development is independent from gonadotropins, but later follicular growth, ovulation, and luteinization are primarily regulated by the pituitary gonadotropins follicle-stimulating hormone (FSH) and luteinizing hormone (LH). However, their actions are also dependent on other peptidergic and non-peptidergic signaling pathways (Mayerhofer et al., 1997; Bodis et al., 2001; Matsuda et al., 2012). Accumulating evidence shows that PACAP is one of the regulatory peptides in the ovary.

ACTIONS OF PACAP ON PRIMORDIAL GERM CELLS

There is evidence for the involvement of PACAP in the proliferation of primordial germ cells (Pesce et al., 1996). The authors showed PACAP immunoreactivity in gonadal ridges, mostly on the germ cell surface. Primordial germ cells intensively proliferate during their migration to the gonadal ridges and PACAP was found to stimulate this proliferation process. The peptide binds to the germ cells and also to gonadal somatic cells (Pesce et al., 1996). These observations show that PACAP plays an important role in reproductive functions from the earliest stage of differentiation and development.

PACAP IN THE OVARY

In rat ovarian cells, PACAP positive cells were found in the preovulatory and ovulatory periods (Gras et al., 1996), with PACAP and PACAP mRNA positivity in granulosa and cumulus cells. Positivity was also found in stroma cells and theca cells and even nerve fibers innervating the ovary showed immunopositivity. These observations suggest that PACAP is involved in a number of processes regulated via hormonal as well as neuronal activity during follicular development in the ovary (Gras et al., 1996). Another group published on the existence of PACAP in the rat ovary the same year (Scaldaferri et al., 1996).

Pituitary adenylate cyclase activating polypeptide expression in the corpus luteum of the rat was subsequently shown by Kotani et al. (1997, 1998). Park et al. (2001) showed that PACAP mRNA was only expressed in the granulosa but not theca cells. This expression has a stage-specific regulation by GnRH in rat granulosa cells. While treatment of preovulatory granulosa cells with GnRH agonist stimulates PACAP mRNA expression, GnRH agonist treatment alone has no effect but reduces the FSH-induced PACAP mRNA levels. GnRH antagonist on the other hand had opposite effects: it inhibited induced PACAP gene expression in preovulatory cells while stimulating expression in immature granulosa cells. These results show that GnRH plays an important role in the regulation of ovarian PACAP expression and that PACAP expression is differentially regulated during the ovarian cycle (Park et al., 2001). The LH and FSH control of the PACAP expression was also confirmed by Lee et al. (1999). The involvement of progesterone receptors have also been shown in LH-induced PACAP gene expression (Ko et al., 1999). In addition, the gonadotropin-dependent regulation of PACAP mRNA has been confirmed in bovine preovulatory follicles (Sayasith et al., 2007). PACAP was found to be expressed in granulosa cells and its expression was found to be dependent on protein kinase A. A recent study has shown that PACAP mRNA expression gradually increases in pregnancy in the corpus luteum, suggesting its involvement in the maintenance of mid-term and late pregnancy (Zhao et al., 2010).

Transient expression of PACAP has also been observed in the mouse ovary within granulosa cells of preovulatory follicles after hCG treatment (Barberi et al., 2007). The contemporary induction of PACAP in preovulatory follicles suggests an important role for PACAP around the time of ovulation (Barberi et al., 2007). In human granulosa cells, it has been found that FSH and LH promote PACAP expression (Morelli et al., 2008). PACAP is synthesized as a preprohormone and is processed by prohormone convertases. It has been shown that in both testis and ovary, prohormone convertase 4 is the enzyme responsible for PACAP processing, supported by the finding that prohormone convertase 4 deficient mice expressed no PACAP in their ovaries (Li et al., 2000).

EXPRESSION OF PACAP RECEPTORS IN THE OVARY

Earlier studies examining binding sites for PACAP have already identified specific binding sites in the ovary (Gottschall et al., 1990). Scaldaferri et al. (1996) identified isoforms of the PAC receptor in the rat ovary. Later, PAC1 receptors were shown in th rat corpus luteum (Kotani et al., 1997, 1998). Park et al. (2000 have demonstrated stage-specific expression of PACAP receptor in the rat ovary. Northern blot analysis shows that the ovarian tran script of the PAC1 receptor appears at day three in the rat ovary followed by a gradual increase later in development. There is marked increase at puberty, at the age of 21 days, when compare to an age of 15 days, when only non-growing small follicles ar present. *In situ* hybridization has revealed that PACAP recepto mRNA is present mainly in the granulosa cells of the large pre antral follicles, while atretic follicles and mural granulosa cells ar devoid of the receptor. The authors have also demonstrated tha the dominant splice variant of the PAC1 receptor was the shor variant in the ovary (Park et al., 2000). Gonadotropin stimula tion has been shown to induce PACAP receptor mRNA expressio in the granulosa cells of the preovulatory follicles (Ko and Park Sarge, 2000; Park et al., 2000). Pregnant mare serum gonadotropi (PMSG), on the other hand, causes reduction of PACAP recepto gene expression. PMSG induces multiple follicular growth to th preovulatory stage. These observations suggest an involvement o PACAP in the follicular growth, and in ovulation, in a stage- an time-dependent manner. The observation that PACAP recepto expression is restricted to granulosa cells of the growing follicle at the time of puberty and to granulosa cells of preovulatory fol licles after gonadotropin treatment indicates that PACAP may ac in a limited time-window in the ovary. Progesterone receptor have been shown to be involved in the induced PAC1 recepto expression (Ko and Park-Sarge, 2000).

A more detailed analysis of the rat ovarian PACAP recepto expression has confirmed the expression of PAC1 receptors in th granulosa cells and, furthermore, the presence of VPAC2 receptor in these cells (Vaccari et al., 2006). Theca cells do not express PAC receptors, only VPAC1 and 2 receptors. Fully developed oocyte only express the PAC1 receptor. hCG stimulation has been found to induce PAC1 receptor expression in granulosa and VPAC2 recepto expression in theca cells. The VPAC receptor expression has bee found to have a lower expression level than the PAC1 receptor. Thi study has also confirmed the previous findings of Park et al. (2000 describing receptor expression at 3 days after birth with a marke increase before puberty. In addition, they found that VPAC1 recep tors decreased with age and VPAC2 receptors remained constant Immunohistochemical analysis revealed the presence of VPAC receptors in association with stromal blood vessels in the vicinity of the follicles, especially at the entrance site of the ovarian arter ies into the medulla. The expression of the VPAC2 receptors wa more ubiquitous in the ovary. Denuded oocytes express only th PAC1 receptor, which could not be detected in Met-I and II phase in oocytes matured *in vivo*. Gras et al. (2000) also described PAC and VPAC2 receptors in preovulatory follicles. All three types o the PACAP receptors have been identified in human granulos cells, although the main receptor types in these cells seem to be th VPAC receptors (Morelli et al., 2008).

All three receptors have also been identified in the mous (Barberi et al., 2007). PAC1 receptors could be stimulated by hCG VPAC2 only mildly stimulated, and VPAC1 downregulated. Th authors suggested that the contemporary induction of PACAI and PAC1 receptors by hCG in granulosa cells of preovulatory follicles indicates an important role for PACAP around the time of ovulation (Barberi et al., 2007).

ACTIONS OF PACAP IN THE OVARY

Follicular development, hormone production, and ovulation

In all mammalian species, the early stages of folliculogenesis, including the initiation of primordial follicle growth, are independent from gonadotropins (Latini et al., 2010). Fine balances between inhibitory and stimulatory signals regulate follicular recruitment. PACAP has been shown to inhibit primordial to primary follicle transition (Latini et al., 2010); PACAP did not influence granulosa cell viability at these stages but inhibited proliferation. PACAP also inhibited the growth of preantral follicles. These observations indicate an important role of PACAP in follicular recruitment (Latini et al., 2010). On the other hand, at later stages, PACAP can prime immature follicles (Gras et al., 2005). A 12-h PACAP priming stimulates FSH-induced estradiol production, which is an important step in cyclic recruitment, when a cohort of antral follicles escapes apoptosis and reaches the preovulatory stage (Gras et al., 2005). These results show a fine balance between factors, including PACAP, that play a role in follicular recruitment. Other studies have also shown that PACAP plays an important role in preantral follicular growth and differentiation (Cecconi et al., 2004). In the mouse ovary, PACAP or VIP alone did not affect follicular growth, but they both inhibited it when added to FSH-stimulated follicles. Both peptides caused a dose-dependent inhibition of follicle growth, antrum formation, granulosa cell proliferation, and estradiol production (Cecconi et al., 2004).

Studies on the endocrine effects of PACAP revealed that PACAP can stimulate cAMP accumulation and steroidogenesis in the rat ovary (Zhong and Kasson, 1994; Heindel et al., 1996; Vaccari et al., 2006). Granulosa cell cultures responded to PACAP treatment with increased production of estrogen, progesterone, and 20alpha-dihydroprogesterone. This effect was dose-dependent and more potent than similar effects of VIP and GHRH (Zhong and Kasson, 1994). The peptide was also able to augment FSH-induced progesterone and 20alpha-dihydroprogesterone accumulation, and in high doses that of estrogen. The PACAP-stimulated progesterone accumulation was minimal in the absence of androstendion and dramatically augmented in the presence of the androgen. This shows that androgens are required for the PACAP to stimulate steroid production and indicate that PACAP might play a role in modulating the production of steroids in the ovary (Zhong and Kasson, 1994). The effects of PACAP depend on the presence of LH. In cultured luteal cells of the rat, PACAP alone stimulates progesterone, 20alpha hydroxyl-4-pregnene-3-one along with cAMP accumulation (Usuki and Kotani, 2001, 2002). However, when LH is present, PACAP in high concentrations inhibits the LH-induced cAMP accumulation and progesterone production, while it enhances the LH-induced stimulation of 20alpha hydroxyl-4-pregnene-3-one production (Kotani et al., 1998). This decreases the ratio of progesterone to 20alpha hydroxyl-4-pregnene-3-one in LH-stimulated cells, which suggests an involvement in luteolysis. This is supported by the finding that PACAP suppresses increases in LH receptors in luteal cells (Usuki and Kotani, 2001). Gras et al. (2000) showed that PACAP can stimulate progesterone production and cAMP synthesis, and the involvement of the PKA pathway. These data together provide evidence for the involvement of PACAP as an autocrine-paracrine regulator of ovarian hormone production, especially in preovulatory follicles (Gras et al., 2000).

Interestingly, one intracerebroventricular PACAP treatment was shown to inhibit ovulation in adult animals (Koves et al., 1998). Injecting PACAP before the critical period of the proestrous stage, blocks the ovulation and prevents the proestrous LH surge (Koves et al., 1996). Furthermore, neonatal administration of PACAP delays onset of puberty in female animals (Szabo et al., 2002).

The effects of PACAP on ovarian steroidogenesis have been confirmed in human studies as well (Apa et al., 1997), where PACAP was found to stimulate progesterone synthesis without synergistic effects with hCG. This was tested in corpora lutea obtained from non-pregnant women undergoing hysterectomy.

PLC was activated by PACAP in granulosa but not theca cells (Vaccari et al., 2006). Plasminogen activators are known to be involved also in ovulation. PACAP has been shown to increase the tissue-type plasminogen activator and to decrease the urokinase-type one (Apa et al., 2002). VIP did not show this effect in granulosa cells, but when entire follicles were exposed to the peptides, both VIP and PACAP exerted similar stimulatory effects on tissue-type plasminogen activator levels, supporting the observations of different PACAP/VIP receptors being expressed in different ovarian compartments (Apa et al., 2002).

Apoptosis

In addition to gonadotropins, factors secreted from granulosa cells, including steroids, growth factors, and cytokines, are essential for granulosa cell survival and follicular growth (Matsuda et al., 2012). Granulosa cells are the initial population to undergo apoptosis in atretic follicles, indicating their role in the initiation of follicular atresia (Matsuda et al., 2012). Besides estradiol, as the main ovarian steroid influencing follicular apoptosis, several other factors play an important role. Among those, insulin-like growth factor, epidermal growth factor, fibroblast-like growth factor, and interleukin-1 beta have prosurvival effects, while the Fas ligand system and the tumor necrosis alpha are proapoptotic. Pro- and antiapoptotic members of the mitochondrial Bcl family have also been described to play an important role (Matsuda et al., 2012). A few papers suggest that PACAP is also one of the factors influencing granulosa cell death and survival.

One of the main effects of PACAP is its cell survival-promoting effects, which was first described in neuronal cells, and thus, PACAP was designated as an important neuroprotective peptide (Vaudry et al., 2002; Somogyvari-Vigh and Reglodi, 2004). However, numerous studies have revealed that the antiapoptotic effects of PACAP are not restricted to neuronal cells, but can be shown in several other cell types, such as lymphocytes (Delgado and Ganea, 2000), prostate cancer cells (Gutierrez-Canas et al., 2003), endothelial cells (Racz et al., 2007), retinal pigment epithelial cells (Fabian et al., 2012), and even in the invertebrate mollusks (Pirger et al., 2008). Therefore, PACAP can be considered as a general cytoprotective peptide. VIP, structurally the closest peptide to PACAP has been described to have antiapoptotic effects in the ovary (Flaws et al., 1995).

Based on these data, it is expected that PACAP can also exert antiapoptotic effects in ovarian cells. Indeed, several studies have shown this in granulosa cells. In isolated granulosa cells, apoptosis can be induced by serum-free culturing. In accordance with the generally known antiapoptotic role of PACAP, the peptide could reduce the granulosa cell apoptosis in a dose-dependent manner, an effect that could be blocked by the PACAP antagonist PACAP6-38 (Vaccari et al., 2006). These results are in accordance with earlier observations showing that PACAP could block the apoptotic cascade in granulosa cells (Lee et al., 1999) and that the LH suppression of follicle apoptosis was partially blocked by PACAP 6-38. The antiapoptotic effect of PACAP was also confirmed in human granulosa-luteal cells (Morelli et al., 2008). Both PACAP and VIP could reverse the decrease in procaspase-3 induced by the serum withdrawal. However, it was found that spontaneous apoptosis was not influenced by PACAP in another study (Gras et al., 2005).

Expression of PACAP in both benign and malignant ovarian tumors has been shown (Odum and Fahrenkrug, 1998). Higher levels were found in cancers than benign tumors. The authors suggest a trophic function of PACAP in ovarian cells (Odum and Fahrenkrug, 1998). Interestingly, PACAP does not influence the cisplatin-induced toxicity in proliferating ovary cells of the CHO ovarian cell line (Aubert et al., 2008). The same treatment, however, does prevent toxicity and related apoptosis in cerebellar granule cells. This dissociation in the antiapoptotic behavior of PACAP could be of high clinical importance: PACAP can decrease the cisplatin-induced neurotoxic side effects while leaving the antitumor therapeutic effect intact (Aubert et al., 2008).

Effects in oocytes

Fully developed oocytes express PAC1 receptor and the addition of nanomolar concentrations of PACAP induces calcium release. However, this answer could not be observed in Met-I and II phase oocytes, supporting that finding that receptors are expressed stage-specifically (Vaccari et al., 2006).

In *Xenopus* oocytes, PACAP has been described to modulate membrane potential by eliciting hyperpolarization-activated chloride current, thereby affecting oocyte physiology (Kato et al., 1997).

Very interesting results have been described by Apa et al. (1997) supporting both a direct and indirect effect of PACAP on oocyte maturation. Mammalian oocytes are known to arrest in the first meiotic division, which is resumed at the time of the preovulatory LH surge. The inhibition of oocyte maturation and its relief is mediated by gonadotropins in conjunct with several other factors, while only a few are known to act directly on oocytes. The authors described that PACAP accelerated meiotic maturation in follicle- and cumulus-enclosed oocytes while inhibiting meiotic maturation in denuded oocytes (Apa et al., 1997). This result was not due to a direct cytotoxic effect because the inhibition on oocyte maturation was reversible when PACAP was removed from the medium. This difference in PACAP action on enclosed and denuded oocytes support the stage-dependent regulatory effects of PACAP. Other studies have also confirmed the effect of PACAP on the meiotic processes. In the mouse ovary, Cecconi et al. (2004) found that PACAP severely impaired meiotic maturation in oocytes isolated from the follicles.

Recently, mass spectrometric and radioimmunoassay analysis have shown that PACAP is present in human follicular fluid obtained from patients undergoing hyperstimulation treatment (Brubel et al., 2011; Koppan et al., 2012). PACAP could be identified in all human samples examined. Correlation was found between retrieved oocytes and PACAP levels in the follicular fluid drawing the attention to PACAP as an important factor in the medium of the developing oocyte and its possible future use as a biomarker in women with fertility problems (Koppan et al., 2012).

EVOLUTIONARY PERSPECTIVES

Recent reports point to the important roles of PACAP in fish reproduction, pointing to the fact that the effects of PACAP on the hypothalamo-pituitary axis, as well as in the gonads, are conserved and biologically ancient functions (Levy and Degani, 2011, 2012). In fish, stage-specific expression of PACAP has also been revealed. For example, higher PACAP expression can be found in female blue gourami, with oocytes in the final maturation stage than in vitellogenic individuals. Also, higher expression was found in mature males that are not reproductively active than in nest builders and juveniles (Levy and Degani, 2012). PACAP is thus differentially expressed in females and males. PACAP acts in close association with GnRH in fish reproduction and the expression and actions of PACAP also depend on environmental factors, such as temperature (Levy et al., 2011; Levy and Degani, 2012). It has been proposed that PACAP is involved in the final oocyte maturation in females and in males it is mainly associated with sexual behavior (Levy et al., 2010). In the zebrafish, a new type of PACAP has been described in the ovary and its role as an ovarian factor mediating gonadotropin action have been suggested (Wang et al., 2003).

ROLE OF ENDOGENOUS PACAP

Given the important functions of PACAP in reproduction outlined above, it would be expected that the lack of endogenous PACAP have major effects on fertility and reproduction. Indeed, PACAP deficient mice have been shown to have lower reproductive rates in several studies (Shintani et al., 2002; Sherwood et al., 2007; Isaac and Sherwood, 2008). To study the exact mechanism, a few studies examined the possible background for this lower reproductive rate. Interestingly, Isaac and Sherwood (2008) found that these mice had normal puberty onset, estrous cycle, and seminal plugs when paired with males. However, the birth rate after mating was only 20% when compared to the 100% in wild type mice. The authors found no defect in ovulation, ovarian histology, or fertilization, but they found major defects in implantation and associated hormone levels (Isaac and Sherwood, 2008). Similarly, low birth rates were found by Shintani et al. (2002), but they also found reduced mating and maternal behaviors. It is possible that in the ovary, compensatory mechanisms counteract the lack of PACAP and thus, no major alterations can be detected under normal circumstances. However, more studies are necessary to elucidate the exact role of endogenous PACAP in the ovary. Furthermore, in several other organs, including intestine, kidney, retina, and central nervous system, PACAP deficient mice do not exhibit major alterations unchallenged conditions (Reglodi et al., 2012). However, in case of stressors or under pathological conditions, PACAP deficient mice react with increased vulnerability and the observed deficits have been shown to be more severe in mice lacking endogenous PACAP (Reglodi et al., 2012). Based on these observations, it is possible that endogenous PACAP has ovarian functions not compensated under challenged or pathological conditions. Further studies are required to shed light on this possibility.

CONCLUDING REMARKS

The present review summarized findings on the presence and effects of PACAP in the ovary. It has to be emphasized that this is only one role in the plethora of actions that PACAP plays in fertility and reproduction and that the detailed discussion of these is beyond the scope of the present review. Briefly, PACAP, at the hypothalamic level, influences receptive behavior in female rodents, in association with GnRH and steroids (Apostolakis et al., 2004, 2005), and plays an important modulatory role in pituitary hormone production. The role of PACAP in the hypothalamo-pituitary-gonadal axis has been reviewed several times previously (Rawlings and Hezareh, 1996; Nussdorfer and Malendowicz, 1998; Sherwood et al., 2000; Koves et al., 2003; Vaudry et al., 2006; Counis et al., 2007).

Pituitary adenylate cyclase activating polypeptide also plays a role in the muscle contraction of the vaginal wall as well as that of the uterus and uterine tube (Steenstrup et al., 1995; Ziessen et al., 2002), and even decreased immunoreactivity has been shown in premenopausal and postmenopausal women in the vaginal wall (Hong et al., 2008). The PACAPergic innervation of the female genital tract has also been shown and has been associated with nerves originating from the paracervical ganglia (Fahrenkrug and Hannibal, 1996; Fahrenkrug et al., 1996).

Effects of PACAP have also been shown in the placenta where PACAP and its receptors are present (Scaldaferri et al., 2000; Koh et al., 2005; Brubel et al., 2010), where the peptide influences blood flow in the utero-placental unit (Steenstrup et al., 1996) and influences survival of trophoblast cells (Boronkai et al., 2009). The serum level of PACAP increases in the third trimester of pregnancy in healthy pregnant women and it markedly decreases during delivery, reaching prebirth levels 3 days after delivery (Reglodi et al., 2010). High concentrations of PACAP have been shown in human and animal milk (Borzsei et al., 2009; Csanaky et al., 2012), which suggests that the peptide is also an important nutritional source for the newborn. However, its exact function in breastfeeding has not been identified yet.

In summary, PACAP is one of the peptides regulating germ cell development in the ovary and it has several other regulatory functions in reproduction. PACAP influences ovarian hormone production, affects meiosis, and is an important local regulator of follicular development. The exact physiological role and its possible clinical importance still awaits further investigation, but the current evidence points to a possible clinical diagnostic or therapeutic use of the peptide in both human and veterinary fertility.

ACKNOWLEDGMENTS

This work was supported by Hungarian National Scientific Grants OTKA104984, CNK 78480, SROP 4.1.2.B-10/2/KONV-20/0-0002, SROP-4.2.2/B-10/1-2010-0029, Bolyai Scholarship, MTA Lendulet Program, TAMOP-4.2.2.A-11/1/KONV-2012-0024, 4.2.2A-11/1konv-2012-0053, Akira Arimura Foundation, Ross University School of Medicine Research Fund, PTE AOK Research Fund AOK KA/34039-81-8000.

REFERENCES

Apa, R., Lanzone, A., Mastrandrea, M., Miceli, F., de Feo, D., Caruso, A., et al. (1997). Control of human luteal steroidogenesis: role of growth hormone-releasing hormone, vasoactive intestinal peptide, and pituitary adenylate cyclase-activating peptide. *Fertil. Steril.* 68, 1097–1102.

Apa, R., Lanzone, A., Miceli, F., Vaccari, S., Macchione, E., Stefanini, M., et al. (2002). Pituitary adenylate cyclase-activating polypeptide modulates plasminogen activator expression in rat granulosa cell. *Biol. Reprod.* 66, 830–835.

Apostolakis, E. M., Lanz, R., and O'Malley, B. W. (2004). Pituitary adenylate cyclase-activating peptide: a pivotal modulator of steroid-induced reproductive behavior in female rodents. *Mol. Endocrinol.* 18, 173–183.

Apostolakis, E. M., Riherd, D. N., and O'Malley, B. W. (2005). PAC1 receptors mediate pituitary adenylate cyclase-activating polypeptide- and progesterone-facilitated receptivity in female rats. *Mol. Endocrinol.* 19, 2798–2811.

Arimura, A. (2007). PACAP: the road to discovery. *Peptides* 28, 1617–1619.

Arimura, A., Somogyvari-Vigh, A., Miyata, A., Mizuno, K., Coy, D. H., and Kitada, C. (1991). Tissue distribution of PACAP as determined by RIA: highly abundant in the rat brain and testes. *Endocrinology* 129, 2787–2789.

Aubert, N., Vaudry, D., Falluel-Morel, A., Desfeux, A., Fisch, C., Ancian, P., et al. (2008). PACAP prevents toxicity induced by cisplatin in rat and primate neurons but not in proliferating ovary cells: involvement of the mitochondrial apoptotic pathway. *Neurobiol. Dis.* 32, 66–80.

Barberi, M., Muciaccia, B., Morelli, M. B., Stefanini, M., Cecconi, S., and Canipari, R. (2007). Expression localisation and functional activity of pituitary adenylate cyclase-activating polypeptide, vasoactive intestinal polypeptide and their receptors in mouse ovary. *Reproduction* 134, 281–292.

Bodis, J., Koppan, M., Kornya, L., Tinneberg, H. R., and Torok, A. (2001). Influence of melatonin on basal and gonadotropin-stimulated progesterone and estradiol secretion of cultured human granulosa cells and in the superfused granulosa cell system. *Gynecol. Obstet. Invest.* 52, 198–202.

Boronkai, A., Brubel, R., Racz, B., Tamas, A., Kiss, P., Horvath, G., et al. (2009). Effects of pituitary adenylate cyclase activating polypeptide (PACAP) on the survival and signal transduction pathways in human choriocarcinoma cells. *Ann. N. Y. Acad. Sci.* 1163, 353–357.

Borzsei, R., Mark, L., Tamas, A., Bagoly, T., Bay, C., Csanaky, K., et al. (2009). Presence of pituitary adenylate cyclase activating polypeptide-38 in human plasma and milk. *Eur. J. Endocrinol.* 160, 561–565.

Brubel, R., Boronkai, A., Reglodi, D., Racz, B., Nemeth, J., Kiss, P., et al. (2010). Changes in the expression of pituitary adenylate cyclase-activating polypeptide in the human placenta during pregnancy and its effects on the survival of JAR choriocarcinoma cells. *J. Mol. Neurosci.* 42, 450–458.

Brubel, R., Reglodi, D., Jambor, E., Koppan, M., Varnagy, A., Biro, Z., et al. (2011). Investigation of pituitary adenylate cyclase activating polypeptide in human gynecological and other biological fluids by using MALDI TOF mass spectrometry. *J. Mass Spectrom.* 46, 189–194.

Cecconi, S., Rossi, G., Barberi, M., Scaldaferri, L., and Canipari, R. (2004). Effect of pituitary adenylate cyclase-activating polypeptide and vasoactive intestinal polypeptide on mouse preantral follicle development in vitro. *Endocrinology* 145, 2071–2079.

Counis, R., Laverriere, J. N., Garrel-Lazayres, G., Cohen-Tannoudji, J., Lariviere, S., Bleux, C., et al. (2007). What is the role of PACAP in gonadotrope function? *Peptides* 28, 1797–1804.

Csanaky, K., Banki, E., Szabadfi, K., Reglodi, D., Tarcai, I., Czegledi, L., et al. (2012). Changes in PACAP immunoreactivity in human milk and presence of PAC1 receptor in mammary gland during lactation. *J. Mol. Neurosci.* 48, 631–637.

Delgado, M., and Ganea, D. (2000). Vasoactive intestinal peptide and pituitary adenylate cyclase activating polypeptide inhibit antigen-induced apoptosis of mature T lymphocytes by inhibiting Fas ligand expression. *J. Immunol.* 164, 1200–1210.

Fabian, E., Reglodi, D., Mester, L., Szabo, A., Szabadfi, K., Tamas, A., et al. (2012). Effects of PACAP on intracellular signaling pathways in human retinal pigment epithelial cells exposed to oxidative stress. *J. Mol. Neurosci.* 48, 493–500.

Fahrenkrug, J., and Hannibal, J. (1996). Pituitary adenylate cyclase activating polypeptide innervation of the rat female reproductive tract and the associated paracervical ganglia: effect of capsaicin. *Neuroscience* 73, 1049–1060.

Fahrenkrug, J., Steenstrup, B. R., Hannibal, J., Alm, P., and Ottesen, B. (1996). Role of PACAP in the female reproductive organs. *Ann. N. Y. Acad. Sci.* 805, 394–407.

Flaws, J. A., DeSanti, A., Tilly, K. I., Kugu, K., Johnson, A. L., Hirschfield, A. N., et al. (1995). Vasoactive intestinal peptide-mediated suppression of apoptosis in the ovary: potential mechanisms of action and evidence of a conserved antiatretogenic role through evolution. *Endocrinology* 136, 4351–4359.

Gottschall, P. E., Tatsuno, I., Miyata, A., and Arimura, A. (1990). Characterization and distribution of binding sites for the hypothalamic peptide, pituitary adenylate cyclase-activating polypeptide. *Endocrinology* 127, 272–277.

Gras, S., Hannibal, J., Georg, B., and Fahrenkrug, J. (1996). Transient periovulatory expression of pituitary adenylate cyclase activating peptide in rat ovarian cells. *Endocrinology* 137, 4779–4785.

Gras, S., Hedetoft, C., Pedersen, S. H., and Fahrenkrug, J. (2000). Pituitary adenylate cyclase-activating peptide stimulates acute progesterone production in rat granulosa/lutein cells via two receptor subtypes. *Biol. Reprod.* 63, 206–212.

Gras, S., Host, E., and Fahrenkrug, J. (2005). Role of pituitary adenylate cyclase-activating peptide (PACAP) in the cyclic recruitment of immature follicles in the rat ovary. *Regul. Pept.* 128, 69–74.

Gutierrez-Canas, I., Rodriguez-Henche, N., Bolanos, O., Carmena, M. J., Prieto, J. C., and Juarranz, M. G. (2003). VIP and PACAP are autocrine factors that protect the androgen-independent prostate cancer cell line PC-3 from apoptosis induced by serum withdrawal. *Br. J. Pharmacol.* 139, 1050–1058.

Heindel, J. J., Sneeden, J., Powell, A. J., Davis, B., and Culler, M. D. (1996). A novel hypothalamic peptide, pituitary adenylate cyclase activating peptide, regulates the function of rat granulose cells in vitro. *Biol. Reprod.* 54, 523–530.

Hong, X., Huang, L., and Song, Y. (2008). Role of vasoactive intestinal peptide and pituitary adenylate cyclase activating polypeptide in the vaginal wall of women with stress urinary incontinence and pelvic organ prolapse. *Int. Urogynecol. J. Pelvic Floor Dysfunct.* 19, 1151–1157.

Isaac, E. R., and Sherwood, N. M. (2008). Pituitary adenylate cyclase-activating polypeptide (PACAP) is important for embryo implantation in mice. *Mol. Cell. Endocrinol.* 280, 13–19.

Kato, M., Hanaoka, Y., Tatemoto, K., and Kimura, C. (1997). Hyperpolarization-activated Cl- current elicited by pituitary adenylate cyclase activating polypeptide in Xenopus oocytes. *Regul. Pept.* 70, 167–172.

Ko, C., In, Y. H., and Park-Sarge, O. K. (1999). Role of progesterone receptor activation in pituitary adenylate cyclase activating polypeptide gene expression in rat ovary. *Endocrinology* 140, 5185–5194.

Ko, C., and Park-Sarge, O. K. (2000). Progesterone receptor activation mediates LH-induced type-I pituitary adenylate cyclase activating polypeptide receptor (PAC1) gene expression in rat granulose cells. *Biochem. Biophys. Res. Commun.* 277, 270–279.

Koh, P. O., Won, C. K., Noh, H. S., Cho, G. J., and Choi, W. S. (2005). Expression of pituitary adenylate cyclase activating polypeptide and its type I receptor mRNAs in human placenta. *J. Vet. Sci.* 6, 1–5.

Koppan, M., Varnagy, A., Reglodi, D., Brubel, R., Nemeth, J., Tamas, A., et al. (2012). Correlation between oocyte number and follicular fluid concentration of pituitary adenylate cyclase-activating polypeptide (PACAP) in women after superovulation treatment. *J. Mol. Neurosci.* 48, 617–622.

Kotani, E., Usuki, S., and Kubo, T. (1997). Rat corpus luteum expresses both PACAP and PACAP type IA receptor mRNAs. *Peptides* 18, 1453–1455.

Kotani, E., Usuki, S., and Kubo, T. (1998). Effect of pituitary adenylate cyclase-activating polypeptide (PACAP) on progestin biosynthesis in cultured granulosa cells from rat ovary and expression of mRNA encoding PACAP type I receptor. *J. Reprod. Fertil.* 112, 107–114.

Koves, K., Kantor, O., Molnar, J., Heinzlmann, A., Szabo, E., Szabo, F., et al. (2003). The role of PACAP in gonadotropic hormone secretion at hypothalamic and pituitary levels. *J. Mol. Neurosci.* 20, 141–152.

Koves, K., Molnar, J., Kantor, O., Lakatos, A., Fogel, K., Kausz, M., et al. (1998). Role of PACAP in the regulation of gonadotroph hormone secretion during ontogenesis: a single neonatal injection of PACAP delays puberty and its intracerebroventricular administration before the critical period of proestrous stage blocks ovulation in adulthood. *Ann. N. Y. Acad. Sci.* 865, 590–594.

Koves, K., Molnar, J., Kantor, O., Lakatos, A., Gorcs, T. J., Somogyvari-Vigh, A., et al. (1996). PACAP participates in the regulation of the hormonal events preceeding the ovulation. *Acta Biol. Hung.* 47, 239–249.

Latini, S., Chiarpotto, M., Muciaccia, B., Vaccari, S., Barberi, M., Guglielmo, M. C., et al. (2010). Inhibitory effect of pituitary adenylate cyclase activating polypeptide on the initial stages of rat follicle development. *Mol. Cell. Endocrinol.* 320, 34–44.

Lee, J., Park, H. J., Choi, H. S., Kwon, H. B., Arimura, A., Lee, B. J., et al. (1999). Gonadotropin stimulation of pituitary adenylate cyclase activating polypeptide (PACAP) messenger ribonucleic acid in the rat ovary and the role of PACAP as a follicle survival factor. *Endocrinology* 140, 818–826.

Levy, G., David, D., and Degani, G. (2011). Effect of environmental temperature on growth- and reproduction-related hormones gene expression in the female blue gourame (Trichogaster trichopterus). *Comp. Biochem. Physiol. Part A Mol. Integr. Physiol.* 160, 381–189.

Levy, G., and Degani, G. (2011). Evidence of a reproduction-related function for pituitary adenylate cyclase activating polypeptide-related peptide in an Anabantidae fish. *J. Mol. Endocrinol.* 46, 101–110.

Levy, G., and Degani, G. (2012). Involvement of GnRH, PACAP and PRP in the reproduction of blue gourami females (Trichogaster trichopterus). *J. Mol. Neurosci.* 48, 603–616.

Levy, G., Jackson, K., and Degani, G. (2010). Association between pituitary adenylate cyclase activating polypeptide and reproduction in the blue gourami. *Gen. Comp. Endocrinol.* 166, 83–93.

Li, M., Mbikay, M., and Arimura, A. (2000). Pituitary adenylate cyclase-activating polypeptide precursor is processed solely by prohormone convertase 4 in the gonads. *Endocrinology* 14[illegible] 3723–3730.

Matsuda, F., Inoue, N., Manabe, N., and Ohkura, S. (2012). Follicular growth and atresia in mammalian ovaries: regulation by survival and death of granulosa cells. *J. Reprod. Dev.* 5[illegible] 44–50.

Mayerhofer, A., Dissen, G. A., Costa, M. E., and Ojeda, S. R. (1997). A role for neurotransmitters in early follicular development: induction of functional follicle-stimulating hormone receptors in newly formed follicles of the rat ovary. *Endocrinology* 13[illegible] 3320–3329.

Miyata, A., Arimura, A., Dahl, R. R., Minamino, N., Uehara, A., Jiang, L., et al. (1989). Isolation of a novel 38 residue-hypothalamic polypeptide which stimulates adenylate cyclase in pituitary cells. *Biochem. Biophys. Res. Commun.* 164, 567–574.

Morelli, M. B., Barberi, M., Gambardella, A., Borini, A., Cecconi, S., Coticchio, G., et al. (2008). Characterization, expression, and functional activity of pituitary adenylate cyclase-activating polypeptide and its receptors in human granulosa-luteal cells. *J. Clin. Endocrinol. Metab.* 93, 4924–3492.

Nussdorfer, G. G., and Malendowicz, L. K. (1998). Role of VIP, PACAP, and related peptides in the regulation of the hypothalamo-pituitary-adrenal axis. *Peptides* 19, 1443–1467.

Odum, L., and Fahrenkrug, J. (1998). Pituitary adenylate cyclase activating polypeptide (PACAP) in human ovarian cancers. *Cancer Lett.* 125, 185–189.

Park, H. J., Lee, J., Wang, L., Park, J. H., Kwon, H. B., and Arimura, A. (2000). Stage-specific expression of pituitary adenylate cyclase activating polypeptide type I receptor messenger ribonucleic acid during ovarian follicle development in the rat. *Endocrinology* 141, 702–709.

Park, J. Y., Park, J. H., Park, H. J., Lee, J. Y., Lee, Y. I., Lee, K., et al. (2001). Stage-dependent regulation of ovarian pituitary adenylate cyclase-activating polypeptide mRNA levels by GnRH in cultured rat granulosa cells. *Endocrinology* 142, 3828–3835.

Pesce, M., Canipari, R., Ferri, G. L., Siracusa, G., and De Felici, M. (1996).

Pituitary adenylate cyclase activating polypeptide (PACAP) stimulates adenylate cyclase and promotes proliferation of mouse primordial germ cells. *Development* 122, 215–221.

Pirger, Z., Nemeth, J., Hiripi, L., Toth, G., Kiss, P., Lubics, A., et al. (2008). PACAP has anti-apoptotic effect in the salivary gland of an invertebrate species, Helix pomatia. *J. Mol. Neurosci.* 36, 105–114.

Racz, B., Gasz, B., Borsiczky, B., Gallyas, F., Jr. Tamas, A., Jozsa, R., et al. (2007). Protective effects of pituitary adenylate cyclase activating polypeptide in endothelial cells against oxidative stress-induced apoptosis. *Gen. Comp. Endocrinol.* 153, 115–123.

Rawlings, S. R., and Hezareh, M. (1996). Pituitary adenylate cyclase activating polypeptide (PACAP) and PACAP/Vasoactive intestinal polypeptide receptors: actions on the anterior pituitary gland. *Endocr. Rev.* 17, 4–29.

Reglodi, D., Gyarmati, J., Ertl, T., Borzsei, R., Bodis, J., Tamas, A., et al. (2010). Alterations of pituitary adenylate cyclase activating polypeptide (PACAP)-like immunoreactivity in the human plasma during pregnancy and after birth. *J. Endocrinol. Invest.* 33, 443–445.

Reglodi, D., Kiss, P., Szabadfi, K., Atlasz, T., Gabriel, R., Horvath, G., et al. (2012). PACAP is an endogenous protective factor – insights from PACAP deficient mice. *J. Mol. Neurosci.* 48, 482–492.

Sadler, T. W. (2012). *Medical Embriology.* Baltimore: Lippincott Williams and Wilkins.

Sayasith, K., Brown, K. A., and Sirois, J. (2007). Gonadotropin-dependent regulation of bovine pituitary adenylate cyclase-activating polypeptide in ovarian follicles prior to ovulation. *Reproduction* 133, 441–453.

Scaldaferri, L., Arora, K., Lee, S. H., Catt, K. J., and Moretti, C. (1996). Expression of PACAP and its type-I receptor isoforms in the rat ovary. *Mol. Cell. Endocrinol.* 117, 227–232.

Scaldaferri, M. L., Modesti, A., Palumbo, C., Ulisse, S., Fabbri, A., Piccione, E., et al. (2000). Pituitary adenylate cyclase-activating polypeptide (PACAP) and PACAP-receptor type 1 expression in rat and human placenta. *Endocrinology* 141, 1158–1167.

Sherwood, N. M., Adams, B. A., Isaac, E. R., Wu, S., and Fradinger, E. A. (2007). Knocked down and out: PACAP in development, reproduction and feeding. *Peptides* 28, 1680–1687.

Sherwood, N. M., Krueckl, S. L., and McRory, J. E. (2000). The origin and function of the pituitary adenylate cyclase-activating polypeptide (PACAP)/glucagon superfamily. *Endocr. Rev.* 21, 619–670.

Shintani, N., Mori, W., Hashimoto, H., Imai, M., Tanaka, K., Tomimoto, S., et al. (2002). Defects in reproductive functions in PACAP-deficient female mice. *Regul. Pept.* 109, 45–48.

Somogyvari-Vigh, A., and Reglodi, D. (2004). Pituitary adenylate cyclase activating polypeptide: a potential neuroprotective peptide. *Curr. Pharm. Des.* 10, 2861–2889.

Steenstrup, B. R., Alm, P., Hannibal, J., Jorgensen, J. C., Palle, C., Junge, J., et al. (1995). Pituitary adenylate cyclase activating polypeptide: occurrence and relaxant effect in female genital tract. *Am. J. Physiol.* 269, E108–E117.

Steenstrup, B. R., Jorgensen, J. C., Alm, P., Hannibal, J., Junge, J., Fahrenkrug, J., et al. (1996). Pituitary adenylate cyclase activating polypeptide (PACAP): occurrence and vasodilatory effect in the human uteroplacental unit. *Regul. Pept.* 61, 197–204.

Szabo, F., Horvath, J., Heinzlmann, A., Arimura, A., and Koves, K. (2002). Neonatal PACAPadministration in rats delays puberty through the influence of the LHRH neuronal system. *Regul. Pept.* 109, 49–55.

Usuki, S., and Kotani, E. (2001). Effect of pituitary adenylate cyclase-activating polypeptide (PACAP) on progestin biosynthesis in cultured luteal cells from rat ovary. *Gynecol. Endocrinol.* 15, 184–191.

Usuki, S., and Kotani, E. (2002). Tokishakuyakusan directly attenuates PACAP's luteolytic action on luteal function in the rat ovary. *Am. J. Chin. Med.* 30, 521–531.

Vaccari, S., Latini, S., Barberi, M., Teti, A., Stefanini, M., and Canipari, R. (2006). Characterization and expression of different pituitary adenylate cyclase-activating polypeptide/vasoactive intestinal polypeptide receptors in rat ovarian follicles. *J. Endocrinol.* 191, 287–299.

Vaudry, D., Falluel-Morel, A., Bourgault, S., Basille, M., Burel, D., Wurtz, O., et al. (2009). Pituitary adenylate cyclase activating polypeptide and its receptors: 20 years after the discovery. *Pharmacol. Rev.* 61, 283–357.

Vaudry, D., Ravni, A., Wurtz, O., Benard, M., Botia, B., and Jolivel, V. (2006). "Effects of PACAP in the local regulation of endocrine glands," in *Handbook of Biologically Active Peptides*, ed. A. J. Kastin (London: Academic Press), 867–874.

Vaudry, D., Rousselle, C., Basille, M., Falluel-Morel, A., Pamantung, T. F., Fontaine, M., et al. (2002). Pituitary adenylate cyclase activating polypeptide protects rat cerebellar granule neurons against ethanol-induced apoptotic cell death. *Proc. Natl. Acad. Sci. U.S.A.* 99, 6398–6403.

Wang, Y., Wong, A. O., and Ge, W. (2003). Cloning, regulation of messenger ribonucleic acid expression, and function of a new isoform of pituitary adenylate cyclase activating polypeptide in the zebrafish ovary. *Endocrinology* 144, 4799–4810.

Zhao, W., Cheng, D. L., Zheng, H. L., Zhu, H., and Ni, J. (2010). Expression and regulation of pituitary adenylate cyclase activating polypeptide mRNA in pregnant rat corpus luteum. *Zhongguo Ying Yong Sheng Li Xue Za Zhi* 26, 313–317.

Zhong, Y., and Kasson, B. G. (1994). Pituitary adenylate cyclase-activating polypeptide stimulates steroidogenesis and adenosine 3',5'-monophosphate accumulation in cultured rat granulosa cells. *Endocrinology* 135, 207–213.

Ziessen, T., Moncada, S., and Cellek, S. (2002). Characterization of the non-nitrergic NANC relaxation responses in the rabbit vaginal wall. *Br. J. Pharmacol.* 135, 546–554.

6

Glucagon-like peptide-1 receptor overexpression in cancer and its impact on clinical applications

Meike Körner[1], Emanuel Christ[2], Damian Wild[3] and Jean Claude Reubi[1]*

[1] Division of Cell Biology and Experimental Research, Institute of Pathology, University of Berne, Berne, Switzerland
[2] Division of Endocrinology, Diabetology and Clinical Nutrition, University Hospital of Berne, Inselspital, Berne, Switzerland
[3] Division of Nuclear Medicine, Department of Radiology, University Basel Hospital, Basel, Switzerland

Edited by:
Jae Young Seong, Korea University, South Korea

Reviewed by:
Jong-Ik Hwang, Korea University, South Korea
Billy K. Chow, University of Hong Kong, China

****Correspondence:***
Jean Claude Reubi, Division of Cell Biology and Experimental Research, Institute of Pathology, University of Berne, Murtenstrasse 31, CH – 3010 Berne, Switzerland.
e-mail: reubi@pathology.unibe.ch

Peptide hormones of the glucagon-like peptide (GLP) family play an increasing clinical role, such as GLP-1 in diabetes therapy. Moreover, GLP receptors are overexpressed in various human tumor types and therefore represent molecular targets for important clinical applications. In particular, virtually all benign insulinomas highly overexpress GLP-1 receptors (GLP-1R). Targeting GLP-1R with the stable GLP-1 analogs ^{111}In-DOTA/DPTA-exendin-4 offers a new approach to successfully localize these small tumors. This non-invasive technique has the potential to replace the invasive localization of insulinomas by selective arterial stimulation and venous sampling. Malignant insulinomas, in contrast to their benign counterparts, express GLP-1R in only one-third of the cases, while they more often express the somatostatin type 2 receptors. Importantly, one of the two receptors appears to be always expressed in malignant insulinomas. The GLP-1R overexpression in selected cancers is worth to be kept in mind with regard to the increasing use of GLP-1 analogs for diabetes therapy. While the functional role of GLP-1R in neoplasia is not known yet, it may be safe to monitor patients undergoing GLP-1 therapy carefully.

Keywords: glucagon-like peptide-1, glucagon-like peptide-1 receptor, insulinoma, ^{111}In-DOTA/DPTA-exendin-4

INTRODUCTION

G protein-coupled peptide hormone receptors play an increasing role as tumor targets in cancer medicine (Reubi, 2003). The underlying molecular basis is primarily an overexpression of a specific peptide receptor on tumor cells, irrespective of receptor functions. This overexpression allows a receptor-targeted scintigraphic imaging and radiotherapy of tumors with adequate radiolabeled peptide analogs (Reubi, 2003). Historically, the somatostatin receptors were the first receptors identified for these purposes (Reubi, 2003). They are expressed in high incidence and at high levels in gastroenteropancreatic neuroendocrine tumors (Reubi, 2003). Somatostatin receptor scintigraphy using the somatostatin analog octreotide (OctreoScan®) represents nowadays a standard imaging procedure for patients with gut neuroendocrine tumors, while PET/CT with ^{68}Ga-labeled somatostatin analogs turns out to be even superior to OctreoScan® (Gabriel et al., 2007). Furthermore, results from clinical studies performing somatostatin receptor-mediated radionuclide therapy are encouraging (Kwekkeboom et al., 2008; Imhof et al., 2011).

The clinical success of somatostatin receptor targeting of gut neuroendocrine tumors has stimulated the search for other peptide receptors suitable for similar applications. A promising candidate is the glucagon-like peptide 1 (GLP-1) receptor (GLP-1R). This receptor has been cloned almost 20 years ago (Thorens et al., 1993). It is a member of the class 2 G protein-coupled receptor family (Gros et al., 1993; Nauck, 2009). Only a single GLP-1R has been identified so far, which is structurally identical in all tissues (Thorens et al., 1993). Receptor activation upon agonist binding stimulates adenylate cyclase and phospholipase C, with subsequent activation of protein kinase A and C, respectively (Thorens et al., 1993).

Physiologically, the GLP-1R is expressed mainly in the alimentary tract, particularly in the pancreatic islet cells (Wei and Mojsov, 1995) where it mediates the actions of GLP-1 released from the small intestines in response to food intake. GLP-1 is considered to be one of the most important glucose-dependent insulin secretagogues (Nauck, 2009). Specifically, it stimulates glucose-dependent insulin synthesis and secretion, inhibits glucagon secretion, decreases β-cell apoptosis and increases differentiation of β-cell precursor cells in the pancreas as well as inhibits gastric emptying and appetite at the hypothalamic level (Nauck et al., 2009). Exploiting GLP-1 pathways therefore represents an ideal therapeutic approach for patients with type 2 diabetes, as this interferes with the main pathophysiological mechanisms of the disease (Nauck et al., 2009). Indeed, synthetic GLP-1 analogs are FDA- and EMEA-approved for the treatment of type 2 diabetes (Nauck et al., 2009).

The GLP-1R is of clinical interest not only due to its physiologic expression and functions in pancreatic islet cells and its potential in diabetes therapy, but also because of its possible role in cancer. Indeed, 10 years ago, the GLP-1R was found to be expressed in insulin-producing islet cell tumors, i.e., insulinomas (Reubi and Waser, 2003). This discovery lead to an extensive evaluation of the potential of the GLP-1R for targeted tumor imaging and therapy analogous to somatostatin receptor targeting of gut neuroendocrine tumors. This evaluation included the characterization of human tumors and normal tissues for their GLP-1R expression, since an important prerequisite for a successful peptide receptor targeting of tumors is a high receptor expression in tumors, but a low receptor expression in normal background tissues. Further activities included the development of adequate radiolabeled GLP-1 analogs, testing of such analogs in *in vivo* animal models and application of selected suitable candidate analogs to tumor patients in preliminary clinical studies. This review summarizes the knowledge on the *in vitro* and *in vivo* basis of GLP-1 receptor targeting of tumors accumulated in the last decade.

GLP-1R IN TUMORS

The GLP-1R expression has been systematically assessed in a broad spectrum of original human tumor tissues using *in vitro* receptor autoradiography (Reubi and Waser, 2003; Korner et al., 2007; Waser et al., 2011). The GLP-1R was thus identified in specific endocrine, embryonal, and brain tumors, but virtually not in carcinomas (**Table 1**). The most striking GLP-1R expression was found in insulinoma. This is an endocrine tumor of the pancreatic islet cells with mostly benign biological behavior, but characterized clinically by severe symptoms of hyperinsulinism due to insulin secretion. Benign insulinomas expressed GLP-1Rs in very high incidence (>90%) and extremely high density (Reubi and Waser, 2003; **Table 1**; **Figure 1**). In fact, no other peptide receptor has been found to exhibit such high expression levels in this tumor type (Reubi and Waser, 2003). On the contrary, malignant, metastasizing insulinomas expressed GLP-1Rs significantly less frequently. High GLP-1R levels were found in only 36% malignant insulinomas (Wild et al., 2011). In insulinoma cells, the GLP-1R may represent a mediator of insulin secretion: in a model of GLP-1R transfected insulinoma cells, glucose-mediated insulin release was increased compared to control cells, in parallel with an increase of the intracellular second messenger of the GLP-1R (cAMP; Montrose-Rafizadeh et al., 1997).

Table 1 | GLP-1R expressing human tumors: receptor incidences and densities.

Tumor type	GLP-1R incidence	GLP-1R density*
Endocrine tumors		
Benign insulinomas	25/27 (93%)	8,133
Malignant insulinomas	4/11 (36%)	8,508†
Gastrinomas	10/10 (100%)	2,461
Glucagonomas	2/4 (50%)	910
VIPomas	1/4 (25%)	3,028
Ileal carcinoids	8/27 (30%)	1,027
Bronchial carcinoid tumors	11/29 (38%)	2,456
Pheochromocytomas	12/20 (60%)	3,970
Paragangliomas	5/18 (28%)	1,353
Medullary thyroid carcinomas	5/18 (28%)	1,326
Embryonal tumors		
Medulloblastomas	3/12 (25%)	1,246
Nephroblastomas	2/9 (22%)	421
Neuroblastomas	3/16 (19%)	932
Brain tumors		
Meningiomas	7/20 (35%)	989
Astrocytomas	4/16 (25%)	1,069
Glioblastomas	2/21 (9%)	790
Ependymomas	1/6 (16%)	1,075
Carcinomas		
Ovarian adenocarcinomas	2/12 (16%)	688
Prostate adenocarcinomas	1/20 (5%)	1,283

**dpm/mg tissue.*
† Mean value of two tumors tested with in vitro GLP-1R autoradiography.

Also several other functioning endocrine tumors of the pancreas expressed GLP-1Rs, in particular gastrinomas, however in lower amounts compared with insulinomas (**Table 1**; Reubi and Waser, 2003). Moreover, GLP-1Rs were discovered in a number of extrapancreatic endocrine tumors, including ileal carcinoids, pheochromocytomas, paragangliomas, bronchial carcinoid tumors, and medullary thyroid carcinomas, while they were not identified in pituitary adenomas or adrenal cortical tumors (Korner et al., 2007). Pheochromocytomas are of particular clinical interest due to their high GLP-1R expression levels (**Table 1**). Furthermore, medullary thyroid carcinomas are noteworthy because of important species differences in their GLP-1R expression. In rats, virtually all medullary thyroid carcinomas expressed GLP-1Rs in high amounts (Waser et al., 2011), while in humans only 28% expressed GLP-1R at low density levels (**Table 1**).

Lower GLP-1R expression levels were found in embryonal tumors, including medulloblastoma, nephroblastoma, and neuroblastoma (**Table 1**). They showed GLP-1Rs in low density in 15–25% of the tumors (Korner et al., 2007). Similarly, tumors of the nervous system such as meningiomas and astrocytomas demonstrated an incidence of GLP-1Rs between 25 and 35%, whereas glioblastomas and ependymomas expressed GLP-1Rs in 9–16% (**Table 1**; Korner et al., 2007). Schwannomas were devoid of GLP-1Rs (Korner et al., 2007).

Conversely, carcinomas exhibited a very low or no GLP-1R expression. Only ovarian and prostate carcinomas rarely showed GLP-1R at low levels, while breast, colorectal, gastric, pancreatic, hepatocellular, and cholangiocellular as well as lung carcinomas (non-small and small cell carcinomas) were negative for GLP-1R (Korner et al., 2007). Likewise, non-Hodgkin lymphomas did not express GLP-1R (Korner et al., 2007).

Among all GLP-1R expressing tumor types, insulinomas are at present of highest clinical interest for an *in vivo* targeting in patients, based on several considerations. First, insulinomas exhibit particularly high GLP-1R expression levels with respect to both incidence and density. Second, benign insulinomas, in contrast to most other gastroenteropancreatic neuroendocrine tumors, show relatively low expression levels of somatostatin receptors. Consequently, OctreoScan® is not a reliable tool to detect these tumors (Plockinger et al., 2004). Third, the exact intraoperative localization of insulinomas is critical in order to minimize the surgical intervention (Rostambeigi and Thompson, 2009). This is, however, difficult due to the small size of benign insulinomas (usually 10–20 mm). Conventional radiological procedures (endosonography, MR-, and CT-imaging) are not always

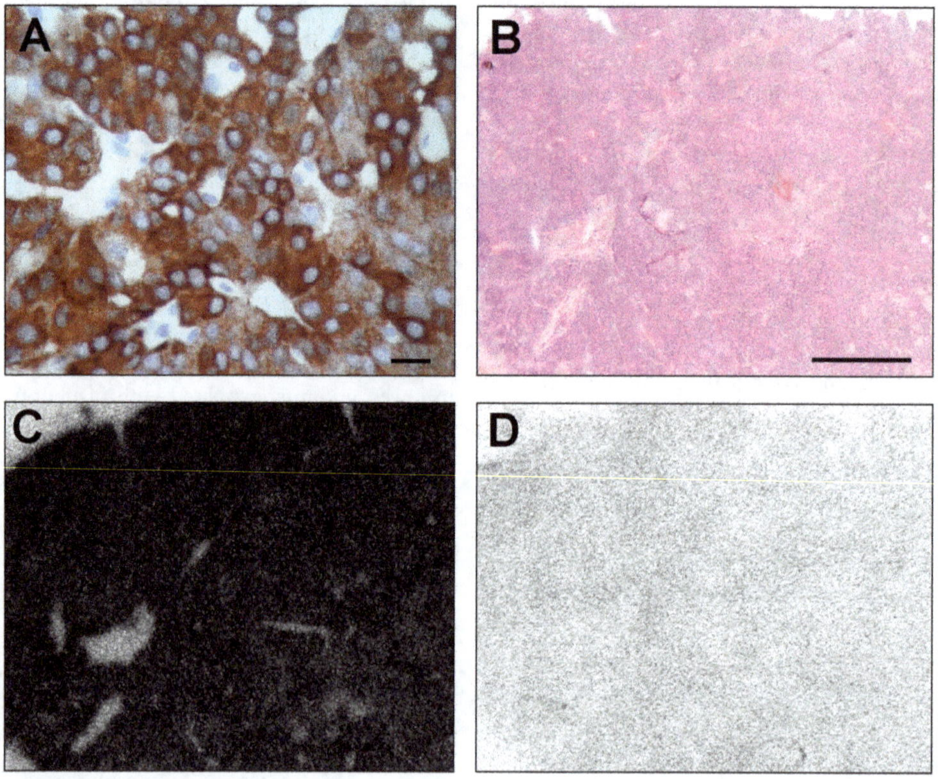

FIGURE 1 | Hormone and receptor determinations *in vitro* in a benign insulinoma. (A) Immunohistochemistry for insulin showing strongly labeled tumor cells. Bar = 0.01 mm. **(B–D)** *In vitro* GLP-1R autoradiography on consecutive insulinoma tissue sections. **(B)** Hematoxylin & eosin (H&E) staining showing the tumor tissue. Bar = 1 mm. **(C)** Autoradiogram showing total binding of ^{125}I-GLP-1(7-36) amide. The entire tumor is strongly positive. **(D)** Autoradiogram showing non-specific binding of ^{125}I-GLP-1(7-36) amide in the presence of 100 nM cold GLP1(7-36) amide. Reprinted from Christ et al. (2010), with permission from Elsevier.

successful in localizing insulinomas (Chatziioannou et al., 2001). Moreover, [^{18}F]DOPA PET shows at present controversial results, with sensitivities ranging between 17 and 90% (Kauhanen et al., 2007; Tessonnier et al., 2010). Although selective arterial stimulation and venous sampling is a reliable intraoperative tool to detect insulinomas in experienced institutions (Wiesli et al., 2004), it is an invasive procedure with the associated risks. Moreover, this procedure identifies only the region of the pancreas – depending on the vasculature – where the insulinoma should be located and not the tumor itself (Wiesli et al., 2004).

GLP-1R IN NON-NEOPLASTIC TISSUES

The GLP-1R expression was similarly characterized in human normal tissues. It has been found in the pancreatic islets and acini, stomach, duodenal Brunner's gland, small and large intestinal myenteric plexus, lung and kidney vasculature, breast parenchyma, heart, brainstem, hypothalamus, neurohypophysis, and meninges (Wei and Mojsov, 1995; Korner et al., 2007). *In vitro* receptor autoradiography revealed that GLP-1R levels were highest in the neurohypophysis, followed by Brunner's glands, meninges, and pancreatic islets (Korner et al., 2007). Of practical importance, with the exception of Brunner's glands, the different tissues in the pancreatic area (i.e., pancreas islets and acini, intestines, and kidney) exhibit far lower GLP-1R density levels than insulinomas. This results in a high tumor-to-background ratio in GLP-1R density levels for insulinomas, which is an important prerequisite for a GLP-1R-targeted scintigraphic imaging of insulinomas.

Prominent species differences in the physiological GLP-1R expression between humans and rodents are noteworthy. Indeed, autoradiography experiments indicate that GLP-1R density levels are considerably higher in the lungs of rats and mice than of humans (Korner et al., 2007). This has to be considered when interpreting results of *in vivo* testing of GLP-1R targeting in rodent models. Likewise, the GLP-1R expression in the thyroid gland is substantial in rodents, but virtually absent in humans (Korner et al., 2007). In rodent thyroids, GLP-1Rs are located in the medullary C-cells. Of interest, treatment with GLP-1 analogs in rats is known to occasionally lead to thyroid C-cell hyperplasia and medullary thyroid carcinoma, whereas in humans there is so far no evidence of such complications. It can be speculated whether the species differences in the GLP-1R density expression in the precursor cells of these tumors, the medullary C-cells, contribute to these controversial findings (Waser et al., 2011).

RADIOLABELED GLP-1 ANALOGS

In general, radioactively labeled peptide analogs represent pharmaceuticals with favorable characteristics. Due to their small size, they show fast diffusion and rapid blood clearance and lack immunogenicity. Moreover, radiopeptides exhibit only rare side effects (Reubi, 2003). In addition, radiolabeling is easily feasible, preferably after attaching a chelator to the peptide (Reubi and Maecke, 2008). However, since peptides are physiologically degraded within minutes in the human blood by potent peptidases such as dipeptidyl-peptidase-4 (DPP-4; Baggio and Drucker, 2007), stable peptide analogs have to be used instead in clinical applications. As for GLP-1, a naturally occurring stable analog exists, namely exendin-4, which is a component of the Gila monster venom. It shares 53% homology with GLP-1 and similarly binds to GLP-1Rs, but is resistant to DPP-4 cleavage (Nauck, 2009). Exendin-4 is, therefore, a good candidate for the development of radiolabeled GLP-1R ligands.

The first radiopeptides tested for *in vivo* GLP-1R targeting were ^{125}I-labeled GLP-1 and the GLP-1 analog exendin-3 (Gotthardt et al., 2002). However, the low peptide stability of GLP-1 and the low efficiency of radio-iodination of exendin-3 limited their clinical use. Further testing resulted in the development of ^{111}In-labeled exendin-4 (Wild et al., 2006): exendin-4 was coupled via the Lys side chain to a chelator (DOTA, tetraazacyclododecane tetraacetic acid or DTPA, diethylenetriaminepentaacetic acid) using a spacer (Ahx, aminohexanoic acid) and then labeled with ^{111}In. This radiopeptide was subsequently extensively tested *in vitro* and *in vivo* in insulinoma models and applied to insulinoma patients (see below). Lately, several studies have been published that describe GLP-1R ligands suitable for PET/CT imaging, such as ^{68}Ga-, ^{64}Cu-, or ^{18}F-labeled exendin-4, or for SPECT/CT imaging like ^{99m}Tc-labeled exendin-4 (Brom et al., 2010; Wild et al., 2010; Wu et al., 2011; Kiesewetter et al., 2012). These novel radiopeptides have not yet been tested in insulinoma patients.

GLP-1R TARGETING IN ANIMAL MODELS

Initially, GLP-1R targeting was performed in the rat insulinoma cell line RINm5F and in a rat insulinoma animal model (NEDH rats) using ^{125}I-labeled GLP-1 and exendin-3 (Gotthardt et al., 2002). Specific uptake was detected in the cell and animal models. This provided the proof of principle for GLP-1R targeting of insulinoma (Gotthardt et al., 2002).

Follow-up experiments were carried out in the Rip1tag2 mouse model with ^{111}In-DTPA-exendin-4. These transgenic mice develop tumors of the pancreatic β-cells in a reproducible multi-stage fashion (Hanahan, 1985) and, therefore, represent an ideal model to study GLP-1R targeting *in vivo* and *in vitro*. Using GLP-1R multipinhole SPECT/MRI and SPECT/CT, *in vivo* GLP-1R imaging was performed in these animals following administration of ^{111}In-DTPA-exendin-4 (Wild et al., 2006). In parallel, GLP-1R autoradiography of the tumors was carried out *in vitro*. Finally, biodistribution and pharmacokinetics as well as internalization and cellular retention of ^{111}In-DTPA-exendin-4 were measured *in vitro* (Wild et al., 2006).

This preclinical study showed the following main findings: First, the GLP-1R density in the tumors was extremely high, resulting in a remarkably high uptake of ^{111}In-DTPA-exendin-4 (287 ± 62% IA/g tissue) already 4 h after injection. Second, excellent visualization of tumors as small as 1 mm by pinhole SPECT/MRI and SPECT/CT was demonstrated. Third, the tumor-to-background ratio was very high (between 13.6 and 299), substantiating the high potential of this radiopeptide to specifically localize GLP-1R positive lesions within the pancreas. Lastly, *in vitro* studies in the cells derived from the tumor model demonstrated a specific internalization of ^{111}In-DTPA-exendin-4, and biochemical investigations confirmed the high metabolic stability of the radiopeptide in the tumor cells as well as in the serum.

The same Rip1tag2 mouse model also provided preliminary data on GLP-1R-targeted therapy of insulinoma. Mice were injected with different doses of ^{111}In-DTPA-exendin-4 (1.1, 5.6, and 28 MBq) and sacrificed 7 days after injection. Most impressively, a single injection lead to a reduction in tumor volume of up to 94% in a dose-dependent manner without significant acute organ toxicity. Histological examination revealed that the decrease in tumor mass was mainly due to an increase in tumor cell apoptosis and decreased proliferation (Wicki et al., 2007).

GLP-1R TARGETING IN HUMANS

The first patient who underwent GLP-1R scintigraphy suffered from severe endogenous hyperinsulinemic hypoglycemia with non-convulsive seizures. MRI, CT scan, and endosonography did not detect any suspicious lesion. However, GLP-1R scintigraphy revealed an increased extrapancreatic uptake in the mesentery supplied by the anterior mesentery artery. Selective arterial stimulation and venous sampling correctly indicated the vascular territory, but since this patient had an ectopic insulinoma, the results of the invasive investigation without GLP-1R imaging would have been misleading for the surgical strategy (Wild et al., 2008).

In a proof of principle study, ^{111}In-DOTA-exendin-4 was prospectively administered to a total of six patients (Christ et al., 2009). All of them presented with neuroglycopenic symptoms lasting for 4–26 months. Biochemical evaluation during a fasting test revealed endogenous hyperinsulinemic hypoglycemia in all patients.

Conventional imaging (CT or MRI) reliably detected the insulinoma in only two patients, whereas endosonography identified a possible lesion in four patients, in keeping with data in the literature (McAuley et al., 2005). In three patients, selective arterial stimulation and venous sampling was performed, with accurate localization in all (Christ et al., 2009). Remarkably, GLP1-R scintigraphy correctly detected the insulinoma in all six consecutive patients (**Figure 2**; Christ et al., 2009). Four patients underwent an enucleation of the insulinoma. In two patients, a Whipple procedure had to be performed due to the localization of the insulinoma. In all patients, a benign insulinoma was confirmed by histology. *In vitro* autoradiography studies showed GLP-1R densities in the range as previously described (between 2,600 to >10,000 dpm/mg tissue; Reubi and Waser, 2003), but low levels of somatostatin receptor type 1 in 2 patients only (Christ et al., 2009). Importantly, within a time frame of 2–14 days after injection of ^{111}In-DOTA-exendin-4, intraoperative utilization of a gamma probe was highly beneficial for the *in situ* localization of the insulinoma in all patients, resulting in a successful enucleation where possible (Christ et al., 2009).

Fortunately, background uptake over the whole body was low with the exceptions of the kidneys, which were strongly labeled due to renal excretion of the radioligand (**Figure 2**). In two

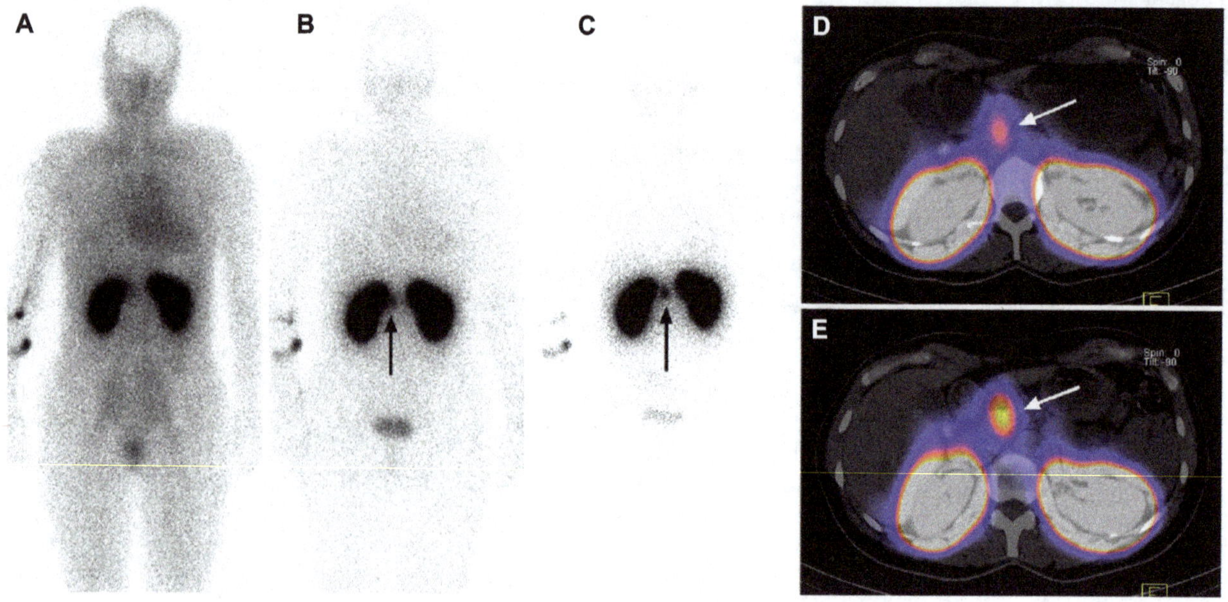

FIGURE 2 | ^{111}In-DOTA-exendin-4 whole-body planar images (A–C) and ^{111}In-DOTA-exendin-4 SPECT/CT images (D,E) from the same patient. Whole-body scans were carried out 20 min **(A)**, 4 h **(B)**, and 3 days **(C)**, and SPECT/CT scans were performed 4 h **(D)** and 3 days **(E)** after injection of 97 MBq ^{111}In-DOTA-exendin-4. Four hours after injection, there was already a focal ^{111}In-DOTA-exendin-4 uptake visible in the head of the pancreas (arrow) on whole-body **(B)** and SPECT/CT **(D)** scans. The tumor-to-pancreas-uptake ratio was 1.9 at 4 h after injection **(D)** and 3.2 at 3 days after injection of the radioligand. The longest residence times of ^{111}In-DOTA-exendin-4 were observed in the tumor (arrow) and kidneys **(C)**. Reprinted from Christ et al. (2009), with permission from The Endocrine Society.

patients demarcation between tumors (maximal diameter of 9–11 mm) and kidneys was only possible after late scans, indicating an improved tumor-to-kidney ratio with time, in keeping with the fact that the effective half-life of ^{111}In-DOTA-exendin-4 was longer in the tumor (38–64 h) than in the kidneys (31.2–31.8 h; **Figure 2**; Christ et al., 2009). This suggests that patients with negative early scans should have additional imaging 3–7 days after the injection.

In humans, ^{111}In-DOTA-exendin-4 was initially administered, but later replaced by ^{111}In-DTPA-exendin-4 due to the four times higher specific activity of the latter (Wild et al., 2009). A higher specific activity permits to reduce the amount of peptide (exendin-4), thereby decreasing the occurrence of possible side effects. In addition, radiolabeling of DTPA-exendin-4 can be performed at room temperature, whereas labeling of DOTA-exendin-4 has to be accomplished at high temperature (95°C; Wild et al., 2006).

By now, data of a prospective, multicenter trial including 30 patients that underwent GLP-1R scanning are available. The inclusion criteria were proven endogenous hyperinsulinemic hypoglycemia and none or maximally one lesion on conventional imaging. Conventional imaging (CT, MRI) and endosonography – where available – was performed locally using a standard protocol. ^{111}In-DTPA-exendin-4 was administered intravenously at a dose of 90–130 MBq over 2 min. Whole-body planar images and SPECT/CT of the abdomen were performed at 4, 24 and in some patients between 72 and 96 up to 168 h post-injection, the most important time point being the scan 24 h after injection. Diagnosis was confirmed by histology after surgical removal (Christ et al., 2012).

Conventional imaging (MRI, CT, endosonography) was positive in 17 patients. ^{111}In-DTPA/DOTA-exendin-4 SPECT/CT detected 23 true positive benign insulinomas and five additional positive lesions (one malignant insulinoma; two islet cell hyperplasias; two uncharacterized lesions). True negative tests were detected in two patients (one malignant insulinoma; one islet cell hyperplasia). Malignant insulinomas were diagnosed based on the histological finding of a positive lymph node, not detected on conventional imaging preoperatively. There was no false negative result. Sensitivity was 100% and the positive predictive value was 82% (Christ et al., 2012). These findings are encouraging and suggest that *in vivo* GLP-1R imaging defines a new non-invasive diagnostic approach to successfully localize small benign insulinomas.

About 90% of insulinomas are benign and only 10% of patients present with malignant disease usually characterized by liver metastasis (Plockinger et al., 2004). Anecdotal evidence suggests that malignant insulinomas exhibit more often somatostatin receptors type 2 than benign ones and can, therefore, be visualized by OctreoScan® (Plockinger et al., 2004). A more extensive study with data from 10 patients with malignant insulinoma showed that somatostatin receptors type 2 were expressed in seven patients, whereas GLP-1R were present in four patients, and both receptors in only one patient (Wild et al., 2011). Importantly, one of the two imaging methods appears always to be positive in a malignant type of insulinoma (Wild et al., 2011). The consequences of the respective receptor expression in an insulinoma with regard to biological behavior (malignant or benign course) remains to be established.

SIDE EFFECTS AND LIMITATIONS

In humans, the injection of ^{111}In-DOTA-exendin-4 and ^{111}In-DPTA-exendin-4 was well tolerated. Due to the small amount of exendin-4, the decrease in plasma glucose concentrations was only 1.4 ± 0.7 mmol/L after 40 min (Christ et al., 2009). By regularly monitoring glucose levels, no severe hypoglycemic episode occurred. One patient experienced a short episode of vomiting only with ^{111}In-DOTA-exendin-4. Otherwise, no further side effects were observed (Christ et al., 2009).

In two patients, there was focal ^{111}In-DOTA-exendin-4 uptake in the proximal duodenum. This may be related to the presence of Brunnner's gland of the duodenum which, as previously mentioned, are known to contain GLP-1Rs in a significant density (Korner et al., 2007). Brunner's glands may become hyperplastic (Levine et al., 1995), as observed in particular in patients with chronic pancreatitis (Stolte et al., 1981). Such hyperplastic glands may possibly be detected by GLP-1R imaging.

A differential diagnosis of endogenous hyperinsulinemic hypoglycemia includes nesidioblastosis, also known as "non-insulinoma pancreatogenous hypoglycemia syndrome" in a clinical setting (Thompson et al., 2000). Histopathologically, this entity is defined as a diffuse hyperplasia of β-cells occurring usually in children (Yakovac et al., 1971). Recent evidence suggests that this pathology can also be demonstrated in adults, in particular after bypass surgery for morbid obesity (Service et al., 2005). In the previously mentioned series of patients (Christ et al., 2012), islet cell hyperplasia was diagnosed in three patients, two were positive on GLP-1R imaging and one was negative. Based on these preliminary data GLP-1R imaging does not appear to be an appropriate tool to diagnose or exclude islet cell hyperplasia. These findings are further supported by the recent evidence that the *in vitro* density of GLP-1R in pancreatic tissues of patients with nesidioblastosis after bypass surgery for morbid obesity is much lower than in benign insulinomas (Reubi et al., 2010). Recently, ^{18}F-DOPA-PET has successfully been used to detect nesidioblastosis and benign insulinoma (Kauhanen et al., 2007). Although ^{18}F-DOPA-PET may be helpful to diagnose nesidioblastosis, in benign insulinomas the tumor-to-background ratios are higher for ^{111}In-DOTA-exendin-4 SPECT than for ^{18}F-DOPA-PET (3.3 vs. 1.4), suggesting an increased sensitivity of targeting GLP-1Rs (Kauhanen et al., 2007; Christ et al., 2009) in benign insulinomas.

SUMMARY AND CONCLUSION

Because of the massive GLP-1R overexpression in selected gastrointestinal tumors, GLP-1 and GLP-1R play an increasing role in endocrine gastrointestinal tumor management. Targeting GLP-1R with ^{111}In-DOTA-exendin-4 or ^{111}In-DPTA-exendin-4 offers a new approach that permits the successful localization of small benign insulinomas pre- and intraoperatively. Since virtually all benign insulinomas express GLP-1Rs and the preliminary clinical data are very encouraging, it is likely that this approach will affect the algorithm of pre- and intraoperative localization of suspected insulinoma.

In contrast to benign insulinomas, where the exact localization of the tumor is the main goal, the clinical challenge in malignant, metastasizing insulinomas is to define the extension of the disease and – if possible – offer a targeted therapy (peptide receptor radionuclide therapy, PRRT). Contrary to benign insulinomas, malignant insulinomas more often express sst2 receptors than GLP-1R. Importantly, one of the two receptors seems to be always expressed.

With regard to the increasing and successful use of GLP-1 analogs for diabetes therapy, it is worth keeping in mind that selected cancers can overexpress GLP-1R. While the functional role of these receptors in these tumors is not known yet, it may be safe to monitor patients with such tumors carefully during their GLP-1-analog-based diabetes therapy.

REFERENCES

Baggio, L. L., and Drucker, D. J. (2007). Biology of incretins: GLP-1 and GIP. *Gastroenterology* 132, 2131–2157.

Brom, M., Oyen, W. J., Joosten, L., Gotthardt, M., and Boerman, O. C. (2010). (68)Ga-labelled exendin-3, a new agent for the detection of insulinomas with PET. *Eur. J. Nucl. Med. Mol. Imaging* 37, 1345–1355.

Chatziioannou, A., Kehagias, D., Mourikis, D., Antoniou, A., Limouris, G., Kaponis, A., et al. (2001). Imaging and localization of pancreatic insulinomas. *Clin. Imaging* 25, 275–283.

Christ, E., Forrer, F., Wild, D., Clerici, T., Braendle, M., Maecke, H., et al. (2012). Glucagon-like peptide 1 receptor (GLP-1R) imaging for the preoperative localization of benign insulinomas in 30 patients. *Neuroendocrinology* 96, 24–24.

Christ, E., Wild, D., Forrer, F., Brandle, M., Sahli, R., Clerici, T., et al. (2009). Glucagon-like peptide-1 receptor imaging for localization of insulinomas. *J. Clin. Endocrinol. Metab.* 94, 4398–4405.

Christ, E., Wild, D., and Reubi, J. C. (2010). Glucagonlike peptide-1 receptor: an example of translational research in insulinomas: a review. *Endocrinol. Metab. Clin. North Am.* 39, 791–800.

Gabriel, M., Decristoforo, C., Kendler, D., Dobrozemsky, G., Heute, D., Uprimny, C., et al. (2007). 68Ga-DOTA-Tyr3-octreotide PET in neuroendocrine tumors: comparison with somatostatin receptor scintigraphy and CT. *J. Nucl. Med.* 48, 508–518.

Gotthardt, M., Fischer, M., Naeher, I., Holz, J. B., Jungclas, H., Fritsch, H. W., et al. (2002). Use of the incretin hormone glucagon-like peptide-1 (GLP-1) for the detection of insulinomas: initial experimental results. *Eur. J. Nucl. Med. Mol. Imaging* 29, 597–606.

Gros, L., Thorens, B., Bataille, D., and Kervran, A. (1993). Glucagon-like peptide-1-(7-36) amide, oxyntomodulin, and glucagon interact with a common receptor in a somatostatin-secreting cell line. *Endocrinology* 133, 631–638.

Hanahan, D. (1985). Heritable formation of pancreatic beta-cell tumours in transgenic mice expressing recombinant insulin/simian virus 40 oncogenes. *Nature* 315, 115–122.

Imhof, A., Brunner, P., Marincek, N., Briel, M., Schindler, C., Rasch, H., et al. (2011). Response, survival, and long-term toxicity after therapy with the radiolabeled somatostatin analogue [90Y-DOTA]-TOC in metastasized neuroendocrine cancers. *J. Clin. Oncol.* 29, 2416–2423.

Kauhanen, S., Seppanen, M., Minn, H., Gullichsen, R., Salonen, A., Alanen, K., et al. (2007). Fluorine-18-L-dihydroxyphenylalanine (18F-DOPA) positron emission tomography as a tool to localize an insulinoma or beta-cell hyperplasia in adult patients. *J. Clin. Endocrinol. Metab.* 92, 1237–1244.

Kiesewetter, D. O., Gao, H., Ma, Y., Niu, G., Quan, Q., Guo, N., et al. (2012). 18F-radiolabeled analogs of exendin-4 for PET imaging of GLP-1 in insulinoma. *Eur. J. Nucl. Med. Mol. Imaging* 39, 463–473.

Korner, M., Stockli, M., Waser, B., and Reubi, J. C. (2007). GLP-1 receptor expression in human tumors and human normal tissues: potential for in vivo targeting. *J. Nucl. Med.* 48, 736–743.

Kwekkeboom, D. J., de Herder, W. W., Kam, B. L., van Eijck, C. H., van Essen, M., Kooij, P. P., et al. (2008). Treatment with the radiolabeled somatostatin analog [177 Lu-DOTA 0,Tyr3]octreotate: toxicity, efficacy, and survival. *J. Clin. Oncol.* 26, 2124–2130.

Levine, J. A., Burgart, L. J., Batts, K. P., and Wang, K. K. (1995). Brunner's gland hamartomas: clinical presentation and pathological features of

27 cases. *Am. J. Gastroenterol.* 90, 290–294.

McAuley, G., Delaney, H., Colville, J., Lyburn, I., Worsley, D., Govender, P., et al. (2005). Multimodality preoperative imaging of pancreatic insulinomas. *Clin. Radiol.* 60, 1039–1050.

Montrose-Rafizadeh, C., Wang, Y., Janczewski, A. M., Henderson, T. E., and Egan, J. M. (1997). Overexpression of glucagon-like peptide-1 receptor in an insulin-secreting cell line enhances glucose responsiveness. *Mol. Cell. Endocrinol.* 130, 109–117.

Nauck, M. A. (2009). Unraveling the science of incretin biology. *Eur. J. Intern. Med.* 20, S303–S308.

Nauck, M. A., Vilsboll, T., Gallwitz, B., Garber, A., and Madsbad, S. (2009). Incretin-based therapies: viewpoints on the way to consensus. *Diabetes Care* 32, S223–S231.

Plockinger, U., Rindi, G., Arnold, R., Eriksson, B., Krenning, E. P., de Herder, W. W., et al. (2004). Guidelines for the diagnosis and treatment of neuroendocrine gastrointestinal tumours. *Neuroendocrinology* 80, 394–424.

Reubi, J. C. (2003). Peptide receptors as molecular targets for cancer diagnosis and therapy. *Endocr. Rev.* 24, 389–427.

Reubi, J. C., and Maecke, H. R. (2008). Peptide-based probes for cancer imaging. *J. Nucl. Med.* 49, 1735–1738.

Reubi, J. C., Perren, A., Rehmann, R., Waser, B., Christ, E., Callery, M., et al. (2010). Glucagon-like peptide-1 (GLP-1) receptors are not overexpressed in pancreatic islets from patients with severe hyperinsulinaemic hypoglycaemia following gastric bypass. *Diabetologia* 53, 2641–2645.

Reubi, J. C., and Waser, B. (2003). Concomitant expression of several peptide receptors in neuroendocrine tumors as molecular basis for in vivo multireceptor tumor targeting. *Eur. J. Nucl. Med.* 30, 781–793.

Rostambeigi, N., and Thompson, G. B. (2009). What should be done in an operating room when an insulinoma cannot be found? *Clin. Endocrinol. (Oxf.)* 70, 512–515.

Service, G. J., Thompson, G. B., Service, F. J., Andrews, J. C., Collazo-Clavell, M. L., and Lloyd, R. V. (2005). Hyperinsulinemic hypoglycemia with nesidioblastosis after gastric-bypass surgery. *N. Engl. J. Med.* 353, 249–254.

Stolte, M., Schwabe, H., and Prestele, H. (1981). Relationship between diseases of the pancreas and hyperplasia of Brunner's glands. *Virchows Arch. A Pathol. Anat. Histol.* 394, 75–87.

Tessonnier, L., Sebag, F., Ghander, C., De Micco, C., Reynaud, R., Palazzo, F. F., et al. (2010). Limited value of 18F-F-DOPA PET to localize pancreatic insulin-secreting tumors in adults with hyperinsulinemic hypoglycemia. *J. Clin. Endocrinol. Metab.* 95, 303–307.

Thompson, G. B., Service, F. J., Andrews, J. C., Lloyd, R. V., Natt, N., van Heerden, J. A., et al. (2000). Non-insulinoma pancreatogenous hypoglycemia syndrome: an update in 10 surgically treated patients. *Surgery* 128, 937–944.

Thorens, B., Porret, A., Buhler, L., Deng, S. P., Morel, P., and Widmann, C. (1993). Cloning and functional expression of the human islet GLP-1 receptor. Demonstration that exendin-4 is an agonist and exendin-(9-39) an antagonist of the receptor. *Diabetes* 42, 1678–1682.

Waser, B., Beetschen, K., Pellegata, N. S., and Reubi, J. C. (2011). Incretin receptors in non-neoplastic and neoplastic thyroid C cells in rodents and humans: relevance for incretin-based diabetes therapy. *Neuroendocrinology* 94, 291–301.

Wei, Y., and Mojsov, S. (1995). Tissue-specific expression of the human receptor for glucagon-like peptide-I: brain, heart and pancreatic forms have the same deduced amino acid sequences. *FEBS Lett.* 358, 219–224.

Wicki, A., Wild, D., Storch, D., Seemayer, C., Gotthardt, M., Behe, M., et al. (2007). [Lys40(Ahx-DTPA-111In)NH2]-exendin-4 is a highly efficient radiotherapeutic for glucagon-like peptide-1 receptor-targeted therapy for insulinoma. *Clin. Cancer Res.* 13, 3696–3705.

Wiesli, P., Brandle, M., Schmid, C., Krahenbuhl, L., Furrer, J., Keller, U., et al. (2004). Selective arterial calcium stimulation and hepatic venous sampling in the evaluation of hyperinsulinemic hypoglycemia: potential and limitations. *J. Vasc. Interv. Radiol.* 15, 1251–1256.

Wild, D., Behe, M., Wicki, A., Storch, D., Waser, B., Gotthardt, M., et al. (2006). [Lys40(Ahx-DTPA-111In)NH2]exendin-4, a very promising ligand for glucagon-like peptide-1 (GLP-1) receptor targeting. *J. Nucl. Med.* 47, 2025–2033.

Wild, D., Caplin, M., Christ, E., Forrer, F., Brändle, M., Seufert, J., et al. (2011). Glucagon-like peptide-1 vs. somatostatin receptor targeting in malignant insulinomas. *J. Nucl. Med.* 52, 1073–1078.

Wild, D., Christ, E., Forrer, F., Reubi, J. C., Maecke, H., Ell, P. J., et al. (2009). 111In-DTPA-exendin-4 SPECT/CT scans localize hardly detectable insulinomas. *J. Nucl. Med.* 50, 1937.

Wild, D., Mäcke, H., Christ, E., Gloor, B., and Reubi, J. C. (2008). Glucagon-like peptide 1-receptor scans to localize occult insulinomas. *N. Engl. J. Med.* 359, 766–768.

Wild, D., Wicki, A., Mansi, R., Béhé, M., Keil, B., Bernhardt, P., et al. (2010). Exendin-4-based radiopharmaceuticals for glucagons-like peptide-1 (GLP-1) receptor PET/CT and SPECT/CT imaging. *J. Nucl. Med.* 51, 1059–1067.

Wu, Z., Todorov, I., Li, L., Bading, J. R., Li, Z., Nair, I., et al. (2011). In vivo imaging of transplanted islets with 64Cu-DO3A-VS-Cys40-exendin-4 by targeting GLP-1 receptor. *Bioconjug. Chem.* 22, 1587–1594.

Yakovac, W. C., Baker, L., and Hummeler, K. (1971). Beta cell nesidioblastosis in idiopathic hypoglycemia of infancy. *J. Pediatr.* 79, 226–231.

7

Structural and molecular conservation of glucagon-like peptide-1 and its receptor confers selective ligand-receptor interaction

Mi Jin Moon[1], Sumi Park[1], Dong-Kyu Kim[1], Eun Bee Cho[1], Jong-Ik Hwang[1], Hubert Vaudry[2] and Jae Young Seong[1]*

[1] _Graduate School of Medicine, Korea University, Seoul, Republic of Korea_
[2] _INSERM U982, Laboratory of Neuronal and Neuroendocrine Differentiation and Communication, University of Rouen, Mont-Saint-Aignan, France_

Edited by:
Billy K. Chow, University of Hong Kong, China

Reviewed by:
Joao Carlos Dos Reis Cardoso, University of Algarve, Portugal
Charlier Dominique Thierry, University of Liege, Belgium

*Correspondence:
Jae Young Seong, Graduate School of Medicine, Korea University, Seoul 136-705, Republic of Korea.
e-mail: jyseong@korea.ac.kr

Glucagon-like peptide-1 (GLP-1) is a major player in the regulation of glucose homeostasis. It acts on pancreatic beta cells to stimulate insulin secretion and on the brain to inhibit appetite. Thus, it may be a promising therapeutic agent for the treatment of type 2 diabetes mellitus and obesity. Despite the physiological and clinical importance of GLP-1, molecular interaction with the GLP-1 receptor (GLP1R) is not well understood. Particularly, the specific amino acid residues within the transmembrane helices and extracellular loops of the receptor that may confer ligand-induced receptor activation have been poorly investigated. Amino acid sequence comparisons of GLP-1 and GLP1R with their orthologs and paralogs in vertebrates, combined with biochemical approaches, are useful to determine which amino acid residues in the peptide and the receptor confer selective ligand-receptor interaction. This article reviews how the molecular evolution of GLP-1 and GLP1R contributes to the selective interaction between this ligand-receptor pair, providing critical clues for the development of potent agonists for the treatment of diabetes mellitus and obesity.

Keywords: GLP-1, GLP1R, G protein-coupled receptors, evolution, paralog, ortholog, ligand-receptor interaction

INTRODUCTION

Glucagon-like peptide-1 (GLP-1) is an intestinal incretin released in response to nutrient ingestion that stimulates insulin secretion in a glucose-dependent manner. The insulinotropic effect of GLP-1 on the pancreas has been demonstrated to be preserved in animal models of diabetes by stimulating insulin exocytosis (Shen et al., 1998; Drucker, 2001; MacDonald et al., 2002), and promoting insulin biosynthesis (Fehmann and Habener, 1992; Perfetti and Merkel, 2000; Moon et al., 2011). Recently, direct effects of GLP-1 on growth, survival (Xu et al., 1999; Stoffers et al., 2000; List and Habener, 2004), and differentiation of β-cells have been reported (Drucker, 2003). Beside its insulinotropic effects, GLP-1 inhibits glucagon (GCG) secretion in pancreatic α-cells (Nauck et al., 2002), attenuates gastric emptying, and ameliorates glucose excursion in the gastrointestinal tract (Nauck et al., 2002).

GLP-1 exerts its action through the G protein-coupled receptor (GPCR), GLP1R. This receptor belongs to the class B (or secretin-like) GPCR family. This GPCR family has only 15 members in humans and is characterized by a relatively long N-terminal extracellular domain (ECD) containing six conserved Cys residues that form a constraint structure necessary for ligand binding (Couvineau et al., 2004). GLP1R is mainly expressed in pancreatic β-cells, and upon stimulation by GLP-1, it induces the accumulation of cAMP and the influx of intracellular calcium which accelerate insulin release from secretory granules (Drucker et al., 1987; Fehmann et al., 1995).

GLP-1 and GLP1R are also expressed in the central nervous system. GLP-1 is synthesized largely in the brainstem and transported along axonal networks to diverse brain regions, including the hypothalamus (Vrang et al., 2007; Hisadome et al., 2010). GLP1R is expressed in cerebral cortex, hypothalamus, hippocampus, thalamus, caudate-putamen, and globus pallidum (Alvarez et al., 2005). In the brain, GLP-1 is known to reduce appetite, leading to significant reductions in body weight (Zander et al., 2002). In addition, GLP-1 is likely neuroprotective and involved in neurite growth and spatial learning ability in the brain (During et al., 2003; Perry et al., 2007).

Due to its combined beneficial effects, GLP-1 has been identified as a potential therapeutic agent for the treatment of diabetes mellitus and obesity. However, the molecular mechanisms leading to high affinity ligand-receptor binding and receptor activation have not been fully understood. Studies using alanine scanning mutagenesis, substitution/modification, and chimeric peptide construction of GLP-1 have explored the bioactive motifs of GLP-1(Adelhorst et al., 1994; Gallwitz et al., 1994; Hinke et al., 2004), yet none have been able to identify the mechanism through which individual residues in the peptide interact with residues in the receptor. Recent studies using X-ray crystallography have demonstrated that residues in the central α-helical region of GLP-1

Abbreviations: Bpa, *p*-benzoyl-L-phenyl alanine; CRFR, CRF receptor; Cys, cysteine; ECD, extracellular domain; ECL, extracellular loop; ER, endoplasmic reticulum; GCG, glucagon; GCGR, glucagon receptor; GIP, glucose-dependent insulinotropic polypeptide; GIPR, GIP receptor; GLP-1, glucagon-like peptide-1; GLP1R, GLP-1 receptor; GPCR, G protein-coupled receptor; PAC1R, PACAP receptor; PTHR, PTH receptor; TMH, transmembrane helix.

interact with residues in the N-terminal ECD of GLP1R (Runge et al., 2008; Underwood et al., 2010). However, as ligand-induced receptor activation is mainly governed by interactions between residues in the N-terminus of the peptide and residues within the transmembrane helices (TMH) and extracellular loops (ECL) of the receptor (Thorens et al., 1993; During et al., 2003), this crystal structure only accounts for the peptide binding to the ECD of the receptor. Indeed, virtually no progress has been made in exploring the receptor binding sites for the N-terminal moiety of the peptide which is responsible for ligand-induced receptor activation.

Peptide ligands and their receptors have become diversified through evolutionary processes that ultimately yield families of related, yet distinct, peptides and receptors (Hoyle, 1999; Cho et al., 2007; Lee et al., 2009; Kim et al., 2011, 2012). Specific diversification of peptides, conservation within orthologs but variation among paralogs, would often confer the selective interaction with their cognate receptors, allowing discrimination of paralogous receptors (Acharjee et al., 2004; Wang et al., 2004; Li et al., 2005). Thus, amino acid sequence comparison of the peptide and receptor with their orthologs and paralogs, along with mutational mapping approaches, are useful tools helping to determine specific residues in the peptide ligands and receptors that are essential for maintaining selective ligand-receptor interaction. Indeed, ligand binding domains identified in mammalian receptors are highly conserved in orthologous non-mammalian receptors, indicating that there is high evolutionary selection pressure to maintain selectivity for their ligands (Acharjee et al., 2004; Wang et al., 2004; Li et al., 2005). Recently, we reported that evolutionarily conserved amino acid residues in GLP-1 and core domains of the GLP1R confer selective ligand-receptor interaction and receptor activation (Moon et al., 2010, 2012). This article reviews how the molecular evolution of GLP-1 and GLP1R contributes to acquiring high affinity interaction between this peptide ligand and receptor.

GENERAL STRUCTURE OF GLP-1 AND ITS FAMILY PEPTIDES

GLP-1 is a product of the *GCG* gene which encodes a common GCG-GLP-1-GLP-2 precursor. All three peptides are encoded by different exons of the *GCG* gene, raising the possibility of exon duplications during early vertebrate evolution (Sherwood et al., 2000). The *GCG* gene produces one or two mature peptides by a tissue-specific alternative post-translational process (Kieffer and Habener, 1999; Irwin, 2001, 2009). For instance, in pancreatic α-cells mature GCG, but not GLP-1 and GLP-2, is produced. In intestinal L cells, however, mature GLP-1 and GLP-2, but not GCG, are generated. One GLP-1 paralog is the glucose-dependent insulinotropic polypeptide (GIP) which is independently encoded by the *GIP* gene (McIntosh et al., 2009). GLP-1 and GIP share a high degree of amino acid sequence identity, particularly in their N-terminal moiety, and function similarly by inducing insulin secretion from β-cells. However, these peptides act through distinct yet related receptors, GLP1R and GIP receptor (GIPR), respectively. In addition, albeit absent in mammals, another GLP-1 paralog is exendin, which was first discovered in Gila monsters (*Heloderma suspectum*; Göke et al., 1993). Recently, the full-length and/or partial cDNAs for exendin were characterized in a few species, such as *Xenopus*, chicken, and Gila monster (Irwin and Prentice, 2011). Although the receptor for exendin has not yet been identified in non-mammals, exendin exhibits high affinity binding for mammalian GLP1R (Göke et al., 1993). Recent evidence suggests that the *GCG*, *GIP*, and *exendin* genes were generated by genome duplication events during early vertebrate evolution, as these genes are flanked by similar neighboring genes in the genomes of vertebrates (Irwin, 2002; Irwin and Prentice, 2011).

GLP-1 and its family peptides are 30 ~ 40 amino acids in length and share similarities in amino acid sequence and secondary structure. All these peptides tend to be disordered in aqueous solutions but exhibit a marked propensity to form α-helices under mild ambient conditions, such as in the presence of organic solvents or lipids (Braun et al., 1983; Gronenborn et al., 1987; Thornton and Gorenstein, 1994; Inooka et al., 2001; Neidigh et al., 2001; Chang et al., 2002; Tan et al., 2006; Alana et al., 2007), or upon crystallization (Sasaki et al., 1975). It is now well known that the N-terminal domains of GLP-1-related peptides form a random coil structure, while the central parts of these peptides have an α-helical structure. In addition, hydrophobic amino acids at positions 6 and 10, and a short-chain polar amino acid at position 7 form a helix N-capping motif through hydrophobic interaction and hydrogen bonding (Neumann et al., 2008). This capping motif is believed to introduce a specific local fold that facilitates receptor activation upon peptide-receptor binding (Neumann et al., 2008).

The N-terminus of GLP-1 and its family peptides share a high degree of sequence identity (**Figure 1**). Particularly, Gly^4, Thr/Ser^5, Phe^6, and Asp/Glu^9 are conserved across all GLP-1 paralogs. Indeed, alanine scanning of these conserved residues of GLP-1 suggest that positions 4, 6, and 9 are crucial for either maintaining secondary structure of the peptide or for interaction with the receptor (Adelhorst et al., 1994; Gallwitz et al., 1994). His^1 and Thr/Ser^7 are common for most GLP-1 paralogs except for GIP, which has Tyr^1 and Ile^7 in these positions. Our recent observation using a chimeric GLP-1/GIP peptide revealed that His/Tyr^1 and Thr/Ile^7 are responsible for the selective interaction toward GLP1R and GIPR (Moon et al., 2010). The second position of the peptides is highly variable across paralogs, even within orthologs of vertebrates, and it is known to be of lesser importance for receptor binding. This residue can be modified to Ser or another amino acid to confer protection against cleavage by dipeptidyl peptidase IV (Hinke et al., 2002). The third position of the peptides is variable across paralogs but conserved within orthologs. Although the importance of this ortholog-specific third residue in receptor binding or peptide structure is not fully understood, Glu^3 of GIP is known to be critical for receptor interaction (Hinke et al., 2003; Gault et al., 2007; Yaqub et al., 2010).

The sequence similarity of the α-helix domain of the peptides is not pronounced among GLP-1 paralogs, and there are also many variable residues within orthologs (**Figure 1**). However, the Phe^{22}, Ile/Val^{23}, and Leu^{26} residues that are part of the hydrophobic surface of the α-helix are highly conserved among GLP-1 and its paralogs. Interestingly, all these residues are known to interact with highly conserved residues in the ECD of the GLP1R and its paralogs (Parthier et al., 2007; Runge et al., 2008; Underwood et al., 2010). Some ortholog-conserved residues, Glu/Asp^{15} of exendin and GIP, along with $Ala^{18/19}$ and Lys^{20} of GLP-1, are found to interact with the receptors as was revealed by the peptide-bound

Peptides	1 10 20 30 40
GLP-1	HAEGTFTSDVSSYLEGQAAKEFIAWLVKGR
Exendin	HGEGTFTSDLSKQMEEEAVRLFIEWLKNGGPSSGAPPPS
GLP-2	HADGSFSDEMNTILDNLAARDFINWLIQTKITD
Glucagon	HSQGTFTSDYSKYLDSRRAQDFVQWLMNT
GIP	YAEGTFISDYSIAMDKIHQQDFVNWLLAQKGKKNDWKHNITQ

conserved across paralogs
conserved within orthologs
variable
interacting with the receptor

FIGURE 1 | Amino acid sequence alignment of GLP-1 and its family peptides. Amino acid sequences of human GLP-1, GLP-2, glucagon, GIP, and Gila monster exendin are aligned. Residues in red are conserved sequences within orthologs of vertebrates including mouse, anole, chicken, *Xenopus tropicalis*, medaka, fugu, tetraodon, stickleback, and zebrafish. The residues colored in blue represent conserved sequences across paralogs. The residues in black are variable sequences. Underlines indicate the α-helical conformation. The residues responsible for interaction with their receptor are shaded.

ECD crystal structures (Parthier et al., 2007; Runge et al., 2008; Underwood et al., 2010).

GENERAL STRUCTURE OF CLASS B GPCRs

The class B GPCR family is composed of 15 members including receptors for VIP, PACAP, secretin, GCG, GLP-1, GLP-2, GHRH, GIP, PTH, calcitonin, calcitonin gene-related peptide, and CRH (Laburthe et al., 2007). This family shares the general GPCR architecture: seven TMH interconnected by intracellular loops with a C-terminal intracellular domain. Class B GPCRs differ from class A rhodopsin-like GPCRs in the structures of their TMH. The TMH of class B GPCRs do not contain conserved amino acid residues such as Asp/Asn$^{2.50}$ in TMH2, Asn/Asp$^{7.49}$-Pro$^{7.50}$-x-x-Tyr$^{7.53}$ (N/DPxxY) motif in TMH7, Asp/Glu$^{3.49}$-Arg$^{3.50}$-Tyr/Trp$^{3.51}$ (D/ERY/W) motif at the junction between TMH3 and intracellular loop 2 that are commonly found in class A rhodopsin-like GPCRs (Oh et al., 2005). Instead, class B receptors share a high degree of amino acid identity in TMH with one another. Further, they possess a large and structured N-terminal ECD of ~120 residues.

Although no experimentally determined full-length class B receptor structure has been achieved to date, the structure elucidation of individual class B GPCR ECDs represents considerable progress toward a molecular understanding of their action. The first structure of the agonist-bound recombinant N-terminal ECD of the CRH2B receptor has been resolved using NMR (Grace et al., 2004). Six representative ECD structures of the class B family of GPCRs have been determined by X-ray crystallography or NMR spectroscopy in complex with bound ligand: the human VPAC1 receptor (Tan et al., 2006), a subtype of human PACAP receptor (PAC1R$_S$; Sun et al., 2007), human GIPR (Parthier et al., 2007), human GLP1R (Runge et al., 2008; Underwood et al., 2010), human PTH receptor (PTH1R; Pioszak and Xu, 2008), the human type-1 CRF receptor (CRFR1; Pioszak et al., 2008), and human GLP2R (Venneti and Hewage, 2011).

Class B GPCRs contain N-terminal signal peptides that are cleaved off by the signal peptidase of the endoplasmic reticulum (ER) during the translocation-mediated receptor insertion into the ER membrane. These signal peptides play a crucial role in the membrane expression of receptors (Couvineau et al., 2004; Alken et al., 2005; Huang et al., 2010). After cleavage of the signal peptide, the N-terminal helix at the beginning of the ECD and four β-strands forming two antiparallel sheets remain (**Figure 2**). Three disulfide bonds formed by a set of six Cys residues lock these secondary structural elements together. Cysteine residues are completely conserved across the receptors. The disulfide bond pattern seems to be conserved in all receptors, suggesting a similar three dimensional structure. There are three disulfide bonds between the first and third, the second and fifth, and the fourth and sixth cysteine residues (Cys^1-Cys^3, Cys^2-Cys^5, Cys^4-Cys^6). The first bond (Cys^1-Cys^3) links the N-terminal α-helix to the first β-sheet. The second (Cys^2-Cys^5) connects the two β-sheets, whereas the third disulfide bond (Cys^4-Cys^6) holds the C-terminus of the domain in close proximity to the central β-sheets (Tan et al., 2006; Parthier et al., 2007, 2009; Sun et al., 2007; Pioszak and Xu, 2008; Pioszak et al., 2008; Runge et al., 2008; Underwood et al., 2010; Venneti and Hewage, 2011).

In addition, this core folding is further stabilized by a salt bridge involving acidic and basic residues flanked by hydrophobic aromatic residues. This fold, called the Sushi domain, is conserved in all class B GPCRs (Grace et al., 2004). Five additional residues, Asp^{67}, Trp^{72}, Pro^{86}, Gly^{108}, and Trp^{110} in GLP1R and the corresponding residues in class B GPCRs, are conserved. Particularly, Asp and the two Trp residues take part in forming the Sushi domain, suggesting that these residues are crucial for domain stability and ligand binding. The strongly conserved fold observed in the ECD of class B GPCRs suggests that a common mechanism underlies ligand recognition.

The crystal structures of the ligand-bound ECD reveal amino acid residues that interact with their cognate ligands (Parthier et al., 2007; Runge et al., 2008; Underwood et al., 2010). It is of interest to note that many ligand-interacting residues are highly conserved between GLP1R and its paralogs. For instance, Trp^{39} in the α1-helix, Asp^{67} in the β1-sheet, Tyr^{69} between the β1- and β2-sheet, Arg^{121} near TMH1 of GLP1R, residues 87–90 (Tyr-Leu-Pro-Trp) between the β3- and β4-sheet, Arg^{101} in the β4-sheet, and Trp^{112} near TMH1 of GIPR are all highly conserved across paralogs (**Figure 2**). There are also ortholog-specific residues that interact with the peptide ligands, such as Leu^{32} in the α1-helix of GLP1R, and Gly^{110} and His^{115} near TMH1 of GIPR.

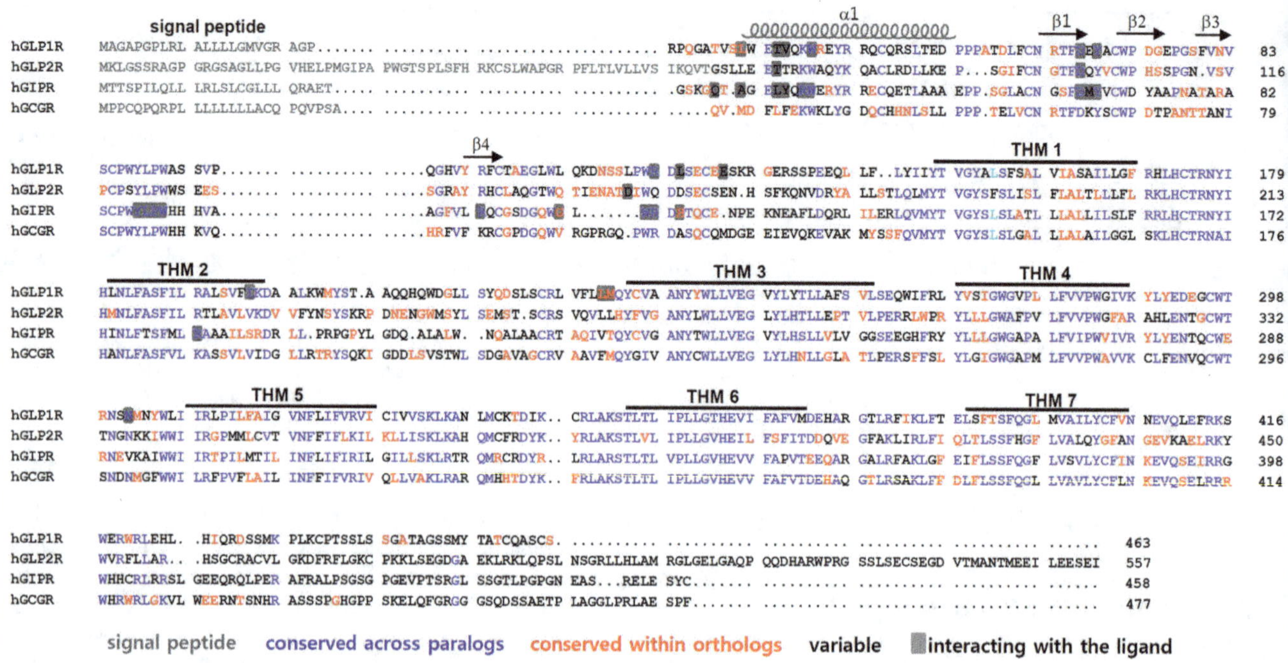

FIGURE 2 | Amino acid sequence alignment of GLP1R and its paralogous receptors. Amino acid sequences of human GLP1R, GLP2R, GCGR, and GIPR are compared. The signal peptides are indicated in gray. The residues colored in blue represent conserved sequences across the GLP-1-related peptide receptors. Residues in red are conserved sequences within orthologs of vertebrates such as mouse, anole, chicken, *Xenopus tropicalis*, medaka, fugu, tetraodon, stickleback, and zebrafish. The residues in black are variable sequences. The amino acid residues that interact with their peptides are shaded. The α-helix, β-sheets, and TMH domains of GLP1R are indicated.

THE TWO-DOMAIN HYPOTHESIS FOR CLASS B GPCR LIGAND BINDING AND ACTIVATION

Class B GPCRs likely share a similar secondary and tertiary structure with long N-terminal ECD and highly conserved TMHs. The orientation and mechanism of interaction of the peptide with their receptors has been investigated in studies using fragmented peptide/receptor, and chimeric peptides and receptors (Holtmann et al., 1995; Stroop et al., 1995; Bergwitz et al., 1996; Laburthe and Couvineau, 2002; Runge et al., 2003). For instance, the GLP1R ECD itself is able to bind with its peptide ligands (Graziano et al., 1996; Van Eyll et al., 1996; Wilmen et al., 1996, 1997; Runge et al., 2003; Parthier et al., 2007). This binding, however, may not account for ligand-induced receptor activation (Buggy et al., 1995; Holtmann et al., 1995, 1996; Hjorth and Schwartz, 1996; Xiao et al., 2000). The N-terminally truncated exendin(9–39) is unable to activate GLP1R even though it binds to the receptor with an affinity that is comparable to that of wild type exendin (Thorens et al., 1993). In contrast, exendin(1–9), a short N-terminal fragment of exendin, is able to activate GLP1R although its affinity to the receptor is quite low (During et al., 2003). Likewise, the GIP fragment, GIP (7–30), is able to bind to GIPR with high affinity but fails to induce receptor activation. In contrast, GIP (1–14) exhibits a very low affinity toward the receptor but fully activates the receptor at a micromolar concentration (Hinke et al., 2001, 2003; Gault et al., 2007). Thus, the two-domain model explaining ligand binding followed by receptor activation has emerged: the central α-helical and C-terminal portion of the peptide binds to the N-terminal ECD of the receptor (Al-Sabah and Donnelly, 2003; Dong et al., 2003; Lopez de Maturana et al., 2003) followed by binding of the N-terminal moiety of the peptide with the core domain – including the TMH and ECL – of the receptor, conferring receptor activation and G protein coupling (Runge et al., 2003; Lopez de Maturana et al., 2004; Castro et al., 2005; Wittelsberger et al., 2006). The two-domain model is generally consistent with photoaffinity crosslinking studies of several class B receptors. With a few exceptions, photoreactive side chains in the C-terminus of the peptide ligand interact with residues in the ECD of the receptor whereas photoreactive side chains in the N-terminus of the ligand bind to the TMH domain (Gensure et al., 2001; Assil-Kishawi and Abou-Samra, 2002; Dong and Miller, 2002; Dong et al., 2004). Most recently, strong corroborating evidence for the two-domain model has been obtained by the structural characterization of the isolated ECDs of several class B GPCRs (Grace et al., 2004; Parthier et al., 2007; Sun et al., 2007; Pioszak and Xu, 2008; Pioszak et al., 2008; Runge et al., 2008; Underwood et al., 2010).

MOLECULAR EVOLUTION OF GLP-1 AND GLP1R FOR THEIR SELECTIVE INTERACTION

Although GLP-1 and its paralogs share a high degree of sequence identity and structural similarly, they generally exhibit specific binding to their own cognate receptors with little cross-reactivity with paralogous receptors (Runge et al., 2003; Moon et al., 2010, 2012). This observation allows us to presume the presence of distinct amino acid residues within each peptide and receptor that allows for the selective interaction with their own partners. Further, these facts indicate that evolutionary selection pressure has exerted a specific diversification of peptide and receptor: variation among paralogs but conservation within orthologs. However, there are some exceptional cross-reactivities among paralogous partners. For instance, exendin, a GLP-1 paralog in non-mammals, has a high affinity for the mammalian GLP1R (Göke et al., 1993). Until now, genetic orthologs for GLP1R have not been found in teleost fish, yet teleost fish have two copies of GLP-1 peptides which have been generated by teleost-specific genome duplication (Plisetskaya and Mommsen, 1996; Irwin and Wong, 2005). Interestingly, GLP-1 is able to activate fish GCG receptor (GCGR) orthologs (Yeung et al., 2002; Irwin and Wong, 2005), indicating that fish GCGRs have achieved functional response to GLP-1 through an evolutionary process. These exceptional cross-reactivities provide a unique opportunity to explore the identification of specific amino acid residues in the peptides and receptors responsible for specific ligand-receptor interaction. For instance, amino acid sequence comparison between GLP-1 and exendin allows us to predict which amino acid residues are important for the activation of GLP1R (Moon et al., 2010). Sequence comparison between tetrapod GLP1Rs and fish GCGRs has led to the identification of residues in these receptors that interact with GLP-1 (Moon et al., 2012).

INTERACTION BETWEEN THE α-HELIX OF THE PEPTIDE AND THE ECD OF THE RECEPTOR

The crystal structures of the ligand-bound ECD revealed that GLP-1 is a continuous α-helix from Thr^{7} to Val^{27}, with a kink around Gly^{16}. Only the residues between Ala^{18} and Val^{27} interact with the ECD. The α-helical segment of GLP-1 is amphiphilic, allowing hydrophilic and hydrophobic interactions through opposite faces of the α-helix (Underwood et al., 2010). The hydrophilic face of GLP-1 comprises residues Gln^{17}, Lys^{20}, Glu^{21}, and Lys^{28}, of which only Lys^{20} interacts directly with the ECD by forming a hydrogen bond with the side chain of Glu^{128}. Interestingly, exendin also possesses a basic residue at position 20 (Arg^{20}), allowing interaction with Glu^{128} of the GLP1R ECD (Runge et al., 2008; Underwood et al., 2010). The hydrophobic face of GLP-1 includes Ala^{18}, Ala^{19}, Phe^{22}, Ile^{23}, Leu^{26}, and Val^{27}. The hydrophobic residues are exposed toward the complementary hydrophobic binding pocket in the ECD. Particularly, Phe^{22}, Ile^{23}, and Leu^{26} of the peptide are found to interact with the highly conserved residues Val^{36}, Trp^{39}, Asp^{67}, Tyr^{69}, Arg^{121}, and Leu^{123} in the ECD of GLP1R (Underwood et al., 2010). The contribution of Phe^{22}, Ile^{23}, and Leu^{26} to GLP1R binding has been demonstrated by Ala substitutions or mutations of these residues (Adelhorst et al., 1994; Wilmen et al., 1997). It is of interest to note that the GLP-1 family peptides exendin, GIP, GLP-2, and GCG also contain hydrophobic residues Phe^{22}, Ile/Va^{23}, and Leu^{26}. Further, residues Trp^{39}, Asp^{67}, Tyr^{69}, and Arg^{121} in the GLP1R ECD are also highly conserved in GLP2R, GIPR, and GCGR (Parthier et al., 2007; Runge et al., 2008; Underwood et al., 2010; Venneti and Hewage, 2011). This observation suggests that these residues are evolutionarily conserved and likely contribute to the primary binding between the α-helix of the peptides and ECD of the receptors. This may also in part account for the cross-interaction of one α-helix of the peptide with the ECD of other partners (Parthier et al., 2007; Runge et al., 2008; Underwood et al., 2010). Indeed, this is supported by the observations that chimeric peptides containing the GLP-1 N-terminus with the α-helix of GIP or GCG can induce GLP1R activation with a relatively high potency (Runge et al., 2003; Moon et al., 2010). However, the specific interaction of the α-helix of the peptide with the ECD of its own receptor may be of higher affinity than those with other related paralogous receptors. For instance, interaction of Ala^{19} of GLP-1 with GLP1R-specific Leu^{32}, and Gln^{19} of GIP with GIPR-specific Ala^{32}, may explain the higher affinity of each peptide toward its own receptor than toward paralogous receptors (Parthier et al., 2007; Underwood et al., 2010).

INTERACTIONS BETWEEN THE N-TERMINUS OF THE PEPTIDE AND THE CORE DOMAIN OF THE RECEPTOR

Specificity of ligand-receptor binding between a peptide and the corresponding receptor can be further conferred by binding between the N-terminus of the peptide and the receptor core domain. In addition, this interaction allows ligand-induced receptor activation (Thorens et al., 1993; Montrose-Rafizadeh et al., 1997; Hinke et al., 2001, 2003; During et al., 2003; Gault et al., 2007). Therefore, many approaches, such as alanine scanning, photoaffinity labeling, and molecular modeling-based approaches have explored the specific residues within the peptide and receptor responsible for ligand-receptor interaction (Adelhorst et al., 1994; Gallwitz et al., 1994; Xiao et al., 2000; Lopez de Maturana and Donnelly, 2002; Lopez de Maturana et al., 2004; Chen et al., 2009, 2010; Lin and Wang, 2009). Alanine scanning of GLP1R demonstrated that residues found between the TMH2 and ECL1 including Lys^{197}, Asp^{198}, Lys^{202}, Met^{204}, Tyr^{205}, Asp^{215}, and Arg^{227} are likely important for the binding of the receptor to the N-terminal moiety of GLP-1, as mutations at these residues lead to a significant decrease in ligand affinity (Xiao et al., 2000; Lopez de Maturana and Donnelly, 2002; Lopez de Maturana et al., 2004). However, these observations did not define how these individual residues interact with in the N-terminal moiety of GLP-1. Further, Ala mutations in these residues can modify the receptor conformation which may interfere with binding to the ligand. Recently, using photoaffinity labeling, Chen et al. (2010) observed that Tyr^{205} in ECL1 is in close proximity to the *p*-benzoyl-L-phenyl alanine (Bpa) at position 6 of GLP-1. However, the mutation of Tyr^{205} to Ala in GLP1R does not alter either receptor activity or ligand binding, indicating that Tyr^{205} is not the direct binding site for the N-terminal moiety of GLP-1. Furthermore, no ligand-bound crystal structure for the core domain of the class B GPCR family is currently available. Thus, our understanding of the molecular mechanism underlying the high affinity interaction between the N-terminal moiety of the peptide and the receptor core domain is primitive.

Recently, by comparing the amino acid sequences of GLP-1 and GLP1R with their orthologs and paralogs in vertebrates, we were able to obtain clues to help determine which amino acid residues may be responsible for ligand-receptor interaction (Moon et al., 2010, 2012). Although the GLP-1-related family of peptides shares a similarity in the amino acid sequence at the N-terminal moiety, there are specific, divergent amino acid sequences. For instance, the N-terminus of GLP-1 and its family peptides starts with either His^{1} (for GCG, GLP-1, GLP-2, and exendin) or Tyr^{1} (for GIP), and most of the peptides contain Thr at position 7 (GCG, GLP-1, and exendin), or Ser (GLP-2); only GIP contains Ile at this position. The first and seventh amino acid residues of each peptide are conserved within orthologs of vertebrate species. Thus, it may be postulated that His/Tyr^1 or Thr/Ile^7 residues of GLP-1 and GIP confer ligand selectivity to their cognate receptors. Indeed, our recent observation using chimeric GLP-1/GIP peptide reveals that the His/Tyr^1 and Thr/Ile^7 residues within these peptides confer differential ligand selectivity toward GIPR and GLP1R, respectively (Moon et al., 2010).

The chimeric GLP1R/GIPR approach together with chimeric GLP-1/GIP peptides offers a new strategy to determine which residues in the core domain are responsible for interacting with His^1 and Thr^7 of GLP-1 (Moon et al., 2012). For example, this approach enables us to determine crude motifs in TMH2, ECL1, and ECL2 of GLP1R which are likely to interact with His^1 and Thr^7 of GLP-1. Amino acid sequence comparison of these regions between those of tetrapod GLP1Rs, fish GCGRs, and vertebrate GIPRs further define amino acid residues that tentatively interact with His^1 and Thr^7 of GLP-1. In this case, we searched for residues which are conserved within GLP1R ortholog and fish GCGR but are different from those of GIPRs. We were able to identify Ile^{196} and Lys^{197} of TMH2, and Met^{233} of ECL1, and Asn^{302} and Met^{30} of ECL2 in GLP1R (Moon et al., 2012). It is noteworthy that fish GCGRs exhibit both a significantly high affinity for GLP-1 (Irwin and Wong, 2005) and these conserved residues, even though other regions are significantly different from tetrapod GLP1R (**Figure 3**). Mutational mapping together with application of chimeric GLP-1/GIP peptides reveals that His^1-harboring peptides are sensitive for Asn^{302} mutations, while Thr^7-containing chimeric peptides are highly sensitive for the Ile^{196} mutation, indicating a possible interaction of His^1 and Thr^7 of GLP-1 with Asn^{302} and Ile^{196} of GLP1R, respectively. Indeed, computer-aided molecular modeling showed interaction of His^1 with Asn^{302} and of Thr^7 with a binding pocket formed by Ile^{196}, Leu^{232}, and Met^{233} of GLP1R (Moon et al., 2012). Interestingly, Asn^{302} is highly conserved at the corresponding position in GCGRs (Asn^{300} for human) and GLP2Rs (Asn^{336} for human), and these receptors have peptide ligands containing His^1. In addition, GCGRs that respond to a Thr^7-containing peptide ligands have conserved Val^{193} and Met^{23} at the corresponding positions of Ile^{196}, and Met^{233} of GLP1R indicating that these residues may have a contact with Thr^7 of GCG. This possibility, however, needs to be further addressed.

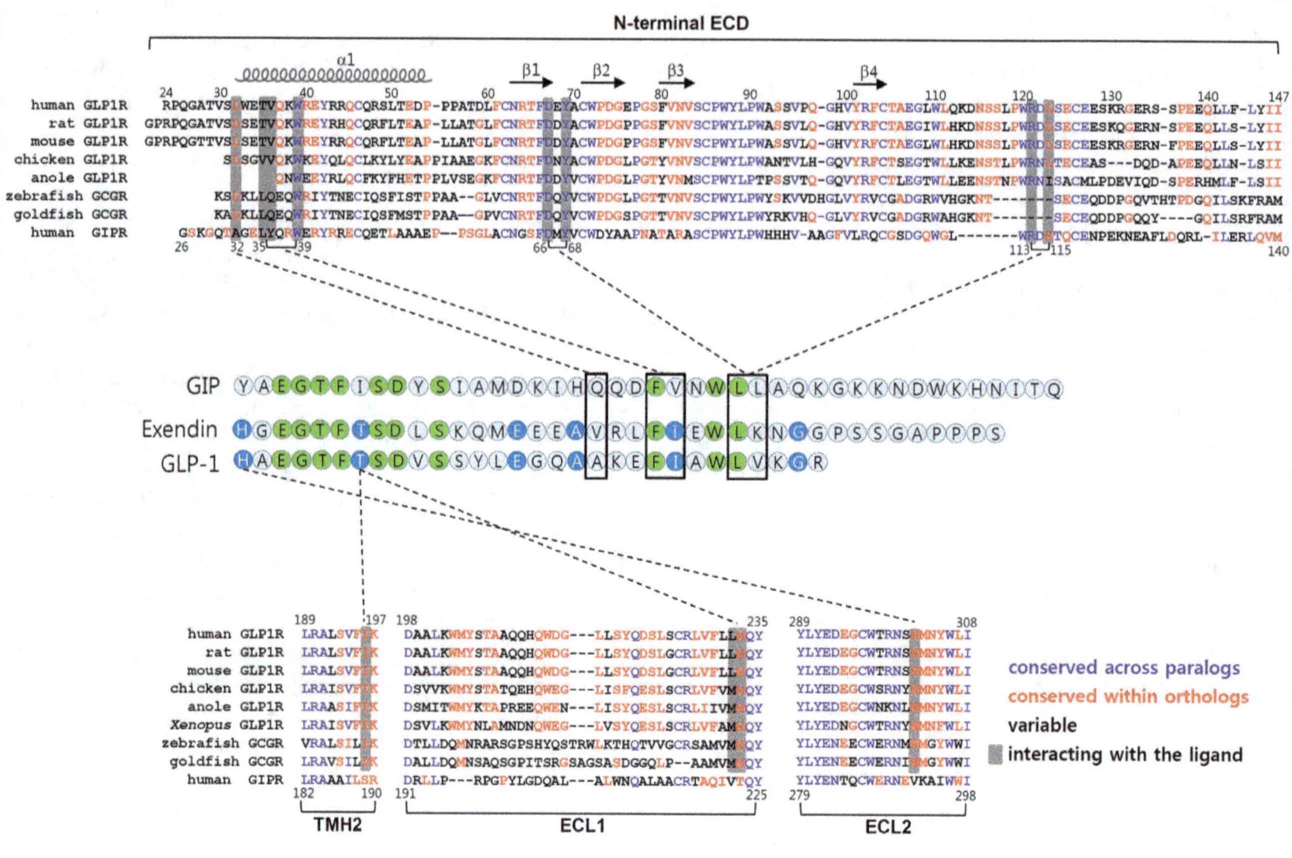

FIGURE 3 | Molecular interaction between GLP-1 and GLP1R. The amino acid sequences of the N-terminal ECD, TMH2, ECL1, and ECL2 of vertebrate GLP1Rs, fish GCGRs (which are known to bind GLP-1), and human GIPR are shown in top and bottom panels. The residues in blue are conserved between GLP1Rs and GIPR. Residues shown in red are conserved sequences within the orthologous receptor of vertebrates. The residues in black are variable sequences. The amino acid residues that interact with their peptides are shaded. Amino acid sequence alignment of GLP-1, exendin, and GIP are shown in the middle. Residues which are identical among three peptides are in green. Residues common for GLP-1 and exendin are in blue. The interaction between peptides and receptors are indicated by dotted lines.

CONCLUSION

Although GLP-1 may become a promising therapeutic agent for the treatment of type 2 diabetes mellitus and obesity, these peptide agonists cannot be administered orally due to their peptide nature. Thus, orally administered small molecules that regulate GLP1R need to be developed. However, a bottleneck slowing the development of these small molecules is the lack of information regarding the molecular structure of the ligand-bound GLP1R. Unfortunately, the crystal structure of the ligand-bound N-terminal ECD of GLP1R may not fully account for the interaction between peptide ligands and receptors. Rather, it is likely that the seven TMHs and ECLs of the receptors are more critical than the N-terminal ECD for peptide binding and receptor activation. Thus, exploring the domains or amino acid residues within TMHs and ECLs that confer ligand binding and receptor activation may greatly contribute to the design of the molecular model for the peptide ligand-receptor complex. In turn, this would facilitate the development of potent small molecules capable of regulating GLP1R. Determination of ligand-receptor interaction points (either by ligand-bound ECD crystal structure or by biochemical analysis using chimeric peptides and receptors) demonstrates that conserved residues across paralogous peptides tend to interact with conserved residues among the paralogous receptors while the same can be said of conserved residues within orthologous peptides that likely interact with conserved residues within orthologous receptors. Thus, evolutionary conservation across ortholog and specific diversification within paralogs may be required for maintaining the selective interaction of a peptide ligand with its cognate receptor. The crystal structure of ligand-bound GLP1R ECD explains how residues between Ala^{18} and Val^{27} interact with the ECD. Biochemical studies using chimeric peptides and receptors reveal receptor contact points only at His^{1} and Thr^{7}. Thus, the residues between the N-terminus through to position 17 of GLP-1 remain to be explored for their impact on binding to the receptor. Comparative biochemical approaches combined with computer-aided molecular modeling will discover additional residues in the peptide and receptor sequences that help understanding the high affinity binding interaction between the ligand-receptor pair.

ACKNOWLEDGMENTS

This work was supported by grants (2011K00277) from the Brain Research Center of the 21st Century Frontier Research Program, the Brain Research Program of the National Research Foundation of Korea (NRF) funded by the Ministry of Education.

REFERENCES

Acharjee, S., Do-Rego, J. L., Oh, D. Y., Ahn, R. S., Choe, H., Vaudry, H., et al. (2004). Identification of amino acid residues that direct differential ligand selectivity of mammalian and nonmammalian V1a type receptors for arginine vasopressin and vasotocin. Insights into molecular coevolution of V1a type receptors and their ligands. *J. Biol. Chem.* 279, 54445–54453.

Adelhorst, K., Hedegaard, B. B., Knudsen, L. B., and Kirk, O. (1994). Structure-activity studies of glucagon-like peptide-1. *J. Biol. Chem.* 269, 6275–6278.

Alana, I., Malthouse, J. P., O'Harte, F. P., and Hewage, C. M. (2007). The bioactive conformation of glucose-dependent insulinotropic polypeptide by NMR and CD spectroscopy. *Proteins* 68, 92–99.

Alken, M., Rutz, C., Kochl, R., Donalies, U., Oueslati, M., Furkert, J., et al. (2005). The signal peptide of the rat corticotropin-releasing factor receptor 1 promotes receptor expression but is not essential for establishing a functional receptor. *Biochem. J.* 390, 455–464.

Al-Sabah, S., and Donnelly, D. (2003). A model for receptor-peptide binding at the glucagon-like peptide-1 (GLP-1) receptor through the analysis of truncated ligands and receptors. *Br. J. Pharmacol.* 140, 339–346.

Alvarez, E., Martinez, M. D., Roncero, I., Chowen, J. A., Garcia-Cuartero, B., Gispert, J. D., et al. (2005). The expression of GLP-1 receptor mRNA and protein allows the effect of GLP-1 on glucose metabolism in the human hypothalamus and brainstem. *J. Neurochem.* 92, 798–806.

Assil-Kishawi, I., and Abou-Samra, A. B. (2002). Sauvagine cross-links to the second extracellular loop of the corticotropin-releasing factor type 1 receptor. *J. Biol. Chem.* 277, 32558–32561.

Bergwitz, C., Gardella, T. J., Flannery, M. R., Potts, J. T. Jr., Kronenberg, H. M., Goldring, S. R., et al. (1996). Full activation of chimeric receptors by hybrids between parathyroid hormone and calcitonin. Evidence for a common pattern of ligand-receptor interaction. *J. Biol. Chem.* 271, 26469–26472.

Braun, W., Wider, G., Lee, K. H., and Wuthrich, K. (1983). Conformation of glucagon in a lipid-water interphase by 1H nuclear magnetic resonance. *J. Mol. Biol.* 169, 921–948.

Buggy, J. J., Livingston, J. N., Rabin, D. U., and Yoo-Warren, H. (1995). Glucagon.glucagon-like peptide I receptor chimeras reveal domains that determine specificity of glucagon binding. *J. Biol. Chem.* 270, 7474–7478.

Castro, M., Nikolaev, V. O., Palm, D., Lohse, M. J., and Vilardaga, J. P. (2005). Turn-on switch in parathyroid hormone receptor by a two-step parathyroid hormone binding mechanism. *Proc. Natl. Acad. Sci. U.S.A.* 102, 16084–16089.

Chang, X., Keller, D., O'Donoghue, S. I., and Led, J. J. (2002). NMR studies of the aggregation of glucagon-like peptide-1: formation of a symmetric helical dimer. *FEBS Lett.* 515, 165–170.

Chen, Q., Pinon, D. I., Miller, L. J., and Dong, M. (2009). Molecular basis of glucagon-like peptide 1 docking to its intact receptor studied with carboxyl-terminal photolabile probes. *J. Biol. Chem.* 284, 34135–34144.

Chen, Q., Pinon, D. I., Miller, L. J., and Dong, M. (2010). Spatial approximations between residues 6 and 12 in the amino-terminal region of glucagon-like peptide 1 and its receptor: a region critical for biological activity. *J. Biol. Chem.* 285, 24508–24518.

Cho, H. J., Acharjee, S., Moon, M. J., Oh, D. Y., Vaudry, H., Kwon, H. B., et al. (2007). Molecular evolution of neuropeptide receptors with regard to maintaining high affinity to their authentic ligands. *Gen. Comp. Endocrinol.* 153, 98–107.

Couvineau, A., Rouyer-Fessard, C., and Laburthe, M. (2004). Presence of a N-terminal signal peptide in class II G protein-coupled receptors: crucial role for expression of the human VPAC1 receptor. *Regul. Pept.* 123, 181–185.

Dong, M., Li, Z., Zang, M., Pinon, D. I., Lybrand, T. P., and Miller, L. J. (2003). Spatial approximation between two residues in the mid-region of secretin and the amino terminus of its receptor. Incorporation of seven sets of such constraints into a three-dimensional model of the agonist-bound secretin receptor. *J. Biol. Chem.* 278, 48300–48312.

Dong, M., and Miller, L. J. (2002). Molecular pharmacology of the secretin receptor. *Recept. Channels* 8, 189–200.

Dong, M., Pinon, D. I., Cox, R. F., and Miller, L. J. (2004). Importance of the amino terminus in secretin family G protein-coupled receptors. Intrinsic photoaffinity labeling establishes initial docking constraints for the calcitonin receptor. *J. Biol. Chem.* 279, 1167–1175.

Drucker, D. J. (2001). Minireview: the glucagon-like peptides. *Endocrinology* 142, 521–527.

Drucker, D. J. (2003). Glucagon-like peptides: regulators of cell proliferation, differentiation, and apoptosis. *Mol. Endocrinol.* 17, 161–171.

Drucker, D. J., Philippe, J., Mojsov, S., Chick, W. L., and Habener, J. F. (1987). Glucagon-like peptide I stimulates insulin gene expression and increases cyclic AMP levels in a rat islet cell line. *Proc. Natl. Acad. Sci. U.S.A.* 84, 3434–3438.

During, M. J., Cao, L., Zuzga, D. S., Francis, J. S., Fitzsimons, H. L., Jiao, X., et al. (2003). Glucagon-like peptide-1 receptor is involved in learning and neuroprotection. *Nat. Med.* 9, 1173–1179.

Fehmann, H. C., and Habener, J. F. (1992). Insulinotropic hormone glucagon-like peptide-I(7-37) stimulation of proinsulin gene expression and proinsulin biosynthesis in insulinoma beta TC-1 cells. *Endocrinology* 130, 159–166.

Fehmann, H. C., Hering, B. J., Wolf, M. J., Brandhorst, H., Brandhorst, D., Bretzel, R. G., et al. (1995). The effects of glucagon-like peptide-I (GLP-I) on hormone secretion from isolated human pancreatic islets. *Pancreas* 11, 196–200.

Gallwitz, B., Witt, M., Paetzold, G., Morys-Wortmann, C., Zimmermann, B., Eckart, K., et al. (1994). Structure/activity characterization of glucagon-like peptide-1. *Eur. J. Biochem.* 225, 1151–1156.

Gault, V. A., McClean, P. L., Cassidy, R. S., Irwin, N., and Flatt, P. R. (2007). Chemical gastric inhibitory polypeptide receptor antagonism protects against obesity, insulin resistance, glucose intolerance and associated disturbances in mice fed high-fat and cafeteria diets. *Diabetologia* 50, 1752–1762.

Gensure, R. C., Gardella, T. J., and Juppner, H. (2001). Multiple sites of contact between the carboxyl-terminal binding domain of PTHrP-(1–36) analogs and the amino-terminal extracellular domain of the PTH/PTHrP receptor identified by photoaffinity cross-linking. *J. Biol. Chem.* 276, 28650–28658.

Göke, R., Fehmann, H. C., Linn, T., Schmidt, H., Krause, M., Eng, J., et al. (1993). Exendin-4 is a high potency agonist and truncated exendin-(9-39)-amide an antagonist at the glucagon-like peptide 1-(7-36)-amide receptor of insulin-secreting beta-cells. *J. Biol. Chem.* 268, 19650–19655.

Grace, C. R., Perrin, M. H., DiGruccio, M. R., Miller, C. L., Rivier, J. E., Vale, W. W., et al. (2004). NMR structure and peptide hormone binding site of the first extracellular domain of a type B1 G protein-coupled receptor. *Proc. Natl. Acad. Sci. U.S.A.* 101, 12836–12841.

Graziano, M. P., Hey, P. J., and Strader, C. D. (1996). The amino terminal domain of the glucagon-like peptide-1 receptor is a critical determinant of subtype specificity. *Recept. Channels* 4, 9–17.

Gronenborn, A. M., Bovermann, G., and Clore, G. M. (1987). A 1H-NMR study of the solution conformation of secretin. Resonance assignment and secondary structure. *FEBS Lett.* 215, 88–94.

Hinke, S. A., Gelling, R., Manhart, S., Lynn, F., Pederson, R. A., Kuhn-Wache, K., et al. (2003). Structure-activity relationships of glucose-dependent insulinotropic polypeptide (GIP). *Biol. Chem.* 384, 403–407.

Hinke, S. A., Kuhn-Wache, K., Hoffmann, T., Pederson, R. A., McIntosh, C. H., and Demuth, H. U. (2002). Metformin effects on dipeptidylpeptidase IV degradation of glucagon-like peptide-1. *Biochem. Biophys. Res. Commun.* 291, 1302–1308.

Hinke, S. A., Manhart, S., Pamir, N., Demuth, H., Gelling, R. W., Pederson, R. A., et al. (2001). Identification of a bioactive domain in the amino-terminus of glucose-dependent insulinotropic polypeptide (GIP). *Biochim. Biophys. Acta* 1547, 143–155.

Hinke, S. A., Manhart, S., Speck, M., Pederson, R. A., Demuth, H. U., and McIntosh, C. H. (2004). In depth analysis of the N-terminal bioactive domain of gastric inhibitory polypeptide. *Life Sci.* 75, 1857–1870.

Hisadome, K., Reimann, F., Gribble, F. M., and Trapp, S. (2010). Leptin directly depolarizes preproglucagon neurons in the nucleus tractus solitarius: electrical properties of glucagon-like Peptide 1 neurons. *Diabetes* 59, 1890–1898.

Hjorth, S. A., and Schwartz, T. W. (1996). Glucagon and GLP-1 receptors: lessons from chimeric ligands and receptors. *Acta Physiol. Scand.* 157, 343–345.

Holtmann, M. H., Ganguli, S., Hadac, E. M., Dolu, V., and Miller, L. J. (1996). Multiple extracellular loop domains contribute critical determinants for agonist binding and activation of the secretin receptor. *J. Biol. Chem.* 271, 14944–14949.

Holtmann, M. H., Hadac, E. M., and Miller, L. J. (1995). Critical contributions of amino-terminal extracellular domains in agonist binding and activation of secretin and vasoactive intestinal polypeptide receptors. Studies of chimeric receptors. *J. Biol. Chem.* 270, 14394–14398.

Hoyle, C. H. (1999). Neuropeptide families and their receptors: evolutionary perspectives. *Brain Res.* 848, 1–25.

Huang, Y., Wilkinson, G. F., and Willars, G. B. (2010). Role of the signal peptide in the synthesis and processing of the glucagon-like peptide-1 receptor. *Br. J. Pharmacol.* 159, 237–251.

Inooka, H., Ohtaki, T., Kitahara, O., Ikegami, T., Endo, S., Kitada, C., et al. (2001). Conformation of a peptide ligand bound to its G-protein coupled receptor. *Nat. Struct. Biol.* 8, 161–165.

Irwin, D. M. (2001). Molecular evolution of proglucagon. *Regul. Pept.* 98, 1–12.

Irwin, D. M. (2002). Ancient duplications of the human proglucagon gene. *Genomics* 79, 741–746.

Irwin, D. M. (2009). Molecular evolution of mammalian incretin hormone genes. *Regul. Pept.* 155, 121–130.

Irwin, D. M., and Prentice, K. J. (2011). Incretin hormones and the expanding families of glucagon-like sequences and their receptors. *Diabetes Obes. Metab.* 13(Suppl. 1), 69–81.

Irwin, D. M., and Wong, K. (2005). Evolution of new hormone function: loss and gain of a receptor. *J. Hered.* 96, 205–211.

Kieffer, T. J., and Habener, J. F. (1999). The glucagon-like peptides. *Endocr. Rev.* 20, 876–913.

Kim, D. K., Cho, E. B., Moon, M. J., Park, S., Hwang, J. I., Do Rego, J. L., et al. (2012). Molecular coevolution of neuropeptides gonadotropin-releasing hormone and kisspeptin with their cognate G protein-coupled receptors. *Front. Neurosci.* 6:3. doi:10.3389/fnins.2012.00003

Kim, D. K., Cho, E. B., Moon, M. J., Park, S., Hwang, J. I., Kah, O., et al. (2011). Revisiting the evolution of gonadotropin-releasing hormones and their receptors in vertebrates: secrets hidden in genomes. *Gen. Comp. Endocrinol.* 170, 68–78.

Laburthe, M., and Couvineau, A. (2002). Molecular pharmacology and structure of VPAC Receptors for VIP and PACAP. *Regul. Pept.* 108, 165–173.

Laburthe, M., Couvineau, A., and Tan, V. (2007). Class II G protein-coupled receptors for VIP and PACAP: structure, models of activation and pharmacology. *Peptides* 28, 1631–1639.

Lee, Y. R., Tsunekawa, K., Moon, M. J., Um, H. N., Hwang, J. I., Osugi, T., et al. (2009). Molecular evolution of multiple forms of kisspeptins and GPR54 receptors in vertebrates. *Endocrinology* 150, 2837–2846.

Li, J. H., Choe, H., Wang, A. F., Maiti, K., Wang, C., Salam, A., et al. (2005). Extracellular loop 3 (EL3) and EL3-proximal transmembrane helix 7 of the mammalian type I and type II gonadotropin-releasing hormone (GnRH) receptors determine differential ligand selectivity to GnRH-I and GnRH-II. *Mol. Pharmacol.* 67, 1099–1110.

Lin, F., and Wang, R. (2009). Molecular modeling of the three-dimensional structure of GLP-1R and its interactions with several agonists. *J. Mol. Model.* 15, 53–65.

List, J. F., and Habener, J. F. (2004). Glucagon-like peptide 1 agonists and the development and growth c pancreatic beta-cells. *Am. J. Physio Endocrinol. Metab.* 286, E875–E881

Lopez de Maturana, R., and Donnelly, D (2002). The glucagon-like peptide 1 receptor binding site for the N terminus of GLP-1 requires polar ity at Asp198 rather than negativ charge. *FEBS Lett.* 530, 244–248.

Lopez de Maturana, R., Treece-Birch, J Abidi, F., Findlay, J. B., and Donnell D. (2004). Met-204 and Tyr-205 ar together important for binding GLP 1 receptor agonists but not thei N-terminally truncated analogues *Protein Pept. Lett.* 11, 15–22.

Lopez de Maturana, R., Willshaw, A Kuntzsch, A., Rudolph, R., and Donnelly, D. (2003). The isolated N terminal domain of the glucagon like peptide-1 (GLP-1) recepto binds exendin peptides with mucl higher affinity than GLP-1. *J. Bio Chem.* 278, 10195–10200.

MacDonald, P. E., El-Kholy, W., Riede M. J., Salapatek, A. M., Light, P. E and Wheeler, M. B. (2002). The multiple actions of GLP-1 on the proces of glucose-stimulated insulin secretion. *Diabetes* 51(Suppl. 3), S434-S442.

McIntosh, C. H., Widenmaier, S. and Kim, S. J. (2009). Glucose dependent insulinotropic polypeptide (Gastric Inhibitory Polypeptide GIP). *Vitam. Horm.* 80, 409–471.

Montrose-Rafizadeh, C., Yang, H. Rodgers, B. D., Beday, A., Pritchette, L. A., and Eng, J. (1997). Higl potency antagonists of the pancreatic glucagon-like peptide-1 receptor. *J. Biol. Chem.* 272, 21201–21206

Moon, M. J., Kim, H. Y., Kim, S G., Park, J., Choi, D. S., Hwang J. I., et al. (2010). Tyr1 and Ile7 of glucose-dependent insulinotropic polypeptide (GIP) confer differential ligand selectivity toward GIP and glucagon-like peptide-1 receptors *Mol. Cells* 30, 149–154.

Moon, M. J., Kim, H. Y., Park, S., Kim D. K., Cho, E. B., Hwang, J.-I., et al (2011). Insulin contributes to fine-tuning of the pancreatic beta-cel response to glucagon-like peptide-1 *Mol. Cells* 32, 389–395.

Moon, M. J., Kim, H. Y., Park, S., Kim D. K., Cho, E. B., Park, C. R., et al. (2012). Evolutionarily conserved residues at glucagon-like peptide-1 (GLP-1) receptor core confer ligand-induced receptor activation. *J. Biol. Chem.* 287, 3873–3884.

Nauck, M. A., Heimesaat, M. M., Behle, K., Holst, J. J., Nauck, M. S., Ritzel, R., et al. (2002). Effects of glucagon-like peptide 1 on counterregulatory hormone responses, cognitive functions, and insulin secretion during hyperinsulinemic, stepped hypoglycemic clamp experiments in healthy volunteers. *J. Clin. Endocrinol. Metab.* 87, 1239–1246.

Neidigh, J. W., Fesinmeyer, R. M., Prickett, K. S., and Andersen, N. H. (2001). Exendin-4 and glucagon-like-peptide-1: NMR structural comparisons in the solution and micelle-associated states. *Biochemistry* 40, 13188–13200.

Neumann, J. M., Couvineau, A., Murail, S., Lacapere, J. J., Jamin, N., and Laburthe, M. (2008). Class-B GPCR activation: is ligand helix-capping the key? *Trends Biochem. Sci.* 33, 314–319.

Oh, D. Y., Song, J. A., Moon, J. S., Moon, M. J., Kim, J. I., Kim, K., et al. (2005). Membrane-proximal region of the carboxyl terminus of the gonadotropin-releasing hormone receptor (GnRHR) confers differential signal transduction between mammalian and nonmammalian GnRHRs. *Mol. Endocrinol.* 19, 722–731.

Parthier, C., Kleinschmidt, M., Neumann, P., Rudolph, R., Manhart, S., Schlenzig, D., et al. (2007). Crystal structure of the incretin-bound extracellular domain of a G protein-coupled receptor. *Proc. Natl. Acad. Sci. U.S.A.* 104, 13942–13947.

Parthier, C., Reedtz-Runge, S., Rudolph, R., and Stubbs, M. T. (2009). Passing the baton in class B GPCRs: peptide hormone activation via helix induction? *Trends Biochem. Sci.* 34, 303–310.

Perfetti, R., and Merkel, P. (2000). Glucagon-like peptide-1: a major regulator of pancreatic beta-cell function. *Eur. J. Endocrinol.* 143, 717–725.

Perry, T., Holloway, H. W., Weerasuriya, A., Mouton, P. R., Duffy, K., Mattison, J. A., et al. (2007). Evidence of GLP-1-mediated neuroprotection in an animal model of pyridoxine-induced peripheral sensory neuropathy. *Exp. Neurol.* 203, 293–301.

Pioszak, A. A., Parker, N. R., Suino-Powell, K., and Xu, H. E. (2008). Molecular recognition of corticotropin-releasing factor by its G-protein-coupled receptor CRFR1. *J. Biol. Chem.* 283, 32900–32912.

Pioszak, A. A., and Xu, H. E. (2008). Molecular recognition of parathyroid hormone by its G protein-coupled receptor. *Proc. Natl. Acad. Sci. U.S.A.* 105, 5034–5039.

Plisetskaya, E. M., and Mommsen, T. P. (1996). Glucagon and glucagon-like peptides in fishes. *Int. Rev. Cytol.* 168, 187–257.

Runge, S., Thogersen, H., Madsen, K., Lau, J., and Rudolph, R. (2008). Crystal structure of the ligand-bound glucagon-like peptide-1 receptor extracellular domain. *J. Biol. Chem.* 283, 11340–11347.

Runge, S., Wulff, B. S., Madsen, K., Brauner-Osborne, H., and Knudsen, L. B. (2003). Different domains of the glucagon and glucagon-like peptide-1 receptors provide the critical determinants of ligand selectivity. *Br. J. Pharmacol.* 138, 787–794.

Sasaki, K., Dockerill, S., Adamiak, D. A., Tickle, I. J., and Blundell, T. (1975). X-ray analysis of glucagon and its relationship to receptor binding. *Nature* 257, 751–757.

Shen, H. Q., Roth, M. D., and Peterson, R. G. (1998). The effect of glucose and glucagon-like peptide-1 stimulation on insulin release in the perfused pancreas in a non-insulin-dependent diabetes mellitus animal model. *Metab. Clin. Exp.* 47, 1042–1047.

Sherwood, N. M., Krueckl, S. L., and McRory, J. E. (2000). The origin and function of the pituitary adenylate cyclase-activating polypeptide (PACAP)/glucagon superfamily. *Endocr. Rev.* 21, 619–670.

Stoffers, D. A., Kieffer, T. J., Hussain, M. A., Drucker, D. J., Bonner-Weir, S., Habener, J. F., et al. (2000). Insulinotropic glucagon-like peptide 1 agonists stimulate expression of homeodomain protein IDX-1 and increase islet size in mouse pancreas. *Diabetes* 49, 741–748.

Stroop, S. D., Kuestner, R. E., Serwold, T. F., Chen, L., and Moore, E. E. (1995). Chimeric human calcitonin and glucagon receptors reveal two dissociable calcitonin interaction sites. *Biochemistry* 34, 1050–1057.

Sun, C., Song, D., Davis-Taber, R. A., Barrett, L. W., Scott, V. E., Richardson, P. L., et al. (2007). Solution structure and mutational analysis of pituitary adenylate cyclase-activating polypeptide binding to the extracellular domain of PAC1-RS. *Proc. Natl. Acad. Sci. U.S.A.* 104, 7875–7880.

Tan, Y. V., Couvineau, A., Murail, S., Ceraudo, E., Neumann, J. M., Lacapere, J. J., et al. (2006). Peptide agonist docking in the N-terminal ectodomain of a class II G protein-coupled receptor, the VPAC1 receptor. Photoaffinity, NMR, and molecular modeling. *J. Biol. Chem.* 281, 12792–12798.

Thorens, B., Porret, A., Buhler, L., Deng, S. P., Morel, P., and Widmann, C. (1993). Cloning and functional expression of the human islet GLP-1 receptor. Demonstration that exendin-4 is an agonist and exendin-(9-39) an antagonist of the receptor. *Diabetes* 42, 1678–1682.

Thornton, K., and Gorenstein, D. G. (1994). Structure of glucagon-like peptide (7-36) amide in a dodecylphosphocholine micelle as determined by 2D NMR. *Biochemistry* 33, 3532–3539.

Underwood, C. R., Garibay, P., Knudsen, L. B., Hastrup, S., Peters, G. H., Rudolph, R., et al. (2010). Crystal structure of glucagon-like peptide-1 in complex with the extracellular domain of the glucagon-like peptide-1 receptor. *J. Biol. Chem.* 285, 723–730.

Van Eyll, B., Goke, B., Wilmen, A., and Goke, R. (1996). Exchange of W39 by A within the N-terminal extracellular domain of the GLP-1 receptor results in a loss of receptor function. *Peptides* 17, 565–570.

Venneti, K. C., and Hewage, C. M. (2011). Conformational and molecular interaction studies of glucagon-like peptide-2 with its N-terminal extracellular receptor domain. *FEBS Lett.* 585, 346–352.

Vrang, N., Hansen, M., Larsen, P. J., and Tang-Christensen, M. (2007). Characterization of brainstem preproglucagon projections to the paraventricular and dorsomedial hypothalamic nuclei. *Brain Res.* 1149, 118–126.

Wang, C., Yun, O., Maiti, K., Oh, D. Y., Kim, K. K., Chae, C. H., et al. (2004). Position of Pro and Ser near Glu7.32 in the extracellular loop 3 of mammalian and nonmammalian gonadotropin-releasing hormone (GnRH) receptors is a critical determinant for differential ligand selectivity for mammalian GnRH and chicken GnRH-II. *Mol. Endocrinol.* 18, 105–116.

Wilmen, A., Goke, B., and Goke, R. (1996). The isolated N-terminal extracellular domain of the glucagon-like peptide-1 (GLP)-1 receptor has intrinsic binding activity. *FEBS Lett.* 398, 43–47.

Wilmen, A., Van Eyll, B., Goke, B., and Goke, R. (1997). Five out of six tryptophan residues in the N-terminal extracellular domain of the rat GLP-1 receptor are essential for its ability to bind GLP-1. *Peptides* 18, 301–305.

Wittelsberger, A., Corich, M., Thomas, B. E., Lee, B. K., Barazza, A., Czodrowski, P., et al. (2006). The mid-region of parathyroid hormone (1-34) serves as a functional docking domain in receptor activation. *Biochemistry* 45, 2027–2034.

Xiao, Q., Jeng, W., and Wheeler, M. B. (2000). Characterization of glucagon-like peptide-1 receptor-binding determinants. *J. Mol. Endocrinol.* 25, 321–335.

Xu, G., Stoffers, D. A., Habener, J. F., and Bonner-Weir, S. (1999). Exendin-4 stimulates both beta-cell replication and neogenesis, resulting in increased beta-cell mass and improved glucose tolerance in diabetic rats. *Diabetes* 48, 2270–2276.

Yaqub, T., Tikhonova, I. G., Lattig, J., Magnan, R., Laval, M., Escrieut, C., et al. (2010). Identification of determinants of glucose-dependent insulinotropic polypeptide receptor that interact with N-terminal biologically active region of the natural ligand. *Mol. Pharmacol.* 77, 547–558.

Yeung, C. M., Mojsov, S., Mok, P. Y., and Chow, B. K. (2002). Isolation and structure-function studies of a glucagon-like peptide 1 receptor from goldfish Carassius auratus: identification of three charged residues in extracellular domains critical for receptor function. *Endocrinology* 143, 4646–4654.

Zander, M., Madsbad, S., Madsen, J. L., and Holst, J. J. (2002). Effect of 6-week course of glucagon-like peptide 1 on glycaemic control, insulin sensitivity, and beta-cell function in type 2 diabetes: a parallel-group study. *Lancet* 359, 824–830.

8

Acting on hormone receptors with minimal side effect on cell proliferation: a timely challenge illustrated with GLP-1R and GPER

Véronique Gigoux * and Daniel Fourmy

Université de Toulouse, Université Paul Sabatier, Toulouse, France

Edited by:
Hubert Vaudry, University of Rouen, France

Reviewed by:
Lisa Chopin, Queensland University of Technology, Australia
Terry Moody, National Cancer Institute, USA

****Correspondence:***
Véronique Gigoux, CHU Rangueil – INSERM, Université de Toulouse, Université Paul Sabatier, EA4552, 1 Avenue Jean Poulhès, BP 84225, 31432 Toulouse Cedex 4, France.
e-mail: veronique.gigoux@inserm.fr

G protein-coupled receptors (GPCRs) constitute a large family of receptors that sense molecules outside the cell and activate inside signal transduction pathways and cellular responses. GPCR are involved in a wide variety of physiological processes, including in the neuroendocrine system. GPCR are also involved in many diseases and are the target of 30% of marketed medicinal drugs. Whereas the majority of the GPCR-targeting drugs have proved their therapeutic benefit, some of them were associated with undesired effects. We develop two examples of used drugs whose therapeutic benefits are tarnished by carcinogenesis risks. The chronic administration of glucagon-like peptide-1 (GLP-1) analogs widely used to treat type-2 diabetes was associated with an increased risk of pancreatic or thyroid cancers. The long-term treatment with the estrogen antagonist tamoxifen, developed to target breast cancer overexpressing estrogen receptors ER, presents agonist activity on the G protein-coupled estrogen receptor which is associated with an increased incidence of endometrial cancer and breast cancer resistance to hormonotherapy. We point out and discuss the need of pharmacological studies to understand and overcome the undesired effects associated with the chronic administration of GPCR ligands. In fact, biological effects triggered by GPCR often result from the activation of multiple intracellular signaling pathways. Deciphering which signaling networks are engaged following GPCR activation appears to be primordial to unveil their contribution in the physiological and physiopathological processes. The development of biased agonists to elucidate the role of the different signaling mechanisms mediated by GPCR activation will allow the generation of new therapeutic agents with improved efficacy and reduced side effects. In this regard, the identification of GLP-1R biased ligands promoting insulin secretion without inducing pro-tumoral effects would offer therapeutic benefit.

Keywords: receptor, G protein, arrestin, GLP-1, estrogen, biased ligands, adverse effects, cancer

INTRODUCTION

Seven transmembrane receptors, also termed G protein-coupled receptors (GPCR), form the largest class of the cell surface membrane receptors, involving 850 members in the human genome. GPCR are generally expressed in several different tissues in the same individual and involved in numerous physiological processes, including in the neuroendocrine system by playing a pivotal role in the control of feeding behavior, reproduction, growth, hydromineral homeostasis and stress response. At the cellular level, biological effects triggered by GPCR often result from the activation of multiple intracellular signaling pathways which are dependent or independent of G protein coupling (Rajagopal et al., 2010a).

Near 30% of therapeutic agents on the pharmaceutical market target GPCR (Hopkins and Groom, 2002). Whereas the majority of the GPCR-targeting drugs have proved their therapeutic benefit, some of them were associated with undesired effects (**Table 1**). Around 70% of the drugs which target GPCR are derived from the natural ligand and the use of agonist mimetics in clinical indication can act on the different tissues expressing the targeted GPCR and potentially induce undesired effects. Notably, prolonged treatment with GPCR-targeting agonist analogs was shown to induce preneoplastic and tumoral side effects. Here, we develop two examples of the use of GPCR-targeting drugs whose therapeutic benefits are tarnished by carcinogenesis risks. As a first example, glucagon-like peptide-1 receptor (GLP-1R) agonists used as anti-diabetic treatment were shown to induce preneoplastic lesions and/or cancers in the pancreas and the thyroid. The second example of ligands that we chose to develop does not initially target a GPCR, but the unexpected undesired effect is associated with a new GPCR target. Indeed, nuclear estrogen receptor antagonists such as tamoxifen are a breakthrough in the therapy and the prevention of breast cancer; however, long-term treatment was shown to be associated with an increased risk in endometrial cancer which was explained by the tamoxifen-induced activation of a GPCR, named G protein-coupled estrogen receptor (GPER).

We point out and discuss the need of more pharmacological studies to understand and overcome the undesired effects associated with the chronic administration of ligands which target GPCR. Deciphering the signaling networks engaged following GPCR activation appears to be primordial to unveil

Table 1 | Examples of ligands used for clinical indication in endocrinology with undesired side effect.

Receptor	Ligand	Clinical indication	Undesired side effects	Reference
Dopamine-R	Antagonist	Schizophrenia/bipolar disorder (*Central nervous system*)	Diabetes (*Pancreatic β-cells:serotonin, histamine, muscarinic antagonism*)	Nasrallah (2008), Medved et al. (2009)
EstrogenR/ GPER	Tamoxifen	Breast cancer/osteoporosis	Endometrial cancer/uterine sarcoma/ovarian cancer Tamoxifen breast cancer resistance	Du et al. (2012a), Ignatov et al. (2010a), He et al. (2012) Wei et al. (2012)
GLP-1R	GLP-1 analogs	Diabetes (*pancreatic β cell*)	Preneoplasia/pancreatitis (*Pancretic duct cell*) Medullary thyroid cancer (*Thyroid C-cell*)	Nachnani et al. (2010), Gier et al. (2012a), Elashoff et al. (2011) Bjerre Knudsen et al. (2010), Madsen et al. (2012), Victoza (Liraglutide) Injection (2012)
GnRH-R	Agonist	Prostate cancer (*anterior pituitary*)	Diabetes	Kintzel et al. (2008), Saylor and Smith (2009)
NPY-R		Eating disorders (*Brain*)	Neuroblastoma	Lu et al. (2010)
PTH-R	Agonist	Osteoporosis (*Osteoblast*)	Osteosarcoma (*Mesenchymal stem cell*)	Subbiah et al. (2010), Hodsman et al. (2005)
Serotonin 5HT4R	Agonist	Gastrointestinal disorder (*enteric nervous system in GI tract*)	Cardiovascular disease	Tack et al. (2012)
SST-R	Somatostatin analogs	Acromegaly (*Pituitary: suppress GH/IGF-1 secretion*) Carcinoid tumors/Vipomas Endocrine tumor	Hypo/hyperglycemia Hypothyroidism (Pituitary: suppress secretion TSH) Pancreatitis	

The cells or organs targeted by the drug in the clinical indication or in the adverse effects are given in parenthesis.

their contribution in the physiological and physiopathological processes.

THE GLUCAGON-LIKE PEPTIDE-1 RECEPTOR

One of the main physiological roles of GLP-1 is to enhance insulin secretion in a glucose-dependent manner. Thus, GLP-1 is an incretin hormone released after meals by L cells in the intestine (**Figure 1**) (Mojsov et al., 1987). GLP-1 exerts its physiological effects through binding to its specific G protein-coupled receptor, GLP-1R, which is primarily and positively coupled to adenylate cyclase, through Gαs-containing heterotrimeric G proteins, leading to the activation of second messenger pathways such as protein kinase A (PKA) and cAMP-regulated guanine nucleotide exchange factor II (cAMP-GEFII, also known as Epac2) signaling pathways (**Figure 2**) (Thorens, 1992; Kashima et al., 2001; Mayo et al., 2003; Holz, 2004; Seino and Shibasaki, 2005; Doyle and Egan, 2007; Holst, 2007). In addition to its stimulatory effect on insulin secretion, GLP-1 suppresses the secretion of glucagon, a counter-hormone to insulin, thus maintaining glucose homeostasis following a meal (Nauck et al., 1993). GLP-1 plays also a key role in the homeostasis of β-cell mass by inducing β-cell proliferation and protecting against apoptosis which favor an expansion of β-cell mass (**Figure 2**) (Doyle and Egan, 2007). These functions are mediated *via* the activation of the cAMP/PKA/CREB (cAMP-responsive element binding protein) and the transactivation of the EGF-R (epidermal growth factor receptor) leading to the activation of phosphatidylinositol-3 kinase (PI3K), Protein Kinase Cζ (PKCζ), Akt-protein kinase B, Extracellular Regulated Kinase (ERK1/2) signaling pathways and to the up-regulation of the expression of the cell cycle regulator cyclin D1 (Buteau et al., 2003; Drucker, 2003; Trumper et al., 2005; Park et al., 2006; Doyle and Egan, 2007). The antiapoptotic effect of GLP-1 in β-cells also involves β-arrestin1 recruitment by GLP-1R which mediates the ERK1/2 activation leading to the phosphorylation and inactivation of the pro-apoptotic protein Bad (Quoyer et al., 2010). The properties of GLP-1 on insulin secretion and β-cell proliferation make GLP-1 one of the most promising therapeutic agent to treat type-2 diabetes. Moreover, GLP-1 analogs offer the advantage of improved glycemic control of type-2 diabetic patients, without inducing severe hypoglycemia (Phillips and Prins, 2011).

On the other hand, GLP-1 receptor activation directly promotes cell proliferation and enhances cell survival in several tissues including neurons, fibroblasts, and cardiomyocytes (Brubaker and Drucker, 2004).

COULD ANTI-DIABETIC TREATMENT WITH GLP-1 ANALOGS INDUCE CANCERS?

Two GLP-1 mimetic drugs are now widely used to treat type-2 diabetes, exendin-4/exenatide and liraglutide, because of their optimal glucose lowering capacity with low risk of hypoglycemia (Chia and Egan, 2008; Buse et al., 2009; Nauck et al., 2009). Preclinical and clinical studies indicated that exenatide and liraglutide

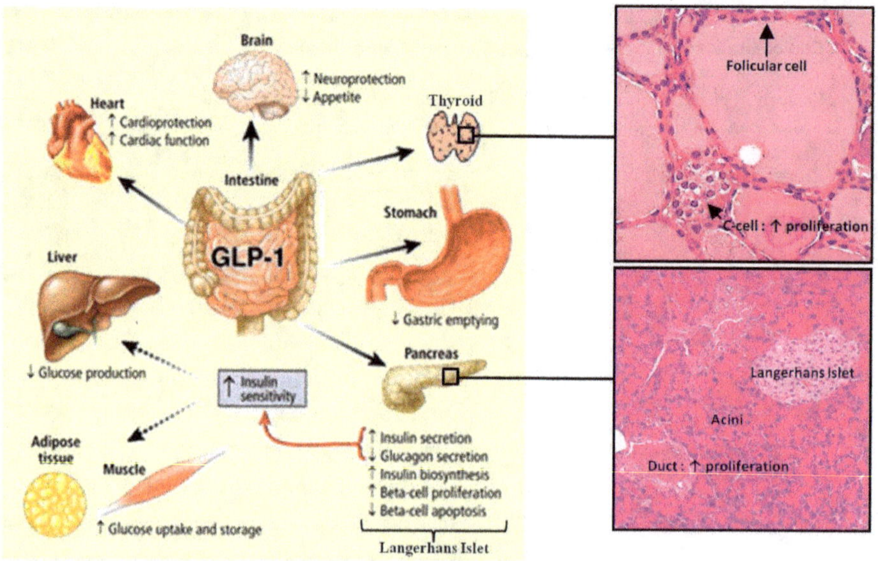

FIGURE 1 | Actions of GLP-1 in peripheral tissues. Most of the effects of GLP-1 are mediated by direct interaction with GLP-1R on specific tissues. However, the actions of GLP-1 in liver, fat, and muscle most likely occur through indirect mechanisms. GLP-1 induces the proliferation of pancreatic duct cells and thyroid C-cells. Reprinted from Gastroenterology (Baggio and Drucker, 2007).

exert a positive effect on insulin secretion, β-cell proliferation, and survival (Goke et al., 1993; Chang et al., 2003; Drucker, 2006; Vilsboll et al., 2007, 2008; Pratley and Gilbert, 2008; Madsbad, 2009; Vilsboll, 2009). On the other hand, recent studies showed that the use of these GLP-1R agonists in anti-diabetic treatment can be associated with an increase of cancer risk. The main organs where concerns exist about the trophic effects of GLP-1 analogs and their potential carcinogenic propensity are the pancreas and the thyroid, both organs expressing GLP-1R.

The pancreas

Recent studies reported that both treatments with exenatide and liraglutide are associated with an increased risk of pancreatitis in humans, a disease which represents a known risk factor for pancreatic cancer (Denker and Dimarco, 2006; Cure et al., 2008; Tripathy et al., 2008; Greer and Whitcomb, 2009). The chronic administration of GLP-1 agonists was also shown to be associated with increased serum lipase and amylase in many patients with type-2 diabetes, suggesting pancreatic damage and inflammation (Lando et al., 2012). Evaluation of the U.S. Food and Drug Administration (FDA) adverse events database by Elashoff et al. (2011), showed 10- and 3-fold increases in the incidence of pancreatitis and pancreatic cancer, respectively, in diabetic patients treated with exenatide as compared to other therapies (rosiglitazone, nateglinide, repaglinide, and glipizide) (Elashoff et al., 2011).

Undesired effects were also observed on different animal models. Indeed, chronic administration of exenatide during 12 weeks increased pancreatic acinar inflammation, sensitized to pancreatitis, and promoted pancreatic duct hyperplasia in rats or in the LSL-Kras$^{G12D/+}$/Pdx1-Cre$^{\pm}$ murine model of pancreatic carcinogenesis (Nachnani et al., 2010; Gier et al., 2012a). The authors of this study related these adverse effects to the expression of GLP-1R in duct cells of the exocrine pancreatic tissue (Gier et al., 2012a). Whereas GLP-1R expression is clearly established in normal β-cells, its expression in the exocrine pancreas raises questions as it could be detected or not in the ductal or acinar cells according to the study (Horsch et al., 1997; Xu et al., 1999; Korner et al., 2007; Tornehave et al., 2008; Gier et al., 2012a). Importantly, inflammation and/or tissue damage can promote neoplasia by altering the fate of acinar and endocrine differentiated cells which can transdifferentiate to ductal cells, thus leading to ductal cell proliferation and preneoplastic lesion formation eventually progressing to pancreatic cancer (Jura et al., 2005; Means et al., 2005; Hernandez-Munoz et al., 2008; Gidekel Friedlander et al., 2009; Logsdon and Ji, 2009; Rebours et al., 2009; Perez-Mancera et al., 2012). Other studies carried on normal and diabetic mice and rats treated with exenatide or liraglutide with or without induction of experimental pancreatic injury did not find any relationship between incretin therapy and the development of pancreatic disease such as pancreatitis and pancreatic tumor (Koehler and Drucker, 2006; Koehler et al., 2009; Tatarkiewicz et al., 2010). But, in these last studies, GLP-1 agonists administration did not exceed 6 days or 4 weeks. Nevertheless, exenatide treatment upregulated PAP/Reg3b (pancreatitis-associated protein) expression as already observed in the course of pancreatic carcinogenesis and pancreatitis (Graf et al., 2006; Gigoux et al., 2008; Koehler et al., 2009; Tatarkiewicz et al., 2010). At last, Nyborg et al. (2012) did not observe pancreatitis in non-diabetic mice, rats, or monkeys after 2 years of liraglutide treatment at exposure levels up to 60 times higher than in humans.

There are very few data on GLP-1R-induced proliferative signaling in pancreatic duct cells. Gier et al. (2012a) showed that

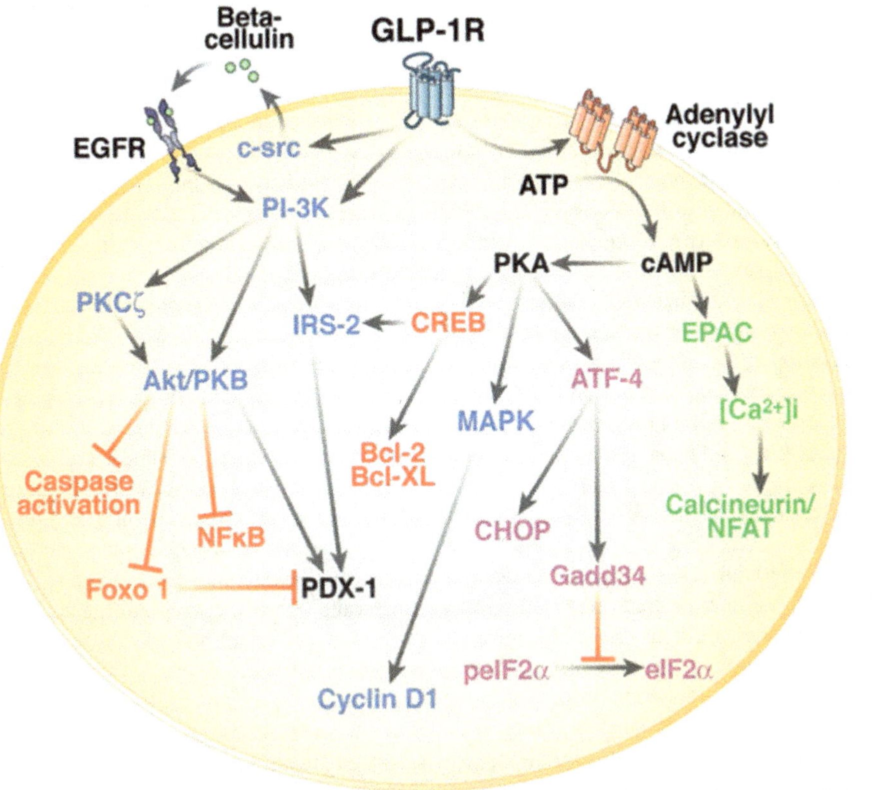

FIGURE 2 | Intracellular signaling pathways of GLP-1R in the pancreatic β-cell. One of the main physiological roles of GLP-1 is to enhance insulin secretion in a glucose-dependent manner. To stimulate insulin secretion and biosynthesis (green), GLP-1R coupled to adenylyl cyclase leading to the activation of cAMP-regulated guanine nucleotide exchange factor II (cAMP-GEFII, also known as Epac2) signaling pathway. GLP-1 plays also a key role in the homeostasis of β-cell mass by inducing β-cell proliferation (blue) and protecting against apoptosis (red). These functions are mediated *via* the activation of the cAMP/PKA/CREB (cAMP-responsive element binding protein) and the transactivation of the epidermal growth factor receptor (EGF-R) leading to the activation of phosphatidylinositol-3 kinase (PI3K), Protein Kinase Cζ (PKCζ), Akt-protein kinase B, ERK1/2 (Extracellular Regulated Kinase, named also MAPK, Mitogen-Activated Protein Kinase) signaling pathways, and to the up-regulation of the expression of the cell cycle regulator cyclin D1. GLP-1R agonists also improve β-cell function and survival during endoplasmic reticulum stress (purple) by enhancing of ATF-4 translation in a cAMP- and PKA-dependent manner, promoting the up-regulation of the endoplasmic reticulum stress markers CHOP and GADD34 expression and the dephosphorylation of eIF2α. Of note, there is considerable overlap between pathways induced by the GLP-1R activation. Reprinted from Gastroenterology (Baggio and Drucker, 2007).

exenatide induced proliferative signaling pathways in human pancreatic duct cell line by increasing CREB and ERK1/2 phosphorylation and cyclin D1 expression. ERK1/2 phosphorylation induced by exenatide is dependent of EGF-R activation (Buteau et al., 2003; MacDonald et al., 2003). Koehler and Drucker (2006) also showed that exenatide increased cAMP or induced ERK1/2 activation in some pancreatic cancer cell lines although the proliferation of these cell lines was not modulated.

The thyroid

Elashoff et al. (2011) showed a 4.7-fold increase in the incidence of thyroid cancer in diabetic patients treated with exenatide as compared to other therapies (rosiglitazone, nateglinide, repaglinide, and glipizide), by analyzing the U.S. FDA's database of reported adverse events. In contrast, Hegedus et al. (2011) reported no significant risk for the activation or growth of C-cell cancer in response to liraglutide over a 2-year period. Nevertheless, GLP-1R expression was found in thyroid glands of 20, 91, and 100% of patients with papillary carcinoma, medullary thyroid cancer (MTC), and C-Cell hyperplasia, respectively (Gier et al., 2012b). GLP-1R could be also detected in human normal thyroids (Bjerre Knudsen et al., 2010; Gier et al., 2012b). Therefore, GLP-1 analogs might increase the risk of thyroid C-cell pathology, but this awaits confirmation in humans.

Preclinical studies carried out on rodents treated with liraglutide or exenatide showed a higher incidence of C-cell neoplasia and tumor formation in the thyroid [European Medicines Agency (EMA), 2006, 2009, 2011; Bjerre Knudsen et al., 2010; U.S. Food and Drug Administration, 2011; Bulchandani et al., 2012; Madsen et al., 2012; Victoza (Liraglutide) Injection, 2012]. Indeed, a continuous exposure to liraglutide or exenatide was associated with marked increases in plasma calcitonin and in the incidence of C-cell hyperplasia. These effects were mediated by the GLP-1R as they were not seen in GLP-1R knockout mice (Bjerre Knudsen et al., 2010; Madsen et al., 2012). C-cell hyperplasia is considered as a preneoplastic lesion that constitutes *in situ* carcinoma of the thyroid C-cells (LiVolsi, 1997) and calcitonin, an hormone secreted by thyroid C-cells, is regarded as an important clinical biomarker for C-cell diseases such as MTC and hereditary C-cell hyperplasia because of its high sensitivity and specificity (Elisei et al., 2004; Costante et al., 2007; Machens et al., 2009). Neoplasms were not observed in monkeys after long-term liraglutide administration, indicating that GLP-1 induced C-cell proliferation in rodents but not in primates and suggesting that possible species-specific differences in GLP-1R expression and activation might occur in the thyroid (Bjerre Knudsen et al., 2010).

There are very few data on GLP-1R-induced proliferative signaling in thyroid C-cells. Chronic administration of liraglutide did not modify ERK phosphorylation, but increased ribosomal S6 phosphorylation, a downstream target of mTor and PI3K activation which plays a role in regulating cell proliferation and survival by growth factors (Sengupta et al., 2010; Madsen et al., 2012).

In conclusion, results obtained from preclinical and clinical studies tend to support a pro-tumoral action of GLP-1 in the pancreas and the thyroid, although few studies contradict this role. The relatively short time of chronic treatment with GLP-1 analogs in some studies could explain the absence of significative pro-tumoral effects. Moreover, this raises the question of whether GLP-1 can induce preneoplastic lesions and cancer alone or enable pre-existing lesions to progress to cancer. Further studies should be conducted to determine whether GLP-1 agonists induce or sensitize to pancreatic and thyroid diseases, by comparing chronic administration of GLP-1 mimetics in rodents presenting or not previous injury in the pancreas and the thyroid. However, it is important to note that diabetes is recognized to increase the incidence of pancreatitis and of a variety of cancers, including breast, pancreas, and colon cancers (Giovannucci et al., 2010; Girman et al., 2010; Pandey et al., 2011). Of note, GLP-1R is overexpressed in neuroendocrine pancreatic tumors, more particularly in insulinomas (Korner et al., 2007; Christ et al., 2010). In the current state of knowledge, GLP-1 agonists remain contra-indicated in patients with a personal or family history of MTC or multiple endocrine neoplasia type-2 (Anonymous, 2010; Victoza (Liraglutide) Injection, 2012). Importantly, Risk Evaluation and Mitigation Strategies program including a FDA safety warning published recommendations regarding the risk of thyroid cancer and pancreatitis after use of liraglutide and after dose increases (U.S. Food and Drug Administration, 2011).

Very few data are available on the proliferative intracellular pathways mediated by GLP-1R in pancreatic ductal cells and thyroid C-cells. Nevertheless, in the current state of knowledge, GLP-1R induces proliferation of these cells by same intracellular pathways as in the pancreatic β-cells. The identification of GLP-1 analogs that promote insulin secretion to treat type-2 diabetes without inducing pro-tumoral effects is therefore a timely challenging issue. Glucose-insulinotropic peptide (GIP) incretin could be also another alternative in type-2 diabetes treatment, especially as the GIP receptor (GIP-R) was not expressed in the normal thyroid and the exocrine pancreas unlike GLP-1R (Ahren, 2009; Waser et al., 2011, 2012). But, these clinical indication of GIP should be effective only after normalization of patient's glycemia which can restore the expression of GIP-R in β-cells (Holst et al., 1997; Vilsboll et al., 2002; Piteau et al., 2007; Younan and Rashed, 2007).

THE ESTROGEN RECEPTORS ER/GPER

Estrogen hormone regulates the growth and the differentiation of many tissues playing a critical role in the development of the reproductive system but also in the nervous, immune, vascular, muscular, skeletal, and endocrine systems. The binding of 17β-estradiol, the natural endogenous estrogen, to the estrogen receptors ERα and ERβ (ER) is the main mechanism responsible for the diverse biological effects of the hormone (Pedram et al., 2006; Meyer and Barton, 2009; Meyer et al., 2009). These highly homologous receptors can shuttle between the cytoplasm and the nucleus and function as ligand-activated nuclear transcription factors that bind *cis*-acting estrogen response elements in the promoter and enhancer regions of hormonally regulated genes (genomic effects of estrogen) (**Figure 3**) (Ring and Dowsett, 2004; Edwards, 2005; Carroll and Brown, 2006). Estrogen also induces some rapid biochemical responses to estrogen stimulation which occur in seconds to minutes, such as the increase in intracellular free calcium and the activation of multiple intracellular kinases including ERK, PI3K, PKA, and PKC (non-genomic effects of estrogen) (Chen et al., 2008).

Estrogen is the one of the risk factors for breast tumors, which accounts for 40% of cancer among the women and approximately 50% of all breast cancers demonstrated elevated levels of ER expression (Pike et al., 2004). Consequently, anti-estrogen therapy has been extended such as the gold standard tamoxifen (**Figure 3**) (Deroo and Korach, 2006; Lorand et al., 2010). Unfortunately, long-term treatment with tamoxifen is associated with adverse effects such as an increased incidence of endometrial cancer and with breast cancer resistance to hormonotherapy. Moreover, these events were shown to be associated with G protein signaling- or growth factor-mediated pathways which were not blocked by tamoxifen antagonist, leading to the prediction that an alternative membrane-bound estrogen receptor exists (Wehling, 1997; Hammes and Levin, 2007; Meyer and Barton, 2009). In fact, an orphan GPCR was identified as an estrogen-binding membrane GPCR from vascular and cancer cells and is now included in the official GPCR nomenclature and was designated GPER or GPR30 by the International Union of Pharmacology (Revankar et al., 2005; Thomas et al., 2005; Prossnitz et al., 2008a; Alexander et al., 2011). Its localization seems to be predominantly intracellular due to the constitutive internalization of plasma membrane GPER (**Figure 3**) (Revankar et al., 2005; Otto et al., 2008; Cheng et al., 2011; Sanden et al., 2011). GPER is widely expressed in cancer cell lines and primary tumors of the breast (Carmeci et al., 1997; Filardo et al., 2000; Revankar et al., 2005; Albanito et al., 2008a), endometrium (Vivacqua et al., 2006a; Leblanc et al., 2007; He et al., 2009), ovaries (Albanito et al., 2007, 2008b; Henic et al., 2009), thyroid (Vivacqua et al., 2006b), lung (Siegfried et al., 2009), prostate (Chan et al., 2010), and testicular germ cells (Franco et al., 2011). GPER does not only bind estrogens but also other substances such as tamoxifen which displays estrogenic agonist activity on GPER notably in the reproductive systems (**Figure 3**) (McDonnell, 1999; Filardo et al., 2000; Thomas and Dong, 2006; Jordan, 2007; Albanito et al., 2008b; Orlando et al., 2010; Chevalier et al., 2012).

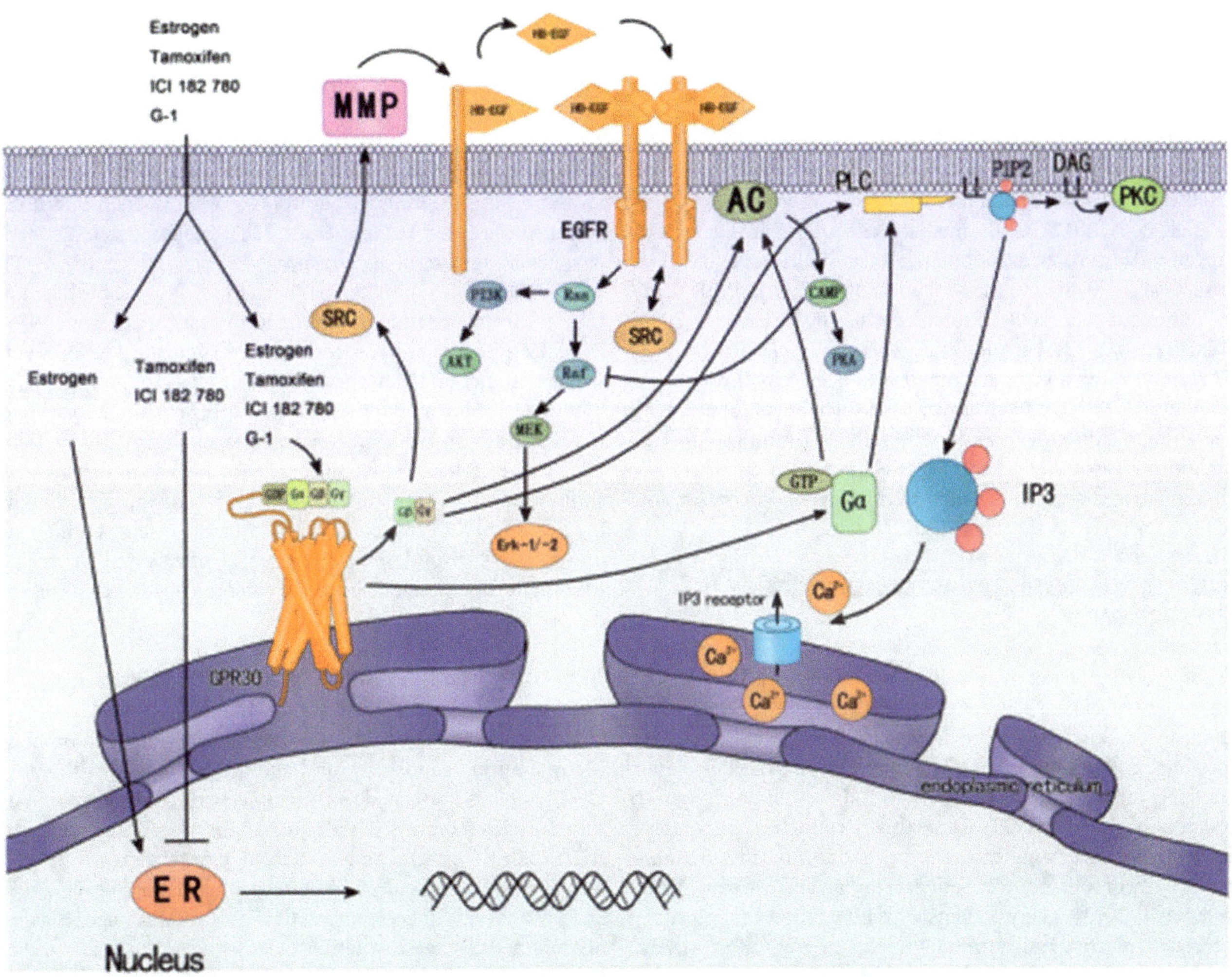

FIGURE 3 | Cellular signaling mechanisms of GPER and classic nuclear estrogen receptors ERs (↓ activate; ⊥ inhibit). ERs are widely accepted as mainly mediating gene transcriptional regulation. Tamoxifen is an ER antagonist in some tissue, such as breast cancer, while has agonistic effects in other tissues, such as endometrium. GPER was found predominantly in the endoplasmic reticulum; estrogen and tamoxifen can bind GPER, and then activate multiple cellular effectors, such as ERK, PI3K, and PLC, and other rapid cellular processes. Most of them are mediated by transactivation of EGF-R. Reprinted from Endocrinology (Wang et al., 2010).

Indeed, tamoxifen stimulates the cell proliferation and growth of cell lines of thyroid, ovarian, endometrial, and breast cancers (Filardo et al., 2000; Thomas et al., 2005; Vivacqua et al., 2006a; Albanito et al., 2007; Prossnitz et al., 2008b; Pandey et al., 2009). The discovery of GPER-selective agents and the elaboration of GPER knockout mice helped to examine GPER signaling pathways and strongly supported that GPER is associated with cancer proliferation, migration, invasion, metastasis, differentiation, prognosis, and drug resistance (Prossnitz et al., 2008b; Wang et al., 2010).

COULD ESTROGEN ANTAGONISTS USED IN BREAST CANCER TREATMENT INDUCE CANCER IN OTHER TISSUES?

An increased incidence of uterine malignancies in association with tamoxifen treatment has been reported. The incidence and severity of endometrial cancer increased by 4- to 6.9-fold in women with 5 years of exposure to tamoxifen (van Leeuwen et al., 1994; Bernstein et al., 1999; Bergman et al., 2000; Goldstein, 2001). Uterine sarcoma has been also reported to occur more frequently among long-term users (≥2 years) of tamoxifen than non-users (Wickerham et al., 2002). In support to these data, tamoxifen has been shown to stimulate the proliferation and the invasion of uterine cells *in vivo* and of human endometrial carcinoma cell lines and these effects were mediated by GPER (Gottardis et al., 1988; Jamil et al., 1991; Schwartz et al., 1997; Du et al., 2012a). Indeed, tamoxifen promoted cell proliferation and invasion of the human endometrial cancer cell lines ISHIKAWA and KLE, while the down-regulation of GPER partly or completely prevented these effects (Du et al., 2012a). GPER is widely expressed in primary tumors of endometrium including ER-negative endometrial carcinomas (He et al., 2009). High levels of GPER expression correlate with an increased incidence of endometrial cancer and with tamoxifen-induced uterine pathology and predict poor survival in endometrial cancer (Smith et al., 2007; Ignatov et al., 2010a). All together, these data strongly support that tamoxifen treatment might have a cancer-promoting effect through GPER.

G protein-coupled estrogen receptor promotes carcinogenesis by endometrial cancer cells as down-regulation of GPER led to reduce growth and invasion by RL95 endometrial cancer cells treated with 17β-estradiol and to decrease tumorigenesis *in vivo* (He et al., 2009, 2012). GPER mediates the proliferative effects of estrogen and tamoxifen in endometrial cancer cells through EGF-R transactivation leading to the activation of ERKs and PI3K pathways (Vivacqua et al., 2006a; Prossnitz et al., 2008b; He et al., 2009, 2012; Du et al., 2012a; Lappano et al., 2012; Wei et al., 2012). GPER also mediates invasion by endometrial cancer cells through the stimulation of ERK pathway, as well as the increase of interleukin-6 secretion, leading to the production and activation of matrix metalloproteinases MMP-2 and MMP-9 known to degrade extracellular matrix components and to be involved in cancer invasion and metastasis (He et al., 2009, 2012; Du et al., 2012a).

COULD GPER BE INVOLVED IN BREAST CANCER RESISTANCE TO HORMONOTHERAPY?

The majority of breast cancers is ER-positive and depends on estrogen for growth. Therefore, blocking estrogen signaling remains the strategy of choice for the treatment and the prevention of breast cancer. Tamoxifen is the prototypical drug that targets ER. It presents potent anti-estrogenic properties and has been used extensively for the past 40 years to treat and prevent breast cancer (Jordan and Morrow, 1999). Tamoxifen treatment is very effective in tumors expressing ER receptors and significantly reduces the mortality of breast cancer patients (Jordan and Morrow, 1999; Powles et al., 2007). Many patients with ER-positive breast cancer have benefited from anti-hormonal treatment, but unfortunately, almost 30–50% of patients with advanced disease did not respond to first-line treatment with tamoxifen. Furthermore, long-term tamoxifen therapy causes the development of acquired resistance (Early Breast Cancer Trialists' Collaborative Group (EBCTCG), 2005). Indeed, development of resistance is very frequent and tamoxifen is not effective for more than 5 years (Saphner et al., 1996; Clarke et al., 2001; Early Breast Cancer Trialists' Collaborative Group (EBCTCG), 2005; Barron et al., 2007; Brewster et al., 2008).

The tumor resistance to tamoxifen treatment is associated to a decrease or a loss of ER expression and to an increase of GPER expression. GPER protein is expressed in ~50% of all breast cancers including half of ER-negative tumors and correlates with increased tumor size and metastasis (Filardo et al., 2006; Ignatov et al., 2011). Moreover, GPER protein expression is increased in breast tumors of patients treated only with tamoxifen and in tamoxifen resistant tumor tissues correlating with a poor relapse-free survival in patients treated with tamoxifen (Filardo et al., 2006; Ignatov et al., 2011). *In vitro* prolonged tamoxifen treatment leads to an increased cell surface expression of GPER and also to clonal selection of GPER-positive MCF-7 breast cancer cells (Ignatov et al., 2010b). Thus, GPER expression is associated with an increased risk of resistance to tamoxifen and patients with breast cancer who have high GPER protein expression should not be treated with tamoxifen alone.

G protein-coupled estrogen receptor mediates the proliferative and tamoxifen-resistance effects through EGF-R transactivation leading to the phosphorylation of ERK and Akt (Filardo et al., 2000; Prossnitz et al., 2008b; Ignatov et al., 2010a,b). Thus, ERK and Akt can further stimulate transcription of different genes (even ER), leading to cell proliferation, and interfere with the activation of Smad proteins, known effectors of the TGF-β signaling, an important intracellular pathway involved in the inhibition of tumor progression (Clarke et al., 2001; Kleuser et al., 2008; Yoo et al., 2008; Ignatov et al., 2010b).

In conclusion, tamoxifen has been the only available hormonal option for the systemic treatment for breast cancer from 1973 to 2000. Despite the clinical success of tamoxifen, the development of drug resistance and endometrial cancers leads to the requirement of alternative hormonal therapy. In this regard, the knowledge of the contribution of GPER-mediated signaling in the undesired effects of estrogenic antagonist uses for breast cancer treatment should allow the future development of new molecules. Moreover, further researches are required to define the role of GPER signaling in estrogen undesired physiological effects and to elucidate the role of non-selective estrogen receptor ligands in health and disease.

NEW HOPES TO OVERCOME UNDESIRED EFFECTS

G protein-coupled receptors are generally expressed in several different tissues and involved in numerous physiological processes. Many natural ligands can bind and activate several subtypes of GPCR. This is illustrated, for example, with cholecystokinin and somatostatin receptors (Guillermet-Guibert et al., 2005; Dufresne et al., 2006). Ligands can also activate different classes of receptors as illustrated before with estrogen (Prossnitz et al., 2008a). Such a diversity of receptors activation following agonist administration can engage multiple intracellular signaling pathways and be responsible for adverse effects in treated patients. Furthermore, biological effects triggered by the same GPCR result from the activation of G protein-dependent and -independent intracellular signaling pathways. Recently, signaling engaged after GPCR recruitment of β-arrestin proteins have emerged as new G protein-independent intracellular signaling pathways (Luttrell and Gesty-Palmer, 2010; Rajagopal et al., 2010a). To increase the complexity, a single GPCR has pleiotropic signaling properties and each signal can crosstalk at different levels with the transactivation of cell surface receptor having tyrosine kinase activity (EGF-R, PDGF-R, FGF-R, for examples) or serine/threonine kinase activity (TGF-β, for example) or with the formation of multimers, thus potentially influencing the signaling pathways of the different receptors (Burch et al., 2012; Wang and Lewis, 2013). Indeed, numerous biochemical and biophysical studies supports that GPCRs can form physiologically relevant homo-, hetero-, or oligo-mers (Angers et al., 2002). Homodimerization of the GLP-1R was shown to be critical for selective coupling of the receptor to physiologically relevant signaling pathways (Harikumar et al., 2012). Indeed, disruption of GLP-1R homodimerization completely abrogated the intracellular calcium mobilization response whereas it slightly reduced cAMP formation and phosphorylation of ERK. Furthermore, GLP-1R dimerization can discriminate between peptide and non-peptide-mediated receptor activation. In the chemokine receptors family, antibodies against the CCR2b promoted the receptor dimerization and second messenger production (Rodriguez-Frade et al., 1999), whereas an antibody directed against CCR5, that induces receptor dimerization, inhibits its function (Vila-Coro et al., 2000). Many studies was also conducted to analyze the role of GPCR heterodimerization and supported that heterodimerization could be the source of additional pharmacological properties which are different from those of the individual receptors. As a first example, the co-expression of the δ- and κ-opioid receptors in the same cell leads to an almost complete loss of binding to selective δ- and κ-ligands while preserving binding to non-selective ligands (Jordan and Devi, 1999). As a second example, somatostatin receptor SSTR1 displays internalization in cells when it is co-expressed with SSTR5, whereas monomeric SSTR1 is resistant to internalization in contrast to monomeric SSTR5, suggesting that the SSTR1 trafficking is modified by its heterodimerization with SSTR5 (Rocheville et al., 2000). Thus, homo- and heterodimerization between GPCR cause complexity in the receptor pharmacological properties that can be responsible of synergistic or antagonistic signaling cross-talks. This GPCR pharmacological and signaling complexity could account for unexpected pharmacological effects and have dramatic impacts on drug development. All together, these hallmarks indicate that undesired adverse effects can be expected with a prolonged agonist administration that targets a GPCR (**Table 1**). Moreover, many GPCR have already been shown to present proliferative and pro-tumoral properties (**Table 2**), suggesting that an increase of preneoplastic lesions and cancer incidence can potentially occur following chronic activation of GPCR. Thus, deciphering which signaling networks are engaged and orchestrated following GPCR receptor activation appears to be primordial to unveil their contribution in the cell fate.

One strategy to overcome these limitations would be to examine the initial steps following receptor activation. The release of X-ray structures of agonist/GPCR complexes (Chung et al., 2011; Lebon et al., 2011; Warne et al., 2011; Xu et al., 2011; Audet and Bouvier, 2012), the numerous biophysical and biochemical studies (Granier et al., 2007; Kahsai et al., 2011; Liu et al., 2012; Rahmeh et al., 2012) have enabled to show that different and selective ligands, named biased ligands, can induce or stabilize distinct receptor conformations and activate one (or several) signaling pathway(s) in contrast to non-biased agonists which activate all the signaling pathways (Vaidehi and Kenakin, 2010). Thus an understanding of the structure and dynamics of the ensemble of receptor conformations would greatly help the design of small molecules with functional selectivity or "biased signaling" properties and would provide more specific and efficient new drugs. Receptor structure/activity relationship studies, structure- and docking-based virtual screening are now widely applied in drug discovery and must take in account the existence of different receptor conformations activating specific signaling pathways.

Although GPCRs can modulate a large variety of distinct signaling pathways, classification of biased ligands are actually restricted to two groups depending on their ability to activate two main transduction pathways (Whalen et al., 2011): (1) G protein-biased ligands which promote G protein activation without β-arrestin recruitment and (2) β-arrestin-biased ligands which recruit β-arrestin to the receptor and initiate consecutive signaling pathways in the absence of G protein activation.

The vast majority of biased ligands identified so far exhibits exclusive β-arrestin activity for a number of receptors (Rajagopal et al., 2010a; Whalen et al., 2011), including the AT1 angiotensin II receptor, β1- and β2-adrenergic receptors, or the CXCR7 decoy receptor (Wei et al., 2003; Wisler et al., 2007; Kim et al., 2008; Rajagopal et al., 2010b). The parathyroid hormone (PTH) analog, D-Trp(12),Tyr(34)-PTH(7-34), binds the PTH receptor 1 (PTHR1) and activates β-arrestin-dependent but not classical G protein-dependent signaling (Gesty-Palmer et al., 2009; Gesty-Palmer and Luttrell, 2011). In mice, this PTH biased agonist induces anabolic bone formation without stimulating bone resorption, comparatively with the non-selective agonist PTH(1-34) which induces both functions. Thus, this PTHR1 biased ligand may present interesting properties for the treatment of metabolic bone diseases such as osteoporosis and is a proof of concept that the exploitation of β-arrestin biased agonism may offer therapeutic benefit.

Few ligands have been yet identified as perfect G protein-biased ligands, namely inducing G protein signal transduction without any β-arrestin recruitment (Whalen et al., 2011). GMME1 ligand binding to the CCR2 chemokine receptor leads to calcium mobilization, caspase-3 activation and consecutive cell death, but does not recruit β-arrestin2 (Rafei et al., 2009). Selective ligands that activate G protein-coupling by FSH-R (follicle-stimulating hormone receptor) and PTH-1R have been also reported (Bisello et al., 2002; Wehbi et al., 2010). Of note, some ligands classified as G protein-biased can induce a weak β-arrestin recruitment by the targeted GPCR (Whalen et al., 2011). For example, oxyntomodulin and glucagon are full agonists in GLP-1R-mediated cAMP accumulation but partial agonists in recruiting β-arrestins to this receptor, suggesting that oxyntomodulin and glucagon are biased ligands on the GLP-1R (Jorgensen et al., 2007).

Interestingly, some ligands are biased in regard to the different G protein families and can trigger opposite cellular responses (Reversi et al., 2005; Sensken et al., 2008). For example, oxytocin receptors (OTR) coupling to Gi inhibits cell proliferation, whereas its coupling to Gq stimulates cell proliferation. Atosiban, an oxytocin derivative, was shown to act as a competitive antagonist on OTR/Gq coupling, and to display agonistic properties on OTR/Gi-coupling, thereby leading to the selective inhibition of cell growth (Reversi et al., 2005; Busnelli et al., 2012). SOM230 which activates the somatostatin receptor sst2A behaves as agonist for Gi coupling and inhibition of adenylyl cyclase, but antagonizes somatostatin's actions on intracellular calcium and ERK phosphorylation which can be activated by a Gi/Go independent process (Cescato et al., 2010).

Biased signaling can also exist with respect to other signaling proteins than G proteins and arrestins. The internalization of apelin receptor takes different signaling pathways depending of the apelin isoforms (Lee et al., 2010). Indeed, apelin-13-activated receptors dissociated rapidly from β-arrestin1 and were recycled to the cell surface through a Rab4-dependent mechanism, while the apelin-36-internalized receptors trafficked with β-arrestin1 to intracellular compartments and were targeted by Rab7 to lysosomes for degradation. CCL19 and CCL21 ligands both induce

Table 2 | Examples of Neuropeptide GPCRs with pro-tumoral activities and properties.

Ligands	Receptors	Target	Activity	Reference
Adrenocorticotropic hormone	MC2R	Prostate	Proliferation	Hafiz et al. (2012)
Angiotensin II	AT1R	Breast	Proliferation, adhesion, migration, invasion	Rodrigues-Ferreira et al. (2012), Du et al. (2012b)
Gastrin	CCK2	Pancreas, stomach	Proliferation, adhesion	Dufresne et al. (2006), Cayrol et al. (2006), Bierkamp et al. (2004), Clerc et al. (2002a,b), Mathieu et al. (2005)
Glucagon-like peptide-1	GLP-1R	Exocine pancreas Thyroid	Pro-tumoral	Nachnani et al. (2010), Gier et al. (2012a), Elashoff et al. (2011), Bjerre Knudsen et al. (2010), Madsen et al. (2012), Victoza (Liraglutide) Injection (2012)
Ghrelin	GHS-R	Breast Prostate Endometrium Stomach	Proliferation, migration Proliferation Proliferation	Jeffery et al. (2005) Yeh et al. (2005), Jeffery et al. (2002) Fung et al. (2010) Tian and Fan (2012)
Melanin-concentrating hormone	MCHR1	colon	Pro-tumoral, apoptosis	Nagel et al. (2012)
Neuromedin B	NMB-R	Colon Breast	Proliferation Apoptosis, proliferation	Matusiak et al. (2005) Park et al. (2011)
Neuromedin U	NMU-R2	Pancreas	Migration, invasion	Ketterer et al. (2009)
Neuropeptide Y	NPY Y5-R NPY Y2-R NPY Y1-R	Breast Neuroblastoma Prostate	Proliferation, migration Proliferation, angiogenesis Proliferation	Medeiros et al. (2012), Sheriff et al. (2010) Lu et al. (2010) Ruscica et al. (2006)
Neurotensin	NTSR1/3	Colon	Proliferation, Pro-tumoral	Muller et al. (2011)
Parathyroid hormone	PTH-R	bone	Pro-tumoral	Subbiah et al. (2010), Hodsman et al. (2005)
Pituitary adenylate cyclase-activating polypeptide	PAC1	Lung	Proliferation	Moody et al. (2012)
Prokineticin 1/2	PROKR1/2	Thyroid	Angiogenesis	Monnier and Samson (2010)
Relaxin	RXFP1	Uterus Prostate	Proliferation, apoptosis Pro-tumoral, metastasis, proliferation	Suzuki et al. (2012) Feng et al. (2010)
Urotensin II	UTR	Prostate Lung	Migration, invasion Proliferation	Grieco et al. (2011) Wu et al. (2010)
Vasoactive intestinal peptide	VPAC1	Prostate Brain (glioblastoma) Breast Lung	Proliferation, migration Migration Angiogenesis Proliferation	Fernandez-Martinez et al. (2010) Cochaud et al. (2010) Valdehita et al. (2012) Moody et al. (2000)
26RFa	GPR103	Prostate	Migration	Alonzeau et al. (2012)

β-arrestin2 recruitment by the receptor CCR7, but activate different GRK (G protein receptor kinase) isoforms (Zidar et al., 2009). Indeed, CCL19 leads to robust CCR7 phosphorylation and β-arrestin2 recruitment catalyzed by both GRK3 and GRK6 whereas CCL21 activates GRK6 alone. The functional consequences are that only CCL19 leads to classical receptor desensitization whereas both agonists are capable of signaling through GRK6 and β-arrestin2 to ERK kinases.

THE GLP-1R

Results obtained from preclinical and clinical studies tend to support a pro-tumoral action of GLP-1 in the pancreas and the thyroid. Deciphering the signaling networks engaged following GLP-1R agonist administration in pancreatic ductal cells and thyroid C-cells comparatively to pancreatic β-cells is critical to unveil their contribution in the different cellular processes. The identification of GLP-1 analogs that promote insulin secretion to treat type-2 diabetes without inducing pro-tumoral effects is therefore a timely challenging issue. Like most GPCRs, the GLP-1R couples to different classes of heterotrimeric G proteins, including Gαs, Gαq, and Gαi, regulatory proteins such as the β-arrestins, and activates multiple signaling pathways such as cAMP production, intracellular calcium mobilization, phosphorylation of ERK1/2. While GLP-1 can activate all of these signaling pathways, some compounds were shown to present biased activity on GLP-1R. Oxyntomodulin and glucagon biased the GLP-1R toward cAMP accumulation over the recruitment of β-arrestins, BMS21 compound toward ERK1/2 activation and cAMP production over β-arrestins recruitment, BETP compound toward calcium mobilization and β-arrestins recruitment over cAMP production and ERK1/2 activation (Jorgensen et al., 2007; Wootten et al., 2013). Moreover, some molecules acting as allosteric modulators were shown to modulate GLP-1R agonist-mediated signaling pathways (Willard et al., 2012; Wootten et al., 2013). For example, BETP increases the affinity of GLP-1R to oxyntomodulin and potentiates the activation of cAMP production induced by oxyntomodulin.

The most crucial GLP-1R signaling pathway for enhancing glucose-dependent insulin secretion involved the receptor coupling to Gαs proteins and the activation of cAMP production (Baggio and Drucker, 2007). While GLP-1 analogs are currently tested for their capacity to activate Gαs protein and cAMP production, their effects on other signaling pathways, particularly those involved in cell proliferation, should be included. Moreover, the analysis of pharmacological ligand properties should be done on the main cellular target, the pancreatic β-cell, but also on cells involved in carcinogenic side effects. This could enable the design and development of improved therapeutics that have the ability to fine-tune receptor signaling leading to beneficial therapeutic outcomes while reducing side effect profiles. The use of allosteric ligands in addition to GLP-1R biased agonists could also provide a therapeutic advantage to target a specific receptor response toward signaling pathways promoting insulin secretion over cell proliferation.

THE GPER

Despite the clinical success of tamoxifen in breast cancer treatment, the development of drug resistance and endometrial cancers involving the GPER leads to the requirement of alternative hormonal therapy. In this regard, the contribution of GPER-mediated responses estrogen antagonists must be considered in the future development of anti-estrogenic molecules. Recent studies based on pharmacological structure/function relationship on ER and/or GPER have identified selective GPER antagonists which completely block uterine epithelial cell proliferation mediated by GPER and which are poorly active or inactive on ER (Dennis et al., 2009, 2011; Burai et al., 2012). Future studies utilizing GPER-selective ligands will further define the role of this receptor *in vivo* and open the door to the generation of diagnostics and therapeutics directed at individual or both estrogen receptors. Such compounds might represent an important new approach for cancer therapy, thus increasing the armamentarium of drugs used to treat estrogen-sensitive and resistant cancers. On the other hand, aromatase inhibitors which act by preventing the enzyme aromatase to convert androgens into estrogen have been also brought forward as a potential alternative (Josefsson and Leinster, 2010; Abdulkareem and Zurmi, 2012).

In conclusion, GPCRs provide huge therapeutic opportunities; some are already in use. The progress in the knowledges of signaling pathways downstream of these receptors and the effects arising, their regulation by pharmacological agents, and the data from the receptor structure provide new opportunities which should lead to new generation of ligands with minimized side effects.

REFERENCES

Abdulkareem, I. H., and Zurmi, I. B. (2012). Review of hormonal treatment of breast cancer. *Niger. J. Clin. Pract.* 15, 9–14.

Ahren, B. (2009). Islet G protein-coupled receptors as potential targets for treatment of type 2 diabetes. *Nat. Rev. Drug Discov.* 8, 369–385.

Albanito, L., Madeo, A., Lappano, R., Vivacqua, A., Rago, V., Carpino, A., et al. (2007). G protein-coupled receptor 30 (GPR30) mediates gene expression changes and growth response to 17beta-estradiol and selective GPR30 ligand G-1 in ovarian cancer cells. *Cancer Res.* 67, 1859–1866.

Albanito, L., Sisci, D., Aquila, S., Brunelli, E., Vivacqua, A., Madeo, A., et al. (2008a). Epidermal growth factor induces G protein-coupled receptor 30 expression in estrogen receptor-negative breast cancer cells. *Endocrinology* 149, 3799–3808.

Albanito, L., Lappano, R., Madeo, A., Chimento, A., Prossnitz, E. R., Cappello, A. R., et al. (2008b). G-protein-coupled receptor 30 and estrogen receptor-alpha are involved in the proliferative effects induced by atrazine in ovarian cancer cells. *Environ. Health Perspect.* 116, 1648–1655.

Alexander, S. P., Mathie, A., and Peters, J. A. (2011). Guide to receptors and channels (GRAC), 5th edition. *Br. J. Pharmacol.* 164(Suppl. 1), S1–S324.

Alonzeau, J., Alexandre, D., Jeandel, L., Courel, M., Hautot, C., Yamani, F. Z., et al. (2012). The neuropeptide 26RFa is expressed in human prostate cancer and stimulates the neuroendocrine differentiation and the migration of androgeno-independent prostate cancer cells. *Eur. J. Cancer.* 49, 511–519.

Angers, S., Salahpour, A., and Bouvier, M. (2002). Dimerization: an emerging concept for G protein-coupled receptor ontogeny and function. *Annu. Rev. Pharmacol. Toxicol.* 42, 409–435.

Anonymous. (2010). Liraglutide (Victoza) for type 2 diabetes. *Med. Lett. Drugs Ther.* 52, 25–27.

Audet, M., and Bouvier, M. (2012). Restructuring G-protein- coupled receptor activation. *Cell* 151, 14–23.

Baggio, L. L., and Drucker, D. J. (2007). Biology of incretins: GLP-1 and GIP. *Gastroenterology* 132, 2131–2157.

Barron, T. I., Connolly, R., Bennett, K., Feely, J., and Kennedy, M. J. (2007). Early discontinuation of tamoxifen: a lesson for oncologists. *Cancer* 109, 832–839.

Bergman, L., Beelen, M. L., Gallee, M. P., Hollema, H., Benraadt, J., and van Leeuwen, F. E. (2000). Risk and prognosis of endometrial cancer after tamoxifen for breast cancer. Comprehensive Cancer Centres' ALERT Group. Assessment of Liver and Endometrial cancer Risk following Tamoxifen. *Lancet* 356, 881–887.

Bernstein, L., Deapen, D., Cerhan, J. R., Schwartz, S. M., Liff, J., McGann-Maloney, E., et al. (1999). Tamoxifen therapy for breast cancer and endometrial cancer risk. *J. Natl. Cancer Inst.* 91, 1654–1662.

Bierkamp, C., Bonhoure, S., Mathieu, A., Clerc, P., Fourmy, D., Pradayrol, L., et al. (2004). Expression of cholecystokinin-2/gastrin receptor in the murine pancreas modulates cell adhesion and cell differentiation in vivo. *Am. J. Pathol.* 165, 2135–2145.

Bisello, A., Chorev, M., Rosenblatt, M., Monticelli, L., Mierke, D. F., and Ferrari, S. L. (2002). Selective ligand-induced stabilization of active and desensitized parathyroid hormone type 1 receptor conformations. *J. Biol. Chem.* 277, 38524–38530.

Bjerre Knudsen, L., Madsen, L. W., Andersen, S., Almholt, K., de Boer, A. S., Drucker, D. J., et al. (2010). Glucagon-like Peptide-1 receptor agonists activate rodent thyroid C-cells causing calcitonin release and C-cell proliferation. *Endocrinology* 151, 1473–1486.

Brewster, A. M., Hortobagyi, G. N., Broglio, K. R., Kau, S. W., Santa-Maria, C. A., Arun, B., et al. (2008). Residual risk of breast cancer recurrence 5 years after adjuvant therapy. *J. Natl. Cancer Inst.* 100, 1179–1183.

Brubaker, P. L., and Drucker, D. J. (2004). Minireview: glucagon-like peptides regulate cell proliferation and apoptosis in the pancreas, gut, and central nervous system. *Endocrinology* 145, 2653–2659.

Bulchandani, D., Nachnani, J. S., Herndon, B., Molteni, A., Pathan, M. H., Quinn, T., et al. (2012). Effect of exendin (exenatide)-GLP 1 receptor agonist on the thyroid and parathyroid gland in a rat model. *Eur. J. Pharmacol.* 691, 292–296.

Burai, R., Ramesh, C., Nayak, T. K., Dennis, M. K., Bryant, B. K., Prossnitz, E. R., et al. (2012). Synthesis and characterization of tricarbonyl-Re/Tc(I) chelate probes targeting the G protein-coupled estrogen receptor GPER/GPR30. *PLoS ONE* 7:e46861. doi:10.1371/journal.pone.0046861

Burch, M. L., Osman, N., Getachew, R., Al-Aryahi, S., Poronnik, P., Zheng, W., et al. (2012). G protein coupled receptor transactivation: extending the paradigm to include serine/threonine kinase receptors. *Int. J. Biochem. Cell Biol.* 44, 722–727.

Buse, J. B., Rosenstock, J., Sesti, G., Schmidt, W. E., Montanya, E., Brett, J. H., et al. (2009). Liraglutide once a day versus exenatide twice a day for type 2 diabetes: a 26-week randomised, parallel-group, multinational, open-label trial (LEAD-6). *Lancet* 374, 39–47.

Busnelli, M., Sauliere, A., Manning, M., Bouvier, M., Gales, C., and Chini, B. (2012). Functional selective oxytocin-derived agonists discriminate between individual G protein family subtypes. *J. Biol. Chem.* 287, 3617–3629.

Buteau, J., Foisy, S., Joly, E., and Prentki, M. (2003). Glucagon-like peptide 1 induces pancreatic beta-cell proliferation via transactivation of the epidermal growth factor receptor. *Diabetes* 52, 124–132.

Carmeci, C., Thompson, D. A., Ring, H. Z., Francke, U., and Weigel, R. J. (1997). Identification of a gene (GPR30) with homology to the G-protein-coupled receptor superfamily associated with estrogen receptor expression in breast cancer. *Genomics* 45, 607–617.

Carroll, J. S., and Brown, M. (2006). Estrogen receptor target gene: an evolving concept. *Mol. Endocrinol.* 20, 1707–1714.

Cayrol, C., Clerc, P., Bertrand, C., Gigoux, V., Portolan, G., Fourmy, D., et al. (2006). Cholecystokinin-2 receptor modulates cell adhesion through beta 1-integrin in human pancreatic cancer cells. *Oncogene* 25, 4421–4428.

Cescato, R., Loesch, K. A., Waser, B., Macke, H. R., Rivier, J. E., Reubi, J. C., et al. (2010). Agonist-biased signaling at the sst2A receptor: the multi-somatostatin analogs KE108 and SOM230 activate and antagonize distinct signaling pathways. *Mol. Endocrinol.* 24, 240–249.

Chan, Q. K., Lam, H. M., Ng, C. F., Lee, A. Y., Chan, E. S., Ng, H. K., et al. (2010). Activation of GPR30 inhibits the growth of prostate cancer cells through sustained activation of Erk1/2, c-jun/c-fos-dependent upregulation of p21, and induction of G(2) cell-cycle arrest. *Cell Death Differ.* 17, 1511–1523.

Chang, A. M., Jakobsen, G., Sturis, J., Smith, M. J., Bloem, C. J., An, B., et al. (2003). The GLP-1 derivative NN2211 restores beta-cell sensitivity to glucose in type 2 diabetic patients after a single dose. *Diabetes* 52, 1786–1791.

Chen, G. G., Zeng, Q., and Tse, G. M. (2008). Estrogen and its receptors in cancer. *Med. Res. Rev.* 28, 954–974.

Cheng, S. B., Graeber, C. T., Quinn, J. A., and Filardo, E. J. (2011). Retrograde transport of the transmembrane estrogen receptor, G-protein-coupled-receptor-30 (GPR30/GPER) from the plasma membrane towards the nucleus. *Steroids* 76, 892–896.

Chevalier, N., Bouskine, A., and Fenichel, P. (2012). Bisphenol A promotes testicular seminoma cell proliferation through GPER/GPR30. *Int. J. Cancer* 130, 241–242.

Chia, C. W., and Egan, J. M. (2008). Incretin-based therapies in type 2 diabetes mellitus. *J. Clin. Endocrinol. Metab.* 93, 3703–3716.

Christ, E., Wild, D., and Reubi, J. C. (2010). Glucagonlike peptide-1 receptor: an example of translational research in insulinomas: a review. *Endocrinol. Metab. Clin. North Am.* 39, 791–800.

Chung, K. Y., Rasmussen, S. G., Liu, T., Li, S., DeVree, B. T., Chae, P. S., et al. (2011). Conformational changes in the G protein Gs induced by the beta2 adrenergic receptor. *Nature* 477, 611–615.

Clarke, R., Skaar, T. C., Bouker, K. B., Davis, N., Lee, Y. R., Welch, J. N., et al. (2001). Molecular and pharmacological aspects of antiestrogen resistance. *J. Steroid Biochem. Mol. Biol.* 76, 71–84.

Clerc, P., Leung-Theung-Long, S., Wang, T. C., Dockray, G. J., Bouisson, M., Delisle, M. B., et al. (2002a). Expression of CCK2 receptors in the murine pancreas: proliferation, transdifferentiation of acinar cells, and neoplasia. *Gastroenterology* 122, 428–437.

Clerc, P., Saillan-Barreau, C., Desbois, C., Pradayrol, L., Fourmy, D., and Dufresne, M. (2002b). Transgenic mice expressing cholecystokinin 2 receptors in the pancreas. *Pharmacol. Toxicol.* 91, 321–326.

Cochaud, S., Chevrier, L., Meunier, A. C., Brillet, T., Chadeneau, C., and Muller, J. M. (2010). The vasoactive intestinal peptide-receptor system is involved in human glioblastoma cell migration. *Neuropeptides* 44, 373–383.

Costante, G., Meringolo, D., Durante, C., Bianchi, D., Nocera, M., Tumino, S., et al. (2007). Predictive value of serum calcitonin levels for preoperative diagnosis of medullary thyroid carcinoma in a cohort of 5817 consecutive patients with thyroid nodules. *J. Clin. Endocrinol. Metab.* 92, 450–455.

Cure, P., Pileggi, A., and Alejandro, R. (2008). Exenatide and rare adverse events. *N. Engl. J. Med.* *358*, 1969–1970; discussion 1971–1972.

Denker, P. S., and Dimarco, P. E. (2006). Exenatide (exendin-4)-induced pancreatitis: a case report. *Diabetes Care* 29, 471.

Dennis, M. K., Burai, R., Ramesh, C., Petrie, W. K., Alcon, S. N., Nayak, T. K., et al. (2009). In vivo effects of a GPR30 antagonist. *Nat. Chem. Biol.* 5, 421–427.

Dennis, M. K., Field, A. S., Burai, R., Ramesh, C., Petrie, W. K., Bologa, C. G., et al. (2011). Identification of a GPER/GPR30 antagonist with improved estrogen receptor counterselectivity. *J. Steroid Biochem. Mol. Biol.* 127, 358–366.

Deroo, B. J., and Korach, K. S. (2006). Estrogen receptors and human disease. *J. Clin. Invest.* 116, 561–570.

Doyle, M. E., and Egan, J. M. (2007). Mechanisms of action of glucagon-like peptide 1 in the pancreas. *Pharmacol. Ther.* 113, 546–593.

Drucker, D. J. (2003). Glucagon-like peptides: regulators of cell proliferation, differentiation, and apoptosis. *Mol. Endocrinol.* 17, 161–171.

Drucker, D. J. (2006). The biology of incretin hormones. *Cell Metab.* 3, 153–165.

Du, G. Q., Zhou, L., Chen, X. Y., Wan, X. P., and He, Y. Y. (2012a). The G protein-coupled receptor GPR30 mediates the proliferative and invasive effects induced by hydroxytamoxifen in endometrial cancer cells. *Biochem. Biophys. Res. Commun.* 420, 343–349.

Du, N., Feng, J., Hu, L. J., Sun, X., Sun, H. B., Zhao, Y., et al. (2012b). Angiotensin II receptor type 1 blockers suppress the cell proliferation effects of angiotensin II in breast cancer cells by inhibiting AT1R signaling. *Oncol. Rep.* 27, 1893–1903.

Dufresne, M., Seva, C., and Fourmy, D. (2006). Cholecystokinin and gastrin receptors. *Physiol. Rev.* 86, 805–847.

Early Breast Cancer Trialists' Collaborative Group (EBCTCG). (2005). Effects of chemotherapy and hormonal therapy for early breast cancer on recurrence and 15-year survival: an overview of the randomised trials. *Lancet* 365, 1687–1717.

Edwards, D. P. (2005). Regulation of signal transduction pathways by estrogen and progesterone. *Annu. Rev. Physiol.* 67, 335–376.

Elashoff, M., Matveyenko, A. V., Gier, B., Elashoff, R., and Butler, P. C. (2011). Pancreatitis, pancreatic, and thyroid cancer with glucagon-like peptide-1-based therapies. *Gastroenterology* 141, 150–156.

Elisei, R., Bottici, V., Luchetti, F., Di Coscio, G., Romei, C., Grasso, L., et al. (2004). Impact of routine measurement of serum calcitonin on the diagnosis and outcome of medullary thyroid cancer: experience in 10,864 patients with nodular thyroid disorders. *J. Clin. Endocrinol. Metab.* 89, 163–168.

European Medicines Agency (EMA). (2006). *Assessment Report for Byetta.* Available at: http://www.ema.europa.eu/docs/en_GB/document_library/EPAR_-_Scientific_Discussion/human/000698/WC500051842.pdf [accessed September 27, 2011].

European Medicines Agency (EMA). (2009). *Assessment report for Victoza.* Available at: http://www.ema.europa.eu/docs/en_GB/document_library/EPAR_-_Public_assessment_report/human/001026/WC500050016. pdf [accessed September 27, 2011].

European Medicines Agency (EMA). (2011). *Assessment Report for By-Dureon.* Available at: http://www.ema.europa.eu/docs/en_GB/document_library/EPAR_-_Public_assessment_report/human/002020/WC500108239.pdf [accessed September 27, 2011].

Feng, S., Agoulnik, I. U., Truong, A., Li, Z., Creighton, C. J., Kaftanovskaya, E. M., et al. (2010). Suppression of relaxin receptor RXFP1 decreases prostate cancer growth and metastasis. *Endocr. Relat. Cancer* 17, 1021–1033.

Fernandez-Martinez, A. B., Bajo, A. M., Isabel Arenas, M., Sanchez-Chapado, M., Prieto, J. C., and Carmena, M. J. (2010). Vasoactive intestinal peptide (VIP) induces malignant transformation of the human prostate epithelial cell line RWPE-1. *Cancer Lett.* 299, 11–21.

Filardo, E. J., Graeber, C. T., Quinn, J. A., Resnick, M. B., Giri, D., DeLellis, R. A., et al. (2006). Distribution of GPR30, a seven membrane-spanning estrogen receptor, in primary breast cancer and its association with clinicopathologic determinants of tumor progression. *Clin. Cancer Res.* 12, 6359–6366.

Filardo, E. J., Quinn, J. A., Bland, K. I., and Frackelton, A. R. Jr. (2000). Estrogen-induced activation of Erk-1 and Erk-2 requires the G protein-coupled receptor homolog, GPR30, and occurs via trans-activation of the epidermal growth factor receptor through release of HB-EGF. *Mol. Endocrinol.* 14, 1649–1660.

Franco, R., Boscia, F., Gigantino, V., Marra, L., Esposito, F., Ferrara, D., et al. (2011). GPR30 is overexpressed in post-puberal testicular germ cell tumors. *Cancer Biol. Ther.* 11, 609–613.

Fung, J. N., Seim, I., Wang, D., Obermair, A., Chopin, L. K., and Chen, C. (2010). Expression and in vitro functions of the ghrelin axis in endometrial cancer. *Horm. Cancer* 1, 245–255.

Gesty-Palmer, D., Flannery, P., Yuan, L., Corsino, L., Spurney, R., Lefkowitz, R. J., et al. (2009). A beta-arrestin-biased agonist of the parathyroid hormone receptor (PTH1R) promotes bone formation independent of G protein activation. *Sci. Transl. Med.* 1, 1ra1.

Gesty-Palmer, D., and Luttrell, L. M. (2011). "Biasing" the parathyroid hormone receptor: a novel anabolic approach to increasing bone mass? *Br. J. Pharmacol.* 164, 59–67.

Gidekel Friedlander, S. Y., Chu, G. C., Snyder, E. L., Girnius, N., Dibelius, G., Crowley, D., et al. (2009). Context-dependent transformation of adult pancreatic cells by oncogenic K-Ras. *Cancer Cell* 16, 379–389.

Gier, B., Matveyenko, A. V., Kirakossian, D., Dawson, D., Dry, S. M., and Butler, P. C. (2012a). Chronic GLP-1 receptor activation by exendin-4 induces expansion of pancreatic duct glands in rats and accelerates formation of dysplastic lesions and chronic pancreatitis in the Kras(G12D) mouse model. *Diabetes* 61, 1250–1262.

Gier, B., Butler, P. C., Lai, C. K., Kirakossian, D., DeNicola, M. M., and Yeh, M. W. (2012b). Glucagon like peptide-1 receptor expression in the human thyroid gland. *J. Clin. Endocrinol. Metab.* 97, 121–131.

Gigoux, V., Clerc, P., Sanchez, D., Coll, M. G., Corominola, H., Leung-Theung-Long, S., et al. (2008). Reg genes are CCK2 receptor targets in ElasCCK2 mice pancreas. *Regul. Pept.* 146, 88–98.

Giovannucci, E., Harlan, D. M., Archer, M. C., Bergenstal, R. M., Gapstur, S. M., Habel, L. A., et al. (2010). Diabetes and cancer: a consensus report. *Diabetes Care* 33, 1674–1685.

Girman, C. J., Kou, T. D., Cai, B., Alexander, C. M., O'Neill, E. A., Williams-Herman, D. E., et al. (2010). Patients with type 2 diabetes mellitus have higher risk for acute pancreatitis compared with those without diabetes. *Diabetes Obes. Metab.* 12, 766–771.

Goke, R., Fehmann, H. C., Linn, T., Schmidt, H., Krause, M., Eng, J., et al. (1993). Exendin-4 is a high potency agonist and truncated exendin-(9-39)-amide an antagonist at the glucagon-like peptide 1-(7-36)-amide receptor of insulin-secreting beta-cells. *J. Biol. Chem.* 268, 19650–19655.

Goldstein, S. R. (2001). The effect of SERMs on the endometrium. *Ann. N. Y. Acad. Sci.* 949, 237–242.

Gottardis, M. M., Robinson, S. P., Satyaswaroop, P. G., and Jordan, V. C. (1988). Contrasting actions of tamoxifen on endometrial and breast tumor growth in the athymic mouse. *Cancer Res.* 48, 812–815.

Graf, R., Schiesser, M., Reding, T., Appenzeller, P., Sun, L. K., Fortunato, F., et al. (2006). Exocrine meets endocrine: pancreatic stone protein and regenerating protein – two sides of the same coin. *J. Surg. Res.* 133, 113–120.

Granier, S., Kim, S., Shafer, A. M., Ratnala, V. R., Fung, J. J., Zare, R. N., et al. (2007). Structure and conformational changes in the C-terminal domain of the beta2-adrenoceptor: insights from fluorescence resonance energy transfer studies. *J. Biol. Chem.* 282, 13895–13905.

Greer, J. B., and Whitcomb, D. C. (2009). Inflammation and pancreatic cancer: an evidence-based review. *Curr. Opin. Pharmacol.* 9, 411–418.

Grieco, P., Franco, R., Bozzuto, G., Toccacieli, L., Sgambato, A., Marra, M., et al. (2011). Urotensin II receptor predicts the clinical outcome of prostate cancer patients and is involved in the regulation of motility of prostate adenocarcinoma cells. *J. Cell. Biochem.* 112, 341–353.

Guillermet-Guibert, J., Lahlou, H., Cordelier, P., Bousquet, C., Pyronnet, S., and Susini, C. (2005). Physiology of somatostatin receptors. *J. Endocrinol. Invest.* 28, 5–9.

Hafiz, S., Dennis, J. C., Schwartz, D., Judd, R., Tao, Y. X., Khazal, K., et al. (2012). Expression of melanocortin receptors in human prostate cancer cell lines: MC2R activation by ACTH increases prostate cancer cell proliferation. *Int. J. Oncol.* 41, 1373–1380.

Hammes, S. R., and Levin, E. R. (2007). Extranuclear steroid receptors: nature and actions. *Endocr. Rev.* 28, 726–741.

Harikumar, K. G., Wootten, D., Pinon, D. I., Koole, C., Ball, A. M., Furness, S. G., et al. (2012). Glucagon-like peptide-1 receptor dimerization differentially regulates agonist signaling but does not affect small molecule allostery. *Proc. Natl. Acad. Sci. U.S.A.* 109, 18607–18612.

He, Y. Y., Cai, B., Yang, Y. X., Liu, X. L., and Wan, X. P. (2009). Estrogenic G protein-coupled receptor 30 signaling is involved in regulation of endometrial carcinoma by promoting proliferation, invasion potential, and interleukin-6 secretion via the MEK/ERK mitogen-activated protein kinase pathway. *Cancer Sci.* 100, 1051–1061.

He, Y. Y., Du, G. Q., Cai, B., Yan, Q., Zhou, L., Chen, X. Y., et al. (2012). Estrogenic transmembrane receptor of GPR30 mediates invasion and carcinogenesis by endometrial cancer cell line RL95-2. *J. Cancer Res. Clin. Oncol.* 138, 775–783.

Hegedus, L., Moses, A. C., Zdravkovic, M., Le Thi, T., and Daniels, G. H. (2011). GLP-1 and calcitonin concentration in humans: lack of evidence of calcitonin release from sequential screening in over 5000 subjects with type 2 diabetes or nondiabetic obese subjects treated with the human GLP-1 analog, liraglutide. *J. Clin. Endocrinol. Metab.* 96, 853–860.

Henic, E., Noskova, V., Hoyer-Hansen, G., Hansson, S., and Casslen, B. (2009). Estradiol attenuates EGF-induced rapid uPAR mobilization and cell migration via the G-protein-coupled receptor 30 in ovarian cancer cells. *Int. J. Gynecol. Cancer* 19, 214–222.

Hernandez-Munoz, I., Skoudy, A., Real, F. X., and Navarro, P. (2008). Pancreatic ductal adenocarcinoma: cellular origin, signaling pathways and stroma contribution. *Pancreatology* 8, 462–469.

Hodsman, A. B., Bauer, D. C., Dempster, D. W., Dian, L., Hanley, D. A., Harris, S. T., et al. (2005). Parathyroid hormone and teriparatide for the treatment of osteoporosis: a review of the evidence and suggested guidelines for its use. *Endocr. Rev.* 26, 688–703.

Holst, J. J. (2007). The physiology of glucagon-like peptide 1. *Physiol. Rev.* 87, 1409–1439.

Holst, J. J., Gromada, J., and Nauck, M. A. (1997). The pathogenesis of NIDDM involves a defective expression of the GIP receptor. *Diabetologia* 40, 984–986.

Holz, G. G. (2004). Epac: a new cAMP-binding protein in support of glucagon-like peptide-1 receptor-mediated signal transduction in the pancreatic beta-cell. *Diabetes* 53, 5–13.

Hopkins, A. L., and Groom, C. R. (2002). The druggable genome. *Nat. Rev. Drug Discov.* 1, 727–730.

Horsch, D., Goke, R., Eissele, R., Michel, B., and Goke, B. (1997). Reciprocal cellular distribution of glucagon-like peptide-1 (GLP-1) immunoreactivity and GLP-1 receptor mRNA in pancreatic islets of rat. *Pancreas* 14, 290–294.

Ignatov, A., Ignatov, T., Weissenborn, C., Eggemann, H., Bischoff, J., Semczuk, A., et al. (2011). G-protein-coupled estrogen receptor GPR30 and tamoxifen resistance in breast cancer. *Breast Cancer Res. Treat.* 128, 457–466.

Ignatov, T., Eggemann, H., Semczuk, A., Smith, B., Bischoff, J., Roessner, A., et al. (2010a). Role of GPR30 in endometrial pathology after tamoxifen for breast cancer. *Am. J. Obstet. Gynecol.* 203, e9–e16.

Ignatov, A., Ignatov, T., Roessner, A., Costa, S. D., and Kalinski, T. (2010b). Role of GPR30 in the mechanisms of tamoxifen resistance in breast cancer MCF-7 cells. *Breast Cancer Res. Treat.* 123, 87–96.

Jamil, A., Croxtall, J. D., and White, J. O. (1991). The effect of anti-oestrogens on cell growth and progesterone receptor concentration in human endometrial cancer cells (Ishikawa). *J. Mol. Endocrinol.* 6, 215–221.

Jeffery, P. L., Herington, A. C., and Chopin, L. K. (2002). Expression and action of the growth hormone releasing peptide ghrelin and its receptor in prostate cancer cell lines. *J. Endocrinol.* 172, R7–R11.

Jeffery, P. L., Murray, R. E., Yeh, A. H., McNamara, J. F., Duncan, R. P., Francis, G. D., et al. (2005). Expression and function of the ghrelin axis, including a novel preproghrelin isoform, in human breast cancer tissues and cell lines. *Endocr. Relat. Cancer* 12, 839–850.

Jordan, B. A., and Devi, L. A. (1999). G-protein-coupled receptor heterodimerization modulates receptor function. *Nature* 399, 697–700.

Jordan, V. C. (2007). SERMs: meeting the promise of multifunctional medicines. *J. Natl. Cancer Inst.* 99, 350–356.

Jordan, V. C., and Morrow, M. (1999). Tamoxifen, raloxifene, and the prevention of breast cancer. *Endocr. Rev.* 20, 253–278.

Jorgensen, R., Kubale, V., Vrecl, M., Schwartz, T. W., and Elling, C. E. (2007). Oxyntomodulin differentially affects glucagon-like peptide-1 receptor beta-arrestin recruitment and signaling through Galpha(s). *J. Pharmacol. Exp. Ther.* 322, 148–154.

Josefsson, M. L., and Leinster, S. J. (2010). Aromatase inhibitors versus tamoxifen as adjuvant hormonal therapy for oestrogen sensitive early breast cancer in post-menopausal women: meta-analyses of monotherapy, sequenced therapy and extended therapy. *Breast* 19, 76–83.

Jura, N., Archer, H., and Bar-Sagi, D. (2005). Chronic pancreatitis, pancreatic adenocarcinoma and the black box in-between. *Cell Res.* 15, 72–77.

Kahsai, A. W., Xiao, K., Rajagopal, S., Ahn, S., Shukla, A. K., Sun, J., et al. (2011). Multiple ligand-specific conformations of the beta2-adrenergic receptor. *Nat. Chem. Biol.* 7, 692–700.

Kashima, Y., Miki, T., Shibasaki, T., Ozaki, N., Miyazaki, M., Yano, H., et al. (2001). Critical role of cAMP-GEFII – Rim2 complex in incretin-potentiated insulin secretion. *J. Biol. Chem.* 276, 46046–46053.

Ketterer, K., Kong, B., Frank, D., Giese, N. A., Bauer, A., Hoheisel, J., et al. (2009). Neuromedin U is overexpressed in pancreatic cancer and increases invasiveness via the hepatocyte growth factor c-Met pathway. *Cancer Lett.* 277, 72–81.

Kim, I. M., Tilley, D. G., Chen, J., Salazar, N. C., Whalen, E. J., Violin, J. D., et al. (2008). Beta-blockers alprenolol and carvedilol stimulate beta-arrestin-mediated EGFR transactivation. *Proc. Natl. Acad. Sci. U.S.A.* 105, 14555–14560.

Kintzel, P. E., Chase, S. L., Schultz, L. M., and O'Rourke, T. J. (2008). Increased risk of metabolic syndrome, diabetes mellitus, and cardiovascular disease in men receiving androgen deprivation therapy for prostate cancer. *Pharmacotherapy* 28, 1511–1522.

Kleuser, B., Malek, D., Gust, R., Pertz, H. H., and Potteck, H. (2008). 17-Beta-estradiol inhibits transforming growth factor-beta signaling and function in breast cancer cells via activation of extracellular signal-regulated kinase through the G protein-coupled receptor 30. *Mol. Pharmacol.* 74, 1533–1543.

Koehler, J. A., Baggio, L. L., Lamont, B. J., Ali, S., and Drucker, D. J. (2009). Glucagon-like peptide-1 receptor activation modulates pancreatitis-associated gene expression but does not modify the susceptibility to experimental pancreatitis in mice. *Diabetes* 58, 2148–2161.

Koehler, J. A., and Drucker, D. J. (2006). Activation of glucagon-like peptide-1 receptor signaling does not modify the growth or apoptosis of human pancreatic cancer cells. *Diabetes* 55, 1369–1379.

Korner, M., Stockli, M., Waser, B., and Reubi, J. C. (2007). GLP-1 receptor expression in human tumors and human normal tissues: potential for in vivo targeting. *J. Nucl. Med.* 48, 736–743.

Lando, H. M., Alattar, M., and Dua, A. P. (2012). Elevated amylase and lipase levels in patients using glucagon-like peptide-1 receptor agonists or dipeptidyl-peptidase-4 inhibitors in the outpatient setting. *Endocr. Pract.* 18, 472–477.

Lappano, R., Rosano, C., Santolla, M. F., Pupo, M., De Francesco, E. M., De Marco, P., et al. (2012). Two novel GPER agonists induce gene expression changes and growth effects in cancer cells. *Curr. Cancer Drug Targets* 12, 531–542.

Leblanc, K., Sexton, E., Parent, S., Belanger, G., Dery, M. C., Boucher, V., et al. (2007). Effects of 4-hydroxytamoxifen, raloxifene and ICI 182 780 on survival of uterine cancer cell lines in the presence and absence of exogenous estrogens. *Int. J. Oncol.* 30, 477–487.

Lebon, G., Warne, T., Edwards, P. C., Bennett, K., Langmead, C. J., Leslie, A. G., et al. (2011). Agonist-bound adenosine A2A receptor structures reveal common features of GPCR activation. *Nature* 474, 521–525.

Lee, D. K., Ferguson, S. S., George, S. R., and O'Dowd, B. F. (2010). The fate of the internalized apelin receptor is determined by different isoforms of apelin mediating differential interaction with beta-arrestin. *Biochem. Biophys. Res. Commun.* 395, 185–189.

Liu, J. J., Horst, R., Katritch, V., Stevens, R. C., and Wuthrich, K. (2012). Biased signaling pathways in beta2-adrenergic receptor characterized by 19F-NMR. *Science* 335, 1106–1110.

LiVolsi, V. A. (1997). C cell hyperplasia/neoplasia. *J. Clin. Endocrinol. Metab.* 82, 39–41.

Logsdon, C. D., and Ji, B. (2009). Ras activity in acinar cells links chronic pancreatitis and pancreatic cancer. *Clin. Gastroenterol. Hepatol.* 7, S40–S43.

Lorand, T., Vigh, E., and Garai, J. (2010). Hormonal action of plant derived and anthropogenic non-steroidal estrogenic compounds: phytoestrogens and xenoestrogens. *Curr. Med. Chem.* 17, 3542–3574.

Lu, C., Everhart, L., Tilan, J., Kuo, L., Sun, C. C., Munivenkatappa, R. B., et al. (2010). Neuropeptide Y and its Y2 receptor: potential targets in neuroblastoma therapy. *Oncogene* 29, 5630–5642.

Luttrell, L. M., and Gesty-Palmer, D. (2010). Beyond desensitization: physiological relevance of arrestin-dependent signaling. *Pharmacol. Rev.* 62, 305–330.

MacDonald, P. E., Wang, X., Xia, F., El-kholy, W., Targonsky, E. D., Tsushima, R. G., et al. (2003). Antagonism of rat beta-cell voltage-dependent K+ currents by exendin 4 requires dual activation of the cAMP/protein kinase A and phosphatidylinositol 3-kinase signaling pathways. *J. Biol. Chem.* 278, 52446–52453.

Machens, A., Hoffmann, F., Sekulla, C., and Dralle, H. (2009). Importance of gender-specific calcitonin thresholds in screening for occult sporadic medullary thyroid cancer. *Endocr. Relat. Cancer* 16, 1291–1298.

Madsbad, S. (2009). Treatment of type 2 diabetes with incretin-based therapies. *Lancet* 373, 438–439.

Madsen, L. W., Knauf, J. A., Gotfredsen, C., Pilling, A., Sjogren, I., Andersen, S., et al. (2012). GLP-1 receptor agonists and the thyroid: C-cell effects in mice are mediated via the GLP-1 receptor and not associated with RET activation. *Endocrinology* 153, 1538–1547.

Mathieu, A., Clerc, P., Portolan, G., Bierkamp, C., Lulka, H., Pradayrol, L., et al. (2005). Transgenic expression of CCK2 receptors sensitizes murine pancreatic acinar cells to carcinogen-induced preneoplastic lesions formation. *Int. J. Cancer* 115, 46–54.

Matusiak, D., Glover, S., Nathaniel, R., Matkowskyj, K., Yang, J., and Benya, R. V. (2005). Neuromedin B and its receptor are mitogens in both normal and malignant epithelial cells lining the colon. *Am. J. Physiol. Gastrointest. Liver Physiol.* 288, G718–G728.

Mayo, K. E., Miller, L. J., Bataille, D., Dalle, S., Goke, B., Thorens, B., et al. (2003). International union of pharmacology. XXXV. The glucagon receptor family. *Pharmacol. Rev.* 55, 167–194.

McDonnell, D. P. (1999). The molecular pharmacology of SERMs. *Trends Endocrinol. Metab.* 10, 301–311.

Means, A. L., Meszoely, I. M., Suzuki, K., Miyamoto, Y., Rustgi, A. K., Coffey, R. J., et al. (2005). Pancreatic epithelial plasticity mediated by acinar cell transdifferentiation and generation of nestin-positive intermediates. *Development* 132, 3767–3776.

Medeiros, P. J., Al-Khazraji, B. K., Novielli, N. M., Postovit, L. M., Chambers, A. F., and Jackson, D. N. (2012). Neuropeptide Y stimulates proliferation and migration in the 4T1 breast cancer cell line. *Int. J. Cancer* 131, 276–286.

Medved, V., Jovanovic, N., and Knapic, V. P. (2009). The comorbidity of diabetes mellitus and psychiatric disorders. *Psychiatr. Danub.* 21, 585–588.

Meyer, M. R., and Barton, M. (2009). ERalpha, ERbeta, and gpER: novel aspects of oestrogen receptor signalling in atherosclerosis. *Cardiovasc. Res.* 83, 605–610.

Meyer, M. R., Haas, E., Prossnitz, E. R., and Barton, M. (2009). Non-genomic regulation of vascular cell function and growth by estrogen. *Mol. Cell. Endocrinol.* 308, 9–16.

Mojsov, S., Weir, G. C., and Habener, J. F. (1987). Insulinotropin: glucagon-like peptide I (7-37) co-encoded in the glucagon gene is a potent stimulator of insulin release in the perfused rat pancreas. *J. Clin. Invest.* 79, 616–619.

Monnier, J., and Samson, M. (2010). Prokineticins in angiogenesis and cancer. *Cancer Lett.* 296, 144–149.
Moody, T. W., Osefo, N., Nuche-Berenguer, B., Ridnour, L., Wink, D., and Jensen, R. T. (2012). Pituitary adenylate cyclase-activating polypeptide causes tyrosine phosphorylation of the epidermal growth factor receptor in lung cancer cells. *J. Pharmacol. Exp. Ther.* 341, 873–881.
Moody, T. W., Walters, J., Casibang, M., Zia, F., and Gozes, Y. (2000). VPAC1 receptors and lung cancer. *Ann. N. Y. Acad. Sci.* 921, 26–32.
Muller, K. M., Tveteraas, I. H., Aasrum, M., Odegard, J., Dawood, M., Dajani, O., et al. (2011). Role of protein kinase C and epidermal growth factor receptor signalling in growth stimulation by neurotensin in colon carcinoma cells. *BMC Cancer* 11:421. doi:10.1186/1471-2407-11-421
Nachnani, J. S., Bulchandani, D. G., Nookala, A., Herndon, B., Molteni, A., Pandya, P., et al. (2010). Biochemical and histological effects of exendin-4 (exenatide) on the rat pancreas. *Diabetologia* 53, 153–159.
Nagel, J. M., Geiger, B. M., Karagiannis, A. K., Gras-Miralles, B., Horst, D., Najarian, R. M., et al. (2012). Reduced intestinal tumorigenesis in APCmin mice lacking melanin-concentrating hormone. *PLoS ONE* 7:e41914. doi:10.1371/journal.pone.0041914
Nasrallah, H. A. (2008). Atypical antipsychotic-induced metabolic side effects: insights from receptor-binding profiles. *Mol. Psychiatry* 13, 27–35.
Nauck, M. A., Heimesaat, M. M., Orskov, C., Holst, J. J., Ebert, R., and Creutzfeldt, W. (1993). Preserved incretin activity of glucagon-like peptide 1 [7-36 amide] but not of synthetic human gastric inhibitory polypeptide in patients with type-2 diabetes mellitus. *J. Clin. Invest.* 91, 301–307.
Nauck, M. A., Vilsboll, T., Gallwitz, B., Garber, A., and Madsbad, S. (2009). Incretin-based therapies: viewpoints on the way to consensus. *Diabetes Care* 32(Suppl. 2), S223–S231.
Nyborg, N. C., Molck, A. M., Madsen, L. W., and Knudsen, L. B. (2012). The human GLP-1 analog liraglutide and the pancreas: evidence for the absence of structural pancreatic changes in three species. *Diabetes* 61, 1243–1249.
Orlando, L., Schiavone, P., Fedele, P., Calvani, N., Nacci, A., Rizzo, P., et al. (2010). Molecularly targeted endocrine therapies for breast cancer. *Cancer Treat. Rev.* 36(Suppl. 3), S67–S71.
Otto, C., Rohde-Schulz, B., Schwarz, G., Fuchs, I., Klewer, M., Brittain, D., et al. (2008). G protein-coupled receptor 30 localizes to the endoplasmic reticulum and is not activated by estradiol. *Endocrinology* 149, 4846–4856.
Pandey, A., Forte, V., Abdallah, M., Alickaj, A., Mahmud, S., Asad, S., et al. (2011). Diabetes mellitus and the risk of cancer. *Minerva Endocrinol.* 36, 187–209.
Pandey, D. P., Lappano, R., Albanito, L., Madeo, A., Maggiolini, M., and Picard, D. (2009). Estrogenic GPR30 signalling induces proliferation and migration of breast cancer cells through CTGF. *EMBO J.* 28, 523–532.
Park, H. J., Kim, S. R., Kim, M. K., Choi, K. S., Jang, H. O., Yun, I., et al. (2011). Neuromedin B receptor antagonist suppresses tumor angiogenesis and tumor growth in vitro and in vivo. *Cancer Lett.* 312, 117–127.
Park, S., Dong, X., Fisher, T. L., Dunn, S., Omer, A. K., Weir, G., et al. (2006). Exendin-4 uses Irs2 signaling to mediate pancreatic beta cell growth and function. *J. Biol. Chem.* 281, 1159–1168.
Pedram, A., Razandi, M., and Levin, E. R. (2006). Nature of functional estrogen receptors at the plasma membrane. *Mol. Endocrinol.* 20, 1996–2009.
Perez-Mancera, P. A., Guerra, C., Barbacid, M., and Tuveson, D. A. (2012). What we have learned about pancreatic cancer from mouse models. *Gastroenterology* 142, 1079–1092.
Phillips, L. K., and Prins, J. B. (2011). Update on incretin hormones. *Ann. N. Y. Acad. Sci.* 1243, E55–E74.
Pike, M. C., Pearce, C. L., and Wu, A. H. (2004). Prevention of cancers of the breast, endometrium and ovary. *Oncogene* 23, 6379–6391.
Piteau, S., Olver, A., Kim, S. J., Winter, K., Pospisilik, J. A., Lynn, F., et al. (2007). Reversal of islet GIP receptor down-regulation and resistance to GIP by reducing hyperglycemia in the Zucker rat. *Biochem. Biophys. Res. Commun.* 362, 1007–1012.
Powles, T. J., Ashley, S., Tidy, A., Smith, I. E., and Dowsett, M. (2007). Twenty-year follow-up of the Royal Marsden randomized, double-blinded tamoxifen breast cancer prevention trial. *J. Natl. Cancer Inst.* 99, 283–290.
Pratley, R. E., and Gilbert, M. (2008). Targeting incretins in Type 2 diabetes: role of GLP-1 receptor agonists and DPP-4 inhibitors. *Rev. Diabet. Stud.* 5, 73–94.
Prossnitz, E. R., Arterburn, J. B., Smith, H. O., Oprea, T. I., Sklar, L. A., and Hathaway, H. J. (2008a). Estrogen signaling through the transmembrane G protein-coupled receptor GPR30. *Annu. Rev. Physiol.* 70, 165–190.
Prossnitz, E. R., Oprea, T. I., Sklar, L. A., and Arterburn, J. B. (2008b). The ins and outs of GPR30: a transmembrane estrogen receptor. *J. Steroid Biochem. Mol. Biol.* 109, 350–353.
Quoyer, J., Longuet, C., Broca, C., Linck, N., Costes, S., Varin, E., et al. (2010). GLP-1 mediates antiapoptotic effect by phosphorylating Bad through a beta-arrestin 1-mediated ERK1/2 activation in pancreatic beta-cells. *J. Biol. Chem.* 285, 1989–2002.
Rafei, M., Berchiche, Y. A., Birman, E., Boivin, M. N., Young, Y. K., Wu, J. H., et al. (2009). An engineered GM-CSF-CCL2 fusokine is a potent inhibitor of CCR2-driven inflammation as demonstrated in a murine model of inflammatory arthritis. *J. Immunol.* 183, 1759–1766.
Rahmeh, R., Damian, M., Cottet, M., Orcel, H., Mendre, C., Durroux, T., et al. (2012). Structural insights into biased G protein-coupled receptor signaling revealed by fluorescence spectroscopy. *Proc. Natl. Acad. Sci. U.S.A.* 109, 6733–6738.
Rajagopal, S., Rajagopal, K., and Lefkowitz, R. J. (2010a). Teaching old receptors new tricks: biasing seven-transmembrane receptors. *Nat. Rev. Drug Discov.* 9, 373–386.
Rajagopal, S., Kim, J., Ahn, S., Craig, S., Lam, C. M., Gerard, N. P., et al. (2010b). Beta-arrestin- but not G protein-mediated signaling by the "decoy" receptor CXCR7. *Proc. Natl. Acad. Sci. U.S.A.* 107, 628–632.
Rebours, V., Boutron-Ruault, M. C., Schnee, M., Ferec, C., Le Marechal, C., Hentic, O., et al. (2009). The natural history of hereditary pancreatitis: a national series. *Gut* 58, 97–103.
Revankar, C. M., Cimino, D. F., Sklar, L. A., Arterburn, J. B., and Prossnitz, E. R. (2005). A transmembrane intracellular estrogen receptor mediates rapid cell signaling. *Science* 307, 1625–1630.
Reversi, A., Rimoldi, V., Marrocco, T., Cassoni, P., Bussolati, G., Parenti, M., et al. (2005). The oxytocin receptor antagonist atosiban inhibits cell growth via a "biased agonist" mechanism. *J. Biol. Chem.* 280, 16311–16318.
Ring, A., and Dowsett, M. (2004). Mechanisms of tamoxifen resistance. *Endocr. Relat. Cancer* 11, 643–658.
Rocheville, M., Lange, D. C., Kumar, U., Sasi, R., Patel, R. C., and Patel, Y. C. (2000). Subtypes of the somatostatin receptor assemble as functional homo- and heterodimers. *J. Biol. Chem.* 275, 7862–7869.
Rodrigues-Ferreira, S., Abdelkarim, M., Dillenburg-Pilla, P., Luissint, A. C., di-Tommaso, A., Deshayes, F., et al. (2012). Angiotensin II facilitates breast cancer cell migration and metastasis. *PLoS ONE* 7:e35667. doi:10.1371/journal.pone.0035667
Rodriguez-Frade, J. M., Vila-Coro, A. J., de Ana, A. M., Albar, J. P., Martinez, A. C., and Mellado, M. (1999). The chemokine monocyte chemoattractant protein-1 induces functional responses through dimerization of its receptor CCR2. *Proc. Natl. Acad. Sci. U.S.A.* 96, 3628–3633.
Ruscica, M., Dozio, E., Boghossian, S., Bovo, G., Martos Riano, V., Motta, M., et al. (2006). Activation of the Y1 receptor by neuropeptide Y regulates the growth of prostate cancer cells. *Endocrinology* 147, 1466–1473.
Sanden, C., Broselid, S., Cornmark, L., Andersson, K., Daszkiewicz-Nilsson, J., Martensson, U. E., et al. (2011). G protein-coupled estrogen receptor 1/G protein-coupled receptor 30 localizes in the plasma membrane and traffics intracellularly on cytokeratin intermediate filaments. *Mol. Pharmacol.* 79, 400–410.
Saphner, T., Tormey, D. C., and Gray, R. (1996). Annual hazard rates of recurrence for breast cancer after primary therapy. *J. Clin. Oncol.* 14, 2738–2746.
Saylor, P. J., and Smith, M. R. (2009). Metabolic complications of androgen deprivation therapy for prostate cancer. *J. Urol.* 181, 1998–2006. discussion 2007–2008.
Schwartz, L. B., Krey, L., Demopoulos, R., Goldstein, S. R., Nachtigall, L. E., and Mittal, K. (1997). Alterations in steroid hormone receptors in the tamoxifen-treated endometrium. *Am. J. Obstet. Gynecol.* 176, 129–137.
Seino, S., and Shibasaki, T. (2005). PKA-dependent and PKA-independent pathways for cAMP-regulated exocytosis. *Physiol. Rev.* 85, 1303–1342.
Sengupta, S., Peterson, T. R., and Sabatini, D. M. (2010). Regulation of the mTOR complex 1 pathway by nutrients, growth factors, and stress. *Mol. Cell* 40, 310–322.

Sensken, S. C., Staubert, C., Keul, P., Levkau, B., Schoneberg, T., and Graler, M. H. (2008). Selective activation of G alpha i mediated signalling of S1P3 by FTY720-phosphate. *Cell. Signal.* 20, 1125–1133.

Sheriff, S., Ali, M., Yahya, A., Haider, K. H., Balasubramaniam, A., and Amlal, H. (2010). Neuropeptide Y Y5 receptor promotes cell growth through extracellular signal-regulated kinase signaling and cyclic AMP inhibition in a human breast cancer cell line. *Mol. Cancer Res.* 8, 604–614.

Siegfried, J. M., Hershberger, P. A., and Stabile, L. P. (2009). Estrogen receptor signaling in lung cancer. *Semin. Oncol.* 36, 524–531.

Smith, H. O., Leslie, K. K., Singh, M., Qualls, C. R., Revankar, C. M., Joste, N. E., et al. (2007). GPR30: a novel indicator of poor survival for endometrial carcinoma. *Am. J. Obstet. Gynecol.* 196, 386.e1–386.e9. discussion 386.e9–386.e11.

Subbiah, V., Madsen, V. S., Raymond, A. K., Benjamin, R. S., and Ludwig, J. A. (2010). Of mice and men: divergent risks of teriparatide-induced osteosarcoma. *Osteoporos. Int.* 21, 1041–1045.

Suzuki, K., Nakabayashi, K., Yamada, A. Y., Lodhi, R. S., Hazama, R., Ebina, Y., et al. (2012). Recombinant H2 relaxin inhibits apoptosis and induces cell proliferation in cultured leiomyoma cells without affecting those in cultured normal myometrial cells. *Fertil. Steril.* 97, 734–741.

Tack, J., Camilleri, M., Chang, L., Chey, W. D., Galligan, J. J., Lacy, B. E., et al. (2012). Systematic review: cardiovascular safety profile of 5-HT(4) agonists developed for gastrointestinal disorders. *Aliment. Pharmacol. Ther.* 35, 745–767.

Tatarkiewicz, K., Smith, P. A., Sablan, E. J., Polizzi, C. J., Aumann, D. E., Villescaz, C., et al. (2010). Exenatide does not evoke pancreatitis and attenuates chemically induced pancreatitis in normal and diabetic rodents. *Am. J. Physiol. Endocrinol. Metab.* 299, E1076–E1086.

Thomas, P., and Dong, J. (2006). Binding and activation of the seven-transmembrane estrogen receptor GPR30 by environmental estrogens: a potential novel mechanism of endocrine disruption. *J. Steroid Biochem. Mol. Biol.* 102, 175–179.

Thomas, P., Pang, Y., Filardo, E. J., and Dong, J. (2005). Identity of an estrogen membrane receptor coupled to a G protein in human breast cancer cells. *Endocrinology* 146, 624–632.

Thorens, B. (1992). Expression cloning of the pancreatic beta cell receptor for the gluco-incretin hormone glucagon-like peptide 1. *Proc. Natl. Acad. Sci. U.S.A.* 89, 8641–8645.

Tian, P. Y., and Fan, X. M. (2012). The proliferative effects of ghrelin on human gastric cancer AGS cells. *J. Dig. Dis.* 13, 453–458.

Tornehave, D., Kristensen, P., Romer, J., Knudsen, L. B., and Heller, R. S. (2008). Expression of the GLP-1 receptor in mouse, rat, and human pancreas. *J. Histochem. Cytochem.* 56, 841–851.

Tripathy, N. R., Basha, S., Jain, R., Shetty, S., and Ramachandran, A. (2008). Exenatide and acute pancreatitis. *J. Assoc. Physicians India* 56, 987–988.

Trumper, J., Ross, D., Jahr, H., Brendel, M. D., Goke, R., and Horsch, D. (2005). The Rap-B-Raf signalling pathway is activated by glucose and glucagon-like peptide-1 in human islet cells. *Diabetologia* 48, 1534–1540.

U.S. Food and Drug Administration. (2011). *Victoza (Liraglutide [rDNA Origin]) Injection: REMS-Risk of Thyroid C-Cell Tumors, Acute Pancreatitis.* Available at: http://www.fda.gov/Safety/MedWatch/Safety Information/SafetyAlertsforHuman MedicalProducts/ucm258826.htm [accessed April 30, 2012].

Vaidehi, N., and Kenakin, T. (2010). The role of conformational ensembles of seven transmembrane receptors in functional selectivity. *Curr. Opin. Pharmacol.* 10, 775–781.

Valdehita, A., Carmena, M. J., Bajo, A. M., and Prieto, J. C. (2012). RNA interference-directed silencing of VPAC1 receptor inhibits VIP effects on both EGFR and HER2 transactivation and VEGF secretion in human breast cancer cells. *Mol. Cell. Endocrinol.* 348, 241–246.

van Leeuwen, F. E., Benraadt, J., Coebergh, J. W., Kiemeney, L. A., Gimbrere, C. H., Otter, R., et al. (1994). Risk of endometrial cancer after tamoxifen treatment of breast cancer. *Lancet* 343, 448–452.

Victoza (Liraglutide) Injection. (2012). *Novo Nordisk.* Available at: http://www.novo-pi.com/victoza.pdf [accessed April 30, 2012].

Vila-Coro, A. J., Mellado, M., Martin de Ana, A., Lucas, P., del Real, G., Martinez, A. C., et al. (2000). HIV-1 infection through the CCR5 receptor is blocked by receptor dimerization. *Proc. Natl. Acad. Sci. U.S.A.* 97, 3388–3393.

Vilsboll, T. (2009). The effects of glucagon-like peptide-1 on the beta cell. *Diabetes Obes. Metab.* 11(Suppl. 3), 11–18.

Vilsboll, T., Brock, B., Perrild, H., Levin, K., Lervang, H. H., Kolendorf, K., et al. (2008). Liraglutide, a once-daily human GLP-1 analogue, improves pancreatic B-cell function and arginine-stimulated insulin secretion during hyperglycaemia in patients with Type 2 diabetes mellitus. *Diabet. Med.* 25, 152–156.

Vilsboll, T., Krarup, T., Madsbad, S., and Holst, J. J. (2002). Defective amplification of the late phase insulin response to glucose by GIP in obese Type II diabetic patients. *Diabetologia* 45, 1111–1119.

Vilsboll, T., Zdravkovic, M., Le-Thi, T., Krarup, T., Schmitz, O., Courreges, J. P., et al. (2007). Liraglutide, a long-acting human glucagon-like peptide-1 analog, given as monotherapy significantly improves glycemic control and lowers body weight without risk of hypoglycemia in patients with type 2 diabetes. *Diabetes Care* 30, 1608–1610.

Vivacqua, A., Bonofiglio, D., Recchia, A. G., Musti, A. M., Picard, D., Ando, S., et al. (2006a). The G protein-coupled receptor GPR30 mediates the proliferative effects induced by 17beta-estradiol and hydroxytamoxifen in endometrial cancer cells. *Mol. Endocrinol.* 20, 631–646.

Vivacqua, A., Bonofiglio, D., Albanito, L., Madeo, A., Rago, V., Carpino, A., et al. (2006b). 17beta-estradiol, genistein, and 4-hydroxytamoxifen induce the proliferation of thyroid cancer cells through the G protein-coupled receptor GPR30. *Mol. Pharmacol.* 70, 1414–1423.

Wang, C. I., and Lewis, R. J. (2013). Emerging opportunities for allosteric modulation of G-protein coupled receptors. *Biochem. Pharmacol.* 85, 153–162.

Wang, D., Hu, L., Zhang, G., Zhang, L., and Chen, C. (2010). G protein-coupled receptor 30 in tumor development. *Endocrine* 38, 29–37.

Warne, T., Moukhametzianov, R., Baker, J. G., Nehme, R., Edwards, P. C., Leslie, A. G., et al. (2011). The structural basis for agonist and partial agonist action on a beta(1)-adrenergic receptor. *Nature* 469, 241–244.

Waser, B., Beetschen, K., Pellegata, N. S., and Reubi, J. C. (2011). Incretin receptors in non-neoplastic and neoplastic thyroid C cells in rodents and humans: relevance for incretin-based diabetes therapy. *Neuroendocrinology* 94, 291–301.

Waser, B., Rehmann, R., Sanchez, C., Fourmy, D., and Reubi, J. C. (2012). Glucose-dependent insulinotropic polypeptide receptors in most gastroenteropancreatic and bronchial neuroendocrine tumors. *J. Clin. Endocrinol. Metab.* 97, 482–488.

Wehbi, V., Decourtye, J., Piketty, V., Durand, G., Reiter, E., and Maurel, M. C. (2010). Selective modulation of follicle-stimulating hormone signaling pathways with enhancing equine chorionic gonadotropin/antibody immune complexes. *Endocrinology* 151, 2788–2799.

Wehling, M. (1997). Specific, nongenomic actions of steroid hormones. *Annu. Rev. Physiol.* 59, 365–393.

Wei, H., Ahn, S., Shenoy, S. K., Karnik, S. S., Hunyady, L., Luttrell, L. M., et al. (2003). Independent beta-arrestin 2 and G protein-mediated pathways for angiotensin II activation of extracellular signal-regulated kinases 1 and 2. *Proc. Natl. Acad. Sci. U.S.A.* 100, 10782–10787.

Wei, Y., Zhang, Z., Liao, H., Wu, L., Wu, X., Zhou, D., et al. (2012). Nuclear estrogen receptor-mediated Notch signaling and GPR30-mediated PI3K/AKT signaling in the regulation of endometrial cancer cell proliferation. *Oncol. Rep.* 27, 504–510.

Whalen, E. J., Rajagopal, S., and Lefkowitz, R. J. (2011). Therapeutic potential of beta-arrestin- and G protein-biased agonists. *Trends. Mol. Med.* 17, 126–139.

Wickerham, D. L., Fisher, B., Wolmark, N., Bryant, J., Costantino, J., Bernstein, L., et al. (2002). Association of tamoxifen and uterine sarcoma. *J. Clin. Oncol.* 20, 2758–2760.

Willard, F. S., Wootten, D., Showalter, A. D., Savage, E. E., Ficorilli, J., Farb, T. B., et al. (2012). Small molecule allosteric modulation of the glucagon-like Peptide-1 receptor enhances the insulinotropic effect of oxyntomodulin. *Mol. Pharmacol.* 82, 1066–1073.

Wisler, J. W., DeWire, S. M., Whalen, E. J., Violin, J. D., Drake, M. T., Ahn, S., et al. (2007). A unique mechanism of beta-blocker action: carvedilol stimulates beta-arrestin signaling. *Proc. Natl. Acad. Sci. U.S.A.* 104, 16657–16662.

Wootten, D., Savage, E. E., Willard, F. S., Bueno, A. B., Sloop, K. W.,

Christopoulos, A., et al. (2013). Differential activation and modulation of the glucagon-like peptide-1 receptor by small molecule ligands. *Mol. Pharmacol.* 83, 822–834.

Wu, Y. Q., Song, Z., Zhou, C. H., Xing, S. H., Pei, D. S., and Zheng, J. N. (2010). Expression of urotensin II and its receptor in human lung adenocarcinoma A549 cells and the effect of urotensin II on lung adenocarcinoma growth in vitro and in vivo. *Oncol. Rep.* 24, 1179–1184.

Xu, F., Wu, H., Katritch, V., Han, G. W., Jacobson, K. A., Gao, Z. G., et al. (2011). Structure of an agonist-bound human A2A adenosine receptor. *Science* 332, 322–327.

Xu, G., Stoffers, D. A., Habener, J. F., and Bonner-Weir, S. (1999). Exendin-4 stimulates both beta-cell replication and neogenesis, resulting in increased beta-cell mass and improved glucose tolerance in diabetic rats. *Diabetes* 48, 2270–2276.

Yeh, A. H., Jeffery, P. L., Duncan, R. P., Herington, A. C., and Chopin, L. K. (2005). Ghrelin and a novel preproghrelin isoform are highly expressed in prostate cancer and ghrelin activates mitogen-activated protein kinase in prostate cancer. *Clin. Cancer Res.* 11, 8295–8303.

Yoo, Y. A., Kim, Y. H., Kim, J. S., and Seo, J. H. (2008). The functional implications of Akt activity and TGF-beta signaling in tamoxifen-resistant breast cancer. *Biochim. Biophys. Acta* 1783, 438–447.

Younan, S. M., and Rashed, L. A. (2007). Impairment of the insulinotropic effect of gastric inhibitory polypeptide (GIP) in obese and diabetic rats is related to the down-regulation of its pancreatic receptors. *Gen. Physiol. Biophys.* 26, 181–193.

Zidar, D. A., Violin, J. D., Whalen, E. J., and Lefkowitz, R. J. (2009). Selective engagement of G protein coupled receptor kinases (GRKs) encodes distinct functions of biased ligands. *Proc. Natl. Acad. Sci. U.S.A.* 106, 9649–9654.

9

The neuroendocrine functions of the parathyroid hormone 2 receptor

Arpád Dobolyi[1]*, Eugene Dimitrov[2], Miklós Palkovits[1] and Ted B. Usdin[2]

[1] Neuromorphological and Neuroendocrine Research Laboratory, Department of Anatomy, Histology and Embryology, Hungarian Academy of Sciences, Semmelweis University, Budapest, Hungary
[2] Section on Fundamental Neuroscience, National Institute of Mental Health, National Institute of Health, Bethesda, MD, USA

Edited by:
Hubert Vaudry, University of Rouen, France

Reviewed by:
Tamas Kozicz, Radboud University Nijmegen, Netherlands
Sarah J. Spencer, Monash University, Australia
Kazuhiro Nakamura, Kyoto University, Japan

***Correspondence:**
Arpád Dobolyi, Neuromorphological and Neuroendocrine Research Laboratory, Department of Anatomy, Histology and Embryology, Hungarian Academy of Sciences, Semmelweis University, Tűzoltó u. 58, Budapest H-1094, Hungary.
e-mail: dobolyi@ana.sote.hu

The G-protein coupled parathyroid hormone 2 receptor (PTH2R) is concentrated in endocrine and limbic regions in the forebrain. Its endogenous ligand, tuberoinfundibular peptide of 39 residues (TIP39), is synthesized in only two brain regions, within the posterior thalamus and the lateral pons. TIP39-expressing neurons have a widespread projection pattern, which matches the PTH2R distribution in the brain. Neuroendocrine centers including the preoptic area, the periventricular, paraventricular, and arcuate nuclei contain the highest density of PTH2R-positive networks. The administration of TIP39 and an antagonist of the PTH2R as well as the investigation of mice that lack functional TIP39 and PTH2R revealed the involvement of the PTH2R in a variety of neural and neuroendocrine functions. TIP39 acting via the PTH2R modulates several aspects of the stress response. It evokes corticosterone release by activating corticotropin-releasing hormone-containing neurons in the hypothalamic paraventricular nucleus. Block of TIP39 signaling elevates the anxiety state of animals and their fear response, and increases stress-induced analgesia. TIP39 has also been suggested to affect the release of additional pituitary hormones including arginine-vasopressin and growth hormone. A role of the TIP39-PTH2R system in thermoregulation was also identified. TIP39 may play a role in maintaining body temperature in a cold environment via descending excitatory pathways from the preoptic area. Anatomical and functional studies also implicated the TIP39-PTH2R system in nociceptive information processing. Finally, TIP39 induced in postpartum dams may play a role in the release of prolactin during lactation. Potential mechanisms leading to the activation of TIP39 neurons and how they influence the neuroendocrine system are also described. The unique TIP39-PTH2R neuromodulator system provides the possibility for developing drugs with a novel mechanism of action to control neuroendocrine disorders.

Keywords: neuropeptide, thermoregulation, stress response, corticotropin-releasing hormone, somatostatin, neuroendocrine hypothalamic regulations, reproductive regulations, maternal adaptation

INTRODUCTION

The parathyroid hormone 2 receptor (PTH2R) is a member of the family B (type II) of G-protein coupled receptors. It was discovered based on its sequence similarity to other proteins belonging to this receptor family (Usdin et al., 1995). The novel receptor was named PTH2R because of its sequence similarity to the parathyroid hormone receptor and also because the human PTH2R can be activated by parathyroid hormone (Usdin et al., 2002). In rat, however, nanomolar concentrations of parathyroid hormone do not cause significant activation of the PTH2R (Hoare et al., 1999a; **Figure 1**). An additional difference between the parathyroid hormone 1 receptor (PTH1R) and the PTH2R is that the distinct polypeptide parathyroid hormone-related peptide is a co-ligand of the PTH1R but does not bind to the PTH2R (Hoare et al., 1999b). A breakthrough in the field of parathyroid hormone receptor research was the discovery of a novel peptide, tuberoinfundibular peptide of 39 residues (TIP39), an endogenous ligand of the PTH2R (Usdin et al., 1999b). TIP39 was purified from bovine hypothalamus based on its ability to elevate cAMP in a PTH2R-expressing cell line (Usdin et al., 1999b). TIP39's sequence has very few amino acid residues in common with parathyroid hormone and parathyroid hormone-related peptide but it does have a similar three-dimensional structure to them (Piserchio et al., 2000). TIP39 is a high affinity and fully potent agonist for both the human and rodent PTH2R (Usdin et al., 1999b). Apart from elevating cAMP (presumably *via* Gs proteins), TIP39 was also shown to elevate intracellular Ca^{2+} levels (presumably *via* Gq proteins) in some cell types (Goold et al., 2001; Della Penna et al., 2003).

PTH2R expression is greater in the brain than in peripheral tissues based on Northern blot, *in situ* hybridization histochemistry and immunohistochemistry (Usdin et al., 1995, 1996, 1999a). In the periphery, its expression pattern was also very different from that of the PTH1R, as only a low level of expression was found distributed in the following places: pancreatic islet somatostatin synthesizing D cells, large vessels in bronchi, and the parenchyma in the lung, cardiac endothelium, a small number of cells associated with the vascular pole of renal glomeruli, spermatids in the

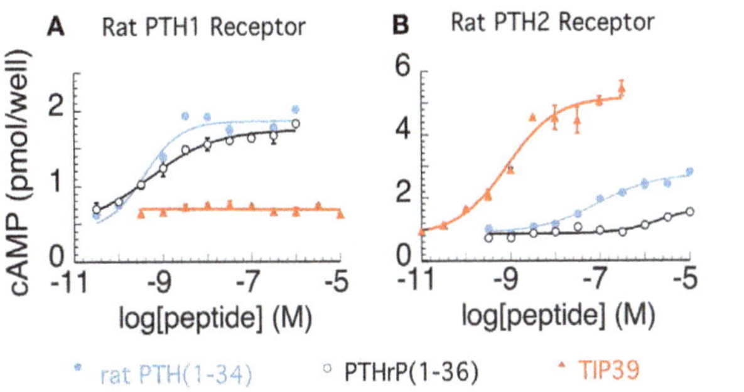

FIGURE 1 | Activation of rat parathyroid hormone 1 (PTH1) and PTH2 receptors. cAMP accumulation is shown in relation to increasing concentrations of PTH, PTH-related peptide, and tuberoinfundibular peptide of 39 residues (TIP39) in COS7 cells expressing the rat PTH1R **(A)** and the rat PTH2R **(B)**, respectively. The figure was created from data presented previously (Hoare and Usdin, 1999; Hoare et al., 1999a; Usdin et al., 1999b).

head of the epididymis, atretic follicles of the ovary, chondrocytes in thyroid cartilage, a small number of cells in bone, and in some endocrine cells including thyroid parafollicular C cells, and some gastrointestinal peptide synthesizing cells. There is relatively little information on the effects of PTH2R signaling outside the brain and potential functions in the periphery are not discussed in this review.

Within the brain, the distributions of TIP39 axon terminals and PTH2R immunoreactivity show remarkable similarities as described below. Therefore, it was suggested that TIP39 is the endogenous ligand of the PTH2R. Consequently, it has been proposed that TIP39 and the PTH2R form a neuromodulator system in many brain regions. This is supported by the very similar phenotypes of mutant mice lacking either functional PTH2Rs or TIP39 or wild type (WT) animals administered a PTH2R antagonist as discussed below.

THE DISTRIBUTION OF THE TIP39-PTH2R SYSTEM

NEURONS EXPRESSING TIP39, THE LIGAND OF THE PTH2R

TIP39-expressing cells in the adult brain are restricted to the subparafascicular area of the thalamus and the medial paralemniscal nucleus of the pons as revealed by immunohistochemistry and *in situ* hybridization histochemistry (Dobolyi et al., 2003b) while the amygdala-hippocampal transitional zone also contains some TIP39 neurons during embryonic development (Brenner et al., 2008). The subparafascicular area TIP39 neurons were subdivided into the medially located group in the periventricular gray of the thalamus (PVG) and a laterally positioned group of the posterior intralaminar complex (PIL) of the thalamus (PIL; Dobolyi et al., 2010; **Figure 2**). Recent evidence supports the idea that the anatomical separation of these cell groups is concomitant with different functions. TIP39 appears in neurons in the PIL earlier during ontogenic development and largely disappears from them immediately after birth (Brenner et al., 2008). In turn, a marked induction of TIP39 in PIL cells but not in PVG cells can be observed in postpartum dams (Cservenak et al., 2010). Although the possibility that the PTH2R has another endogenous ligand apart from TIP39 is theoretically not excluded, the similarity in their distributions argues that TIP39 is available to activate PTH2Rs wherever they are present in the brain. Thus, neurons in the three sites of TIP39 expression would provide all information necessary to act *via* the PTH2R in the brain. Some evidence is available from lesion and tracer studies that TIP39 neurons in the subparafascicular area project to forebrain limbic and hypothalamic regions while TIP39 neurons in the medial paralemniscal nucleus provides TIP39 fibers to the hindbrain and spinal cord potentially affecting auditory and nociceptive functions (Dobolyi et al., 2003a; Wang et al., 2006b; Palkovits et al., 2010).

TIP39 AND THE PTH2R IN THE PITUITARY AND MEDIAN EMINENCE

Neither TIP39 nor PTH2R mRNA or protein were found in the pituitary (Usdin et al., 1999a; Dobolyi et al.; 2002). In contrast, PTH2R-containing fibers were abundant in the external zone of the median eminence. PTH2R was found here in somatostatin fibers but not in fibers containing growth hormone (GH)-, gonadotropin-, or corticotropin-releasing hormones (CRH), or arginine-vasopressin (AVP; Dobolyi et al., 2006a). As opposed to the PTH2R, only a few TIP39-ir fibers were present in the median eminence. This is in fact the most striking difference between the otherwise very similar distributions of TIP39 axon terminals and the PTH2R.

THE SIMILARITIES BETWEEN THE DISTRIBUTION OF THE PTH2R AND TIP39 IN THE BRAIN

The distribution of PTH2R fibers and PTH2R-expressing cells is generally similar in the brain and particularly so in the neuroendocrine hypothalamus (Wang et al., 2000; Faber et al., 2007). However, it has to be pointed out that while the labeling pattern of cell bodies provided by immunocytochemistry and *in situ* hybridization histochemistry was very similar in the rat (Wang et al., 2000), PTH2R-labeled cell bodies were mostly not visible by immunohistochemistry in the mouse, non-human primate and human (Faber et al., 2007; Bago et al., 2009). Nevertheless, *in situ* hybridization histochemistry and X-Gal histochemistry in mice expressing beta-galactosidase driven by the promoter of the PTH2R revealed a similar expression pattern of the PTH2R in these species as well (Faber et al., 2007; Bago et al., 2009). The finding that PTH2R-immunopositive fibers are often localized in the vicinity of PTH2R-expressing neurons suggests that these fibers may represent either axons or dendrites of local PTH2R-expressing neurons. Colocalization of the PTH2R with vesicular glutamate transporters suggests its axonal localization as described below in Section "Development of Fear." Interestingly, the distributions, and even the subregional distributions of TIP39- and PTH2R-containing axon terminals are remarkably similar (Dobolyi et al., 2006a; Faber et al., 2007). Thus, TIP39 axon terminals and the PTH2R are co-distributed in the very same brain structures allowing the presynaptic modulation of PTH2R axon terminals. Therefore, an axo-axonal action of TIP39 is plausible (Dobolyi et al., 2010). However, there is no evidence available at present based on which the dendritic localization of the PTH2R can be excluded. In particular, electron microscopic investigation of the PTH2R has not been reported yet.

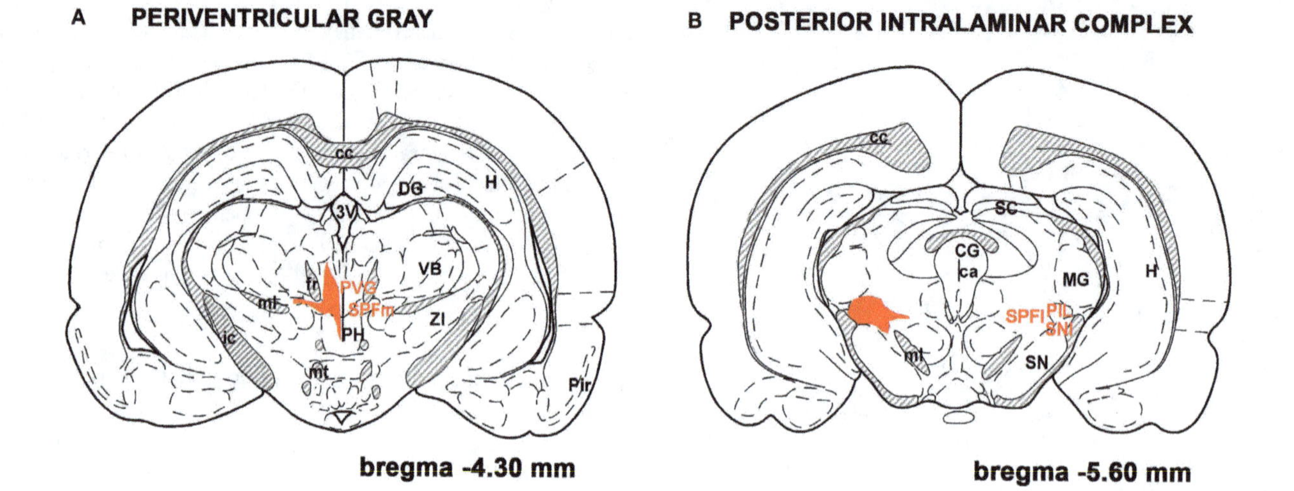

FIGURE 2 | TIP39 neurons in the subparafascicular area. The subparafascicular area is a mediolaterally and to some degree rostrocaudally elongated region. Most TIP39 cells are located in its mediorostral portion, the periventricular gray of the thalamus **(A)** and in its caudolateral part, the posterior intralaminar complex of the thalamus **(B)**. The area where TIP39 neurons are distributed is shown in red. A few TIP39 neurons are scattered between these two regions below the fasciculus retroflexus and above the medial lemniscus. Additional abbreviations: ca, cerebral aqueduct; cc, corpus callosum; CG, central gray; DG, dentate gyrus; fr, fasciculus retroflexus; H, hippocampus; ic, internal capsule; MG, medial geniculate body; ml, medial lemniscus; mt, mamillothalamic tract; PH, posterior hypothalamus; Pir, piriform cortex; PVG, periventricular gray; SC, superior colliculus;SN, substantia nigra; SNl, substantia nigra, lateral subdivision; SPFl, lateral (parvocellular) subparafascicular nucleus; SPFm, magnocellular subparafascicular nucleus; VB, ventrobasal thalamus. The original drawings are modifications of panels from a rat brain atlas (Paxinos and Watson, 2007).

THE TIP39-PTH2R NEUROMODULATOR SYSTEM IN HYPOTHALAMIC AREAS EXPRESSING NEUROENDOCRINE HORMONES

A high density of PTH2R-expressing cells and TIP39- and PTH2R-containing fibers is present in the medial preoptic nucleus and some surrounding parts of the medial preoptic area (Dobolyi et al., 2006a; Faber et al., 2007). A TIP39-PTH2R neuromodulator system is also abundant in the paraventricular and periventricular nuclei while other parts of the anterior hypothalamic region contain a lower density of labeling. Thus, TIP39 terminals are ideally positioned to influence somatostatin and CRH neurons. It has indeed been demonstrated that somatostatin neurons express the PTH2R (Wang et al., 2000; Dobolyi et al., 2006a) and that both TIP39- and PTH2R-containing terminals approximate CRH-expressing neurons in the parvicellular subdivision of the hypothalamic paraventricular nucleus (PVN; Bago et al., 2009; Dimitrov and Usdin, 2010). Similarly, in the tuberal region of the hypothalamus, the arcuate nucleus contains the highest density of PTH2R-expressing cells and TIP39- and PTH2R-containing fibers, providing an anatomical basis for influencing GH and prolactin release *via* GH-releasing hormone (GHRH) and dopamine neurons in the arcuate nucleus (**Table 1**).

TIP39 AND THE PTH2R IN HYPOTHALAMIC, LIMBIC, AND SENSORY BRAIN REGIONS THAT POTENTIALLY EXERT INFLUENCE ON THE NEUROENDOCRINE SYSTEM

In the nervous system, TIP39 fibers and the PTH2R have a widespread distribution pattern (Wang et al., 2000; Dobolyi et al., 2003b; Faber et al., 2007; Bago et al., 2009). A number of brain regions known to affect the neuroendocrine system *via* neuronal projections to hypophysiotropic neurons were shown to contain a high density of PTH2R-expressing cell bodies as well as TIP39- and PTH2R-containing fibers. These brain regions include the medial prefrontal, especially the infralimbic cortex, the lateral septal nucleus, the bed nucleus of the stria terminalis, the amygdala, especially its medial and central nuclei, some midline and intralaminar thalamic nuclei, several hypothalamic nuclei, the periaqueductal gray, the lateral parabrachial nuclei, the locus coeruleus and subcoeruleus areas, and the nucleus of the solitary tract. Within the hypothalamus, the following nuclei contained a high level of TIP39 and PTH2R apart from the above mentioned neuroendocrine regions: the MnPO, the vascular organ of the lamina terminalis, the dorsomedial and perifornical hypothalamic nuclei, and some parts of the lateral hypothalamic area including the so-called far-lateral hypothalamus immediately next to the internal capsule, the medial subdivision of the supramamillary nucleus, the ventral, and dorsal premamillary nuclei, and the posterior hypothalamic nucleus, (Wang et al., 2000; Dobolyi et al., 2003b; Faber et al., 2007; Bago et al., 2009). In contrast, TIP39 and the PTH2R are scarce in a number of hypothalamic nuclei including the lateral preoptic area, the supraoptic, suprachiasmatic, and lateroanterior hypothalamic nuclei, the medial magnocellular part of the paraventricular nucleus, the ventromedial nucleus, and the medial and lateral nuclei of the mamillary body (**Table 1**).

TIP39 AND THE PTH2R IN REGIONS OF THE NERVOUS SYSTEM NOT INVOLVED IN NEUROENDOCRINE REGULATIONS

Elements of the TIP39-PTH2R neuromodulator system are also expressed in some brain regions that are not known to be directly or indirectly involved in neuroendocrine regulation. Thus, TIP39 as well as PTH2R fibers were abundant in the fundus striati, the medial geniculate body, tegmental areas of the midbrain and pons, the deep layers of the superior colliculus, the external cortex of the

Table 1 | The distribution of TIP39 axon terminals and the PTH2R in the nervous system.

	Areas containing a high density of TIP39 fibers and PTH2R
Neuroendocrine hypothalamic areas	Medial preoptic area, paraventricular nucleus, periventricular nucleus, arcuate nucleus
Brain regions that potentially exert influence on the neuroendocrine system	Infralimbic cortex, lateral septal nucleus, the bed nucleus of the stria terminalis, medial and central amygdaloid nuclei, the vascular organ of the lamina terminalis, dorsomedial and perifornical hypothalamic nuclei, far-lateral and posterior hypothalamic areas, the medial subdivision of the supramamillary nucleus, premamillary nuclei, paraventricular, reuniens, posterior intralaminar, and subparafascicular thalamic nuclei, periaqueductal gray, lateral parabrachial nuclei, the locus coeruleus and subcoeruleus areas, and the nucleus of the solitary tract
Regions of the nervous system not directly involved in neuroendocrine regulations	Fundus striati, the medial subdivision of the medial geniculate body, tegmental areas of the midbrain and pons, deep layers of the superior colliculus, the external cortex of the inferior colliculus, the periolivary area, the nucleus of the trapezoid body, the superficial layers of the dorsal horn, the lateral cervical nucleus of the spinal cord, and some primary sensory neurons

inferior colliculus, the periolivary area, the nucleus of the trapezoid body, the superficial layers of the dorsal horn and the lateral cervical nucleus of the spinal cord, and some cells in the dorsal root ganglia (Wang et al., 2000; Dobolyi et al., 2003b; Faber et al., 2007; Bago et al., 2009; Matsumoto et al., 2010). Several of these brain regions may participate in sensory, especially auditory information processing, which could represent non-neuroendocrine-related functions of the TIP39-PTH2R neuromodulator system. However, a potential role of TIP39 in the auditory stress pathway will be discussed later.

NEUROENDOCRINE FUNCTIONS THAT MAY INVOLVE THE TIP39-PTH2R SYSTEM

Based on the distribution of the TIP39-PTH2R system in the brain, its involvement in endocrine, limbic, nociceptive, and auditory functions have been hypothesized (Dobolyi et al., 2003a). These functions can of course be interrelated with each other. Initial studies in which PTH2Rs were activated with exogenous TIP39 as well as *in vitro* approaches provided some insights into the possible functions of the TIP39-PTH2R system. More recently, a selective and potent peptide antagonist of the PTH2R (Kuo and Usdin, 2007) and transgenic mice lacking functional TIP39 and PTH2R genes were developed (Fegley et al., 2008), which accelerated functional studies. It has indeed been established that the peptide neuromodulator system is involved in a variety of neuroendocrine functions including the stress response, thermoregulation, and prolactin release. Some evidence is also available for a role of the TIP39-PTH2R system in the regulation of AVP and GH release.

STRESS RESPONSE

The stress response is a complex reaction of the organism to stimuli that threaten homeostasis. The stress response includes an altered psychological state called anxiety and physiological effects that include catecholamine and glucocorticoid release as final common pathways (Kvetnansky et al., 2009). The anxiety level and the hormone secretions interact to provide the organisms stress response.

The regulation of CRH function

The first functional evidence that the PTH2R might be involved in the regulation of CRH release came from an *in vitro* study. TIP39 increased CRH secretion from medial basal hypothalamic explants (Ward et al., 2001). In addition, intracerebroventricular injection of TIP39 dose-dependently increased the plasma adrenocorticotropin (ACTH) level at 10 min after injection in rat (Ward et al., 2001). In another study, local injection of TIP39 above the paraventricular hypothalamic nucleus (PVN) in mice also elevated plasma corticosterone levels in addition to increasing the number of pCREB-containing activated cells in and around the PVN (Dimitrov and Usdin, 2010). Most importantly, these effects of local TIP39 were not present in PTH2R knockout (KO) animals (Dimitrov and Usdin, 2010) excluding non-specific actions of TIP39 injection. These results suggest that the TIP39-PTH2R system is positioned and available to potentially modulate activation of the hypothalamus-pituitary-adrenal (HPA) axis. In fact, the activation of TIP39 neurons has been reported in some stress situations as described below in Section "The Activation of TIP39 Neurons." Furthermore, the daily peak of the basal plasma corticosterone level was reduced in TIP39 KO mice suggesting that endogenous TIP39 plays a role in the circadian regulation of corticosterone levels (Dimitrov and Usdin, 2010). These findings are consistent with a high density of TIP39 fibers, PTH2R-expressing cells, and PTH2R-containing fiber terminals in the parvicellular subdivisions of the PVN (Faber et al., 2007). In fact, close apposition between CRH neurons and PTH2R-containing fibers has been demonstrated in mice (Dimitrov and Usdin, 2010) as well as in human (Bago et al., 2009).

The regulation of noradrenergic function

The involvement of the PTH2R in the regulation of the catecholamine systems is less well established even though TIP39 fibers are abundant in the locus coeruleus and subcoeruleus areas (Dobolyi et al., 2003b) where rostrally projecting noradrenergic neurons reside. Recent evidence brings up the possibility that TIP39 may interact with some noradrenergic pathways. TIP39 KO mice and WT mice injected with a PTH2R antagonist demonstrated selective impairment of memory performance during novelty-induced arousal (Coutellier et al., 2011a). Noradrenergic signaling has a biphasic, inverted U shaped, effect on cognitive functions (Arnsten, 2009). The impaired performance of mice without TIP39/PTH2R signaling was restored by propranolol, an antagonist of beta adrenoceptors, suggesting that PTH2R signaling influences the effect of novelty stress *via* an interaction with noradrenergic mechanisms (Coutellier et al., 2011a).

Stress-induced analgesia

In an experiment addressing the role of PTH2R signaling in stress-induced analgesia (SIA), hotplate tests were performed before and after an inescapable foot shock, used as the stressful stimulus (Dimitrov et al., 2010). As discussed in a later section, TIP39 KO and PTH2R KO mice as well as WT mice injected with a PTH2R antagonist had somewhat elevated pre-shock response latencies in the hotplate test. Following the foot shock, the response latencies increased in the WT mice as expected based on the phenomenon of SIA. Unexpectedly, a larger and dramatic increase was found in the response latency in mice without PTH2R signaling (Dimitrov et al., 2010). These findings suggest that signaling through the TIP39-PTH2R system may normally limit SIA.

Stress-induced analgesia induced by high intensity stressful stimuli, including inescapable foot shock, has been shown to have a predominant non-opioid component (Lewis et al., 1980; Terman et al., 1984). Indeed the opioid antagonist naloxone did not, but the CB1 cannabinoid receptor antagonist rimonabant did, decrease the SIA in WT mice (Dimitrov et al., 2010). The inhibitory effect of rimonabant on the SIA was much greater in the KO mice suggesting that the KO mice have greater endocannabinoid release or sensitivity and that endogenous TIP39, *via* the PTH2R, may negatively modulate release or an effect of endogenous cannabinoids during SIA.

RELEASE OF ARGININE-VASOPRESSIN

The role of the PTH2R on the release of AVP was investigated by intracerebroventricular injection of TIP39 in rats (Sugimura et al., 2003). Reduced AVP levels were found in plasma 5 min following TIP39 administration. TIP39 also suppressed the plasma AVP increase following dehydration by water deprivation for 48h, hyperosmolality following i.p. injection of hypertonic saline, and hypovolemia following i.p. injection of polyethylene glycol. These inhibitory effects cannot be attributed to a decrease in the level of osmotic or hypovolemic stimulation because plasma Na^+ and plasma total protein were not affected by the injection of TIP39 (Sugimura et al., 2003). The effect of TIP39 was also not a consequence of a change in blood pressure because injection of TIP39 produced a fall in mean arterial blood pressure, which would rather stimulate AVP secretion. In turn, the opioid receptor antagonist naloxone significantly reversed the inhibitory effect of TIP39 on dehydration-induced AVP release while it had no significant effect on the plasma AVP level when injected alone (Sugimura et al., 2003). These results suggest that TIP39 inhibits AVP release by central action – possibly *via* an opioid system but without hemodynamic or osmotic influence. The effect was rapid and did not last long suggesting that TIP39 may play a role in the dynamic regulation of AVP release. TIP39 and PTH2R are scarce in the supraoptic nucleus and the part of the PVN where magnocellular AVP neurons are located. Thus, TIP39 may exert its AVP release-inhibitory effect by acting through other hypothalamic nuclei. The hypothalamic arcuate nucleus is a candidate as it contains a high density of TIP39 and PTH2R immunoreactivity (Faber et al., 2007) as well as many opioid neurons, which are involved in the regulation of AVP release (Haaf et al., 1987; Heijning et al., 1991). Indirect action of TIP39 *via* hypothalamic angiotensin and atrial natriuretic peptide neurons affecting AVP release (Antunes-Rodrigues et al., 2004) is also conceivable.

GROWTH HORMONE SECRETION

In a preliminary experiment, TIP39 injection into the lateral ventricle of male rats blocked the appearance of GH almost completely in plasma for the next 3 h (Usdin et al., 2003). This finding is consistent with anatomical data showing a high density of TIP39-containing fibers around somatostatin neurons in the periventricular hypothalamic nucleus. Somatostatin neurons in this area project to the median eminence and inhibit the release of GH (Luque et al., 2008). PTH2R expression was demonstrated on many of these somatostatin neurons in the rat (Usdin et al., 1999b) as well as in human (Bago et al., 2009) providing the anatomical basis for TIP39 stimulating the release of somatostatin, which in turn inhibits GH secretion (Luque et al., 2008).

PHYSIOLOGICAL ACTIONS OF TIP39 NOT DIRECTLY RELATED TO ITS NEUROENDOCRINE EFFECTS

EFFECTS ON THE ANXIETY LEVEL

The anxiety levels of animals may also be affected by the TIP39-PTH2R system. In the elevated plus maze, a test of anxiety, intracerebroventricular injections of TIP39 in rats resulted in increased open arm entries and duration as compared to controls (animals receiving the inactive TIP (7–39) or saline) while no differences were observed between groups in the number of closed arm entries or total arm entries, suggesting an anxiolytic-like effect of TIP39 (LaBuda et al., 2004). The TIP39-PTH2R system in the infralimbic cortex, lateral hypothalamus, preoptic area, lateral septum, and the paraventricular thalamic nucleus could be involved in this action because TIP39 administration induced Fos activation in these brain regions (LaBuda et al., 2004). In the forced-swim test, a similar TIP39 administration reduced the duration of immobility, and increased the amount of climbing behavior (LaBuda et al., 2004) suggesting an anti-depressant-like action of TIP39. The phenotype of TIP39 KO mice is also consistent with an anxiolytic role of endogenous TIP39. TIP39 KO mice demonstrated increased anxiety in the shock-probe defensive burying test as compared to WT controls. In "standard/low stress" testing conditions, TIP39 KO mice did not differ from WT controls in the arm entries in the elevated plus maze or in the dark-light emergence test of spontaneous anxiety-like behaviors (Fegley et al., 2008). However, an increase in anxiety-like behavior became apparent in TIP39 KO mice that were tested in the elevated plus maze under conditions of mildly increased stress evoked by either brief prior restraint or bright illumination. These results are consistent with a role of endogenous TIP39 in limiting the consequences of stressful perturbations. Furthermore, mice lacking TIP39 or the PTH2R demonstrated increased anxiety- and depression-like behaviors 16–17 days but not 7–9 days after a foot shock in elevated-zero maze, open field, light-dark box and forced-swim tests (Coutellier and Usdin, 2011).

DEVELOPMENT OF FEAR

Closely related to anxiety, fear has also been investigated in relation with the TIP39-PTH2R system using Pavlovian fear conditioning (Fegley et al., 2008). TIP39 KO mice showed more freezing than WT controls after only one tone-shock pairing during conditioning and, subsequently, more freezing during both tone- and context-recall tests (Fegley et al., 2008). However, based on a similar rate of decline in freezing responses to repeated tone presentation and a similar level of freezing during subsequent tone presentation, there did not appear to be an effect of TIP39 deletion on fear extinction learning or extinction recall, respectively (Fegley et al., 2008). Furthermore, foot shock conditioned fear recall was enhanced 14 days but not 6 days after the aversive stimulus in both TIP39 KO and PTH2R KO mice as compared to WT controls (Coutellier and Usdin, 2011). These results suggest that normal TIP39 signaling lessens the long-term consequences of a traumatic event while the absence of signaling *via* the PTH2R delays recovery. Since the amygdala is known to be involved in the fear response (LeDoux, 2003), the abundant TIP39-PTH2R system in the amygdala, especially in its central and medial nuclei (Faber et al., 2007), might be involved in these effects.

THERMOREGULATION

Body temperature regulation is a fundamental homeostatic function that in homeothermic animals. Thermal information on environmental temperature sensed by skin thermoreceptors ascends to the MnPO in the hypothalamic preoptic area. GABAergic inhibitory neurons in the MnPO integrate this input with local thermal influences and project to the dorsomedial hypothalamic nucleus and the rostral medullary raphe region to restore homeostasis (Nakamura, 2011). Injection of TIP39 into the lateral ventricle increased the core temperature of WT mice while TIP39 injection had no effect in PTH2R KO mice, excluding the possibility of non-specific inflammatory actions (Dimitrov et al., 2011). Furthermore, PTH2R KO mice had impaired heat production upon cold exposure, but no change in basal temperature and no impairment in response to a hot environment suggesting that the TIP39-PTH2R system plays a specific role in temperature conservation in a cold environment (Dimitrov et al., 2011). Since temperature sensation was normal in PTH2R KO mice, the PTH2R may play a role in the heat production signal or heat production ability. Both seem to be the case because acute intracerebral PTH2R antagonist administration also impaired the heat production response to a cold environment, though to a smaller extent. In addition, the weight of brown adipose tissue (BAT), and its capacity to increase body temperature were reduced. PTH2Rs in the MnPO seem to be involved in the thermoregulatory action of TIP39 because TIP39 injected locally into the MnPO produced a larger body temperature increase (2°C) for longer periods of time than injection of the same amount of TIP39 into the lateral ventricle. Furthermore, local injection of TIP39 into the dorsomedial hypothalamic nucleus had no effect on the body temperature. The MnPO as a site of action is consistent with its high density of TIP39 terminals and PTH2R immunoreactivity (Faber et al., 2007; Dimitrov et al., 2011) as well as with the known role of MnPO neurons in the control body temperature (Baffi and Palkovits, 2000; Bratincsak and Palkovits, 2004) *via* descending systems regulating BAT thermogenesis and cutaneous vascular tone (Morrison and Nakamura, 2011). The action of TIP39 on the HPA axis and in central thermoregulation allows associations with fever. Although no data are available in this regard, this potential role of the TIP39-PTH2R system will be an interesting line of research in the future.

NOCICEPTIVE FUNCTIONS

The TIP39-PTH2R system may play a role at several levels of nociceptive processing. Its role in nociceptive sensation and spinal cord processing has been revealed by intrathecal administration of TIP39 and antagonizing its actions with the injection of an anti-TIP39 antibody (Dobolyi et al., 2002). Intrathecal injection of TIP39 stimulated a dose-dependent nocifensive response, caudally directed scratching, biting, and licking and decreased the tail-flick and paw-pressure withdrawal latencies. Intrathecal injection of the TIP39 antibody increased the response latency in the thermal tail-flick assay and in the paw-pressure test, corresponding to decreased sensitivity (Dobolyi et al., 2002). These actions are likely related to the facilitation of nociceptive transmission from the DRG to neurons in the spinal cord dorsal horn as intense PTH2R immunoreactivity is present in superficial layers of the spinal cord dorsal horn where most nociceptive afferents terminate (Wang et al., 2000).

The TIP39-PTH2R system may also be involved in the supraspinal regulation of pain processing. Intracerebroventricular injection of TIP39 reduced the latencies in tail-flick and hotplate tests while injection of a PTH2R antagonist had the opposite, anti-nociceptive effect in these tests as well as in the formalin test (Dimitrov et al., 2010). Furthermore, TIP39 and PTH2R KO mice also demonstrated reduced nociceptive responses in these tests, arguing for a pro-nociceptive function of endogenous TIP39 *via* the PTH2R (Dimitrov et al., 2010). These findings are consistent with the distribution of TIP39 and the PTH2R in a variety of brain regions known to be involved in the processing of nociceptive information, including the nucleus of the solitary tract, the parabrachial nuclei, the periventricular gray, the midline thalamic nuclei, the PVN, and the insular and infralimbic cortices. These areas are thought to be components of autonomic-limbic pain-related pathways including the ascending reticular activating system (Benarroch, 2006).

REGULATION OF POSTPARTUM EVENTS IN MOTHERS

TIP39 expression is decreased in neurons in both the subparafascicular area and the MPL during the period of pubertal development in rat (Dobolyi et al., 2006b). Since the level of the PTH2R did not decrease, it was hypothesized that TIP39 is induced under some circumstances to act on the already available PTH2Rs. Indeed, a dramatic increase in the TIP39 mRNA levels was demonstrated in the postpartum period using real-time PCR. Upon removal of the pups, the level of TIP39 mRNA decreased to its basal level. *In situ* hybridization histochemistry confirmed the induction of TIP39 and revealed that within the subparafascicular area, TIP39 neurons in the PIL but not in the PVG demonstrated an increase in TIP39 expression (Cservenak et al., 2010). The elevated mRNA of TIP39 in the PIL and MPL is translated into increased peptide levels, as demonstrated by immunohistochemistry (Varga et al., 2008; Cservenak et al., 2010). The functional significance of the elevated TIP39 was tested on the release of prolactin because pathway transections revealed projection of TIP39 neurons in the PIL toward tyrosine hydroxylase-containing neurons in the mediobasal hypothalamic regions known to regulate prolactin secretion. Retrograde labeling in nulliparous female rats also demonstrated a projection of subparafascicular TIP39 neurons to the arcuate nucleus (Szabo et al., 2010). In rodents, removal of the pups from the dams for 4h results in a decrease in prolactin level, which is in turn dramatically increased upon the return of the litter and the immediate onset of nursing. Injection of a PTH2R antagonist into the lateral ventricle 5 min before uniting the mothers with pups potently and dose-dependently inhibited suckling induced prolactin release in the rat (Cservenak et al., 2010). The physiological significance of this is supported by the observation that in a similar pup removal/return paradigm the weight increase (a measure of milk consumed) of pups suckling PTH2R KO mice was reduced 30 min after the onset of nursing as compared to pups suckling WT mice (Coutellier et al., 2011b). Also consistent with less effective suckling by PTH2R KO dams, pups reared by PTH2R KO mice had a lower body weight at the time of weaning than pups reared by WT mice (Coutellier et al., 2011b). To eliminate the effect of the genotype of the pups from the analysis, WT females were mated with PTH2R KO males while PTH2R KO females were mated with WT males so that all pups were heterozygous in these experiments (Coutellier et al., 2011b).

Additional influences of subparafascicular TIP39 neurons on reproductive neuroendocrine function cannot be excluded. TIP39 fibers and PTH2Rs are ideally positioned to affect gonadotropin-releasing hormone (GnRH) neurons, whose activity is suppressed during lactation. In addition, the TIP39-PTH2R neuromodulator system might also play a role in conveying the effect of suckling on other systems adapted in the postpartum period. PTH2Rs in the preoptic area, the lateral septum, and the periaqueductal gray could be involved in the control of maternal behaviors (Dobolyi, 2011). Emotional changes that take place in the postpartum period could also be affected by TIP39 based on the localization of the TIP39-PTH2R system in the infralimbic cortex, the medial, and central amygdaloid nuclei, the amygdalo-hippocampal transitional zone, the premamillary nuclei, the ventral subiculum, and the periaqueductal gray, which are parts of the circuitry of reproductive and emotional regulation (Lonstein and Stern, 1997; Lin et al., 1998; Li et al., 1999; Simerly, 2002; Numan and Insel, 2003; Hasen and Gammie, 2005).

POSSIBLE MODELS FOR ACTIONS *VIA* THE TIP39-PTH2R SYSTEM

THE ACTIVATION OF TIP39 NEURONS

There is limited information available showing that TIP39 neurons are activated in stress situations. At present, only the effects of an h-long high intensity noise stress have been reported. Medial paralemniscal and posterior intralaminar TIP39 neurons demonstrate Fos induction together with CRH neurons in response to noise stress, suggesting that TIP39 neurons could be involved in the transmission of acoustic stress derived information to CRH neurons in the PVN (Palkovits et al., 2009). In agreement with these findings, medial paralemniscal and possibly also posterior intralaminar TIP39 neurons have afferent neuronal connections with the primary auditory cortex and the external cortex of the inferior colliculus (Varga et al., 2008) providing the anatomical basis for an auditory influence on the CRH neurons in the PVN.

Cold exposure but not warm ambient temperature induced *c-fos* in some PVG neurons (Kiyohara et al., 1995; Miyata et al., 1995; Baffi and Palkovits, 2000; Bratincsak and Palkovits, 2004) providing the possibility that TIP39 neurons in this region could be activated by cold exposure leading to both stress responses and temperature regulation. It has also been reported that the *c-fos* expression in the PVG significantly outlasts the cold exposure (Miyata et al., 1995), suggesting that it may have a role in the maintenance of homeostasis during adaptation to cold stress (Baffi and Palkovits, 2000).

The PVG is a site of stimulation-induced analgesia (Rhodes and Liebeskind, 1978; Peschanski and Mantyh, 1983). Potent analgesia is obtained in rats following electrical stimulation in the gray matter surrounding the caudal portion of the third ventricle and the midline area of the caudal thalamus that is comparable to that produced by stimulation of the caudal periaqueductal gray. Analgesia outlasts the period of brain stimulation, and is not due to a generalized motor debilitation of the animal (Rhodes and Liebeskind, 1978). In addition, some neurons in the area are activated by noxious stimuli (Dong et al., 1978; Sugiyama et al., 1992) providing the possibility that TIP39 neurons in this region could be activated by noxious stimuli leading to both stress and nociceptive responses.

The TIP39-PTH2R neuromodulator system is present in several brain areas that are activated in males following mating (Sachs and Meisel, 1988; Coolen et al., 1997; Veening and Coolen, 1998) including the PIL, the medial preoptic nucleus, the posteromedial part of the medial subdivision of the bed nucleus of the stria terminalis, and the posterodorsal subdivision of the medial amygdaloid nuclei. In addition, the PIL, which contains TIP39 neurons, has also been implicated in sexual functions *via* the facilitation of copulatory behavior by current injection into the area (Shimura and Shimokochi, 1991), by the decreased sexual behavior following lesion in the area (Maillard and Edwards, 1991), and by the demonstration of the activation of neurons in the area following sexual behavior using the Fos technique in rats (Coolen et al., 1997) and imaging techniques in human (Holstege et al., 2003). Indeed, TIP39 neurons in the PIL have been shown to exhibit *Fos* expression following ejaculation (Wang et al., 2006a). This suggests that these TIP39 neurons are part of the afferent circuits that process genital-somatosensory information related to ejaculation contributing to mating and mating-induced changes in reproductive behaviors.

Another reproductive influence reaching TIP39 neurons in the PIL was reported in mother rats. Dams deprived of their pups for a day demonstrated *c-fos* expression in the PIL but not in the PVG in response to reunion with their litter (Cservenak et al., 2010). Almost all TIP39 neurons in the PIL were involved in this response. Since the pups start to suckle very soon after they are returned to their mothers, it was hypothesized that suckling results in the activation of TIP39 neurons in the PIL (Cservenak et al., 2010).

THE POTENTIAL MECHANISMS OF ACTION OF TIP39

There are no indications at present that TIP39 would have any action apart from activating the PTH2R. The PTH2R elevates cAMP and in some cells also increases Ca^{2+} levels (Goold et al., 2001; Della Penna et al., 2003) suggesting an excitatory influence of TIP39 on the target cells. In some cases, the PTH2R may be located in cell bodies and dendrites, there is evidence for this for the somatostatin neurons in the rat periventricular nucleus. Most typically, the PTH2R may be located in axon terminals. Apart from the somatostatin terminals in the median eminence (Dobolyi et al., 2006a), a presynaptic location of the PTH2R at excitatory synapses has been demonstrated in several hypothalamic areas (**Figure 3**). In the PVN, vesicular glutamate transporter 2 (VGluT2)-containing terminals closely apposed to CRH neurons were shown to also contain the PTH2R (Dimitrov and Usdin, 2010). In addition, the close apposition by TIP39-containing terminals suggested that TIP39 from the subparafascicular area might also contribute to the activation of CRH neurons by increasing the efficacy of the excitatory input to the CRH neurons (Dimitrov and Usdin, 2010). In a similar fashion, median preoptic neurons projecting to the dorsomedial hypothalamic nucleus for the potential transfer of thermoregulatory information were also suggested to be modulated by TIP39 *via* presynaptic excitation of their afferents (Dimitrov et al., 2011). Expression of the PTH2R by glutamatergic neurons in several brain regions is supported by data from *in situ* hybridization histochemistry (**Figure 4**). In other cases, the effect of TIP39 on inhibitory neurons has also been postulated based on functional data (Sugimura et al., 2003; Cservenak et al., 2010). Thus, the inhibition of AVP neurons and dopaminergic neurons is expected from the actions of TIP39 on the serum levels of AVP and prolactin, respectively. This inhibition could be carried out *via* potentiation of excitatory inputs to inhibitory interneurons acting on the AVP and dopaminergic neurons, respectively.

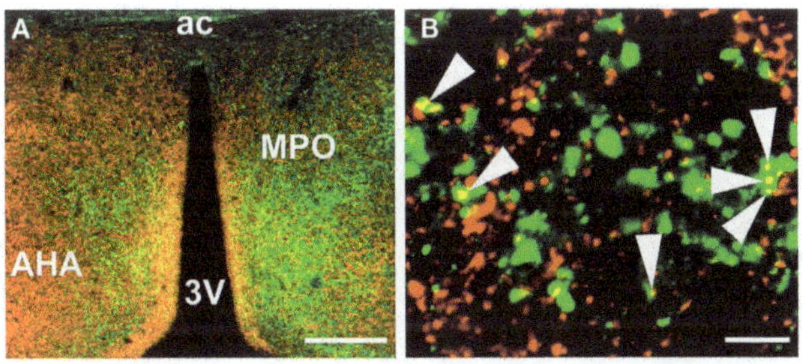

FIGURE 3 | Colocalization of PTH2R fibers and VGluT2 punctae in the anterior hypothalamus as detected by immunohistochemistry. (A) a low magnification image of PTH2R (green) and VGluT2 (red) expression in the region of the medial preoptic area. **(B)** a high magnification image of PTH2R/VGluT2 colocalization, where some of the colocalized points are indicated with arrowheads. Abbreviations: 3V, third ventricle; ac, anterior commissural; AHA, anterior hypothalamic area; MPO, medial preoptic nucleus of the hypothalamus. Scale bars = 200 μm for A and 10 μm for B.

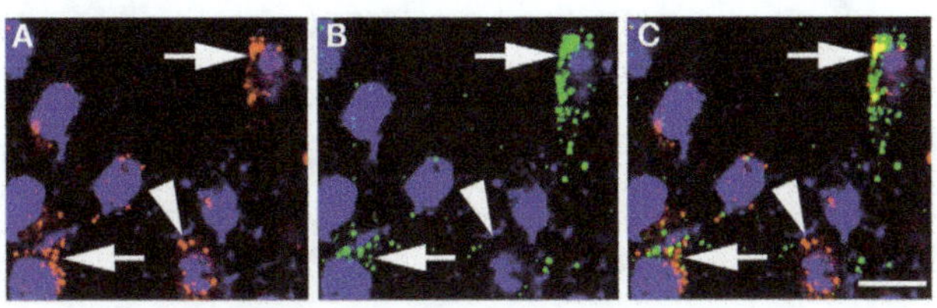

FIGURE 4 | Colocalization of VGluT2 mRNA and PTH2R mRNA in the anterior hypothalamus as detected by fluorescent *in situ* hybridization. (A) VGluT2 mRNA (red puncta) over cell nuclei (blue, DAPI). **(B)** PTH2R mRNA (green puncta) over cell nuclei (blue, DAPI). **(C)** a merged image, where the arrows point to cells expressing both PTH2R/VGluT2 mRNAs and the arrowhead points to a neuron with only VGluT2 signal. Scale bar = 10 μm.

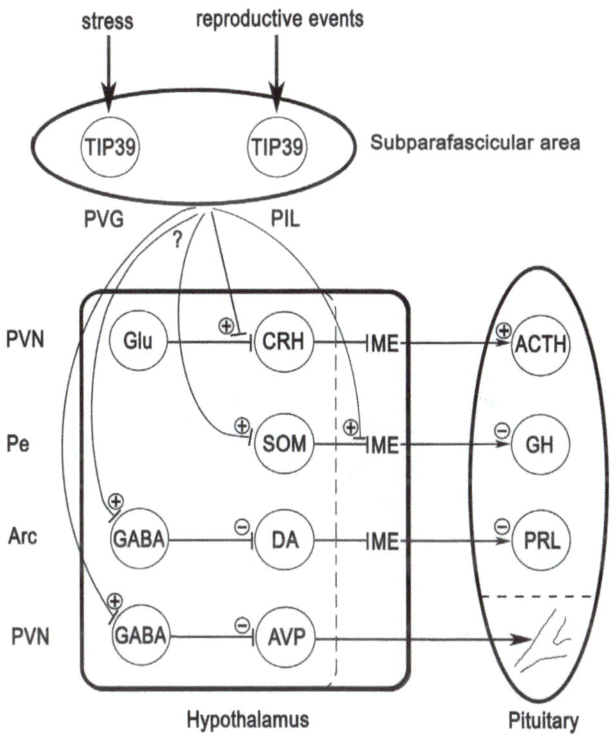

FIGURE 5 | Potential mechanisms of actions of TIP39 *via* the PTH2R. TIP39 neurons in the PVG receive information on threats to homeostasis while those in the PIL receive various inputs related to reproduction. Axon terminals arising from these TIP39 neurons may facilitate excitatory synapses by presynaptic actions. A well-documented example is the action of TIP39 on glutamatergic synapses terminating on CRH neurons in the PVN. Another possible route to influence hypothalamic hormone release is *via* terminals of hypophysiotropic neurons in the median eminence (ME) as has been suggested for somatostatin. Neurons that express PTH2Rs in their cell bodies may be directly affected by TIP39. Some actions of TIP39 including those on prolactin and AVP release, seem to be mediated by inhibitory neurons. TIP39 terminals might innervate cell bodies of GABAergic cells or alternatively, presynaptic terminals leading to the activation of inhibitory neurons (not shown). Additional abbreviations: ACTH, adrenocorticotropin; Arc, arcuate nucleus; DA, dopamine; GH, growth hormone; Glu, glutamate; Pe, periventricular hypothalamic nucleus; PRL, prolactin; SOM, somatostatin.

CONCLUSION

The TIP39-PTH2R neuromodulator system may play an important role in the regulation of several different aspects of neuroendocrine functions. TIP39 neurons in the PVG may be stimulated by stress inputs compromising the homeostasis of the animal while TIP39 neurons in the PIL may be stimulated by various reproductive events (**Figure 5**). Additional, as yet unexplored inputs to the TIP39 neurons are also plausible. These TIP39 neurons in the posterior thalamus relay their input toward neurons located in neuroendocrine and limbic brain areas to exert direct and indirect effects on neuroendocrine systems. So far, substantial evidence is available for the involvement of the TIP39-PTH2R system in the regulation of corticosterone, AVP, and prolactin. These actions of TIP39 suggest that the PTH2R may be a future target to develop drugs for the treatment of some neuroendocrine abnormalities and disorders.

ACKNOWLEDGMENTS

Support was provided by the Bolyai János Fellowship Grant of the Hungarian Academy of Sciences, the Hungarian Science Foundation OTKA K100319 and NFM-OTKA NNF85612 Research Grants for AD, and the Intramural Research Program of the NIH, National Institute of Mental Health for TBU.

REFERENCES

Antunes-Rodrigues, J., de Castro, M., Elias, L. L., Valenca, M. M., and McCann, S. M. (2004). Neuroendocrine control of body fluid metabolism. *Physiol. Rev.* 84, 169–208.

Arnsten, A. F. (2009). Stress signalling pathways that impair prefrontal cortex structure and function. *Nat. Rev. Neurosci.* 10, 410–422.

Baffi, J. S., and Palkovits, M. (2000). Fine topography of brain areas activated by cold stress. A fos immunohistochemical study in rats. *Neuroendocrinology* 72, 102–113.

Bago, A. G., Dimitrov, E., Saunders, R., Seress, L., Palkovits, M., Usdin, T. B., et al. (2009). Parathyroid hormone 2 receptor and its endogenous ligand tuberoinfundibular peptide of 39 residues are concentrated in endocrine, viscerosensory and auditory brain regions in macaque and human. *Neuroscience* 162, 128–147.

Benarroch, E. E. (2006). Pain-autonomic interactions. *Neurol. Sci.* 27(Suppl 2), S130–S133.

Bratincsak, A., and Palkovits, M. (2004). Activation of brain areas in rat following warm and cold ambient exposure. *Neuroscience* 127, 385–397.

Brenner, D., Bago, A. G., Gallatz, K., Palkovits, M., Usdin, T. B., and Dobolyi, A. (2008). Tuberoinfundibular peptide of 39 residues in the embryonic and early postnatal rat brain. *J. Chem. Neuroanat.* 36, 59–68.

Coolen, L. M., Peters, H. J., and Veening, J. G. (1997). Distribution of Fos immunoreactivity following mating versus anogenital investigation in the male rat brain. *Neuroscience* 77, 1151–1161.

Coutellier, L., Logemann, A., Kuo, J., Rusnak, M., and Usdin, T. B. (2011a). TIP39 modulates effects of novelty-induced arousal on memory. *Genes Brain Behav.* 10, 90–99.

Coutellier, L., Logemann, A., Rusnak, M., and Usdin, T. B. (2011b). Maternal absence of the parathyroid hormone 2 receptor affects postnatal pup development. *J. Neuroendocrinol.* 23, 612–619.

Coutellier, L., and Usdin, T. B. (2011). Enhanced long-term fear memory and increased anxiety and depression-like behavior after exposure to an aversive event in mice lacking TIP39 signaling. *Behav. Brain Res.* 222, 265–269.

Cservenak, M., Bodnar, I., Usdin, T. B., Palkovits, M., Nagy, G. M., and Dobolyi, A. (2010). Tuberoinfundibular peptide of 39 residues is activated during lactation and participates in the suckling-induced prolactin release in rat. *Endocrinology* 151, 5830–5840.

Della Penna, K., Kinose, F., Sun, H., Koblan, K. S., and Wang, H. (2003). Tuberoinfundibular peptide of 39 residues (TIP39): molecular structure and activity for parathyroid hormone 2 receptor. *Neuropharmacology* 44, 141–153.

Dimitrov, E., and Usdin, T. B. (2010). Tuberoinfundibular peptide of 39 residues modulates the mouse hypothalamic-pituitary-adrenal axis via paraventricular glutamatergic neurons. *J. Comp. Neurol.* 518, 4375–4394.

Dimitrov, E. L., Kim, Y. Y., and Usdin, T. B. (2011). Regulation of hypothalamic signaling by tuberoinfundibular peptide of 39 residues is critical for the response to cold: a novel peptidergic mechanism of thermoregulation. *J. Neurosci.* 31, 18166–18179.

Dimitrov, E. L., Petrus, E., and Usdin, T. B. (2010). Tuberoinfundibular peptide of 39 residues (TIP39) signaling modulates acute and tonic nociception. *Exp. Neurol.* 226, 68–83.

Dobolyi, A. (2011). Novel potential regulators of maternal adaptations during lactation: tuberoinfundibular peptide 39 and amylin. *J. Neuroendocrinol.* 23, 1002–1008.

Dobolyi, A., Irwin, S., Wang, J., and Usdin, T. B. (2006a). The distribution and neurochemistry of the parathyroid hormone 2 receptor in the rat hypothalamus. *Neurochem. Res.* 31, 227–236.

Dobolyi, A., Wang, J., Irwin, S., and Usdin, T. B. (2006b). Postnatal development and gender-dependent expression of TIP39 in the rat brain. *J. Comp. Neurol.* 498, 375–389.

Dobolyi, A., Palkovits, M., Bodnar, I., and Usdin, T. B. (2003a). Neurons containing tuberoinfundibular peptide of 39 residues project to limbic, endocrine, auditory and spinal areas in rat. *Neuroscience* 122, 1093–1105.

Dobolyi, A., Palkovits, M., and Usdin, T. B. (2003b). Expression and distribution of tuberoinfundibular peptide of 39 residues in the rat central nervous system. *J. Comp. Neurol.* 455, 547–566.

Dobolyi, A., Palkovits, M., and Usdin, T. B. (2010). The TIP39-PTH2 receptor system: unique peptidergic cell groups in the brainstem and their interactions with central regulatory mechanisms. *Prog. Neurobiol.* 90, 29–59.

Dobolyi, A., Ueda, H., Uchida, H., Palkovits, M., and Usdin, T. B. (2002). Anatomical and physiological evidence for involvement of tuberoinfundibular peptide of 39 residues in nociception. *Proc. Natl. Acad. Sci. U.S.A.* 99, 1651–1656.

Dong, W. K., Ryu, H., and Wagman, I. H. (1978). Nociceptive responses of neurons in medial thalamus and their relationship to spinothalamic pathways. *J. Neurophysiol.* 41, 1592–1613.

Faber, C. A., Dobolyi, A., Sleeman, M., and Usdin, T. B. (2007). Distribution of tuberoinfundibular peptide of 39 residues and its receptor, parathyroid hormone 2 receptor, in the mouse brain. *J. Comp. Neurol.* 502, 563–583.

Fegley, D. B., Holmes, A., Riordan, T., Faber, C. A., Weiss, J. R., Ma, S., et al. (2008). Increased fear- and stress-related anxiety-like behavior in mice lacking tuberoinfundibular peptide of 39 residues. *Genes Brain Behav.* 7, 933–942.

Goold, C. P., Usdin, T. B., and Hoare, S. R. (2001). Regions in rat and human parathyroid hormone (PTH) 2 receptors controlling receptor interaction with PTH and with antagonist ligands. *J. Pharmacol. Exp. Ther.* 299, 678–690.

Haaf, J. A., Maigret, C., Andringa-Bakker, E. A., and van Wimersma Greidanus, T. B. (1987). Dynorphin-(1–13) is a potent in vivo suppressor of vasopressin levels in the rat. *Acta Endocrinol.* 114, 96–101.

Hasen, N. S., and Gammie, S. C. (2005). Differential fos activation in virgin and lactating mice in response to an intruder. *Physiol. Behav.* 84, 681–695.

Heijning, B. J., Herik, I. K., Rots, N. Y., and Greidanus, T. B. (1991). Enhanced neurohypophyseal vasopressin release is associated with increased opioid inhibition of oxytocin release. *J. Neuroendocrinol.* 3, 57–64.

Hoare, S. R., Bonner, T. I., and Usdin, T. B. (1999a). Comparison of rat and human parathyroid hormone 2 (PTH2) receptor activation: PTH is a low potency partial agonist at the rat PTH2 receptor. *Endocrinology* 140, 4419–4425.

Hoare, S. R., de Vries, G., and Usdin, T. B. (1999b). Measurement of agonist and antagonist ligand-binding parameters at the human parathyroid hormone type 1 receptor: evaluation of receptor states and modulation by guanine nucleotide. *J. Pharmacol. Exp. Ther.* 289, 1323–1333.

Hoare, S. R., and Usdin, T. B. (1999). Quantitative cell membrane-based radioligand binding assays for parathyroid hormone receptors. *J. Pharmacol. Toxicol. Methods* 41, 83–90.

Holstege, G., Georgiadis, J. R., Paans, A. M., Meiners, L. C., van der Graaf, F. H., and Reinders, A. A. (2003). Brain activation during human male ejaculation. *J. Neurosci.* 23, 9185–9193.

Kiyohara, T., Miyata, S., Nakamura, T., Shido, O., Nakashima, T., and Shibata, M. (1995). Differences in Fos expression in the rat brains between cold and warm ambient exposures. *Brain Res. Bull.* 38, 193–201.

Kuo, J., and Usdin, T. B. (2007). Development of a rat parathyroid hormone 2 receptor antagonist. *Peptides* 28, 887–892.

Kvetnansky, R., Sabban, E. L., and Palkovits, M. (2009). Catecholaminergic systems in stress: structural and molecular genetic approaches. *Physiol. Rev.* 89, 535–606.

LaBuda, C. J., Dobolyi, A., and Usdin, T. B. (2004). Tuberoinfundibular peptide of 39 residues produces anxiolytic and antidepressant actions. *Neuroreport* 15, 881–885.

LeDoux, J. (2003). The emotional brain, fear, and the amygdala. *Cell. Mol. Neurobiol.* 23, 727–738.

Lewis, J. W., Cannon, J. T., and Liebeskind, J. C. (1980). Opioid and nonopioid mechanisms of stress analgesia. *Science* 208, 623–625.

Li, C., Chen, P., and Smith, M. S. (1999). Neural populations in the rat forebrain and brainstem activated by the suckling stimulus as demonstrated by cFos expression. *Neuroscience* 94, 117–129.

Lin, S. H., Miyata, S., Matsunaga, W., Kawarabayashi, T., Nakashima, T., and Kiyohara, T. (1998). Metabolic mapping of the brain in pregnant, parturient and lactating rats using fos immunohistochemistry. *Brain Res.* 787, 226–236.

Lonstein, J. S., and Stern, J. M. (1997). Role of the midbrain periaqueductal gray in maternal nurturance and aggression: c-fos and electrolytic lesion studies in lactating rats. *J. Neurosci.* 17, 3364–3378.

Luque, R. M., Park, S., and Kineman, R. D. (2008). Role of endogenous somatostatin in regulating GH output under basal conditions and in response to metabolic extremes. *Mol. Cell. Endocrinol.* 286, 155–168.

Maillard, C. A., and Edwards, D. A. (1991). Excitotoxin lesions of the zona incerta/lateral tegmentum continuum: effects on male sexual behavior in rats. *Behav. Brain Res.* 46, 143–149.

Matsumoto, M., Kondo, S., Usdin, T. B., and Ueda, H. (2010). Parathyroid hormone 2 receptor is a functional marker of nociceptive myelinated fibers responsible for neuropathic pain. *J. Neurochem.* 112, 521–530.

Miyata, S., Ishiyama, M., Shido, O., Nakashima, T., Shibata, M., and Kiyohara, T. (1995). Central mechanism of neural activation with cold acclimation of rats using Fos immunohistochemistry. *Neurosci. Res.* 22, 209–218.

Morrison, S. F., and Nakamura, K. (2011). Central neural pathways for thermoregulation. *Front. Biosci.* 16, 74–104.

Nakamura, K. (2011). Central circuitries for body temperature regulation and fever. *Am. J. Physiol. Regul. Integr. Comp. Physiol.* 301, R1207–R1228.

Numan, M., and Insel, T. R. (2003). *The Neurobiology of Parental Behavior.* New York: Springer.

Palkovits, M., Helfferich, F., Dobolyi, A., and Usdin, T. B. (2009). Acoustic stress activates tuberoinfundibular peptide of 39 residues neurons in the rat brain. *Brain Struct. Funct.* 214, 15–23.

Palkovits, M., Usdin, T. B., Makara, G. B., and Dobolyi, A. (2010). Tuberoinfundibular peptide of 39 residues-immunoreactive fibers in the zona incerta and the supraoptic decussations terminate in the neuroendocrine hypothalamus. *Neurochem. Res.* 35, 2078–2085.

Paxinos, G., and Watson, C. (2007). *The Rat Brain in Stereotaxic Coordinates.* San Diego: Academic Press.

Peschanski, M., and Mantyh, P. W. (1983). Efferent connections of the subfascicular area of the mesodiencephalic junction and its possible involvement in stimulation-produced analgesia. *Brain Res.* 263, 181–190.

Piserchio, A., Usdin, T., and Mierke, D. F. (2000). Structure of tuberoinfundibular peptide of 39 residues. *J. Biol. Chem.* 275, 27284–27290.

Rhodes, D. L., and Liebeskind, J. C. (1978). Analgesia from rostral brain stem stimulation in the rat. *Brain Res.* 143, 521–532.

Sachs, B. D., and Meisel, R. L. (1988). "The physiology of male sexual behavior," in *The Physiology of Reproduction,* eds E. Knobil and J. Meill (New York: Raven Press), 1393–1485.

Shimura, T., and Shimokochi, M. (1991). Modification of male rat copulatory behavior by lateral midbrain stimulation. *Physiol. Behav.* 50, 989–994.

Simerly, R. B. (2002). Wired for reproduction: organization and development of sexually dimorphic circuits in the mammalian forebrain. *Annu. Rev. Neurosci.* 25, 507–536.

Sugimura, Y., Murase, T., Ishizaki, S., Tachikawa, K., Arima, H., Miura, Y., et al. (2003). Centrally administered tuberoinfundibular peptide of 39 residues inhibits arginine vasopressin release in conscious rats. *Endocrinology* 144, 2791–2796.

Sugiyama, K., Ryu, H., and Uemura, K. (1992). Identification of nociceptive neurons in the medial thalamus: morphological studies of nociceptive neurons with intracellular injection of horseradish peroxidase. *Brain Res.* 586, 36–43.

Szabo, F. K., Snyder, N., Usdin, T. B., and Hoffman, G. E. (2010). A direct neuronal connection between the subparafascicular and ventrolateral arcuate nuclei in non-lactating female rats. Could this pathway play a role in the suckling-induced prolactin release? *Endocrine* 37, 62–70.

Terman, G. W., Shavit, Y., Lewis, J. W., Cannon, J. T., and Liebeskind, J. C. (1984). Intrinsic mechanisms of pain inhibition: activation by stress. *Science* 226, 1270–1277.

Usdin, T. B., Bonner, T. I., Harta, G., and Mezey, E. (1996). Distribution of parathyroid hormone-2 receptor messenger ribonucleic acid in rat. *Endocrinology* 137, 4285–4297.

Usdin, T. B., Bonner, T. I., and Hoare, S. R. (2002). The parathyroid hormone 2 (PTH2) receptor. *Recept. Channels* 8, 211–218.

Usdin, T. B., Dobolyi, A., Ueda, H., and Palkovits, M. (2003). Emerging functions for tuberoinfundibular peptide of 39 residues. *Trends Endocrinol. Metab.* 14, 14–19.

Usdin, T. B., Gruber, C., and Bonner, T. I. (1995). Identification and functional expression of a receptor selectively recognizing parathyroid hormone, the PTH2 receptor. *J. Biol. Chem.* 270, 15455–15458.

Usdin, T. B., Hilton, J., Vertesi, T., Harta, G., Segre, G., and Mezey, E. (1999a). Distribution of the parathyroid hormone 2 receptor in rat: immunolocalization reveals expression by several endocrine cells. *Endocrinology* 140, 3363–3371.

Usdin, T. B., Hoare, S. R., Wang, T., Mezey, E., and Kowalak, J. A. (1999b). TIP39: a new neuropeptide and PTH2-receptor agonist from hypothalamus. *Nat. Neurosci.* 2, 941–943.

Varga, T., Palkovits, M., Usdin, T. B., and Dobolyi, A. (2008). The medial paralemniscal nucleus and its afferent neuronal connections in rat. *J. Comp. Neurol.* 511, 221–237.

Veening, J. G., and Coolen, L. M. (1998). Neural activation following sexual behavior in the male and female rat brain. *Behav. Brain Res.* 92, 181–193.

Wang, J., Coolen, L. M., Brown, J. L., and Usdin, T. B. (2006a). Neurons containing tuberoinfundibular peptide of 39 residues are activated following male sexual behavior. *Neuropeptides* 40, 403–408.

Wang, J., Palkovits, M., Usdin, T. B., and Dobolyi, A. (2006b). Forebrain projections of tuberoinfundibular peptide of 39 residues (TIP39)-containing subparafascicular neurons. *Neuroscience* 138, 1245–1263.

Wang, T., Palkovits, M., Rusnak, M., Mezey, E., and Usdin, T. B. (2000). Distribution of parathyroid hormone-2 receptor-like immunoreactivity and messenger RNA in the rat nervous system. *Neuroscience* 100, 629–649.

Ward, H. L., Small, C. J., Murphy, K. G., Kennedy, A. R., Ghatei, M. A., and Bloom, S. R. (2001). The actions of tuberoinfundibular peptide on the hypothalamo-pituitary axes. *Endocrinology* 142, 3451–3456.

10

Sex differences in behavioral circadian rhythms in laboratory rodents

Jessica A. Krizo[1] ***and Eric M. Mintz***[1,2]*******

[1] *Department of Biological Sciences, Kent State University, Kent, OH, USA*
[2] *School of Biomedical Sciences, Kent State University, Kent, OH, USA*

Edited by:
Hubert Vaudry, University of Rouen, France

Reviewed by:
Jacques Epelbaum, Université Paris Descartes, France
Michael Antle, University of Calgary, Canada

****Correspondence:***
Eric M. Mintz, Department of Biological Sciences, Kent State University, Kent, OH 44242, USA
e-mail: emintz@kent.edu

There is a strong bias in basic research on circadian rhythms toward the use of only male animals in studies. Furthermore, of the studies that use female subjects, many use only females and do not compare results between males and females. This review focuses on behavioral aspects of circadian rhythms that differ between the sexes. Differences exist in the timing of daily onset of activity, responses to both photic and non-photic stimuli, and in changes across the lifespan. These differences may reflect biologically important traits that are ecologically relevant and impact on a variety of responses to behavioral and physiological challenges. Overall, more work needs to be done to investigate differences between males and females as well as differences that are the result of hormonal changes across the lifespan.

Keywords: estrogens, testosterone, locomotor activity, ovariectomy, castration

INTRODUCTION

There has been a longstanding bias against the use of females in basic research involving common animal models, arising out of the belief that females show higher variability in results due to the influence of hormonal cycles (1). However, a recent meta-analysis of publications involving the use of mice across a variety of biomedical research areas concluded that this assumption was without merit (2). The failure to include both females and males, therefore, can result in researchers missing important information on sex differences in biology without any resulting gains from limiting themselves to the use of a single sex. The study of biological rhythms is no exception to this critique, as a large majority of recent work in this area has failed to include females (3). In this review, we look at sex differences in basic parameters of circadian rhythms and hypothesize about their underlying mechanisms and biological relevance.

CIRCADIAN PERIOD

The period of the circadian clock represents the time it takes to complete one cycle under constant environmental conditions, and is usually close to but not exactly 24 h. Sex differences in period are highly species-specific, but even when present the differences are generally modest. Free-running period in rats and golden hamsters is longer in males than females (4, 5); however, the differences in period are very small, whereas in *Octodon degus* period is longer in females by approximately half an hour (6, 7). In mice with a C57BL/6J background, there does not appear to be a sex difference in free-running period (3).

Despite the limited nature of the sex differences, gonadal hormones have a significant impact on circadian period. Ovariectomy lengthens circadian period in rats and hamsters, and period is then shortened by replacement of estradiol (8, 9). However, no change in period is apparent in mice after ovariectomy (3), though estradiol, an estrogen receptor α (ERα) agonist, or an estrogen receptor β (ERβ) agonist shorten period in ovariectomized mice (10). In contrast, reports on the effect of castration on period are more varied. While one study showed no effect in mice (11), others indicate that it lengthens period in this species (12–14). It appears that this effect may be dependent on the presence of constant dim red light (as opposed to true constant darkness) (14). Castration does not result in a change in period in hamsters (15) or adult degus (16).

Given the modest, if any, sex differences in circadian period, it is appropriate to ask whether the differences that are seen are biologically relevant. There is natural variation in circadian period across species and individuals, but circadian period must be under stabilizing selection to keep it close to 24 h. Period length does influence the amplitude of responses of the circadian clock to stimuli (17), so average period for a species may reflect an optimization for responses to external stimuli rather than an optimization for period length. There does not seem to be an overarching theory that explains interspecies variation in period. It is likely that sex differences in period reflect the influence of gonadal steroids, either through direct action on the central circadian clock in the suprachiasmatic nucleus (SCN) or via actions that modify behavioral feedback on the SCN. Organizational effects of gonadal hormones may also play an important role, but in this review we are focusing on potential activational effects. That said, it is remarkable that sex differences are so small, given the considerable influence of gonadal steroids on circadian period.

ONSET OF ACTIVITY

The timing of activity onset represents the most obvious difference in circadian rhythms between the sexes. Variability in activity onset is considerably greater in females than in males, and this variability is closely tied to the phase of the estrous cycle in mice (3), hamsters (8, 18, 19), and rats (20, 21). Variability in the onset of activity in females appears to be largely mediated by ERβ, at least in mice (10, 22). Activity onset is most advanced before ovulation, corresponding to elevated estradiol levels, and then delayed afterward. The functional significance, if any, of this variation is unknown. These effects could be caused by direct effects of estrogens on the phase of the underlying circadian clock and/or by changes in effector systems that cause the threshold for onset of locomotor activity to occur slightly earlier or later depending on the hormonal environment. The idea that the underlying clock in the SCN shifts a little on each day of the estrous cycle under the direct influence of estradiol is supported by the fact that period is shortened by replacement of estradiol in ovariectomized animals (8, 9, 23). However, it is also possible that clock output is unchanged, but downstream brain regions responsible for generating the motivation for locomotor activity are slightly more or less sensitive depending on the level of estrogens present. For example, estrogens upregulate dopamine receptor 1 in the striatum (24, 25), which could result in increased motivation for wheel-running activity, resulting in a slightly earlier onset of activity.

PHOTIC RESPONSES

There are a number of potential mechanisms by which biological sex, via gonadal steroids, can influence the photic sensitivity of the circadian clock. However, it is not known if the effects that have been found thus far are biologically important, and these effects may vary dramatically by species. In *Octodon degus*, females adjust to a 6-h advance of the light–dark cycle significantly faster than males (26). In mice, females have larger phase shifts to light (3), while gonadectomized male mice have larger phase shifts than gonadally intact male mice (27). The lengthening of period that occurs when animals are housed in increasing intensities of constant light is also potentiated in gonadectomized animals (14). Female mice lacking estrogen receptor alpha show increased phase shifting responses to light (28). These data are consistent with the idea that both estradiol and testosterone act to reduce the phase shifting effects of light. The functional significance of this is unknown.

NON-PHOTIC RESPONSES

There has been little work done investigating sex differences in non-photic influences on entrainment. A couple of studies have been done on the influence of the estrous cycle on circadian responses in Syrian hamsters, but not with direct comparisons to male animals. Females show an estrous-cycle dependent modulation of activity level in response to a non-photic stimulus such as a cage change or novel wheel exposure, but this difference in behavioral activation results in only modest variability in the size of non-photic phase shifts (29). However, they did note that large shifts during proestrus caused a 1-day delay in the estrous cycle. A similar delay was observed in response to phenobarbital treatment on proestrus, suggesting that large phase shifts caused the circadian clock to "miss" generating the daily signal needed for the GnRH surge (30). However, in order to demonstrate a true sex difference in non-photic responses, it will be necessary to conduct experiments with direct comparisons between males and females, and it is important that this be done in additional species to see if there are common responses. In degus, there are sex differences in the effect of odor on circadian reentrainment rates to shifts in the light/dark cycle, and these effects are influenced by estrogen, progesterone, and testosterone (31, 32).

FOOD ENTRAINMENT

There has been very little research on sex differences in food entrainment. When rodents are placed on a restricted feeding schedule, such that food is only available for a limited period of time each day during an animal's normal sleep period, they show a behavioral response known as food anticipatory activity (FAA). This FAA generally takes the form of increased behavioral activation for a period of about 3 h prior to food availability. FAA is particularly notable when animals are provided with a running wheel, as wheel-running during FAA can be more intense than normal nocturnal running. This activity is thought to be stimulated by the action of a circadian clock, as food availability that is timed in non-circadian intervals (e.g., 18 h) does not result in FAA (33). In addition, FAA persists for several cycles under conditions of total food deprivation after entrainment to timed restricted feeding, and also does so in the absence of the SCN (34, 35). Little work has been published concerning female responses to timed restricted feeding. Rats will entrain their activity rhythms to restricted feeding if in constant dark, but there is no evidence for or against a sex difference in the ability to entrain to restricted feeding. A few studies have investigated the role of the reward system on entrainment to feeding using palatable foods. To date sex differences in FAA have only been identified in mice. When receiving a high fat food as a snack, male mice exhibit anticipatory activity and females do not (36). However, females show activity at the time of previous food delivery on subsequent days, suggesting that the females are still timing the arrival of the food but are not showing the anticipatory activity. There is some evidence to suggest that female motivation for sugary/fat foods is modulated by the estrous cycle (37). This could impact the response of female mice to a palatable food cue during *ad libitum* conditions. The fact that circadian clock-driven anticipatory activity can occur under both normocaloric and hypocaloric conditions suggests that there are multiple drivers of FAA, a motivational circuit and a homeostatic circuit (38).

PUBERTAL EFFECTS ON RHYTHMS

Puberty represents a period of substantial changes in physiology and endocrine profiles. Given that gonadal steroids have an impact on adult circadian behavior it is reasonable to hypothesize that the circadian system would be responsive to this dynamic endocrine environment. Pubertal changes in circadian phase have been noted in mice (39, 40) and rats (41, 42). However, these studies were limited to male or female subjects and therefore do not address the issues of sex differences. The role of gonadal steroids during the pubertal period on circadian development has been investigated in the rat and the degus (43–47). During the pubertal period, rats and degus (both male and female) have a bimodal distribution of locomotor activity during their active phase. By adulthood, activity in intact male rats and degus changes to a unimodal activity pattern. Pre-pubertal GDX in rats leads to a less extreme bimodal distribution that is maintained into adulthood, suggesting that gonadal steroids are responsible for the consolidation of activity to the beginning of the active phase. In males, GDX results in a loss or reduction in pubertal-related changes in circadian parameters, whereas GDX in females results in a more variable response (45). In degus, pre-pubertal GDX of both males and females stabilizes circadian phase and the bimodal distribution of activity persists into adulthood as seen in intact female degus (46). These studies taken together provide evidence for the developmental role of gonadal steroids during puberty in setting circadian behavioral rhythm parameters.

SITE OF ACTION

A direct action of gonadal steroids on the SCN would be most likely be mediated by one or more of the steroid hormone receptors: ERα, ERβ, androgen receptor (AR), progesterone receptor (PR), or G protein-coupled estrogen receptor 1 (GPER1). ERα, ERβ, and AR are all expressed in the SCN (13, 48–51), with sexual dimorphisms present in ERβ, and AR (51). For a full review of the neuroanatomical aspects of sexual dimorphism in the circadian system, see (52). In addition, the SCN receives input from other estrogen receptor-positive regions of the brain (53), providing another potential mechanism for steroid-modulation of SCN function. Finally, it is possible that signals from some peripheral organs may be sexually dimorphic, and when activated they may alter rhythmic function in a sex-specific manner.

CONCLUSION

There is a clear need for further research to understand how biological sex and gonadal hormones can regulate behavioral rhythmicity. Sex differences in basic behavioral activity rhythms are modest in scope; however, this may not be the case if the system is challenged. For example, there are substantial sex differences in the brain's reward system (54) that could interact with circadian clocks in such a way that result in differential responses of the circadian clock to addictive drugs.

In general, the data reviewed in this article suggests that most initial research studies on the circadian system should be carried out using both male and female animals. If no sex differences in the results are observed, researchers can then decide whether their approach will work best using a single or mixed sex approach. For example, in experiments where precision of the onset of activity is critical, it may be appropriate to conduct studies in males, though modern mathematical techniques for ascertaining rhythm phase make this less of an issue than when activity rhythms were assessed by visual inspection of actograms. Failure to make use of both males and females in studies may result in important physiological and behavioral phenomenon remaining undiscovered.

Finally, most studies that look at female steroid hormone effects on circadian rhythms make use of experimental methods involving gonadectomy and hormone replacement. While such studies yield valuable information about the mechanisms of hormone influences on rhythms, they do not represent the normal physiological variation that occurs across a normal estrous cycle. It is understandable that this has occurred, given the increase in animal numbers needed and workload involved in measuring estrous cycle phase, however, such studies will become increasingly important as we learn more about the potential influence of gonadal hormones on behavioral circadian outputs.

ACKNOWLEDGMENTS

Support for this article was provided by Kent State University and National Science Foundation grant IOS-1021957.

REFERENCES

Beery AK, Zucker I. Sex bias in neuroscience and biomedical research. *Neurosci Biobehav Rev* (2011) 35:565–72. doi:10.1016/j.neubiorev.2010.07.002

Prendergast BJ, Onishi KG, Zucker I. Female mice liberated for inclusion in neuroscience and biomedical research. *Neurosci Biobehav Rev* (2014) 40:1–5. doi:10.1016/j.neubiorev.2014.01.001

Kuljis DA, Loh DH, Truong D, Vosko AM, Ong ML, Mcclusky R, et al. Gonadal- and sex-chromosome-dependent sex differences in the circadian sys- tem. *Endocrinology* (2013) 154:1501–12. doi:10.1210/en.2012-1921

Davis FC, Darrow JM, Menaker M. Sex differences in the circadian control of hamster wheel-running activity. *Am J Physiol* (1983) 244:R93–105.

Schull J, Walker J, Fitzgerald K, Hiilivirta L, Ruckdeschel J, Schumacher D, et al. Effects of sex, thyro-parathyroidectomy, and light regime on levels and circadian rhythms of wheel-running in rats. *Physiol Behav* (1989) 46:341–6. doi:10.1016/0031-9384(89)90001-2

Labyak SE, Lee TM. Estrus- and steroid-induced changes in circadian rhythms in a diurnal rodent, *Octodon degus. Physiol Behav* (1995) 58:573–85. doi:10.1016/ 0031-9384(95)00096-2

Lee TM, Labyak SE. Free-running rhythms and light- and dark-pulse phase response curves for diurnal *Octodon degus* (Rodentia). *Am J Physiol* (1997) 273:R278–86.

Morin LP, Fitzgerald KM, Zucker I. Estradiol shortens the period of hamster circadian rhythms. *Science* (1977) 196:305–7. doi:10.1126/science.557840

Albers HE. Gonadal hormones organize and modulate the circadian system of the rat. *Am J Physiol* (1981) 241:R62–6.

Royston SE, Yasui N, Kondilis AG, Lord SV, Katzenellenbogen JA, Mahoney MM. ESR1 and ESR2 differentially regulate daily and circadian activity rhythms in female mice. *Endocrinology* (2014) 155:2613–23. doi:10.1210/en.2014-1101

Schwartz WJ, Zimmerman P. Circadian timekeeping in BALB/c and C57BL/6 inbred mouse strains. *J Neurosci* (1990) 10:3685–94.

Daan S, Damassa D, Pittendrigh CS, Smith ER. An effect of castration and testos- terone replacement on a circadian pacemaker in mice (*Mus musculus*). *Proc Natl Acad Sci U S A* (1975) 72:3744–7. doi:10.1073/pnas.72.9.3744

Karatsoreos IN, Wang A, Sasanian J, Silver R. A role for androgens in regulat- ing circadian behavior and the suprachiasmatic nucleus. *Endocrinology* (2007) 148:5487–95. doi:10.1210/en.2007-0775

Butler MP, Karatsoreos IN, Lesauter J, Silver R. Dose-dependent effects of andro- gens on the circadian timing system and its response to light. *Endocrinology* (2012) 153:2344–52. doi:10.1210/en.2011-1842

Morin LP, Cummings LA. Effect of surgical or photoperiodic castration, testos- terone replacement or pinealectomy on male hamster running rhythmicity. *Physiol Behav* (1981) 26:825–38. doi:10.1016/0031-9384(81)90106-2

Jechura TJ, Walsh JM, Lee TM. Testicular hormones modulate circadian rhythms of the diurnal rodent, *Octodon degus. Horm Behav* (2000) 38:243–9. doi:10.1006/hbeh.2000.1624

Daan S, Pittendrigh CS. Functional-analysis of circadian pacemakers in noc- turnal rodents. II. Variability of phase response curves. *J Comp Physiol* (1976) 106:253–66. doi:10.1007/BF01417857

Takahashi JS, Menaker M. Interaction of estradiol and progesterone: effects on circadian locomotor rhythm of female golden hamsters. *Am J Physiol* (1980) 239:R497–504.

Widmaier EP, Campbell CS. Interaction of estradiol and photoperiod on activity patterns in the female hamster. *Physiol Behav* (1980) 24:923–30. doi:10.1016/0031-9384(80)90151-1

Albers HE, Gerall AA, Axelson JF. Effect of reproductive state on circadian peri- odicity in the rat. *Physiol Behav* (1981) 26:21–5. doi:10.1016/0031-9384(81)90073-1

Wollnik F, Turek FW. Estrous correlated modulations of circadian and ultra- dian wheel-running activity rhythms in LEW/Ztm rats. *Physiol Behav* (1988) 43:389–96. doi:10.1016/0031-9384(88)90204-1

Blattner MS, Mahoney MM. Estrogen receptor 1 modulates circadian rhythms in adult female mice. *Chronobiol Int* (2014) 31:637–44. doi:10.3109/07420528.2014.885528

Morin LP, Fitzgerald KM, Rusak B, Zucker I. Circadian organization and neural mediation of hamster reproductive rhythms. *Psychoneuroendocrinology* (1977) 2:73–98. doi:10.1016/0306-4530(77)90035-X

Di Paolo T. Modulation of brain dopamine transmission by sex steroids. *Rev Neurosci* (1994) 5:27–41. doi:10.1515/REVNEURO.1994.5.1.27

Lammers CH, D'souza U, Qin ZH, Lee SH, Yajima S, Mouradian MM. Reg- ulation of striatal dopamine receptors by estrogen. *Synapse* (1999) 34:222–7. doi:10.1002/(SICI)1098-2396(19991201)34:3<222::AID-SYN6>3.0.CO;2-J

Goel N, Lee TM. Sex differences and effects of social cues on daily rhythms following phase advances in *Octodon degus*. *Physiol Behav* (1995) 58:205–13. doi:10.1016/0031-9384(95)00051-J

Karatsoreos IN, Butler MP, Lesauter J, Silver R. Androgens modulate structure and function of the suprachiasmatic nucleus brain clock. *Endocrinology* (2011) 152:1970–8. doi:10.1210/en.2010-1398

Blattner MS, Mahoney MM. Photic phase-response curve in 2 strains of mice with impaired responsiveness to estrogens. *J Biol Rhythms* (2013) 28:291–300. doi:10.1177/0748730413497190

Young Janik L, Janik D. Nonphotic phase shifting in female *Syrian* ham- sters: interactions with the estrous cycle. *J Biol Rhythms* (2003) 18:307–17. doi:10.1177/0748730403254005

Legan SJ, Donoghue KM, Franklin KM, Duncan MJ. Phenobarbital block- ade of the preovulatory luteinizing hormone surge: association with phase- advanced circadian clock and altered suprachiasmatic nucleus Period1 gene expression. *Am J Physiol Regul Integr Comp Physiol* (2009) 296:R1620–30. doi:10.1152/ajpregu.90914.2008

Jechura TJ, Walsh JM, Lee TM. Testosterone suppresses circadian responsive- ness to social cues in the diurnal rodent *Octodon degus*. *J Biol Rhythms* (2003) 18:43–50. doi:10.1177/0748730402239675

Jechura TJ, Lee TM. Ovarian hormones influence olfactory cue effects on reen- trainment in the diurnal rodent, *Octodon degus*. *Horm Behav* (2004) 46:349–55. doi:10.1016/j.yhbeh.2004.06.001

Petersen CC, Patton DF, Parfyonov M, Mistlberger RE. Circadian food antic- ipatory activity: entrainment limits and scalar properties re-examined. *Behav Neurosci* (2014) 128:689–702. doi:10.1037/bne0000017

Stephan FK, Swann JM, Sisk CL. Anticipation of 24-Hr feeding schedules in rats with lesions of the suprachiasmatic Nucleus. *Behav Neural Biol* (1979) 25:346–63. doi:10.1016/S0163-1047(79)90415-1

Stephan FK, Swann JM, Sisk CL. Entrainment of circadian-rhythms by feed- ing schedules in rats with suprachiasmatic lesions. *Behav Neural Biol* (1979) 25:545–54. doi:10.1016/S0163-1047(79)90415-1

Hsu CT, Patton DF, Mistlberger RE, Steele AD. Palatable meal anticipation in mice. *PLoS One* (2010) 5:e12903. doi:10.1371/journal.pone.0012903

Clarke SN, Ossenkopp KP. Taste reactivity responses in rats: influence of sex and the estrous cycle. *Am J Physiol* (1998) 274:R718–24.

Gallardo CM, Gunapala KM, King OD, Steele AD. Daily scheduled high fat meals moderately entrain behavioral anticipatory activity, body temperature, and hypothalamic c-Fos activation. *PLoS One* (2012) 7:e41161. doi:10.1371/journal.pone.0041161

Weinert D, Eimert H, Erkert HG, Schneyer U. Resynchronization of the circa- dian corticosterone rhythm after a light/dark shift in juvenile and adult mice. *Chronobiol Int* (1994) 11:222–31. doi:10.3109/07420529409067791

Weinert D, Waterhouse J. Daily activity and body temperature rhythms do not change simultaneously with age in laboratory mice. *Physiol Behav* (1999) 66:605–12. doi:10.1016/S0031-9384(98)00342-4

Melanie E, Kittrell W, Satinoff E. Development of the circadian rhythm of body temperature in rats. *Physiol Behav* (1986) 38:99–104. doi:10.1016/0031-9384(86)90138-1

McGinnis MY, Lumia AR, Tetel MJ, Molenda-Figueira HA, Possidente B. Effects of anabolic androgenic steroids on the development and expression of run- ning wheel activity and circadian rhythms in male rats. *Physiol Behav* (2007) 92:1010–8. doi:10.1016/j.physbeh.2007.07.010

Lee TM, Hummer DL, Jechura TJ, Mahoney MM. Pubertal development of sex differences in circadian function: an animal model. *Ann N Y Acad Sci* (2004) 1021:262–75. doi:10.1196/annals.1308.031

Hummer DL, Jechura TJ, Mahoney MM, Lee TM. Gonadal hormone effects on entrained and free-running circadian activity rhythms in the developing diurnal rodent *Octodon degus*. *Am J Physiol Regul Integr Comp Physiol* (2007) 292:R586–97. doi:10.1152/ajpregu.00043.2006

Hagenauer MH, King AF, Possidente B, Mcginnis MY, Lumia AR, Peckham EM, et al. Changes in circadian rhythms during puberty in *Rattus norvegicus*: devel- opmental time course and gonadal dependency. *Horm Behav* (2011) 60:46–57. doi:10.1016/j.yhbeh.2011.03.001

Hagenauer MH, Ku JH, Lee TM. Chronotype changes during puberty depend on gonadal hormones in the slow-developing rodent, *Octodon degus*. *Horm Behav* (2011) 60:37–45. doi:10.1016/j.yhbeh.2011.02.004

Hummer DL, Peckham EM, Lee TM. Estradiol acts during a post-pubertal sen- sitive period to shorten free-running circadian period in male *Octodon degus*. *Eur J Neurosci* (2012) 36:3051–8. doi:10.1111/j.1460-9568.2012.08228.x

Ehret G, Buckenmaier J. Estrogen-receptor occurrence in the female mouse brain: effects of maternal experience, ovariectomy, estrogen and anosmia. *J Phys- iol Paris* (1994) 88:315–29. doi:10.1016/0928-4257(94)90012-4

Zhou L, Blaustein JD, De Vries GJ. Distribution of androgen receptor immunore- activity in vasopressin- and oxytocin-immunoreactive neurons in the male rat brain. *Endocrinology* (1994) 134:2622–7. doi:10.1210/en.134.6.2622

Shughrue PJ, Lane MV, Merchenthaler I. Comparative distribution of estrogen receptor-alpha and -beta mRNA in the rat central nervous system. *J Comp Neurol* (1997) 388:507–25. doi:10.1002/(SICI)1096-9861(19971201)388:4<507::AID-CNE1>3.0.CO;2-6

Vida B, Hrabovszky E, Kalamatianos T, Coen CW, Liposits Z, Kallo I. Oestro- gen receptor alpha and beta immunoreactive cells in the suprachiasmatic nucleus of mice: distribution, sex differences and regulation by gonadal hor- mones. *J Neuroendocrinol* (2008) 20:1270–7. doi:10.1111/j.1365-2826.2008.01787.x

Bailey M, Silver R. Sex differences in circadian timing systems: implications for disease. *Front Neuroendocrinol* (2014) 35:111–39. doi:10.1016/j.yfrne.2013. 11.003

De La Iglesia HO, Blaustein JD, Bittman EL. Oestrogen receptor-alpha- immunoreactive neurones project to the suprachiasmatic nucleus of the female *Syrian* hamster. *J Neuroendocrinol* (1999) 11:481–90. doi:10.1046/j.1365-2826.1999.00341.x

Bobzean SA, Denobrega AK, Perrotti LI. Sex differences in the neurobiology of drug addiction. *Exp Neurol* (2014) 259:64–74. doi:10.1016/j.expneurol.2014.01.022

11

Response of the nitrergic system to activation of the neuroendocrine stress axis

Hsiao-Jou Cortina Chen *, Jereme G. Spiers, Conrad Sernia and Nickolas A. Lavidis

School of Biomedical Sciences, The University of Queensland, Brisbane, QLD, Australia

Edited by:
Hubert Vaudry, University of Rouen, France

Reviewed by:
Charles W. Wilkinson, University of Washington, USA
Alline C. Campos, Max-Planck-Institute for Experimental Medicine, Germany

****Correspondence:***
Hsiao-Jou Cortina Chen, School of Biomedical Sciences, The University of Queensland, St. Lucia, Brisbane, QLD 4072, Australia
e-mail: h.chen6@uq.edu.au

Exposure to stressful stimuli causes activation of the hypothalamic-pituitary-adrenal axis which rapidly releases high concentrations of glucocorticoid stress hormones, resulting in increased cellular metabolism and spontaneous oxygen and nitrogen radical formation. High concentrations of nitrogen radicals, including nitric oxide, cause damage to cellular proteins in addition to inhibiting components of the mitochondrial transport chain, leading to cellular energy deficiency. During stress exposure, pharmacological inhibition of nitric oxide production reduces indicators of anxiety- and depressive-like behavior in animal models. Therefore, the purpose of this review is to present an overview of the current literature on stress-evoked changes in the nitrergic system, particularly within neural tissue.

Keywords: anxiety, depression, hypothalamic-pituitary-adrenal axis, glucocorticoids, nitrergic system, nitric oxide, peroxynitrite, reactive nitrogen species

INTRODUCTION

An acute stress response is mediated by the tripartite activation of the sympatho-adrenal-medullary (SAM), hypothalamic-spinal-adrenal (HSA), and hypothalamic-pituitary-adrenal (HPA) axes. The first of these axes to respond is the autonomic SAM system, consisting of several hypothalamic and brainstem nuclei, notably including the locus ceruleus (Jansen et al., 1995). The locus ceruleus is the primary source of central noradrenergic signaling, functioning via the ascending noradrenergic bundle and descending through preganglionic neurons in the intermediolateral cell column (IML) of the spinal cord to innervate the adrenal medulla (Sara, 2009; Ulrich-Lai and Herman, 2009). Through the combined action of catecholamines, this system promotes increased arousal and vigilance and is responsible for the rapid generation of the "fight-or-flight" response (Jansen et al., 1995). The paraventricular nucleus (PVN) of the hypothalamus is considered the apex of the HPA stress response as release of corticotropin-releasing hormone from the parvocellular neurosecretory neurons triggers anterior pituitary corticotrophs to release the pro-opiomelanocortin fragment, adrenocorticotropic hormone (ACTH), into the circulation. However, the PVN also facilitates corticosterone release directly through the HSA stress axis via adrenocortical innervation from the IML, and indirectly via an alternative stress pathway involving prolactin release (Buijs et al., 1999; Lowry, 2002; Ulrich-Lai et al., 2006; Jaroenporn et al., 2009). This ultimately sensitizes the adrenal gland to ACTH, resulting in corticosterone release from the *zona fasciculata* of the adrenal cortex thereby exerting the characteristics downstream cellular and metabolic effects of stress (Buijs et al., 1999; Lowry, 2002; Weiser et al., 2011). Adrenal glucocorticoids accelerate cellular metabolism to increase available energy which consequently increases free radical formation in specific regions of the central nervous system (Spiers et al., 2013). This stress-induced increase in radical production, including nitric oxide (NO) formation, leads to oxidative and nitrosative stress (Chen et al., 2014). Furthermore, the toxic metabolite of NO, peroxynitrite, is capable of inhibiting components of the mitochondrial respiratory chain, leading to cellular energy deficiency (Sarti et al., 2012). Since dysfunction of the nitrergic system has been implicated in the neuropathogenesis of several stress-related disease states, the present review summarizes our current understanding and advances relating to the impact of stress on the nitrergic system.

NITRIC OXIDE BIOSYNTHESIS AND FUNCTIONS

Nitric oxide, a gaseous free radical belonging to the family of reactive nitrogen species (RNS), is synthesized through the conversion of L-arginine to L-citrulline by nitric oxide synthase (NOS) in the presence of oxygen, NADPH, and cofactors such as tetrahydrobiopterin (Andrew and Mayer, 1999). There are three main isoforms, each with a specific distribution profile; neuronal NOS (nNOS, type I), inducible NOS (iNOS, type II), and endothelial NOS (eNOS, type III) (Stuehr, 1999). Though nNOS is predominantly active in the cytosol of central and peripheral neurons for signaling and regulation, it has also been found in the sarcolemma and cytoplasm of all muscle fibers (Frandsen et al., 1996). Interestingly, nNOS is present in the hippocampus, hypothalamus, pituitary, and adrenal gland, suggesting co-localization with the HPA axis (Lai et al., 2005; Gadek-Michalska et al., 2012). Furthermore, several studies have demonstrated transcriptional regulation of nNOS by glucocorticoids in the hippocampus, implicating its importance in the stress response, although the upstream promoter of NOS1 does not carry a glucocorticoid responsive element (López-Figueroa et al., 1998; Reagan et al., 1999; Zhou et al., 2011). There are four nNOS splice variants, α, β, γ, and μ, with nNOSα being the most dominant and therefore being physically and functionally coupled to the glutamate receptors of the N-methyl-D-aspartate (NMDA) subtype through their mutual post-synaptic density-95/discs-large/zona occludens-1 (PDZ) binding motif (Eliasson et al., 1997). Within the hippocampus, local calcium influx through NMDA receptors can trigger the production of NO, which subsequently activates its receptor, soluble guanylyl cyclase, leading to release of second messenger cyclic guanosine monophosphate (cGMP) (**Figure 1**). This NO-cGMP signaling has been implicated in the induction of hippocampal long-term potentiation which is known to be one of the principal mechanisms in learning and memory (Schuman and Madison, 1991; Arancio et al., 1996; Kelley et al., 2010). The nNOSμ mainly localizes in the skeletal muscles, with nNOSμ-deficient muscles being myopathic (Percival et al., 2008). The β variant lacks the PDZ domain while nNOSγ has very little to no enzymatic activity (Eliasson et al., 1997). Endothelial NOS contains a putative shear stress responsive element in the promoter region of the NOS3 gene while the protein is membrane-bound to the golgi apparatus and caveolae, producing NO mainly in the endothelium of blood vessels responsible for vasodilation and smooth muscle relaxation (Smith et al., 2006). The inducible form of NOS responds at the transcriptional level to inflammatory factors (Zamora et al., 2000; Aktan, 2004). Within the central nervous system, the iNOS-mediated release of NO by astrocytes and microglia has a major role in antimicrobial and tumoricidal activity in response to various inflammatory signals (Hua et al., 2002; Brantley et al., 2010). Moreover, upon transcriptional activation, this soluble subtype can produce micromolar levels of NO and is known to be associated with diseases such as artherosclerosis, rheumatoid arthritis, diabetes, septic shock,

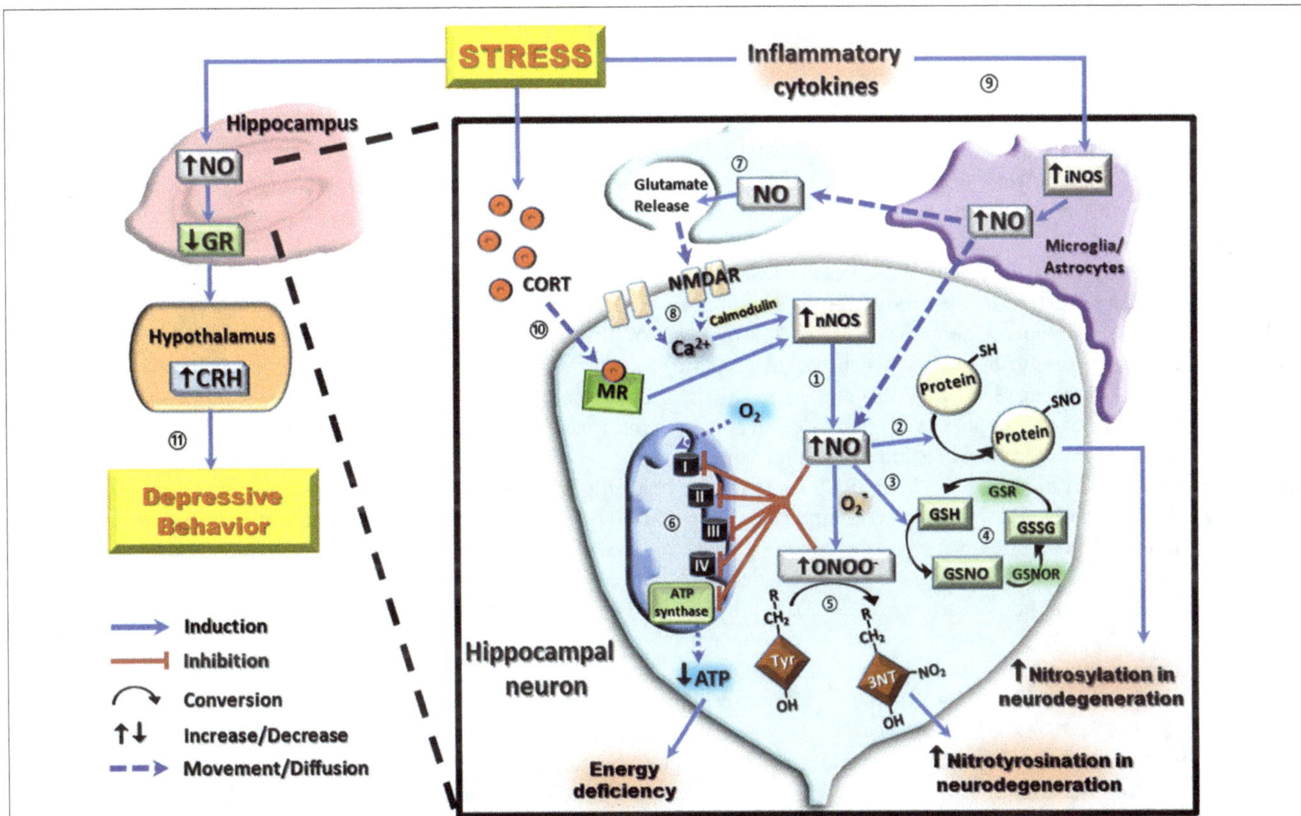

FIGURE 1 | A schematic representation of the nitrergic system and its downstream effects in hippocampal neurons following stress exposure. In hippocampal neurons, the majority of nitric oxide (NO) production occurs via the conversion of L-arginine to L-citrulline by the neuronal isoform of nitric oxide synthase (nNOS) ①. High concentrations of NO can then covalently bond with protein thiol groups (protein-SH) to form S-nitroso-proteins (protein-SNO) ② or interact with the reduced form of glutathione (GSH) forming S-nitrosoglutathione (GSNO) ③. This can be regenerated back to GSH via an initial conversion to oxidized glutathione (GSSG) by S-nitrosoglutathione reductase (GSNOR), and subsequent reduction of GSSG by glutathione reductase (GSR) ④. Interaction of NO with the superoxide radical (O_2^-) results in the formation of the neurotoxic radical, peroxynitrite ($ONOO^-$) which irreversibly reacts with protein tyrosine (Tyr) residues to form 3-nitrotyrosine (3-NT) ⑤. Increased NO and $ONOO^-$ are capable of causing cellular energy deficiency by inhibition of all components of the electron transport chain (Complex I–IV), including ATP synthase, resulting in decreased ATP production ⑥. Both post-synaptically produced NO, and NO produced by the inducible isoform of nitric oxide synthase (iNOS), can act as a neurotransmitter on pre-synaptic neurons ⑦. This pre-synaptic NO causes glutamate release, which activates post-synaptic NMDA receptors (NMDAR) to increase calcium (Ca^{2+}) concentration and, in the presence of calmodulin, further potentiate nNOS-derived NO ⑧. Stress exposure increases NO by activating inflammatory cytokines to potentiate glial/astrocyte iNOS activity ⑨, and by increasing circulating corticosterone (CORT) which induces nNOS activity via a mineralocorticoid receptor (MR)-mediated pathway ⑩. This increase in NO results in downregulation of hippocampal glucocorticoid receptors (GR) and subsequently increases hypothalamic corticotropin-releasing hormone (CRH) to induce depressive-like behaviors ⑪.

and multiple sclerosis (Kuhlencordt et al., 2001; Hill et al., 2004; Maki-Petaja et al., 2008; Heemskerk et al., 2009; Soskic et al., 2011). Both nNOS and eNOS are constitutively active isoforms producing low concentrations of NO (in the nanomolar range) over long periods and are activated by calcium ions though transient binding to the calcium-binding protein, calmodulin (Knott and Bossy-Wetzel, 2009). Comparatively, the inducible form of NOS can produce high concentrations of NO in relatively short periods and is calcium independent due to a high binding affinity to calmodulin (Aktan, 2004). The inorganic ions, nitrate and nitrite (NO*x*), were previously thought to be the end products of NO metabolism. However, recent studies have demonstrated a NOS-independent pathway in which NO can be produced by reducing NO*x*, a reaction catalyzed by xanthine reductase under low oxygen tension and low pH environment. The NO produced by this nitrate-nitrite-NO pathway may have similar roles to NO generated from the L-arginine-NOS pathway representing an important secondary pool (see review by Lundberg et al., 2008).

NITROSATIVE STRESS

High levels of NO and its derivatives are destructive to cellular components such as proteins, lipids and DNA. Nitric oxide can react directly with molecular oxygen to produce two relatively strong oxidants, nitrogen dioxide and dinitrogen trioxide. However, at physiological levels of NO these reactions are relatively slow. A primary reaction in the production of RNS is the combination of NO and superoxide anions to form the highly reactive metabolite, peroxynitrite, a potent neurotoxin (Lipton et al., 1993). It has been suggested that NO and peroxynitrite can disrupt adenosine 5′-triphosphate (ATP) synthase and almost all components of the mitochondrial respiratory chain (Almeida and Bolanos, 2001; Sarti et al., 2012). These RNS reversibly or irreversibly inhibit mitochondrial oxygen consumption, particularly at complex IV (also known as cytochrome *c* oxidase), and may lead to cellular energy deficiency and ultimately cell death in pathological conditions (Sarti et al., 2012). Inhibition of cytochrome *c* oxidase by NO and peroxynitrite causes neuronal dysfunction and, in addition to high iNOS expression, has been observed in the cortex of Alzheimer's patients (Mutisya et al., 1994; Haas et al., 2002).

S-nitrosylation is the covalent attachment of NO to the thiol side chain of the amino acid cysteine, forming other NO derivatives termed *S*-nitroso-proteins. Under physiological conditions, it has been demonstrated that NO is converted to the nitrosonium ion which subsequently S-nitrosylates the NMDA receptor, thereby preventing glutamate excitotoxicity by blocking calcium influx, promoting cell survival (Lipton and Stamler, 1994). Excessive production of NO can be counteracted by conjugation with reduced glutathione, forming the stable adduct *S*-nitrosoglutathione which has important role in signal transduction and regulation of a variety of protein functions (Klatt and Lamas, 2000; Anand and Stamler, 2012). Abnormal *S*-nitrosylation to proteins such as apolipoprotein E, cyclin-dependent kinase 5, dynamin-related protein 1, parkin, peroxiredoxin 2, protein disulfide isomerase, heat-shock protein 90, and X-linked inhibitor of apoptosis have all being linked to neurodegenerative conditions such as Alzheimer's and Parkinson's diseases (Anand and Stamler, 2012). Lastly, peroxynitrite provokes protein nitrotyrosination, an irreversible chemical addition of a nitro group to the tyrosine residue in target proteins generating 3-nitrotyrosine. This post-translational modification usually impairs the normal physiological function of the proteins and therefore nitrotyrosination has been used as a marker in several neurodegenerative conditions such as amyotrophic lateral sclerosis (Peluffo et al., 2004). These aspects of the nitrergic system have been summarized in **Figure 1**.

STRESS-EVOKED MODULATION OF THE NITRERGIC SYSTEM

It has been generally accepted that psychophysiological stress is associated with upregulation of NOS mRNA expression and enzymatic activity. For example, a single 6 h acute immobilization stress induces upregulation of iNOS expression and activity in the cerebral cortex which is mediated by the NMDA receptor and subsequent activation of the transcriptional factor, nuclear factor kappa-light-chain-enhancer of activated B cells (NF-κB) (Madrigal et al., 2001). The acute stress-induced activation of the NMDA receptor also increases tumor necrosis factor-alpha (TNFα) via upregulation of TNFα-convertase. Antagonism of TNFα-convertase prevents the stress-induced translocation of NF-κB and subsequent iNOS expression, thus confirming the involvement of TNFα (Madrigal et al., 2002). This is also supported by Shirakawa et al. (2004) who demonstrated glutamatergic activation and not catecholaminergic drive of the hypothalamic paraventricular nucleus to be responsible for the acute stress-induced increase in NO metabolites. Interestingly, biting activity is capable of suppressing the stress-induced increase in hypothalamic nNOS mRNA expression in rats (Hori et al., 2005). A single 2 h acute restraint stress significantly increases the density of neurons expressing nNOS visualized by nicotinamide adenine dinucleotide phosphate-diaphorase (NADPH-d) histochemistry in the amygdaloid nucleus, an effect delayed by 5 days in the hippocampus and entorhinal cortex (Echeverry et al., 2004). Predator-induced post-traumatic stress significantly increases nNOS positive neurons and total NO*x* in the medial prefrontal cortex 7 days after the 10 min predator stress treatment (Campos et al., 2013). Conversely, Chakraborti et al. (2014) demonstrated that acute restraint stress causes a reduction in total NO*x* and an increase in the major endogenous NOS inhibitor, asymmetric dimethylarginine, in whole brain homogenates. This suggests that the stress-induced NO*x* increases in regions such as the hippocampus and hypothalamus may hold a high degree of functional significance. These biochemical changes in NO*x* and asymmetric dimethylarginine were observed alongside anxiety-like behavior and were more pronounced in male compared to female rats. The pharmacological blockade of estrogen biosynthesis exacerbated these biochemical and behavioral changes in females, suggesting that the observed sex differences are due to a protective role of estrogen. Interestingly, bilateral injection of an NMDA receptor antagonist, NOS inhibitor, or NO scavenger into the dorsal hippocampus attenuated autonomic responses such as hypertension and tachycardia following a 60 min acute restraint stress, suggesting that NMDA/NOS activation within the hippocampus plays a role in autonomic modulation during stress (Moraes-Neto et al., 2014). Another study from the same group proposed a glutamatergic NMDA receptor-NO-cGMP signaling pathway in modulating contextual fear conditioning within the dorsal hippocampus, where intra-hippocampal injection of NMDA receptor antagonist DL-AP7, NO scavenger 2-(4-carboxyphenyl)-4,4,5,5-tetramethylimidazoline-1-oxyl-3-oxide (CPTIO), and cGMP inhibitor 1H-[1,2,4]oxadiazolo[4,3-a]quinoxalin-1-one (ODQ), attenuated the fear-conditioned response (Fabri et al., 2014).

Chronic immobilization stress has been shown to increase NO*x*, iNOS activity, and peroxynitrite-induced 3-nitrotyrosine accumulation in cortical neurons (Olivenza et al., 2000). Notably, de Pablos et al. (2014) recently found a degree of regional specificity associated with this chronic stress-induced iNOS expression, with little to no constitutive expression in the substantia nigra following 9 days of unpredictable stress exposure. However, this same unpredictable stress model potentiates iNOS expression following exposure to exogenous immunostimulatory stressors such as lipopolysaccharides. Recent studies in several animal paradigms have demonstrated that inhibitors of NOS significantly modulate stress-related behaviors. In support of these findings, the commercially available antidepressant paroxetine, a selective serotonin reuptake inhibitor, also possesses NOS inhibition capability (Finkel et al., 1996). Wegener and Volke (2010) have reviewed and summarized these studies including data on each of the NOS inhibitor's specificity and potency, and their anxiolytic- and antidepressant-like properties. Chronic unpredictable mild stress increases plasma nitrite levels and iNOS mRNA expression in the cortex, in addition to damaging cortical neurons and inducing depressive-like behavior (Wang et al., 2008; Peng et al., 2012). These effects can be attenuated or prevented using NOS inhibitors, which was demonstrated by intra-hippocampal injection of the selective iNOS inhibitor, aminoguanidine, resulting in suppression of the chronic unpredictable mild stress-induced depressive-like behavior in rats (Wang et al., 2008). Regional infusion of a selective nNOS inhibitor 7-nitroindazole (7-NI) into the hippocampus showed antidepressant-like effects similar to those with the iNOS inhibitor, aminoguanidine (Joca and Guimaraes, 2006). Likewise, the anxiogenic-like behavior observed in rats during ethanol withdrawal is inhibited by administration of the selective iNOS inhibitor, 1400W, into the dorsolateral periaqueductal gray (Bonassoli et al., 2013). The data with intra-cerebral NOS inhibition is further supported by studies using systemic treatment. Intraperitoneal injection of 1400W increases survival of cortical neurons and decreases the depressive-like behavior in mice (Peng et al., 2012). The nNOS inhibitor 1-(-2-trifluoromethylphenyl)-imidazole (TRIM) given systemically 30 min prior to testing induces anxiolytic-like behavior shown by increased time spent in the light compartment of a light-dark compartment test (Volke et al., 2003). Furthermore, TRIM administration decreased the immobility time in the forced swimming test, demonstrating an antidepressant-like effect comparable to the tricyclic antidepressant imipramine. In agreement with these observations, Ulak et al. (2008) injected TRIM intraperitoneally 50 min before a forced swim test and showed the involvement of the serotonergic system in the antidepressant-like actions of TRIM. This was further clarified in a later study in which the serotonin type II receptors were found to be responsible for this effect (Ulak et al., 2010). Furthermore, Joung et al. (2012) demonstrated that following a 2 h immobilization stress, the selective inhibitor 7-NI produced its anxiolytic-like effects shown by an increase in the time spent on the open arms of the elevated plus-maze through the direct reduction of NO metabolites in the PVN and locus ceruleus. A less specific NOS inhibitor, L-N^G-Nitroarginine methyl ester (L-NAME), injected systemically 30 min prior to testing shows protective effects against chronic swim stress-induced impairment of passive avoidance learning and hyperalgesia in rats (Nazeri et al., 2014). In a similar vein, Ferreira et al. (2012) performed behavioral, genomic, and proteomic analyses in rats and suggested that the antidepressant-like effects of NOS inhibition may involve the expression of additional factors including members of the glutathione redox system.

Genetic animal models have also contributed to the current understanding of nitrergic changes in stress. Thus, inhibition of NO production by nNOS gene deletion in mice suppressed hippocampal neurogenesis and exhibited antidepressant-like properties while nNOS over-expression in the hippocampus was essential for chronic stress-induced depression (Zhou et al., 2007). Recently, a number of studies have proposed a regulatory role of NO on the limbic HPA stress axis. Zhang et al. (2010) used mice lacking the nNOS gene to demonstrate an anxiolytic-like phenotype when tested using an elevated plus-maze, similar to normal mice treated with intra-hippocampal microinjection of the selective nNOS inhibitor 7-NI. The authors proposed a signaling pathway involving the activation of serotonin type IA receptors which mediate, via an unknown mechanism, the down-regulation of hippocampal nNOS, leading to a decrease in NO and subsequent inhibition of cAMP response element-binding (CREB) protein phosphorylation. A follow up study elucidated further the link between NO and the HPA axis by showing that chronic mild stress and glucocorticoid exposure lead to hippocampal nNOS overexpression via activating hippocampal mineralocorticoid receptor (MR) (Zhou et al., 2011). The excessive nNOS-derived NO significantly downregulated local glucocorticoid receptor (GR) expression through either the soluble guanylyl cyclase/cGMP or peroxynitrite/extracellular signal-regulated kinase (ERK) signaling pathways. The significant downregulation of GR in the hippocampus leads to an elevation in hypothalamic corticotropin-releasing hormone and the depressive-like behaviors in mice as illustrated in **Figure 1**. It is important to note that nNOS deletion, infusion of intrahippocampal nNOS inhibitor, and NO-cGMP signaling blockade prevented the chronic mild stress-evoked behavioral modification. Interestingly, this chronic glucocorticoid-induced MR-nNOS-NO pathway is exclusive to the MR-rich hippocampus and drives HPA axis hyperactivity through impaired negative feedback (Zhu et al., 2014).

The considerable body of evidence from animal models is progressively expanding and supported by modest but significant clinical studies. Several reports have shown that increased levels of NO metabolites are present in depressed and autistic patients (Suzuki et al., 2001; Sogut et al., 2003; Lee et al., 2006). Patients with recurrent depressive behavior displayed higher plasma NO*x* concentrations which were associated with cognitive impairment

(Talarowska et al., 2012). Galecki et al. (2010, 2011) discovered single nucleotide polymorphisms in exon 22 of the NOS2A gene (iNOS) and exon 29 of the NOSI gene (nNOS) in depressed Caucasian individuals. Furthermore, three single nucleotide polymorphisms located at the regulatory region of NOSI gene are responsible for the susceptibility of an individual to depressive disorders (Sarginson et al., 2014).

SUMMARY

A growing body of evidence suggests that the etiology of anxiety and depression-related conditions can be derived from the sensitization of particular stress-related circuits that are "primed" following exposure to a short-term stressor. The duration for stress-related circuitry priming far exceeds responses to adrenergic and glucocorticoid-mediated stress responses. Understanding the mechanisms underlying the induction of this long latency will provide a significant link between stress and the pathogenesis of anxiety and depressive disorders. The nitrergic system has been implicated in regulating both short and long-term activation of the stress response, with a variety of NOS inhibitors demonstrating potent anxiolytic and antidepressant activity. The intrinsic cross talk between neuroendocrine stress and nitrergic system activation is now an important physiological consideration. Further understanding the role of this system is important in identifying early players in stress-induced pathological conditions.

AUTHOR CONTRIBUTIONS

Author Hsiao-Jou Cortina Chen managed the literature searches, wrote the first draft of the manuscript, and produced the graphic. Author Jereme G. Spiers, Conrad Sernia and Nickolas A. Lavidis critically revised the manuscript. All authors have approved the final version of the manuscript for journal submission.

ACKNOWLEDGMENT

We would like to thank Szu-Ju Patricia Chen for assistance in graphical design and production.

REFERENCES

Aktan, F. (2004). iNOS-mediated nitric oxide production and its regulation. *Life Sci.* 75, 639–653. doi: 10.1016/j.lfs.2003.10.042

Almeida, A., and Bolanos, J. P. (2001). A transient inhibition of mitochon- drial ATP synthesis by nitric oxide synthase activation triggered apoptosis in primary cortical neurons. *J. Neurochem.* 77, 676–690. doi: 10.1046/j.1471-4159.2001.00276.x

Anand, P., and Stamler, J. S. (2012). Enzymatic mechanisms regulating protein S-nitrosylation: implications in health and disease. *J. Mol. Med.* 90, 233–244. doi: 10.1007/s00109-012-0878-z

Andrew, P. J., and Mayer, B. (1999). Enzymatic function of nitric oxide synthases. *Cardiovasc. Res.* 43, 521–531. doi: 10.1016/S0008-6363(99)00115-7

Arancio, O., Kiebler, M., Lee, C. J., Lev-Ram, V., Tsien, R. Y., Kandel, E. R., et al. (1996). Nitric oxide acts directly in the presynaptic neuron to produce long- term potentiation in cultured hippocampal neurons. *Cell* 87, 1025–1035. doi: 10.1016/S0092-8674(00)81797-3

Bonassoli, V. T., Contardi, E. B., Milani, H., and de Oliveira, R. M. (2013). Effects of nitric oxide synthase inhibition in the dorsolateral periaqueduc- tal gray matter on ethanol withdrawal-induced anxiety-like behavior in rats. *Psychopharmacology (Berl).* 228, 487–498. doi: 10.1007/s00213-013-3049-1

Brantley, E. C., Guo, L., Zhang, C., Lin, Q., Yokoi, K., Langley, R. R., et al. (2010). Nitric oxide-mediated tumoricidal activity of murine microglial cells. *Transl. Oncol.* 3, 380–388. doi: 10.1593/tlo.10208

Buijs, R. M., Wortel, J., Van Heerikhuize, J. J., Feenstra, M. G., Ter Horst, G. J., Romijn, H. J., et al. (1999). Anatomical and functional demonstration of a mul- tisynaptic suprachiasmatic nucleus adrenal (cortex) pathway. *Eur. J. Neurosci.* 11, 1535–1544. doi: 10.1046/j.1460-9568.1999.00575.x

Campos, A. C., Piorino, E. M., Ferreira, F. R., and Guimaraes, F. S. (2013). Increased nitric oxide-mediated neurotransmission in the medial prefrontal cortex is asso- ciated with the long lasting anxiogenic-like effect of predator exposure. *Behav. Brain Res.* 256, 391–397. doi: 10.1016/j.bbr.2013.08.006

Chakraborti, A., Gulati, K., and Ray, A. (2014). Possible role of nitric oxide (NO) in the regulation of gender related differences in stress induced anxiogenesis in rats. *Nitric Oxide* 43, 74–80. doi: 10.1016/j.niox.2014.08.005

Chen, H. J. C., Spiers, J. G., Sernia, C., Anderson, S. T., and Lavidis, N. A. (2014). Reactive nitrogen species contribute to the rapid onset of redox changes induced by acute immobilization stress in rats. *Stress* 17, 520–527. doi: 10.3109/10253890.2014.966264

de Pablos, R. M., Herrera, A. J., Espinosa-Oliva, A. M., Sarmiento, M., Munoz, M. F., Machado, A., et al. (2014). Chronic stress enhances microglia activa- tion and exacerbates death of nigral dopaminergic neurons under conditions of inflammation. *J. Neuroinflammation* 11, 34. doi: 10.1186/1742-2094-11-34

Echeverry, M. B., Guimaraes, F. S., and Del Bel, E. A. (2004). Acute and delayed restraint stress-induced changes in nitric oxide producing neurons in limbic regions. *Neuroscience* 125, 981–993. doi: 10.1016/j.neuroscience.2003.12.046

Eliasson, M. J., Blackshaw, S., Schell, M. J., and Snyder, S. H. (1997). Neuronal nitric oxide synthase alternatively spliced forms: prominent functional local- izations in the brain. *Proc. Natl. Acad. Sci. U.S.A.* 94, 3396–3401. doi: 10.1073/pnas.94.7.3396

Fabri, D. R. S., Hott, S. C., Reis, D. G., Biojone, C., Corrêa, F. M. A., and Resstel, L. B. M. (2014). The expression of contextual fear conditioning involves activation of a NMDA receptor-nitric oxide-cGMP pathway in the dorsal hippocampus of rats. *Eur. Neuropsychopharmacol.* 24, 1676–1686. doi: 10.1016/j.euroneuro.2014.08.002

Ferreira, F. R., Oliveira, A. M., Dinarte, A. R., Pinheiro, D. G., Greene, L. J., Silva, W. A., et al. (2012). Changes in hippocampal gene expression by 7-nitroindazole in rats submitted to forced swimming stress. *Genes Brain Behav.* 11, 303–313. doi: 10.1111/j.1601-183X.2011.00757.x

Finkel, M. S., Laghrissi-Thode, F., Pollock, B. G., and Rong, J. (1996). Paroxetine is a novel nitric oxide synthase inhibitor. *Psychopharmacol. Bull.* 32, 653–658.

Frandsen, U., Lopez-Figueroa, M., and Hellsten, Y. (1996). Localization of nitric oxide synthase in human skeletal muscle. *Biochem. Biophys. Res. Commun.* 227, 88–93. doi: 10.1006/bbrc.1996.1472

Gadek-Michalska, A., Tadeusz, J., Rachwalska, P., Spyrka, J., and Bugajski, J. (2012). Effect of repeated restraint on homotypic stress-induced nitric oxide synthases expression in brain structures regulating HPA axis. *Pharmacol. Rep.* 64, 1381–1390. doi: 10.1016/S1734-1140(12)70935-0

Galecki, P., Maes, M., Florkowski, A., Lewinski, A., Galecka, E., Bienkiewicz, M., et al. (2010). An inducible nitric oxide synthase polymorphism is associated with the risk of recurrent depressive disorder. *Neurosci. Lett.* 486, 184–187. doi: 10.1016/j.neulet.2010.09.048

Galecki, P., Maes, M., Florkowski, A., Lewinski, A., Galecka, E., Bienkiewicz, M., et al. (2011). Association between inducible and neuronal nitric oxide syn- thase polymorphisms and recurrent depressive disorder. *J. Affect. Disord.* 129, 175–182. doi: 10.1016/j.jad.2010.09.005

Haas, J., Storch-Hagenlocher, B., Biessmann, A., and Wildemann, B. (2002). Inducible nitric oxide synthase and argininosuccinate synthetase: co-induction in brain tissue of patients with Alzheimer's dementia and following stim- ulation with beta-amyloid 1-42 *in vitro*. *Neurosci. Lett.* 322, 121–125. doi: 10.1016/S0304-3940(02)00095-2

Heemskerk, S., Masereeuw, R., Russel, F. G., and Pickkers, P. (2009). Selective iNOS inhibition for the treatment of sepsis-induced acute kidney injury. *Nat. Rev. Nephrol.* 5, 629–640. doi: 10.1038/nrneph.2009.155

Hill, K. E., Zollinger, L. V., Watt, H. E., Carlson, N. G., and Rose, J.

W. (2004). Inducible nitric oxide synthase in chronic active multiple sclerosis plaques: distribution, cellular expression and association with myelin damage. *J. Neuroimmunol.* 151, 171–179. doi: 10.1016/j.jneuroim.2004.02.005

Hori, N., Lee, M. C., Sasaguri, K., Ishii, H., Kamei, M., Kimoto, K., et al. (2005). Suppression of stress-induced nNOS expression in the rat hypothalamus by biting. *J. Dent. Res.* 84, 624–628. doi: 10.1177/154405910508400708

Hua, L. L., Kim, M. O., Brosnan, C. F., and Lee, S. C. (2002). Modulation of astrocyte inducible nitric oxide synthase and cytokine expression by interferon beta is associated with induction and inhibition of interferon gamma-activated sequence binding activity. *J. Neurochem.* 83, 1120–1128. doi: 10.1046/j.1471-4159.2002.01226.x

Jansen, A. S., Nguyen, X. V., Karpitskiy, V., Mettenleiter, T. C., and Loewy, A. D. (1995). Central command neurons of the sympathetic nervous system: basis of the fight-or-flight response. *Science* 270, 644–646. doi: 10.1126/science.270.5236.644

Jaroenporn, S., Nagaoka, K., Ohta, R., Shirota, M., Watanabe, G., and Taya, K. (2009). Differences in adrenocortical secretory and gene expression responses to stimulation *in vitro* by ACTH or prolactin between high- and low-avoidance Hatano rats. *Stress* 12, 22–29. doi: 10.1080/10253890801976652

Joca, S. R., and Guimaraes, F. S. (2006). Inhibition of neuronal nitric oxide synthase in the rat hippocampus induces antidepressant-like effects. *Psychopharmacology (Berl).* 185, 298–305. doi: 10.1007/s00213-006-0326-2

Joung, H. Y., Jung, E. Y., Kim, K., Lee, M. S., Her, S., and Shim, I. (2012). The differential role of NOS inhibitors on stress-induced anxiety and neu- roendocrine alterations in the rat. *Behav. Brain Res.* 235, 176–181. doi: 10.1016/j.bbr.2012.07.037

Kelley, J. B., Anderson, K. L., and Itzhak, Y. (2010). Pharmacological modu- lators of nitric oxide signaling and contextual fear conditioning in mice. *Psychopharmacology (Berl).* 210, 65–74. doi: 10.1007/s00213-010-1817-8

Klatt, P., and Lamas, S. (2000). Regulation of protein function by S-glutathiolation in response to oxidative and nitrosative stress. *Eur. J. Biochem.* 267, 4928–4944. doi: 10.1046/j.1432-1327.2000.01601.x

Knott, A. B., and Bossy-Wetzel, E. (2009). Nitric oxide in health and disease of the nervous system. *Antioxid. Redox Signal.* 11, 541–554. doi: 10.1089/ars.2008.2234

Kuhlencordt, P. J., Chen, J., Han, F., Astern, J., and Huang, P. L. (2001). Genetic deficiency of inducible nitric oxide synthase reduces atherosclerosis and low- ers plasma lipid peroxides in apolipoprotein E-knockout mice. *Circulation* 103, 3099–3104. doi: 10.1161/01.CIR.103.25.3099

Lai, F. J., Huang, S. S., Hsieh, M. C., Hsin, S. C., Wu, C. H., Hsin, Y. C., et al. (2005). Upregulation of neuronal nitric oxide synthase mRNA and protein in adrenal medulla of water-deprived rats. *J. Histochem. Cytochem.* 53, 45–53. doi: 10.1177/002215540505300106

Lee, B. H., Lee, S. W., Yoon, D., Lee, H. J., Yang, J. C., Shim, S. H., et al. (2006). Increased plasma nitric oxide metabolites in suicide attempters. *Neuropsychobiology* 53, 127–132. doi: 10.1159/000092542

Lipton, S. A., Choi, Y. B., Pan, Z. H., Lei, S. Z., Chen, H. S., Sucher, N. J., et al. (1993). A redox-based mechanism for the neuroprotective and neurodestructive effects of nitric oxide and related nitroso-compounds. *Nature* 364, 626–632. doi: 10.1038/364626a0

Lipton, S. A., and Stamler, J. S. (1994). Actions of redox-related congeners of nitric oxide at the NMDA receptor. *Neuropharmacology* 33, 1229–1233. doi: 10.1016/0028-3908(94)90021-3

López-Figueroa, M. O., Itoi, K., and Watson, S. J. (1998). Regulation of nitric oxide synthase messenger RNA expression in the rat hippocampus by glucocorticoids. *Neuroscience* 87, 439–446. doi: 10.1016/S0306-4522(98)00075-X

Lowry, C. A. (2002). Functional subsets of serotonergic neurones: implications for control of the hypothalamic-pituitary-adrenal axis. *J. Neuroendocrinol.* 14, 911–923. doi: 10.1046/j.1365-2826.2002.00861.x

Lundberg, J. O., Weitzberg, E., and Gladwin, M. T. (2008). The nitrate-nitrite- nitric oxide pathway in physiology and therapeutics. *Nat. Rev. Drug Discov.* 7, 156–167. doi: 10.1038/nrd2466

Madrigal, J. L., Hurtado, O., Moro, M. A., Lizasoain, I., Lorenzo, P., Castrillo, A., et al. (2002). The increase in TNF-alpha levels is implicated in NF- kappaB activation and inducible nitric oxide synthase expression in brain cortex after immobilization stress. *Neuropsychopharmacology* 26, 155–163. doi: 10.1016/S0893-133X(01)00292-5

Madrigal, J. L., Moro, M. A., Lizasoain, I., Lorenzo, P., Castrillo, A., Bosca, L., et al. (2001). Inducible nitric oxide synthase expression in brain cortex after acute restraint stress is regulated by nuclear factor kappaB-mediated mechanisms. *J. Neurochem.* 76, 532–538. doi: 10.1046/j.1471-4159.2001.00108.x

Maki-Petaja, K. M., Cheriyan, J., Booth, A. D., Hall, F. C., Brown, J., Wallace, S. M., et al. (2008). Inducible nitric oxide synthase activity is increased in patients with rheumatoid arthritis and contributes to endothelial dysfunction. *Int. J. Cardiol.* 129, 399–405. doi: 10.1016/j.ijcard.2008.02.011

Moraes-Neto, T. B., Scopinho, A. A., Biojone, C., Correa, F. M., and Resstel, L. B. (2014). Involvement of dorsal hippocampus glutamatergic and nitrergic neurotransmission in autonomic responses evoked by acute restraint stress in rats. *Neuroscience* 258, 364–373. doi: 10.1016/j.neuroscience.2013.11.022

Mutisya, E. M., Bowling, A. C., and Beal, M. F. (1994). Cortical cytochrome oxi- dase activity is reduced in Alzheimer's disease. *J. Neurochem.* 63, 2179–2184. doi: 10.1046/j.1471-4159.1994.63062179.x

Nazeri, M., Razavinasab, M., Abareghi, F., and Shabani, M. (2014). Role of nitric oxide in altered nociception and memory following chronic stress. *Physiol. Behav.* 129, 214–220. doi: 10.1016/j.physbeh.2014.02.054

Olivenza, R., Moro, M. A., Lizasoain, I., Lorenzo, P., Fernandez, A. P., Rodrigo, J., et al. (2000). Chronic stress induces the expression of inducible nitric oxide synthase in rat brain cortex. *J. Neurochem.* 74, 785–791. doi: 10.1046/j.1471-4159.2000.740785.x

Peluffo, H., Shacka, J. J., Ricart, K., Bisig, C. G., Martìnez-Palma, L., Pritsch, O., et al. (2004). Induction of motor neuron apoptosis by free 3-nitro-l-tyrosine. *J. Neurochem.* 89, 602–612. doi: 10.1046/j.1471-4159.2004.02363.x

Peng, Y.-L., Liu, Y.-N., Liu, L., Wang, X., Jiang, C.-L., and Wang, Y.-X. (2012). Inducible nitric oxide synthase is involved in the modulation of depressive behaviors induced by unpredictable chronic mild stress. *J. Neuroinflammation* 9:75. doi: 10.1186/1742-2094-9-75

Percival, J. M., Anderson, K. N., Gregorevic, P., Chamberlain, J. S., and Froehner, S. C. (2008). Functional deficits in nNOSmu-deficient skeletal muscle: myopathy in nNOS knockout mice. *PLoS ONE* 3:e3387. doi: 10.1371/jour- nal.pone.0003387

Reagan, L. P., McKittrick, C. R., and McEwen, B. S. (1999). Corticosterone and phenytoin reduce neuronal nitric oxide synthase messenger RNA expres- sion in rat hippocampus. *Neuroscience* 91, 211–219. doi: 10.1016/S0306-4522(98)00615-0

Sara, S. J. (2009). The locus coeruleus and noradrenergic modulation of cognition. *Nat. Rev. Neurosci.* 10, 211–223. doi: 10.1038/nrn2573

Sarginson, J. E., Deakin, J. W., Anderson, I. M., Downey, D., Thomas, E., Elliott, R., et al. (2014). Neuronal Nitric Oxide Synthase (NOS1) polymorphisms interact with financial hardship to affect depression risk. *Neuropsychopharmacology* 39, 2857–2866. doi: 10.1038/npp.2014.137

Sarti, P., Forte, E., Mastronicola, D., Giuffre, A., and Arese, M. (2012). Cytochrome c oxidase and nitric oxide in action: molecular mechanisms and pathophysiological implications. *Biochim. Biophys. Acta* 1817, 610–619. doi: 10.1016/j.bbabio.2011.09.002

Schuman, E. M., and Madison, D. V. (1991). A requirement for the intercellular messenger nitric oxide in long-term potentiation. *Science* 254, 1503–1506. doi: 10.1126/science.1720572

Shirakawa, T., Mitome, M., Kikuiri, T., Nakamura, W., Oshima, S., Hasegawa, T., et al. (2004). Immobilization induces acute nitric oxide production in the rat hypothalamus: a role of ionotropic glutamate receptors in the paraventricular nucleus. *Endocrinology* 145, 3603–3607. doi: 10.1210/en.2004-0068

Smith, A. R., Visioli, F., and Hagen, T. M. (2006). Plasma membrane-associated endothelial nitric oxide synthase and activity in aging rat aortic vascular endothelia markedly decline with age. *Arch. Biochem. Biophys.* 454, 100–105. doi: 10.1016/j.abb.2006.02.017

Sogut, S., Zoroglu, S. S., Ozyurt, H., Yilmaz, H. R., Ozugurlu, F., Sivasli, E., et al. (2003). Changes in nitric oxide levels and antioxidant enzyme activities may have a role in the pathophysiological mechanisms involved in autism. *Clin. Chim. Acta* 331, 111–117. doi: 10.1016/S0009-8981(03)00119-0

Soskic, S. S., Dobutovic, B. D., Sudar, E. M., Obradovic, M. M., Nikolic, D. M., Djordjevic, J. D., et al. (2011). Regulation of Inducible Nitric Oxide Synthase (iNOS) and its potential role in insulin resistance, diabetes and heart failure. *Open Cardiovasc. Med. J.* 5, 153–163. doi: 10.2174/18741924011050 10153

Spiers, J. G., Chen, H. J., Bradley, A. J., Anderson, S. T., Sernia, C., and Lavidis, N. A. (2013). Acute restraint stress induces rapid and prolonged changes in erythrocyte and hippocampal redox status. *Psychoneuroendocrinology* 38, 2511–2519. doi: 10.1016/j.psyneuen.2013.05.011

Stuehr, D. J. (1999). Mammalian nitric oxide synthases. *Biochim. Biophys. Acta* 1411, 217–230. doi: 10.1016/S0005-2728(99)00016-X

Suzuki, E., Yagi, G., Nakaki, T., Kanba, S., and Asai, M. (2001). Elevated plasma nitrate levels in depressive states. *J. Affect. Disord.* 63, 221–224. doi: 10.1016/S0165-0327(00)00164-6

Talarowska, M., Galecki, P., Maes, M., Orzechowska, A., Chamielec, M., Bartosz, G., et al. (2012). Nitric oxide plasma concentration associated with cognitive impairment in patients with recurrent depressive disorder. *Neurosci. Lett.* 510, 127–131. doi: 10.1016/j.neulet.2012.01.018

Ulak, G., Mutlu, O., Akar, F. Y., Komsuoglu, F. I., Tanyeri, P., and Erden, B. F. (2008). Neuronal NOS inhibitor 1-(2-trifluoromethylphenyl)-imidazole augment the effects of antidepressants acting via serotonergic system in the forced swimming test in rats. *Pharmacol. Biochem. Behav.* 90, 563–568. doi: 10.1016/j.pbb.2008.04.016

Ulak, G., Mutlu, O., Tanyeri, P., Komsuoglu, F. I., Akar, F. Y., and Erden, B. F. (2010). Involvement of serotonin receptor subtypes in the antidepressant-like effect of TRIM in the rat forced swimming test. *Pharmacol. Biochem. Behav.* 95, 308–314. doi: 10.1016/j.pbb.2010.02.006

Ulrich-Lai, Y. M., Arnhold, M. M., and Engeland, W. C. (2006). Adrenal splanchnic innervation contributes to the diurnal rhythm of plasma corticosterone in rats by modulating adrenal sensitivity to ACTH. *Am. J. Physiol. Regul. Integr. Comp. Physiol.* 290, R1128–R1135. doi: 10.1152/ajpregu.00042.2003

Ulrich-Lai, Y. M., and Herman, J. P. (2009). Neural regulation of endocrine and autonomic stress responses. *Nat. Rev. Neurosci.* 10, 397–409. doi: 10.1038/nrn2647

Volke, V., Wegener, G., Bourin, M., and Vasar, E. (2003). Antidepressant- and anxiolytic-like effects of selective neuronal NOS inhibitor 1-(2- trifluoromethylphenyl)-imidazole in mice. *Behav. Brain Res.* 140, 141–147. doi: 10.1016/S0166-4328(02)00312-1

Wang, D., An, S. C., and Zhang, X. (2008). Prevention of chronic stress-induced depression-like behavior by inducible nitric oxide inhibitor. *Neurosci. Lett.* 433, 59–64. doi: 10.1016/j.neulet.2007.12.041

Wegener, G., and Volke, V. (2010). Nitric oxide synthase inhibitors as antidepres- sants. *Pharmaceuticals* 3, 273–299. doi: 10.3390/ph3010273

Weiser, M. J., Osterlund, C., and Spencer, R. L. (2011). Inhibitory effects of corti- costerone in the hypothalamic paraventricular nucleus (PVN) on stress-induced adrenocorticotrophic hormone secretion and gene expression in the PVN and anterior pituitary. *J. Neuroendocrinol.* 23, 1231–1240. doi: 10.1111/j.1365-2826.2011.02217.x

Zamora, R., Vodovotz, Y., and Billiar, T. R. (2000). Inducible nitric oxide synthase and inflammatory diseases. *Mol. Med.* 6, 347–373.

Zhang, J., Huang, X. Y., Ye, M. L., Luo, C. X., Wu, H. Y., Hu, Y., et al. (2010). Neuronal nitric oxide synthase alteration accounts for the role of 5-HT1A receptor in modulating anxiety-related behaviors. *J. Neurosci.* 30, 2433–2441. doi: 10.1523/JNEUROSCI.5880-09.2010

Zhou, Q. G., Hu, Y., Hua, Y., Hu, M., Luo, C. X., Han, X., et al. (2007). Neuronal nitric oxide synthase contributes to chronic stress-induced depression by suppressing hippocampal neurogenesis. *J. Neurochem.* 103, 1843–1854. doi: 10.1111/j.1471-4159.2007.04914.x

Zhou, Q. G., Zhu, L. J., Chen, C., Wu, H. Y., Luo, C. X., Chang, L., et al. (2011). Hippocampal neuronal nitric oxide synthase mediates the stress-related depres- sive behaviors of glucocorticoids by downregulating glucocorticoid receptor. *J. Neurosci.* 31, 7579–7590. doi: 10.1523/JNEUROSCI.0004-11.2011

Zhu, L. J., Liu, M. Y., Li, H., Liu, X., Chen, C., Han, Z., et al. (2014). The different roles of glucocorticoids in the hippocampus and hypothalamus in chronic stress-induced HPA axis hyperactivity. *PLoS ONE* 9:e97689. doi: 10.1371/jour- nal.pone.0097689

12

Activation of the hypothalamic-pituitary-adrenal stress axis induces cellular oxidative stress

Jereme G. Spiers*, Hsiao-Jou Cortina Chen, Conrad Sernia and Nickolas A. Lavidis

School of Biomedical Sciences, The University of Queensland, Brisbane, QLD, Australia

Edited by:
Hubert Vaudry, University of Rouen, France

Reviewed by:
Jacques Epelbaum, Université Paris Descartes, France
Julie A. Chowen, Hospital Infantil Universitario Niño Jesús, Spain

***Correspondence:**
Jereme G. Spiers, School of Biomedical Sciences, The University of Queensland, St. Lucia, Brisbane, QLD 4072, Australia
e-mail: j.spiers@uq.edu.au

Glucocorticoids released from the adrenal gland in response to stress-induced activation of the hypothalamic-pituitary-adrenal (HPA) axis induce activity in the cellular reduction-oxidation (redox) system. The redox system is a ubiquitous chemical mechanism allowing the transfer of electrons between donor/acceptors and target molecules during oxidative phosphorylation while simultaneously maintaining the overall cellular environment in a reduced state. The objective of this review is to present an overview of the current literature discussing the link between HPA axis-derived glucocorticoids and increased oxidative stress, particularly focussing on the redox changes observed in the hippocampus following glucocorticoid exposure.

Keywords: corticosterone, hypothalamic-pituitary-adrenal axis, oxidative stress, reactive oxygen species, redox status, stress

INTRODUCTION

The acute neuroendocrine response to adverse stress stimuli is characterized by the tripartite activation of the three stress axes including the autonomic sympathetic nervous system, the direct neural innervation of the adrenal cortex, and a cascade of hypothalamic hormonal messengers. Both the sympathetic system and the hypothalamic spinal adrenal axis utilize direct neural innervations of the adrenal medulla and cortex respectively to release adrenal catecholamines and prime the adrenal cortex for subsequent hormonal activation (Jansen et al., 1995; Buijs et al., 1999). This is initiated by neurosecretory neurons in the paraventricular nucleus of the hypothalamus, which release both corticotropin-releasing hormone and arginine vasopressin into the portal circulation of the pituitary gland. These two factors synergistically act on pituitary corticotroph cells to stimulate the release of the pro-opiomelanocortin peptide fragment, adrenocorticotropic hormone, into the circulation. Adrenocorticotropic hormone activates the melanocortin 2 receptor in the *zona fasciculata* of the adrenal cortex to initiate *de novo* synthesis and release of glucocorticoids, primarily cortisol in humans and corticosterone in rodents (Spiga et al., 2011). Together, this hormone cascade constitutes the hypothalamic-pituitary-adrenal (HPA) axis and is the primary system underlying stress physiology.

The physiological effects of corticosterone in the brain are canonically mediated through a near-ubiquitously expressed (with the exception of the suprachiasmatic nucleus of the hypothalamus) low affinity (KD $\approx$ 5.0 nM) glucocorticoid receptor (GR), and a regionally specific high affinity (KD $\approx$ 0.5 nM) mineralocorticoid receptor (MR) (Reul and de Kloet, 1985; Rose et al., 2012). Typically, these receptors reside in the cytoplasm heterocomplexed with heat shock proteins and immunophilins, which maintain the affinity of the hormone-binding domain (Pratt and Toft, 1997). The lipophilic steroid hormones are cell membrane permeable and bind these receptors, causing the dissociation of the chaperone proteins and translocation into the nucleus where the activated receptor complex forms GR and MR homo- or hetero-dimers that interact with specific glucocorticoid responsive elements in the promoter regions of genomic DNA. Both GR and MR elicit equivalent activity at glucocorticoid responsive elements and these interactions can result in transcriptional activation or repression of target genes depending on the cellular context (De Kloet et al., 1998). Transcriptional repression can also be mediated through protein-protein interactions specifically with activated GR and transcription factors such as NFκB, offering a possible mechanism through which delineation of receptor function occurs between the GR and MR (van der Burg and van der Saag, 1996; De Kloet et al., 1998). Termination of the HPA response to stress is mediated through multiple negative feedback loops and utilizes both genomic and non-genomic actions of the GR (Calogero et al., 1988; Groeneweg et al., 2011). In circulation, adrenal glucocorticoids reach peak total plasma concentrations approximately 30 min after activation of the HPA axis (Qian et al., 2011). At the cellular level, these hormones act in conjunction with catecholamines to facilitate glucose availability and increase metabolic rate, which in turn increases spontaneous production of free radicals (Teague et al., 2007; Du et al., 2009).

FREE RADICAL PRODUCTION

The process of aerobic metabolism utilizes oxygen to generate ATP in the mitochondrial electron transport chain (Halliwell and Gutteridge, 1989). During this process, 1–3% of all electrons "leak" from the electron transport chain to react with oxygen, generating superoxide radicals instead of being reduced to water (Liu et al., 2002; Muller et al., 2004; Cash et al., 2007). Although this occurs at both complex I and complex III of the electron transfer chain, the majority occurs at complex I where it is facilitated by succinate (Liu et al., 2002) (**Figure 1**). Most of the cellular superoxide is produced inside the inner mitochondrial membrane where the mitochondrial concentration of superoxide can be between 5–10 times that of the cytosol or nucleus

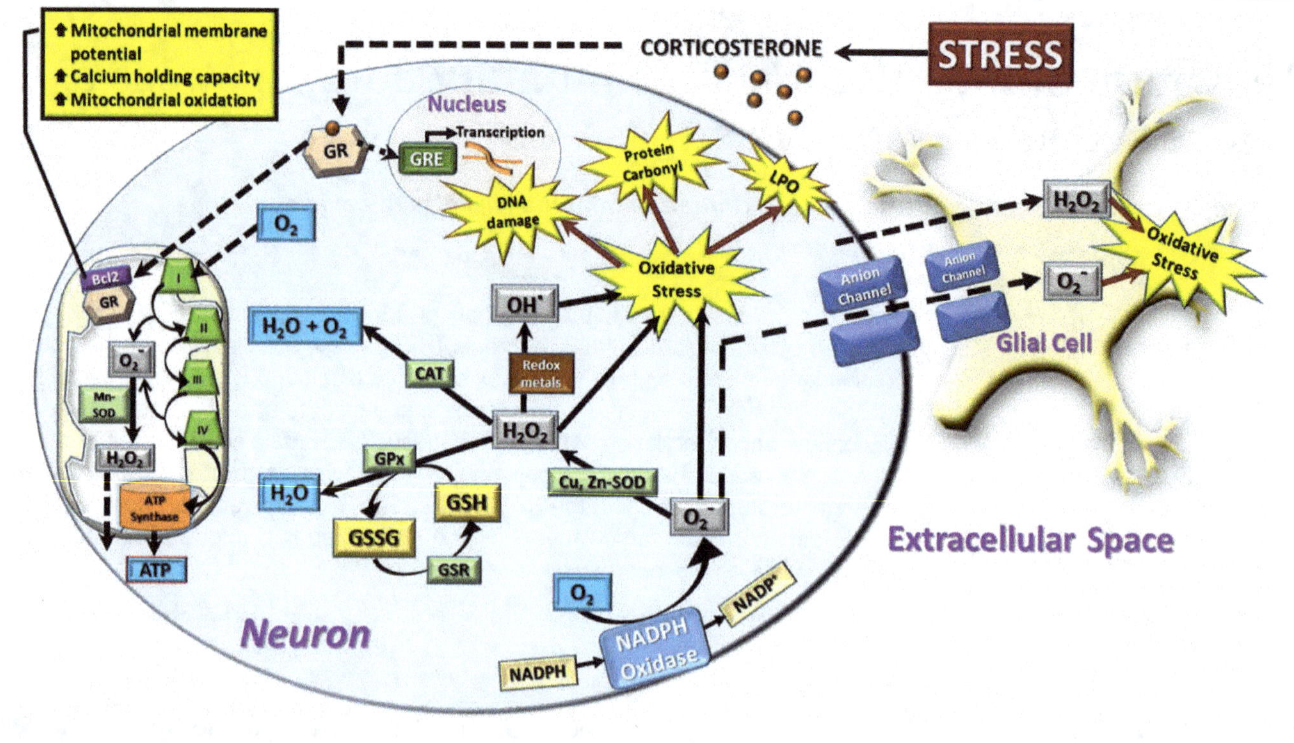

FIGURE 1 | Schematic representation of neural redox reactions. Stress causes an increase in corticosterone which activates cytosolic glucocorticoid receptors (GR). These translocate into the nucleus to modulate gene transcription through glucocorticoid responsive elements (GRE), or co-localize with the anti-apoptotic Bcl-2 protein and translocate into the mitochondria. This increases mitochondrial membrane potential, calcium holding capacity, and mitochondrial oxidation. The increase in cellular metabolic rate promotes ATP synthesis in addition to spontaneous superoxide (O_2^-) production via complex I and III of the electron transport chain. This is dismutated to hydrogen peroxide (H_2O_2) by manganese superoxide dismutase (Mn-SOD) and can be further converted to hydroxyl radical (OH^-) or reduced to water by the mitochondrial antioxidant pathway. In the cytosol, a major source of superoxide production is via the oxidation of NADPH via NADPH oxidase. Cytosolic superoxide is dismutated to hydrogen peroxide by copper, zinc-superoxide dismutase (Cu, Zn-SOD). Hydrogen peroxide is neutralized by catalase (CAT) or glutathione peroxidase (GPx) which oxidizes the reduced form of glutathione (GSH) to oxidized glutathione (GSSG). GSH is then regenerated from GSSG via the glutathione reductase (GSR) enzymatic system. Hydrogen peroxide can also interact with superoxide radicals and/or transition metals such as Fe^{2+} or Cu^{2+} to produce the highly toxic hydroxyl radical by Haber-Weiss and Fenton chemistry. An increase in the production of superoxide, hydrogen peroxide, and hydroxyl radicals leads to a state of cellular oxidative stress which causes oxidative damage to DNA, protein carbonyl formation, and membrane lipid peroxidation (LPO). Hydrogen peroxide is membrane permeable and moves freely from mitochondrial to cytosolic compartments, in addition to traversing the extracellular space to affect neighboring neurons and glial cells. Superoxide radicals can also induce oxidative stress in neighboring cells by diffusing through membrane-bound anion channels. The majority of neuronal and astrocytic reactive oxygen species are produced by mitochondrial oxidation, while other cell types such as microglia rely heavily on the cytosolic NADPH-oxidase system to produce a respiratory burst in response to invading pathogens. However, in comparison to glial cells, neurons display a relatively poor expression of endogenous antioxidants, making them more vulnerable to oxidative stress.

(Cadenas and Davies, 2000). The remainder of mitochondrial superoxide is primarily formed by complex III on both sides of the mitochondrial membrane and by extra-mitochondrial flavoenzymes (Zimmerman and Granger, 1994; Cadenas and Sies, 1998; Brand et al., 2004). Superoxide then undergoes spontaneous or enzymatic dismutation via superoxide dismutase (SOD) to generate hydrogen peroxide. Although hydrogen peroxide is relatively stable, subsequent interactions with superoxide radicals and/or transition metals such as Fe^{2+} or Cu^{2+} induce production of the highly toxic hydroxyl radical by Haber-Weiss and Fenton chemistry. This radical has been suggested to cause more damage to biological systems than any other reactive oxygen species (ROS) due to the extreme reactivity and very short *in vivo* half-life of $\approx$9–10 ms (Pastor et al., 2000).

Outside the mitochondrion, there are three major processes responsible for the production of free radicals, principally in the form of reactive oxygen and nitrogen species. The first process involves the production of hydrogen peroxide as a by-product of fatty acid catabolism by peroxisomes (Ames et al., 1993; Wanders and Waterham, 2006). Although technically not a free radical, hydrogen peroxide is still classed as a ROS for its role in Fenton and Haber-Weiss chemistry (Cimen, 2008). Within the peroxisome, the majority of hydrogen peroxide is neutralized via canonical catalase activity or peroxidation to another catalase substrate (Wanders and Waterham, 2006; Valko et al., 2007). However, under some conditions hydrogen peroxide can avoid degradation and escape the peroxisome, ultimately leading to cellular and nucleic acid damage (Kasai et al., 1989). The second process involves the reliance of the innate immune system on the ability of phagocytic cells such as neutrophils to engulf and digest foreign pathogens. Following the encapsulation of the foreign body into a phagosome, neutrophils increase their oxygen consumption specifically to supply the dormant NADPH-oxidase with molecular oxygen (Dahlgren and Karlsson, 1999). This enzyme catalyzes the oxidation of NADPH to form two superoxide radicals which, together with reactive metabolites of superoxide including hydrogen peroxide and hypochlorite, constitutes the respiratory burst responsible for killing the pathogen (Ames et al., 1993; Dahlgren and Karlsson, 1999; Stadtman et al., 2007; Valko et al., 2007). Hayashi et al. (2008) have also demonstrated that NADPH-oxidase derived ROS can also be produced via a non-genomic mechanism following aldosterone administration in rat cardiac myocytes. The third process involves redox metals such as $Fe^{2/3+}$, Cu^{2+}, and Mn^{2+} which are essential for electron transfer in many enzymatic reactions, including the antioxidant enzymes of the oxidative cascade. However, these transitional metal ions can also undergo reactions resulting in the production of hydroxyl radicals (Rovira et al., 2007).

THE ENDOGENOUS ANTIOXIDANT SYSTEM

In order to neutralize ROS, cells use a suite of enzymatic and non-enzymatic antioxidants, ultimately attempting to neutralize the radical by reduction to water. In the typical ROS reduction cascade, SOD is the top-tier antioxidant, catalyzing the dismutation of this radical to hydrogen peroxide. This is achieved through the transfer of electrons across the catalytic metal core of the enzymes to reduce the superoxide radicals. In mammals, the two main isoforms of SOD are the copper, zinc-SOD which are found throughout most cell compartments, and the manganese-SOD that is specific for mitochondria. Catalase enzymes are centered around an iron-containing ferriheme group that acts as the transition metal during the reduction of hydrogen peroxide. Access to this active site is fairly specific as the channel opening is narrow and does not allow the passage of large molecules. High concentrations of superoxide anions are able to inactivate catalase by oxidizing the heme group in the active site. To prevent this, catalase binds NADPH to maintain this group in the reduced state (Nordberg and Arner, 2001; Fridovich et al., 2007). Hydrogen peroxide can also be reduced directly by both peroxiredoxins, which allow the oxidation of an active cysteine thiol group to degrade one molecule of hydrogen peroxide into two molecules of water, and the glutathione-glutathione peroxidase system. Reduced glutathione (GSH) is the most abundant intracellular thiol-based antioxidant which protects cells against oxidative stress by acting as a substrate for the selenium-containing glutathione peroxidase, subsequently forming oxidized glutathione disulphide (GSSG). In turn, GSSG is regenerated to GSH by glutathione reductase in a NADPH-dependent mechanism (Barycki et al., 2007) (**Figure 1**). The cellular concentrations of this soluble tripeptide range from 1 to 11 mM in the cytosol, 3–15 mM in the nucleus, and 5–11 mM in the mitochondria, although mitochondrial GSH requires membrane transport even against a concentration gradient (Shen et al., 2005; Valko et al., 2007). Glutathione also acts as a substrate for the glutaredoxins, which reduce proteins that have been glutathionylated by reducing GSSG to a mixed disulphide protein and GSH. As the occurrence of mixed disulphides increases with increasing concentrations of GSSG, the ratio of the reduced to oxidized fractions (GSH/GSSG) of GSH within cells is often used as a reliable indicator of redox imbalance and has been shown to strongly influence cell cycle progression in proliferating cells (Menon et al., 2003; Öztürk and Gümüslü, 2004; Rose et al., 2012). The transcription factor nuclear factor-erythroid-2-related factor 2 (Nrf2) is essential for the coordinated induction of cytoprotective enzymes and related proteins in response to oxidative and electrophilic stresses (Itoh et al., 1999; Uruno and Motohashi, 2011). This transcription factor regulates a battery of redox genes such as the glutathione synthesis enzyme gamma-glutamylcysteine synthetase, glutathione peroxidase, glutathione disulphide reductase, glutathione *S*-transferase, thioredoxin-1, and heme oxygenase-1 through their antioxidant response element (Rushmore et al., 1990; Inamdar et al., 1996; Moinova and Mulcahy, 1999; Kim et al., 2003; Kwak et al., 2003). Under basal conditions, Nrf2 activity is sequestered in part by the actin-associated Keap1 protein within the cytoplasm. Activation of Nrf2 in response to oxidative and electrophilic agents is thought to be initiated by disruption of this Nrf2-Keap1 complex, releasing Nrf2, which translocates into the nucleus to regulate the expression of downstream targets.

PHYSIOLOGICAL ROLE OF REACTIVE OXYGEN SPECIES

Although there is a general negative connotation associated with ROS production, they have important cellular functions under normal physiological conditions. Even low levels of the extremely reactive hydroxyl radical have been shown to activate guanylate cyclase, stimulating the production of a cGMP second messenger cascade (Mittal and Murad, 1977). In fact, the physiological roles of ROS vary significantly, ranging from specific oxidations of cysteine groups affecting enzyme activity and function, to cellular redox sensing in the determination of cell differentiation fate (Nicotera et al., 1985; Dalton et al., 1999; Wang et al., 2011). Progression of the cell cycle itself has demonstrated dependence on radicals produced by NADPH-oxidase modulating mitogenic pathways (Burhans and Heintz, 2009). Several transcription factors are also regulated directly by ROS-induced modifications, thereby modulating the downstream expression of several gene families (Dalton et al., 1999). Notably, the dimerized protein products of immediate-early response genes FOS and JUN, AP-1, is activated by ROS through redox reactions and post-translational modification of the individual FOS and JUN proteins (Buscher et al., 1988; Abate et al., 1991; Devary et al., 1991). Under normal conditions, any excessive ROS not participating in these physiological functions are reduced by the antioxidant system. However, an imbalance between the production of ROS and the ability of the antioxidant defense system to readily detoxify the reactive intermediates, termed oxidative stress, leads to damage of biological macromolecules and dysregulation of normal metabolism (Sies, 1997; Nordberg and Arner, 2001).

ADRENAL GLUCOCORTICOIDS AND OXIDATIVE STRESS

Increased secretion of adrenal glucocorticoids following physical and/or psychological stress exposure subsequently liberates glucose through gluconeogenesis, glycogenolysis, and lipolysis (Teague et al., 2007). Although increased metabolism alone generates ROS, glucocorticoids have demonstrated both direct and indirect modulatory roles in the onset of oxidative stress.

Furthermore, both chronic oxidative stress and glucocorticoid exposure promote gliogenesis over neurogenesis in hippocampal neural stem cell progenitors and may be the direct result of accumulated mitochondrial oxidative stress (Wang et al., 2011; Chetty et al., 2014). Glial cells play an important but poorly understood role in the modulation of neuronal redox state. It has recently been shown that astrocyte-derived L-lactate potentiates NMDA receptor activity by modulating neuronal redox status (Yang et al., 2014). This neuron-glia interaction can also increase noradrenaline release from the locus ceruleus and hypothalamic ATP production (Cortes-Campos et al., 2011; Tang et al., 2014). Furthermore, Reyes et al. (2012) have demonstrated that neuronal NADPH oxidase-derived superoxide can traverse the extracellular space to modulate the redox state in neighboring neurons and astrocytes (**Figure 1**). However, in comparison to astrocytes, neurons are known to have relatively poor expression of endogenous antioxidants, making them highly susceptible to oxidative stress.

Glucocorticoids induce neuronal oxidative stress directly through enhanced mitochondrial respiration and oxidative phosphorylation. This was demonstrated clearly in a study by Du et al. (2009), showing that acute incubation of cortical neurons with corticosterone increased mitochondrial oxidation, membrane potential, and calcium-holding capacity in a dose and time-dependent manner (**Figure 1**). This was further clarified by You et al. (2009) using the oxidation product dichlorofluorescien as a ROS indicator in organotypic hippocampal slice cultures exposed to the synthetic glucocorticoid, dexamethasone, and the glucocorticoid receptor antagonist, RU486. The single and combination use of these compounds demonstrated that hippocampal neuronal death, marked by propidium iodide, was selectively induced by glucocorticoid exposure, while other steroid hormones had no effect. Acute incubation with dexamethasone increased the hippocampal oxidative status by approximately 200% in a dose dependent manner, an effect that was ameliorated with pre-treatment of RU486 or the ROS-scavenger, N-acetyl-L-cysteine. Furthermore, 4 h of dexamethasone incubation, induced the highest increase in oxidative status, with concurrent gene expression up-regulation of the ROS-producing enzyme NADPH-oxidase, while the antioxidant enzyme glutathione peroxidase was significantly down-regulated (You et al., 2009). This indicates that the increase in oxidative status is produced by a glucocorticoid-dependent and transcriptional increase in pro-oxidative drive, with concurrent inhibition of the antioxidant defense system, ultimately leading to increased neuronal cell death. Cortical and hippocampal neural cultures have also established that 24 h of glucocorticoid exposure increases basal ROS production and exacerbates the concomitant ROS produced by adriamycin redox cycling, which negatively affects survival in hippocampal neurons (McIntosh and Sapolsky, 1996). This is supported by *in vivo* evidence that administration of exogenous corticosterone over a 14 day period increases hippocampal oxidative indicators including lipid peroxidation and protein carbonyls, while the enzymatic antioxidants SOD, catalase, and glutathione peroxidase activities are all decreased (Sato et al., 2010). This study, performed by Sato et al. (2010), also demonstrated increased apoptosis and decreased glucocorticoid receptor expression, a hallmark of chronically high glucocorticoids, in the hippocampus. Interestingly, this study also utilized a serum measurement of iron-induced superoxide formation in blood serum, establishing that this peripheral marker increased with chronic corticosterone administration. Further *in vivo* studies have shown that both corticosterone administration and restraint stress for 21 days induce an overall decrease in GSH in addition to SOD, catalase, glutathione transferase, and glutathione reductase activities in whole brain, liver, and heart tissues (Zafir and Banu, 2009). This study, by Zafir and Banu (2009), also demonstrated that these treatments increased lipid peroxidation and oxidized protein carbonyl groups in the same tissues. However, in the brain, this overall oxidative increase is likely due to increases in specific subregions. For example, Mendez-Cuesta et al. (2011) used an acute immobilization stress to induce increased lipid peroxidation and decreased SOD activity in a highly oxidative-vulnerable region, the striatum. Interestingly, they found that the decrease in SOD activity was exclusively due to the mitochondrial isoform, manganese-SOD, while the copper, zinc-SOD showed little change. Furthermore, Lucca et al. (2009) used a chronic mild stress regime to show that SOD decreased and oxidized protein carbonyl groups increased in several cerebral regions including the striatum and hippocampus, while the cerebellum remained largely unaffected. We have also observed the induction of regional specific oxidative stress in the hippocampus but not the amygdala following an acute restraint stress, demonstrating that this process is not exclusive to chronic stress exposure (Spiers et al., 2013). Recently, exposure to glucocorticoids or dexamethasone demonstrated inhibitory action over the Nrf2-dependent antioxidant pathway, causing an increase in hepatic and osteoblastic cell ROS, an effect attenuated by exogenous sulforaphane (Kratschmar et al., 2012; Lin et al., 2014).

Interestingly, ROS attenuate the glucocorticoid-induced down-regulation of pro-opiomelanocortin in pituitary corticotrophs, thereby promoting an increase in HPA axis activity via reduced negative feedback (Asaba et al., 2004). The expression and nuclear internalization of GR have also demonstrated susceptibility to highly pro-oxidative environments (Okamoto et al., 1999; Zhou et al., 2011). Using a cultured fluorescently labeled chimeric GR, Okamoto et al. (1999) demonstrated that nuclear translocation of GR following acute dexamethasone treatment is impaired in the presence of hydrogen peroxide. This effect was reduced in the presence of exogenous antioxidants or following substitution of serine for a redox-sensitive cysteine residue. The dissociation of heat shock proteins from the cytosolic GR was also impaired in a pro-oxidative environment, indicating that there may be multiple redox regulatory roles involved in the cellular response to glucocorticoids (Okamoto et al., 1999 reviewed in Tanaka et al., 1999). These observations highlight that maintenance of a balanced redox state is critical for normal cellular homeostatic function within the neuroendocrine system.

CONCLUSIONS

Although oxidative stress and elevated glucocorticoids are both observed in a number of chronic pathologies, the delineation between physiological function and pathological insult is complex and remains unclear. In particular, the role of ROS in neuron-neuron and neuron-glia interactions is an area that requires attention. Based on the observations of increased gliogenesis in the presence of high levels of glucocorticoids, the mobility of ROS in the extracellular space, and the relative paucity of neuronal endogenous antioxidants, we suggest that glia may be playing an active role in response to neuronal oxidative stress. This may have important implications for neurodegenerative conditions involving redox-sensitive regions such as the hippocampus. These observations highlight that maintenance of a balanced redox state is critical for normal cellular homeostatic function and relies heavily on hormonal cues from the neuroendocrine stress system.

AUTHOR CONTRIBUTIONS

Author Jereme G. Spiers managed the literature searches and wrote the first draft of the manuscript. Author Hsiao-Jou Cortina Chen produced the graphic and revised the manuscript. Author Conrad Sernia and Nickolas A. Lavidis critically revised the manuscript. All authors have approved the final version of the manuscript for journal submission.

ACKNOWLEDGMENTS

We would like to thank Szu-Ju Patricia Chen for the assistance on graphical design and production.

REFERENCES

Abate, C., Luk, D., and Curran, T. (1991). Transcriptional regulation by Fos and Jun *in vitro*: interaction among multiple activator and regulatory domains. *Mol. Cell. Biol.* 11, 3624–3632.

Ames, B. N., Shigenaga, M. K., and Hagen, T. M. (1993). Oxidants, antioxi- dants, and the degenerative diseases of aging. *Proc. Natl. Acad. Sci. U.S.A.* 90, 7915–7922.

Asaba, K., Iwasaki, Y., Yoshida, M., Asai, M., Oiso, Y., Murohara, T., et al. (2004). Attenuation by reactive oxygen species of glucocorticoid suppression on proo- piomelanocortin gene expression in pituitary corticotroph cells. *Endocrinology* 145, 39–42. doi: 10.1210/en.2003-0375

Barycki, J. J., Asard, H., Stone, J. M., Wilson, M. A., Banerjee, R., and Becker, D. F. (2007). *Antioxidant Molecules and Redox Cofactors, Redox Biochemistry*. (Hoboken, NJ: John Wiley & Sons, Inc).

Brand, M. D., Affourtit, C., Esteves, T. C., Green, K., Lambert, A. J., Miwa, S., et al. (2004). Mitochondrial superoxide: production, biological effects, and activation of uncoupling proteins. *Free Radic. Biol. Med.* 37, 755–767. doi: 10.1016/j.freeradbiomed.2004.05.034

Buijs, R. M., Wortel, J., Van Heerikhuize, J. J., Feenstra, M. G., Ter Horst, G. J., Romijn, H. J., et al. (1999). Anatomical and functional demonstration of a mul- tisynaptic suprachiasmatic nucleus adrenal (cortex) pathway. *Eur. J. Neurosci.* 11, 1535–1544.

Burhans, W. C., and Heintz, N. H. (2009). The cell cycle is a redox cycle: link- ing phase-specific targets to cell fate. *Free Radic. Biol. Med.* 47, 1282–1293. doi: 10.1016/j.freeradbiomed.2009.05.026

Buscher, M., Rahmsdorf, H. J., Litfin, M., Karin, M., and Herrlich, P. (1988). Activation of the c-fos gene by UV and phorbol ester: different signal transduc- tion pathways converge to the same enhancer element. *Oncogene* 3, 301–311.

Cadenas, E., and Davies, K. J. (2000). Mitochondrial free radical generation, oxida- tive stress, and aging. *Free Radic. Biol. Med.* 29, 222–230. doi: 10.1016/S0891-5849(00)00317-8

Cadenas, E., and Sies, H. (1998). The lag phase. *Free Radic. Res.* 28, 601–609. Calogero, A. E., Gallucci, W. T., Gold, P. W., and Chrousos, G. P. (1988). Multiple feedback regulatory loops upon rat hypothalamic corticotropin-releasing hormone-secretion - potential clinical implications. *J. Clin. Invest.* 82, 767–774.

Cash, T. P., Pan, Y., and Simon, M. C. (2007). Reactive oxygen species and cellular oxygen sensing. *Free Radic. Biol. Med.* 43, 1219–1225. doi: 10.1016/j.freeradbiomed.2007.07.001

Chetty, S., Friedman, A. R., Taravosh-Lahn, K., Kirby, E. D., Mirescu, C., Guo, F., et al. (2014). Stress and glucocorticoids promote oligodendrogenesis in the adult hippocampus. *Mol. Psychiatry* 19, 1275–1283. doi: 10.1038/mp.2013.1190

Cimen, M. Y. (2008). Free radical metabolism in human erythrocytes. *Clin. Chim. Acta* 390, 1–11. doi: 10.1016/j.cca.2007.12.025

Cortes-Campos, C., Elizondo, R., Llanos, P., Uranga, R. M., Nualart, F., and Garcia, M. A. (2011). MCT expression and lactate influx/efflux in tanycytes involved in glia-neuron metabolic interaction. *PLoS ONE* 6:e16411. doi: 10.1371/jour- nal.pone.0016411

Dahlgren, C., and Karlsson, A. (1999). Respiratory burst in human neutrophils. *J. Immunol. Methods* 232, 3–14.

Dalton, T. P., Shertzer, H. G., and Puga, A. (1999). Regulation of gene expression by reactive oxygen. *Annu. Rev. Pharmacol. Toxicol.* 39, 67–101.

De Kloet, E. R., Vreugdenhil, E., Oitzl, M. S., and Joels, M. (1998). Brain corticos- teroid receptor balance in health and disease. *Endocr. Rev.* 19, 269–301.

Devary, Y., Gottlieb, R. A., Lau, L. F., and Karin, M. (1991). Rapid and preferential activation of the c-jun gene during the mammalian UV response. *Mol. Cell. Biol.* 11, 2804–2811.

Du, J., Wang, Y., Hunter, R., Wei, Y., Blumenthal, R., Falke, C., et al. (2009). Dynamic regulation of mitochondrial function by glucocorticoids. *Proc. Natl. Acad. Sci. U.S.A.* 106, 3543–3548. doi: 10.1073/pnas.0812671106

Fridovich, I., Poole, L. B., Holmgren, A., Lou, M. F., Gladyshev, V. N., David, S. S., et al. (2007). *Antioxidant Enzymes, Redox Biochemistry*. (Hoboken, NJ: John Wiley & Sons, Inc).

Groeneweg, F. L., Karst, H., de Kloet, E. R., and Joels, M. (2011). Rapid non- genomic effects of corticosteroids and their role in the central stress response. *J. Endocrinol.* 209, 153–167. doi: 10.1530/JOE-10-0472

Halliwell, B., and Gutteridge, J. M. C. (1989). *Free radicals in biology and medicine, 2nd ed.* New York: Clarendon Press; Oxford: Oxford University Press.

Hayashi, H., Kobara, M., Abe, M., Tanaka, N., Gouda, E., Toba, H., et al. (2008). Aldosterone nongenomically produces NADPH oxidase-dependent reactive oxygen species and induces myocyte apoptosis. *Hypertens. Res.* 31, 363–375. doi: 10.1291/hypres.31.363

Inamdar, N. M., Ahn, Y. I., and Alam, J. (1996). The heme-responsive element of the mouse heme oxygenase-1 gene is an extended AP-1 binding site that resembles the recognition sequences for MAF and NF-E2 transcription factors. *Biochem. Biophys. Res. Commun.* 221, 570–576.

Itoh, K., Wakabayashi, N., Katoh, Y., Ishii, T., Igarashi, K., Engel, J. D., et al. (1999). Keap1 represses nuclear activation of antioxidant responsive elements by Nrf2 through binding to the amino-terminal Neh2 domain. *Genes. Dev.* 13, 76–86.

Jansen, A. S., Nguyen, X. V., Karpitskiy, V., Mettenleiter, T. C., and Loewy, A. D. (1995). Central command neurons of the sympathetic nervous system: basis of the fight-or-flight response. *Science* 270, 644–646.

Kasai, H., Okada, Y., Nishimura, S., Rao, M. S., and Reddy, J. K. (1989). Formation of 8-hydroxydeoxyguanosine in liver DNA of rats following long-term exposure to a peroxisome proliferator. *Cancer Res.* 49, 2603–2605.

Kim, Y. C., Yamaguchi, Y., Kondo, N., Masutani, H., and Yodoi, J. (2003). Thioredoxin-dependent redox regulation of the antioxidant responsive element (ARE) in electrophile response. *Oncogene* 22, 1860–1865. doi: 10.1038/sj.onc.1206369

Kratschmar, D. V., Calabrese, D., Walsh, J., Lister, A., Birk, J., Appenzeller-Herzog, C., et al. (2012). Suppression of the Nrf2-dependent antioxidant response by glucocorticoids and 11beta-HSD1-mediated glucocorticoid activation in hepatic cells. *PLoS ONE* 7:e36774. doi: 10.1371/journal.pone.0036774

Kwak, M. K., Wakabayashi, N., Itoh, K., Motohashi, H., Yamamoto, M., and Kensler, T. W. (2003). Modulation of gene expression by cancer chemopreventive dithiolethiones through the Keap1-Nrf2 pathway. Identification of novel gene clusters for cell survival. *J. Biol. Chem.* 278, 8135–8145. doi: 10.1074/jbc.M211898200

Lin, H., Wei, B., Li, G., Zheng, J., Sun, J., Chu, J., et al. (2014). Sulforaphane reverses glucocorticoid-induced apoptosis in osteoblastic cells through regulation of the Nrf2 pathway. *Drug Des. Devel. Ther.* 8, 973–982. doi: 10.2147/DDDT.S65410

Liu, Y., Fiskum, G., and Schubert, D. (2002). Generation of reactive oxygen species by the mitochondrial electron transport chain. *J. Neurochem.* 80, 780–787. doi: 10.1046/j.0022-3042.2002.00744.x

Lucca, G., Comim, C. M., Valvassori, S. S., Réus, G. Z., Vuolo, F., Petronilho, F., et al. (2009). Effects of chronic mild stress on the oxidative parameters in the rat brain.

Neurochem. Int. 54, 358–362. doi: 10.1016/j.neuint.2009.01.001

McIntosh, L. J., and Sapolsky, R. M. (1996). Glucocorticoids increase the accumu- lation of reactive oxygen species and enhance adriamycin-induced toxicity in neuronal culture. *Exp. Neurol.* 141, 201–206.

Mendez-Cuesta, L. A., Marquez-Valadez, B., Perez-De la Cruz, V., Maldonado, P. D., Santana, R. A., Escobar-Briones, C., et al. (2011). Early changes in oxidative stress markers in a rat model of acute stress: effect of l-carnitine on the striatum. *Basic Clin. Pharmacol. Toxicol.* 109, 123–129. doi: 10.1111/j.1742-7843.2011.00691.x

Menon, S. G., Sarsour, E. H., Spitz, D. R., Higashikubo, R., Sturm, M., Zhang, H., et al. (2003). Redox regulation of the G1 to S phase transition in the mouse embryo fibroblast cell cycle. *Cancer Res.* 63, 2109–2117.

Mittal, C. K., and Murad, F. (1977). Activation of guanylate cyclase by super- oxide dismutase and hydroxyl radical: a physiological regulator of guanosine 3',5'-monophosphate formation. *Proc. Natl. Acad. Sci. U.S.A.* 74, 4360–4364.

Moinova, H. R., and Mulcahy, R. T. (1999). Up-regulation of the human gamma- glutamylcysteine synthetase regulatory subunit gene involves binding of Nrf- 2 to an electrophile responsive element. *Biochem. Biophys. Res. Commun.* 261, 661–668.

Muller, F. L., Liu, Y., and Van Remmen, H. (2004). Complex III releases super- oxide to both sides of the inner mitochondrial membrane. *J. Biol. Chem.* 279, 49064–49073. doi: 10.1074/jbc.M407715200

Nicotera, P., Moore, M., Mirabelli, F., Bellomo, G., and Orrenius, S. (1985). Inhibition of hepatocyte plasma membrane Ca2+-ATPase activity by mena- dione metabolism and its restoration by thiols. *FEBS Lett.* 181, 149–153.

Nordberg, J., and Arner, E. S. J. (2001). Reactive oxygen species, antioxidants, and the mammalian thioredoxin system. *Free Radic. Biol. Med.* 31, 1287–1312. doi: 10.1016/S0891-5849(01)00724-9

Öztürk, O., Gümüslü, S. (2004). Age-related changes of antioxidant enzyme activ- ities, glutathione status and lipid peroxidation in rat erythrocytes after heat stress. *Life Sci.* 75, 1551–1565. doi: 10.1016/j.lfs.2004.03.020

Okamoto, K., Tanaka, H., Ogawa, H., Makino, Y., Eguchi, H., Hayashi, S., et al. (1999). Redox-dependent regulation of nuclear import of the glucocorticoid receptor. *J. Biol. Chem.* 274, 10363–10371.

Pastor, N., Weinstein, H., Jamison, E., and Brenowitz, M. (2000). A detailed inter- pretation of OH radical footprints in a TBP-DNA complex reveals the role of dynamics in the mechanism of sequence-specific binding. *J. Mol. Biol.* 304, 55–68. doi: 10.1006/jmbi.2000.4173

Pratt, W. B., and Toft, D. O. (1997). Steroid receptor interactions with heat shock protein and immunophilin chaperones. *Endocr. Rev.* 18, 306–360.

Qian, X., Droste, S. K., Gutierrez-Mecinas, M., Collins, A., Kersante, F., Reul, J. M., et al. (2011). A rapid release of corticosteroid-binding globulin from the liver restrains the glucocorticoid hormone response to acute stress. *Endocrinology* 152, 3738–3748. doi: 10.1210/en.2011-1008

Reul, J. M., and de Kloet, E. R. (1985). Two receptor systems for corticosterone in rat brain: microdistribution and differential occupation. *Endocrinology* 117, 2505–2511.

Reyes, R. C., Brennan, A. M., Shen, Y., Baldwin, Y., and Swanson, R. A. (2012). Activation of neuronal NMDA receptors induces superoxide-mediated oxidative stress in neighboring neurons and astrocytes. *J. Neurosci.* 32, 12973–12978. doi: 10.1523/JNEUROSCI.1597-12.2012

Rose, S., Melnyk, S., Trusty, T. A., Pavliv, O., Seidel, L., Li, J., et al. (2012). Intracellular and extracellular redox status and free radical generation in pri- mary immune cells from children with autism. *Autism Res. Treat.* 2012:986519. doi: 10.1155/2012/986519

Rovira, I. I., Finkel, T., Masters, B. S., Dickman, M. B., Lee, J., Ragsdale, S. W., et al. (2007). *Redox Regulation of Physiological Processes, Redox Biochemistry.* (Hoboken, NJ: John Wiley & Sons, Inc).

Rushmore, T. H., King, R. G., Paulson, K. E., and Pickett, C. B. (1990). Regulation of glutathione S-transferase Ya subunit gene expression: identification of a unique xenobiotic-responsive element controlling inducible expression by planar aro- matic compounds. *Proc. Natl. Acad. Sci. U.S.A.* 87, 3826–3830.

Sato, H., Takahashi, T., Sumitani, K., Takatsu, H., and Urano, S. (2010). Glucocorticoid generates ROS to induce oxidative injury in the hippocampus, leading to impairment of cognitive function of rats. *J. Clin. Biochem. Nutr.* 47, 224–232. doi: 10.3164/jcbn.10-58

Shen, D., Dalton, T. P., Nebert, D. W., and Shertzer, H. G. (2005). Glutathione redox state regulates mitochondrial reactive oxygen production. *J. Biol. Chem.* 280, 25305–25312. doi: 10.1074/jbc.M500095200

Sies, H. (1997). Oxidative stress: oxidants and antioxidants. *Exp. Physiol.* 82, 291–295.

Spiers, J. G., Chen, H. J., Bradley, A. J., Anderson, S. T., Sernia, C., and Lavidis, N. A. (2013). Acute restraint stress induces rapid and prolonged changes in erythrocyte and hippocampal redox status. *Psychoneuroendocrinology* 38, 2511–2519. doi: 10.1016/j.psyneuen.2013.05.011

Spiga, F., Waite, E. J., Liu, Y., Kershaw, Y. M., Aguilera, G., and Lightman, S. L. (2011). ACTH-dependent ultradian rhythm of corticosterone secretion. *Endocrinology* 152, 1448–1457. doi: 10.1210/en.2010-1209

Stadtman, E. R., Lou, M. F., Crabb, J. W., Rozanski, G. J., Veeramani, S., Lin, M.-F., et al. (2007). *Pathological Processes Related to Redox, Redox Biochemistry.* (Hoboken, NJ: John Wiley & Sons, Inc).

Tanaka, H., Makino, Y., Okamoto, K., Iida, T., Yan, K., and Yoshikawa, N. (1999). Redox regulation of the glucocorticoid receptor. *Antioxid. Redox Signal.* 1, 403–423.

Tang, F., Lane, S., Korsak, A., Paton, J. F., Gourine, A. V., Kasparov, S., et al. (2014). Lactate-mediated glia-neuronal signalling in the mammalian brain. *Nat. Commun.* 5, 3284. doi: 10.1038/ncomms4284

Teague, C. R., Dhabhar, F. S., Barton, R. H., Beckwith-Hall, B., Powell, J., Cobain, M., et al. (2007). Metabonomic studies on the physiological effects of acute and chronic psychological stress in Sprague-Dawley rats. *J. Proteome. Res.* 6, 2080–2093. doi: 10.1021/pr060412s

Uruno, A., and Motohashi, H. (2011). The Keap1-Nrf2 system as an *in vivo* sensor for electrophiles. *Nitric Oxide* 25, 153–160. doi: 10.1016/j.niox.2011.02.007

Valko, M., Leibfritz, D., Moncol, J., Cronin, M. T., Mazur, M., and Telser, J. (2007). Free radicals and antioxidants in normal physiological functions and human disease. *Int. J. Biochem. Cell Biol.* 39, 44–84. doi: 10.1016/j.biocel.2006.07.001

van der Burg, B., and van der Saag, P. T. (1996). Nuclear factor-kappa-B/steroid hormone receptor interactions as a functional basis of anti-inflammatory action of steroids in reproductive organs. *Mol. Hum. Reprod.* 2, 433–438.

Wanders, R. J., and Waterham, H. R. (2006). Biochemistry of mam- malian peroxisomes revisited. *Annu. Rev. Biochem.* 75, 295–332. doi: 10.1146/annurev.biochem.74.082803.133329

Wang, W., Esbensen, Y., Kunke, D., Suganthan, R., Rachek, L., Bjoras, M., et al. (2011). Mitochondrial DNA damage level determines neural stem cell dif- ferentiation fate. *J. Neurosci.* 31, 9746–9751. doi: 10.1523/JNEUROSCI.0852-11.2011

Yang, J., Ruchti, E., Petit, J. M., Jourdain, P., Grenningloh, G., Allaman, I., et al. (2014). Lactate promotes plasticity gene expression by potentiating NMDA signaling in neurons. *Proc. Natl. Acad. Sci. U.S.A.* 111, 12228–12233. doi: 10.1073/pnas.1322912111

You, J. M., Yun, S. J., Nam, K. N., Kang, C., Won, R., and Lee, E. H. (2009). Mechanism of glucocorticoid-induced oxidative stress in rat hippocampal slice cultures. *Can. J. Physiol. Pharmacol.* 87, 440–447. doi: 10.1139/Y09-027

Zafir, A., and Banu, N. (2009). Modulation of *in vivo* oxidative status by exoge- nous corticosterone and restraint stress in rats. *Stress* 12, 167–177. doi: 10.1080/10253890802234168

Zhou, Q. G., Zhu, L. J., Chen, C., Wu, H. Y., Luo, C. X., Chang, L., et al. (2011). Hippocampal neuronal nitric oxide synthase mediates the stress-related depres- sive behaviors of glucocorticoids by downregulating glucocorticoid receptor. *J. Neurosci.* 31, 7579–7590. doi: 10.1523/JNEUROSCI.0004-11.2011

Zimmerman, B. J., and Granger, D. N. (1994). Mechanisms of reperfusion injury. *Am. J. Med. Sci.* 307, 284–292.

13

Early social environment affects the endogenous oxytocin system

Emily Alves[1]*, Andrea Fielder[2], Nerelle Ghabriel[2,3], Michael Sawyer[4,5] and Femke T.A. Buisman-Pijlman[1]*

[1] School of Medical Sciences, University of Adelaide, Adelaide, SA, Australia
[2] School of Midwifery, University of South Australia, Adelaide, SA, Australia
[3] School of Psychology, University of South Australia, Adelaide, SA, Australia
[4] School of Paediatrics and Reproductive Health, University of Adelaide, Adelaide, SA, Australia
[5] Research and Evaluation Unit, Women's and Children's Health Network, Adelaide, SA, Australia

Edited by:
Hubert Vaudry, University of Rouen, France

Reviewed by:
Charles W. Wilkinson, University of Washington, USA
Thiago Pereira Henriques, Universidade Federal do Rio Grande do Sul, Brazil

****Correspondence:***
Emily Alves and Femke T.A. Buisman-Pijlman, Adelaide University, 30 Frome Road, Adelaide, SA 5000, Australia
e-mail: emily.alves@student.adelaide.edu.au; femke.buisman-pijlman@adelaide.edu.au

Endogenous oxytocin plays an important role in a wide range of human functions including birth, milk ejection during lactation, and facilitation of social interaction. There is increasing evidence that both variations in the oxytocin receptor (OXTR) and concentrations of oxytocin are associated with differences in these functions. The causes for the differences that have been observed in tonic and stimulated oxytocin release remain unclear. Previous reviews have suggested that across the life course, these differences may be due to individual factors, e.g., genetic variation (of the OXTR), age or sex, or be the result of early environmental influences, such as social experiences, stress, or trauma partly by inducing epigenetic changes. This review has three aims. First, we briefly discuss the endogenous oxytocin system, including physiology, development, individual differences, and function. Second, current models describing the relationship between the early life environment and the development of the oxytocin system in humans and animals are discussed. Finally, we describe research designs that can be used to investigate the effects of the early environment on the oxytocin system, identifying specific areas of research that need further attention.

Keywords: oxytocin, early-life environment, research design, individual differences, mother–infant bonding

THE ENDOGENOUS OXYTOCIN SYSTEM

Oxytocin, a mammalian hormone, is a naturally produced neuropeptide with nine amino acids. Oxytocin is mainly produced in magnocellular neurons in the hypothamalic paraventricular and supraoptic nuclei (1). The magnocellular neurons release oxytocin into circulating blood via the pituitary gland, while the parvocellular oxytocin neurons release oxytocin in other areas of the central nervous system (CNS). Recent evidence has demonstrated that oxytocinergic axons ending in forebrain regions including the central amygdala and nucleus accumbens may originate exclusively in the magnocellular neurons of the paraventricular nucleus (2). Evidence also indicates that central projections of hypothalamic oxytocin neurons may be widespread, and that oxytocin release from local axonal endings may be able to control region-associated behaviors (2). Oxytocin is also produced in a number of peripheral tissues and organs, such as the uterus, ovaries, testis, vascular endothelium, and the heart (3). For a review of the anatomy and functional aspects of the oxytocin system, see Kiss and Mikkelson (4).

Oxytocin is released in response to a range of internal and external stimuli. Historically, it is known that oxytocin is released in response to vaginocervical and nipple stimulation and plays important roles in mammalian uterine contraction and lactation. Oxytocin also plays a crucial role in the milk ejection reflex. In lactating women, oxytocin peaks during the morning and then declines until the beginning of the afternoon, and it is released in a cyclic manner, with salivary oxytocin concentrations at their highest within 30 min before feeding begins (5). This indicates that the brain may be able to release oxytocin in anticipation of future behaviors and interactions.

More recent data demonstrate the pro-social role of oxytocin, including its role in social and emotional regulation (6), orgasm (7), regulating stress, and anxiety and facilitation of pair, maternal and infant bonding (8–12). Interestingly, the release of oxytocin is dependent on the social context. For example, calves more readily release oxytocin when suckling milk directly from their mother's udder than when drinking the same milk from a bucket (13). Another example shows that oxytocin administration combined with psychological support of a friend lowered salivary cortisol concentrations and was correlated with decreased anxiety and increased calmness in human males (8).

Large individual differences exist in basal concentrations of oxytocin and in response to stimulation [for a review, see Ref. (12)]. Basal individual oxytocin concentrations in humans have been found to vary by thousands of pg/ml within the same study (14). Individual differences, such as genetic variation of the oxytocin receptor (OXTR) may explain some of the variation. Expression of the OXTR also varies in a sex-specific way. It is therefore possible that an interaction with the estrogen system plays a role that warrants further attention and investigation (15).

OXYTOCIN AND THE EARLY SOCIAL ENVIRONMENT

The early-life environment is critical for development in humans and other mammals [for a review on the long-term impact of early-life events, see Ref. (16)]. A significant component of the early-life environment is mother–infant bonding. Social experiences in the early-life period and bonding form the basis for healthy social and emotional development, possibly of the mechanism that manages stress and resilience (11). The well-documented protective associations between secure attachments and later social functioning and behavior underscore the need to understand the origins of attachments and identify the specific individual differences that influence attachment and development (17). Current research highlights the link between oxytocin concentrations and a specific set of maternal bonding behaviors and attitudes in humans (18–24). There is evidence to suggest that oxytocin plays an important role in facilitation of mother–infant bonding [for reviews, see Ref. (10, 25)] and that the early social environment can shape the developing oxytocin system. There is substantial literature documenting the relationship between oxytocin and the early-life environment in animals (26–28); however, minimal research has focused on this area in humans. Importantly, there is only limited data about the normal development of the oxytocin system in humans over time (11).

Oxytocin plays an important role in priming mammals to form social bonds, but in turn, the early social environment may also be able to shape the development of the oxytocin system [for a review, see Ref. (11)]. Interestingly, studies have demonstrated correlations between infant and parental oxytocin concentrations and parenting behaviors in child–parent interactions (14, 29). The following section will review the influence of prenatal and postnatal environment on the oxytocin system. Additionally, maternal mental health problems will be addressed as they can negatively affect the mother–infant bond.

PRENATAL ENVIRONMENT

In humans, prenatal stressors (including substance use, maternal depression, and chronic stress) can lead to a range of abnormal neurodevelopmental outcomes for infants [for a review, see Ref. (30)]. A recent human study found that male and female fetuses respond differentially to chronic maternal stress, indicating that sex may be an important factor influencing fetal development (31).

Lee and colleagues (32) demonstrated that a regime of prenatal stressors in pregnant rats caused numerous changes in the oxytocin systems of adult male offspring (less oxytocin mRNA in the paraventricular nucleus, but increased OXTR binding in the central amygdala). Prenatally stressed rats showed disturbed social behavior, which could be normalized with local oxytocin administration in the central amygdala. Cross fostering the pups did not normalize the behavior.

Drug abuse, including smoking, heavy consumption of alcohol, and illegal substances, can adversely affect fetal development and can also impair infant health and development. Alcohol can cause numerous growth impairments, and is especially well known for its harmful effects on the developing nervous system. Tobacco and cannabis smoking are also notorious for fetal growth-restricting and gestation-shortening effects (33). There is ample evidence on the long-term effects of prenatal drug use (ethanol, stimulants, and nicotine) on rodent offspring, focusing on social behavior and drug use and changes to the oxytocin system (33). Exposure to cocaine in the prenatal period in rats affects both the oxytocin system and social behavior and increases susceptibility to addiction later in life (34, 35).

POSTNATAL ENVIRONMENT

The oxytocin system continues to develop after birth, and this development may be critical for providing humans with the skills for healthy social functioning (25). There is extensive research focusing on the long-term effects of early-life adversity and social environment on the oxytocin system; however, most of these studies use animal models. Differences in rearing conditions and bonding behavior can influence adult social and parental behavior in prairie voles (9). Additionally, quality of maternal behavior has been linked to differences in oxytocin concentrations and OXTR expression observed in animal models (9, 36). For example, high levels of maternal licking resulted in increased plasma oxytocin concentrations in neonatal rats (37). Furthermore, Kojima and colleagues (38) found that maternal skin-to-skin contact stimulates rat pups' central oxytocin concentrations. Early-life adversity and differences in the early social environment may also adversely affect the expression and concentration of the OXTR. Veenema (26) provides a thorough review on the effects of early-life manipulations in rodents on the distribution and expression of oxytocin and vasopressin receptors. Bales and Perkeybile (39) also provide a good review of the effect of early experience on the OXTR system.

Human studies with infants and their parents have demonstrated how oxytocin levels rise in response to social interaction and how infant and parental oxytocin concentrations correlate (39). These findings have been supported in previous research measuring cerebrospinal fluid (CSF) oxytocin concentrations, which have shown that higher infant CSF oxytocin concentrations were positively correlated with active initiation and interest in parental social interaction (40). The human oxytocin system seems to be receptive to both positive and negative early social experiences, such as separation (41). Infants who experienced high affect parent–infant synchrony (i.e., monitoring and responding) showed increase oxytocin saliva measures compared to infants reared in the presence of low affect parent–infant synchrony (42). This suggests that the early environment may directly affect peripheral oxytocin concentrations in humans. Importantly, a study by Wismer Fries and colleagues (43) reported significant social deficiencies and low oxytocin concentrations in children reared in extremely aberrant social environments. These results indicate that the early environment may influence cross-generation transmission of human social attachments and behavior. They also support the notion that peripheral oxytocin measurements may be correlated to social behavior in both infants and adults.

MATERNAL ANXIETY, STRESS, AND DEPRESSION

Maternal mental health problems can greatly influence the mother–child bond as they affect the way they perceive their child's needs and cues, their stress resilience, and their general emotional availability.

Research has shown that mothers with postpartum anxiety report significantly lower bonding with their infants than healthy mothers (44). Depressed mothers are more likely to perceive their infant's behavior negatively than healthy mothers (45). Depression can also play an important role in influencing the early-life environment through its effect on maternal behavior and mother–infant bonding. Research shows that the most significant predictor of lower postnatal maternal attachment was depressive symptoms experienced during the final stages of pregnancy and in the postnatal period (18, 46). Despite this emerging evidence, a recent review of the literature (47) identifies that mechanisms underlying maternal stress, depression and anxiety, and their effects on infant outcomes are poorly understood. Due to its important role in mother–infant bonding, oxytocin could be involved in these mechanisms; however, further study is needed.

Interestingly, a recent pilot study found that exogenous administration of oxytocin stimulated protective behavior in mothers with postnatal depression (48). Eapen and colleagues (49) also found an association between lower plasma oxytocin levels in the post partum period and separation anxiety and depression during pregnancy. Further study is needed to determine the relationship between maternal depression and oxytocin, how this relationship may affect infants, and the potential role of exogenous oxytocin in treating depression.

CONSIDERATIONS FOR RESEARCH

The previous sections have introduced the endogenous oxytocin system and its relationship to early environmental and social factors. The present section will identify limitations in the current literature and provide suggestions for future research.

This review has established that there is evidence showing that early social environment in animals is correlated with altered oxytocin concentrations. Particular attention to maternal behaviors during the postnatal period is warranted given the established link between mother–infant dyadic interactions and later physical, emotional, and social health. Studies by Feldman and colleagues (14, 18, 41, 42) have provided insight into the range of saliva and plasma oxytocin concentrations that should be expected in both mothers and babies. However, very little is still known about the normal development of the oxytocin system into childhood and adolescence.

Additionally, a proposed direction of research would be to determine how an early adverse social environment in humans affects the oxytocin system. Of interest are changes in basal concentrations, differences in reactivity of the oxytocin system under stress or social interaction and changes in OXTR characteristics (e.g., investigation of epigenetics, binding affinity, up- or downregulation of receptors, and methylation).

Up- or downregulation of the number of OXTRs, localization and sensitivity of OXTRs are currently difficult to research in humans, as there is no radio-active ligand that can be used in this process. Therefore, a number of different research techniques are needed to investigate these changes through other means, including the collection of biological samples during observational studies and psychological testing undertaken in large cohort studies, and further refinements of assay methodologies.

Epigenetic changes will be of interest to investigate when determining positive or negative effects of early social environment on the developing oxytocin system. Epigenetics refers to the regulation of DNA transcription without alteration of the original sequence. DNA methylation is an important epigenetic modification in response to, e.g., oxygen deprivation, trauma, or drug use. A recent study found that traumatic experiences and stressful life events in early life were associated with higher methylation of the NR3C1 gene (50). Although the topic of epigenetics has not been thoroughly explored in the present review, there is promising research indicating its importance (28, 51–53).

SAMPLE COLLECTION AND MEASUREMENT

Extensive discussion in the field addresses the most suitable and reliable method of collecting and analyzing oxytocin samples, both from the periphery and centrally. Different methods of sample collection and measurement contribute to the large range in oxytocin concentrations reported in the literature (54).

Human research into oxytocin is significantly more difficult than animals due to the inability to non-invasively assess brain oxytocin pathways and concentration. However, peripheral oxytocin concentrations can be tested through plasma, urine or saliva. These measures possibly may not directly correspond with brain concentrations; however, research has shown that changes in behavior are linked to changes in peripheral oxytocin concentrations (14, 54). There is also increasing evidence suggesting that peripheral oxytocin is reflective of changes in central concentrations. For example, a recent study of human children found that plasma oxytocin concentrations significantly and positively predicted CSF oxytocin concentrations (55).

Collecting samples of oxytocin from infants provide an additional challenge to researchers. CSF, urine, and plasma samples are generally unsuitable in these situations as the collection method is invasive and painful; furthermore, it is unlikely that parents will provide consent for their infant's participation in a study with these extraction methods. Finding correlations between oxytocin concentrations in urine and social behavior has shown some success in both animal and human studies (56, 57). However, this collection method may still not be appropriate when attempting to determine an acute infant increase in oxytocin in response to a parent-infant interaction, as urine concentrations represent accumulated oxytocin concentrations and are not always readily available for collection, especially in infants. Saliva, therefore, would appear to be the most ideal method of measuring oxytocin concentrations in infants, with adoption of this method resulting in significant associations between infant and parent oxytocin concentrations and social behavior (42). Recent research from our group (unpublished) has supported previous studies, finding that oxytocin concentrations can be determined from both adult and infant saliva samples. Adults are able to provide this sample by simply spitting into a tube. Saliva from infants can be collected by collecting passive drool from the baby's mouth with a syringe and then dispensing into a tube. Parents have also willingly provided infant consent for this form of collection as it is a minimally invasive and completely painless extraction method. A limitation of this process, however, is that some infants are more accepting of syringing than others, influencing the collection time. This process of collection could also potentially be difficult if the infant is distressed.

Further refinement of oxytocin assay methodologies is also needed. A comparison of enzyme immunoassays (EIA) and radio immunoassays (RIA) of human plasma samples with and without extraction found that without extraction, plasma measured by EIA was more than 100 times higher than in extracted plasma, and the correlation between them was minimal ($p = 0.54$) (58). The same study found that when using an RIA, the majority of samples (90%) were below the level of detection. This could provide some insight into the general inconsistency of results across different studies, indicating the need to refine oxytocin assay methodologies. Currently, comparing group differences within experiments is the most reliable approach.

Specificity of the role of oxytocin provides a challenge in determining the link with early adversity. Oxytocin and vasopressin are very similar in structure, and the two hormones have a high affinity for each other's receptors (59). It is suggested that early social experiences influence sensitivity to both the oxytocin and vasopressin systems (28). This emphasizes the need for further understanding of the systems interacting with oxytocin and the relationship they may have with early adversity and development in humans.

While focusing on the effect of early life social experiences on infants and their developing oxytocin system, it is important to acknowledge that the oxytocin system has numerous bilateral interactions (e.g., dopamine and HPA-axis) that are likely to affect behavior [for a review, see Ref. (12)]. Changes to the oxytocin system will also influence these systems and vice versa. Additionally, systems like the HPA-axis will be affected by environmental influences as well. Researchers focusing on long-term effects of early social environments need to keep these considerations in mind and try to address all the dimensions.

CHARACTERIZATION AND MEASUREMENT OF EARLY ADVERSITY

Another research challenge is measuring early adversity itself. First, there is little consensus on the term, and second, it is conceptualized differently across different disciplines, i.e., neglect, abuse, toxic stress, disorganized attachment, reduced bonding, etc. Detecting and quantifying early adversity is challenging when relying on questionnaires. Observing single mother–child interactions in a laboratory setting or home environment can provide great insight into the early social environment. Assessing attachment status is often not an option, as extensive training is needed. Mothers of infants who may be experiencing early adversity may be reluctant to participate in behavioral observations, although large cohort studies may be able to incorporate this in sub-groups. The next challenge is selecting a tool that can be used to score behavior in a dyad and quality of the interaction (e.g., reciprocity), which is objective, intuitive, and has large inter-rater reliability. There are few scales that have been validated for this purpose meeting all these criteria.

CONCLUDING REMARKS

Review of the literature indicates that the early-life is a vital period for healthy development in humans, and that oxytocin is an important regulator of emotional development. Specifically, investigating the effect of early adversity on the endogenous oxytocin system is important in understanding normal behavior and social disorders. Understanding this effect can increase knowledge of how the early environment appears to change the way humans are hardwired to respond in social and stressful situations. A number of animal studies have been conducted; however, more human research specifically focusing on this relationship is necessary incorporating a large range of study designs. Future studies must consider the obstacles that prevent conducting this research, such as collecting appropriate peripheral oxytocin measures and selecting a suitable tool to score both infant and maternal behavior.

REFERENCES

Lim MM, Young LJ. Neuropeptidergic regulation of affiliative behaviour and social bonding in animals. *Horm Behav* (2006) 50(4):506–17. doi:10.1016/j. yhbeh.2006.06.028

Knobloch HS, Charlet A, Hoffman LC, Eliava M, Khrulev S, Cetin AH, et al. Evoked axonal oxytocin release in the central amygdala attenuates fear response. *Neuron* (2012) 73(3):553–66. doi:10.1016/j.neuron.2011.11.030

Nishimori K, Takayanagi Y, Yoshida M, Kasahara Y, Young LJ, Kawamata M. New aspects of oxytocin receptor function revealed by knockout mice: sociosex- ual behaviour and control of energy balance. *Prog Brain Res* (2008) 170:79–90. doi:10.1016/S0079-6123(08)00408-1

Kiss A, Mikkelson JD. Oxytocin – anatomy and functional assignments: a minire- view. *Endocr Regul* (2005) 39(3):97–105.

White-Traut R, Watanabe K, Pournajafi-Nazarloo H, Schwertz D, Bell A, Carter S. Detection of salivary oxytocin levels in lactating women. *Dev Psychobiol* (2009) 51(1):367–73. doi:10.1002/dev.20376

Neumann ID. Brain oxytocin: a key regulator of emotional and social behaviour in both females and males. *J Neuroendocrinol* (2008) 6:858–65. doi:10.1111/j. 1365-2826.2008.01726.x

Magon N, Kalra S. The orgasmic history of oxytocin: love, lust, and labor. *Indian J Endocrinol Metab* (2011) 15(Suppl 3):S156–61. doi:10.4103/2230-8210.84851

Heinrichs M, Baumgartner T, Kirschbaum C, Ehlert U. Social support and oxy- tocin interact to suppress cortisol and subjective responses to psychosocial stress. *Biol Psychiatry* (2003) 54(12):1389–98. doi:10.1016/S0006-3223(03)00465-7

Ahern TH, Young LJ. The impact of early life family structure on adult social attachment, allopa-rental behaviour, and the neuropeptide systems regulating affiliative behaviours in the monogamous prairie vole (microtus ochrogaster). *Front Behav Neurosci* (2009) 3:17. doi:10.3389/neuro.08.017.2009

Olff M, Frijling JL, Kubzansky LD, Bradley B, Ellenbogen MA, Cardoso C, et al.The role of oxytocin in social bonding, stress regulation and mental health: an update on the moderating effects of context and interindividual differences. *Psychoneuroendocrinology* (2013) 38(9):1883–94. doi:10.1016/j.psyneuen.2013.06.019

Tops M, Koole SL, IJzerman H, Buisman-Pijlman FTA. Why social attachment and oxytocin protect against addiction and stress: insights from the dynamics between ventral and dorsal corticostriatal systems. *Pharmacol Biochem Behav* (2014) 119:39–48. doi:10.1016/j.pbb.2013.07.015

Buisman-Pijlman FT, Sumracki NM, Gordon JJ, Hull PR, Carter CS, Tops M. Individual differences underlying susceptibility to addiction: role for the endogenous oxytocin system. *Pharmacol Biochem Behav* (2014) 119(1):22–38. doi:10.1016/j.pbb.2013.09.005

Lupoli B, Johansson B, Uvnäs-Moberg K, Svennersten-Sjaunja K. Effect of suck- ling on the release of oxytocin, prolactin, cortisol, gastrin, cholecystokinin, somatostatin and insulin in dairy cows and their calves. *J Dairy Res* (2001) 68(2):175–87. doi:10.1017/S0022029901004721

Feldman R, Gordon I, Zagoory-Sharon O. Maternal and paternal plasma sali- vary and urinary oxytocin and parent-infant synchrony: considering stress and affiliation components of human bonding. *Dev Sci* (2011) 14(4):752–61. doi:10.1111/j.1467-7687.2010.01021.x

Murakami G, Hunter RG, Fontaine C, Ribeiro A, Pfaff D. Relationships among estrogen receptor, oxytocin and vasopressin gene expression and social inter- action in male mice. *Eur J Neurosci* (2011) 34(3):469–77. doi:10.1111/j.1460-9568.2011.07761.x

Boersma GJ, Bale TL, Casanello P, Lara HE, Lucion AB, Suchecki D, et al. Long- term impact of early-life events on physiology and behaviour. *J Neuroendocrinol* (2014) 26(9):587–602. doi:10.1111/jne.12153

Wong MS, Mangelsdorf SC, Brown GL, Neff C, Schoppe-Sullivan

SJ. Parental beliefs, infant temperament, and marital quality: associations with infant- mother and infant-father attachment. *J Fam Psychol* (2009) 23(6):828–38. doi:10.1037/a0016491

Feldman R, Weller A, Zagoory-Sharon O, Levine A. Evidence for a neuroen- docrinological foundation of human affiliation: plasma oxytocin levels across pregnancy and the postpartum period predict mother-infant bonding. *Psychol Sci* (2007) 18(11):965–70. doi:10.1111/j.1467-9280.2007.02010.x

Strathearn L, Fonagy P, Amico J, Montague PR. Adult attachment predicts mater- nal brain and oxytocin response to infant cues. *Neuropsychopharmacology* (2009) 34(13):2655–6. doi:10.1038/npp.2009.103

Gordon I, Zagoory-Sharon O, Leckman JF, Feldman R. Oxytocin, cortisol, and triadic family interactions. *Physiol Behav* (2010) 101(5):679–84. doi:10.1016/j.physbeh.2010.08.008

Atzil S, Hendler T, Feldman R. Specifying the neurobiological basis of human attachment: brain, hormones, and behavior in synchronous and intrusive mothers. *Neuropsychopharmacology* (2011) 36(13):2603–15. doi:10.1038/npp.2011.172

Atzil S, Hendler T, Zagoory-Sharon O, Winetraub Y, Feldman R. Synchrony and specificity in the maternal and the paternal brain: relations to oxytocin and vasopressin. *J Am Acad Child Adolesc Psychiatry* (2012) 51(8):798–811. doi:10.1016/j.jaac.2012.06.008

Feldman R, Gordon I, Influs M, Gutbir T, Ebstein RP. Parental oxytocin and early care giving jointly shape children's oxytocin response and social reciprocity. *Neuropsychopharmacology* (2013) 38(7):1154–62. doi:10.1038/npp.2013.22

Kim S, Fonagy P, Koos O, Dorsett K, Strathearn L. Maternal oxytocin response predicts mother-to-infant gaze. *Brain Res* (2014) 1580:133–42. doi:10.1016/j.brainres.2013.10.050

Taylor AE, Lee HE, Buisman-Pijlman FTA. Oxytocin treatment in paediatric populations. *Front Behav Neurosci* (2014) 8:360. doi:10.3389/fnbeh.2014.00360

Veenema AH. Toward understanding how early-life social experiences alter oxytocin- and vasopressin-regulated social behaviours. *Horm Behav* (2011) 61(3):304–12. doi:10.1016/j.yhbeh.2011.12.002

Bales KL, Boone E, Epperson P, Hoffman G, Carter C. Are behavioural effects of early experience mediated by oxytocin? *Front Psychiatry* (2011) 2:24. doi:10.3389/fpsyt.2011.00024

Cushing BS, Kramer KM. Mechanisms underlying epigenetic effects of early social experience: the role of neuropeptides and steroids. *Neurosci Biobehav Rev* (2005) 29(7):1089–105. doi:10.1016/j.neubiorev.2005.04.001

Levine A, Zagoory-Sharon O, Feldman R, Weller A. Oxytocin during pregnancy and early postpartum: individual patterns and maternal-foetal attachment. *Pep- tides* (2007) 28(6):1162–9. doi:10.1016/j.peptides.2007.04.016

O'Donnell K, O'Connor TG, Glover V. Prenatal stress and neurodevelopment of the child: focus on the HPA axis and role of the placenta. *Dev Neurosci* (2009) 31:285–92. doi:10.1159/000216539

Wainstock T, Shoham-Vardi I, Glasser S, Anteby E, Lerner-Geva L. Fetal sex modifies effects of prenatal stress exposure and adverse birth outcomes. *Stress* (2014):1–8. doi:10.3109/10253890.2014.974153

Lee PR, Brady DL, Shapiro RA, Dorsa DM, Koenig JI. Prenatal stress gen- erates deficits in rat social behaviour: reversal by oxytocin. *Brain Res* (2007) 2(1156):152–67. doi:10.1016/j.brainres.2007.04.042

Vaiserman AM. Long-term health consequences of early-life exposure to substance abuse: an epigenetic perspective. *J Dev Orig Health Dis* (2013) 4(4):269–79. doi:10.1017/S2040174413000123

Johns JM, Noonan LR, Zimmerman LI, McMillen BA, Means LW, Walker CH, et al. Chronic cocaine treatment alters social/aggressive behaviour in Sprague- Dawley rat dams and in their prenatally exposed offspring. *Ann N Y Acad Sci* (1998) 846:399–404. doi:10.1111/j.1749-6632.1998.tb09765.x

Williams SK, Johns JM. Prenatal and gestational cocaine exposure: effects on the oxytocin system and social behaviour with implications for addiction. *Pharma- col Biochem Behav* (2013) 119:10–21. doi:10.1016/j.pbb.2013.07.004

Francis DD, Champagne FC, Meaney MJ. Variations in maternal behaviour are associated with differences in oxytocin receptor levels in the rat. *J Neuroen- docrinol* (2000) 12(1):1145–8. doi:10.1046/j.1365-2826.2000.00599.x

Henriques TP, Szawka RE, Diehl LA, de Souza MA, Correa CN, Aranda BC, et al. Stress in neonatal rats with different maternal care backgrounds: monoamin- ergic and hormonal responses. *Neurochem Res* (2014) 39(12):2531–9. doi:10.1007/s11064-014-1434-8

Kojima S, Stewart RA, Demas GE, Alberts JR. Maternal contact differentially modulates central and peripheral oxytocin in rat pups during a brief regime of mother-pup interaction that induces a filial huddling preference. *J Neuroen- docrinol* (2012) 5:831–40. doi:10.1111/j.1365-2826.2012.02280.x

Bales KL, Perkeybile AM. Developmental experiences and the oxytocin receptor system. *Horm Behav* (2012) 61(3):313–9. doi:10.1016/j.yhbeh.2011.12.013

Clark CL, St John N, Pasca AM, Hyde SA, Hornbeak K, Abramova M, et al. Neonatal CSF oxytocin levels are associated with parent report of infant soothability and sociability. *Psychoneuroendocrinology* (2013) 38(7):1208–12. doi:10.1016/j.psyneuen.2012.10.017

Feldman R. Oxytocin and social affiliation in humans. *Horm Behav* (2012) 61(3):380–91. doi:10.1016/j.yhbeh.2012.01.008

Feldman R, Gordon I, Zagoory-Sharon O. The cross-generation transmission of oxytocin in humans. *Horm Behav* (2010) 58(4):669–76. doi:10.1016/j.yhbeh. 2010.06.005

Wismer Fries AB, Ziegler TE, Kurian JR, Jacoris S, Pollak SD. Early experi- ence in humans is associated with changes in neuropeptides critical for regulating social behaviour. *Proc Natl Acad Sci U S A* (2005) 102(47):17237–40. doi:10.1073/pnas.0504767102

Tietz A, Zietlow AL, Reck C. Maternal bonding in mothers with postpar- tum anxiety disorder: the crucial role of subclinical depressive symptoms and maternal avoidance behaviour. *Arch Womens Ment Health* (2014) 17(5):433–42. doi:10.1007/s00737-014-0423-x

Forman DR, O'Hara MW, Stuart S, Gorman LL, Larsen KE, Coy KC. Effective treatment for postpartum depression is not sufficient to improve the developing mother–child relationship. *Dev Psychopathol* (2007) 19(2):585–602.

Perry DF, Ettinger AK, Mendelson T, Le HN. Prenatal depression predicts post- partum maternal attachment in low-income Latina mothers with infants. *Infant Behav Dev* (2011) 34(2):339–50. doi:10.1016/j.infbeh.2011.02.005

Glover V. Maternal depression, anxiety and stress during preg nancy and child outcome; what needs to be done. *Best Pract Res Clin Obstet Gynaecol* (2014) 28(1):25–35. doi:10.1016/j.bpobgyn.2013.08.017

Mah BL, Bakermans-Kranenburg MJ, Van Ijzendoorn MH, Smith R. Oxy- tocin promotes protective behaviour in depressed mothers: a pilot study with the enthusiastic stranger paradigm. *Depress Anxiety* (2014) 32(2):76–81. doi:10.1002/da.22245

Eapen V, Dadds M, Barnett B, Kohlhoff J, Khan F, Radom N, et al. Separation anxiety, attachment and interpersonal representations: disentangling the role of oxytocin in the perinatal period. *PLoS One* (2014) 17:9. doi:10.1371/journal.pone.0107745

van der Knaap LJ, Riese H, Hudziak JJ, Verbiest MM, Verhulst FC, Oldehinkel AJ, et al. Glucocorticoid receptor gene (NR3C1) methylation following stress- ful events between birth and adolescence. The TRAILS study. *Transl Psychiatry* (2014) 4:e381. doi:10.1038/tp.2014.22

Champagne FA. Epigenetic mechanisms and the transgenerational effects of maternal care. *Front Neuroendocrinol* (2008) 29(3):386–97. doi:10.1016/j.yfrne.2008.03.003

Gregory SG, Connelly JJ, Towers AJ, Johnson J, Biscocho D, Markunas CA, et al. Genomic and epigenetic evidence for oxytocin receptor deficiency in autism. *BMC Med* (2009) 7:62. doi:10.1186/1741-7015-7-62

Cecil CA, Lysenko LJ, Jaffee SR, Pingault JB, Smith RG, Relton CL, et al. Environmental risk, oxytocin receptor gene (OXTR) methylation and youth callous-unemotional traits: a 13-year longitudinal study. *Mol Psychiatry* (2014) 19(10):1071–7. doi:10.1038/mp.2014.95

Crockford C, Deschner T, Ziegler TE, Wittig RM. Endogenous periph- eral oxytocin measures can give insight into the dynamics of social relationships: a review. *Front Behav Neurosci* (2014) 8:68. doi:10.3389/fnbeh. 2014.00068

Carson DS, Berquist SW, Trujillo TH, Garner JP, Hannah SL, Hyde SA, et al. Cerebrospinal fluid and plasma oxytocin concentrations are positively cor- related and negatively predict anxiety in children. *Mol Psychiatry* (2014). doi:10.1038/mp.2014.132

Wittig RM, Crockford C, Deschner

T, Langergraber KE, Ziegler TE, Zuber- bühler K. Food sharing is linked to urinary oxytocin levels and bonding in related and unrelated wild chimpanzees. *Proc Biol Sci* (2014) 281:1778. doi:10.1098/rspb.2013.3096

Saito A, Hamada H, Kikusui T, Mogi K, Nagasawa M, Mitsui S, et al. Urinary oxytocin positively correlates with performance in facial visual search in unmar- ried males, without specific reaction to infant face. *Front Neurosci* (2014) 8:217. doi:10.3389/fnins.2014.00217

Szeto A, McCabe PM, Nation DA, Tabak BA, Rossetti MA, McCullough ME, et al. Evaluation of enzyme immunoassay and radioimmunoassay methods for the measurement of plasma oxytocin. *Psychosom Med* (2011) 73(5):393–400. doi:10.1097/PSY.0b013e31821df0c2

Neumann ID, Landgraf R. Balance of brain oxytocin and vasopressin: impli- cations for anxiety, depression, and social behaviours. *Trends Neurosci* (2012) 35(11):649–59. doi:10.1016/j.tins.2012.08.004

14

Vasopressin proves essensetial: vasopressin and the modulation of sensory processing in mammals

Janet K. Bester-Meredith*, Alexandria P. Fancher and Grace E. Mammarella

Department of Biology, Seattle Pacific University, Seattle, WA, USA

Edited by:
Hubert Vaudry, University of Rouen, France

Reviewed by:
Aldo Lucion, Universidade Federal do Rio Grande do Sul, Brazil
Nicole Kime, Edgewood College, USA

***Correspondence:**
Janet K. Bester-Meredith, Department of Biology, Seattle Pacific University, 3307 3rd Avenue W, Seattle, WA 98119, USA
e-mail: bestej@spu.edu

As mammals develop, they encounter increasing social complexity in the surrounding world. In order to survive, mammals must show appropriate behaviors toward their mates, offspring, and same-sex conspecifics. Although the behavioral effects of the neuropeptide arginine vasopressin (AVP) have been studied in a variety of social contexts, the effects of this neuropeptide on multimodal sensory processing have received less attention. AVP is widely distributed through sensory regions of the brain and has been demonstrated to modulate olfactory, auditory, gustatory, and visual processing. Here, we review the evidence linking AVP to the processing of social stimuli in sensory regions of the brain and explore how sensory processing can shape behavioral responses to these stimuli. In addition, we address the interplay between hormonal and neural AVP in regulating sensory processing of social cues. Because AVP pathways show plasticity during development, early life experiences may shape life-long processing of sensory information. Furthermore, disorders of social behavior such as autism and schizophrenia that have been linked with AVP also have been linked with dysfunctions in sensory processing. Together, these studies suggest that AVP's diversity of effects on social behavior across a variety of mammalian species may result from the effects of this neuropeptide on sensory processing.

Keywords: vasopressin, sensory, olfaction, social behavior, hearing, gustation, social learning

INTRODUCTION

In social species, survival depends on navigating complex social cues. An individual must be able to use sensory cues to distinguish between familiar and unfamiliar individuals. These sensory cues must then be filtered in a way that directs the animal to make an appropriate behavioral response. Although interpretation of sensory cues is influenced by many neural pathways, the neuropeptide arginine vasopressin (AVP) appears to be critical for making these key social distinctions in mammals. This neuropeptide has been associated with pair bonding, aggression, parental care, social memory formation, and stress responses in multiple species of rodents [reviewed in Ref. (1)], possibly due to its broader role in integrating sensory input. In addition, the distribution of AVP and its receptors changes throughout the lifespan. During development, AVP immunoreactivity and receptors show remarkable plasticity in response to environmental influences, such as the quality and quantity of interactions with peers and parents (2–10). Therefore, early developmental experiences may shape how an animal interprets sensory cues related to social behavior throughout its lifespan.

The focus of this article is to review evidence that links AVP with the processing of sensory information and to explore whether this alteration of sensory processing leads to diverse behavioral effects across different mammalian species. This paper describes the distribution of AVP and its receptors within sensory organs and within brain areas that receive direct sensory input. We also describe anatomical pathways containing AVP and its receptors that connect the primary sensory cortices with brain areas that process social cues and that direct complex forms of social behavior. We are proposing that the sex-specificity and species-specificity of AVP effects on behavior in mammals result from the variation in the pattern of distribution of AVP and its receptors in sensory pathways. The convergence of sensory input with vasopressin pathways that travel both within the brain and outside of the brain suggests that the effects of AVP on behavior may be mediated by both central pathways that alter the valence of social stimuli and peripheral pathways that alter physiological responses to social stimuli.

BACKGROUND

SEXUAL DIMORPHISM IN AVP: DIFFERENCES BETWEEN PARVOCELLULAR AND MAGNOCELLULAR NEURONS

Arginine vasopressin has been localized in parvocellular and magnocellular neurons that are widely distributed in the central nervous system (11). AVP within a pathway that originates in the medial amygdala (MA) and bed nucleus of the stria terminalis (BNST) and projects to the lateral septum (LS) has been associated with complex social behavior in mammals [reviewed in Ref. (1)]. Early exploration into the association between this pathway and sex-specific patterns of social behavior originated with the identification of sexual dimorphism in AVP immunohistochemistry. In rats (*Rattus rattus*), prairie voles (*Microtus ochrogaster*), meadow voles (*Microtus pennsylvanicus*), and CD1 mice (*Mus musculus*), males show more AVP-immunoreactive (AVP-ir) staining in the BNST and its projections to the LS than do females (12–14). The sexual dimorphism in AVP appears to be testosterone-dependent because castration reduces AVP immunoreactivity in male rats and testosterone implants increase AVP immunoreactivity in female rats (15–17). Although AVP is found only in mammals, similar sexual dimorphism has been observed in the homologous arginine vasotocin (AVT) pathways of birds, reptiles, and amphibians (18). Although the role of AVT in regulating sensorimotor processing in the amphibian *Taricha granulosa* has been explored elsewhere (19), the role of AVP in regulating sensory processing in mammals has received less attention.

Because AVP immunoreactivity is more pronounced in the male brain, it has been suggested that AVP may regulate male social behavior, and that oxytocin may serve a similar role in the female brain. Early evidence supported the contention that AVP was a key regulator of male social behavior during pair-bonding and aggressive encounters, but more recent evidence also implicates AVP in regulating female social behavior (9, 20–30). The role of AVP in regulating species-specific social behavior in both males and females in different ways in a variety of mammalian species suggests that this neuropeptide serves a broader function in behavioral regulation.

Although behavioral studies usually focus on AVP in the parvocellular pathway described above, AVP produced within magnocellular neurons of the hypothalamus also regulates physiological functions that may indirectly influence an animal's behavioral responses to social stimuli. After its release from the posterior pituitary gland, AVP also enters into the bloodstream where it produces hormonal effects on a variety of peripheral tissues. The magnocellular neurons of the paraventricular nucleus (PVN) of the hypothalamus and of the supraoptic nucleus (SON) appear to be the main sites of AVP production in this pathway and can be distinguished from the parvocellular neurons by measuring their voltage-gated currents (31). Within the bloodstream, AVP is more commonly known as anti-diuretic hormone (ADH), a hormone that increases blood pressure and decreases ion concentrations within the blood by lowering the amount of water that is excreted in urine. AVP also modulates cardiac function by increasing activity of the sympathetic neurons that innervate the heart and decreasing activity of parasympathetic neurons [reviewed in Ref. (32)]. Although the changes in blood pressure and heart rate produced by AVP in response to activation of magnocellular neurons are often overlooked in studies of social behavior, the coupling of these effects with central effects can be critical for normal emotional responses (33). Appropriate responses to social stimuli may be more likely to occur when alterations in heart rate and blood pressure create an optimal level of arousal that allows the animal to focus on subtle social cues.

DISTRIBUTION OF THREE TYPES OF AVP RECEPTORS

Arginine vasopressin produces different effects within the central and peripheral nervous systems because it binds to three main categories of receptors: V1a, V1b, and V2 receptors. Although V2 receptors and both subtypes of V1 receptors are found within the peripheral nervous system, only V1 receptors are found within the central nervous system. Despite the early suggestion that binding of AVP to V1a receptors was responsible for all of the behavioral effects of this neuropeptide, more recent evidence using receptor knockouts indicates that central V1b receptors also are critical for social behavior [(1); for review of V1b receptors, see Ref. (34, 35); for review of V1a receptors, see Ref. (36–38)]. Adding an additional layer of complexity to our understanding of the central effects of AVP is the observation that AVP can bind to oxytocin receptors and that oxytocin may act as an agonist at AVP receptors because of the similarities between the structures of these peptides and their G-protein linked receptors [(39); reviewed in Ref. (40)]. However, the impact of this potential peptide cross-reactivity on social behavior is unclear as it has not been well studied.

Although V1a receptor distribution often varies between closely related species with different mating systems [e.g., Ref. (41–44)], consistent patterns of differences between monogamous and non-monogamous species have not yet been identified. Monogamous California mice (*Peromyscus californicus*) show elevated V1a receptor binding in the LS in comparison to non-monogamous white-footed mice (*Peromyscus leucopus*), but studies in voles have found an opposite pattern with higher V1a receptor binding in the non-monogamous species (42, 45, 46). Despite the lack of consistency in patterns of variability across species, social behaviors related to monogamy can be altered using manipulations of AVP within a single species. In prairie voles, a monogamous species, reduction of V1a gene activity using RNA interference reduces partner preference and other behaviors related to monogamy (47). However, the lack of consistency in V1a receptor distribution patterns between closely related species has led to multiple hypotheses about the reasons for these differences. Although it has been suggested that interspecies variation in V1a receptor distribution may result from differences in aggression, different ecological pressures that alter spatial distributions of animals within their habitats, and/or other social pressures, none of these explanations seem to fit all of the existing data (38, 42, 44, 48, 49). Therefore, it seems reasonable to hypothesize that AVP pathways may serve a broader function related to social behavior because of the large amount of sex and species variation in this system.

VASOPRESSIN AND SENSORY SIGNALING

VASOPRESSIN AND OLFACTION

Olfactory brain circuitry: overview

Two separate olfactory systems exist within the rodent brain that process socially relevant olfactory information. Both of these pathways contain AVP and its receptors (**Figure 1**). In the main olfactory system, input travels from the main olfactory bulb (MOB) to the anterior olfactory nucleus, piriform cortex (PC), and amygdala for additional processing (50). This multi-step pathway brings olfactory information to be processed in multiple areas of the cerebral cortex, including the anterior olfactory nucleus and PC. The anterior olfactory nucleus, a cortical area adjacent to the olfactory bulb that is part of the main olfactory pathway, contains AVP neurons that are activated by the exposure to social odors in rats but not by exposure to other odor cues (51). A parallel system, the accessory olfactory system, brings information from the vomeronasal organ (VNO) into the accessory olfactory bulb (AOB), which innervates the MA, BNST, and cortical amygdala (52). Although it was originally assumed that only the accessory olfactory system processed pheromones and other socially relevant odors, more recent evidence suggests that social information is processed by both pathways (52).

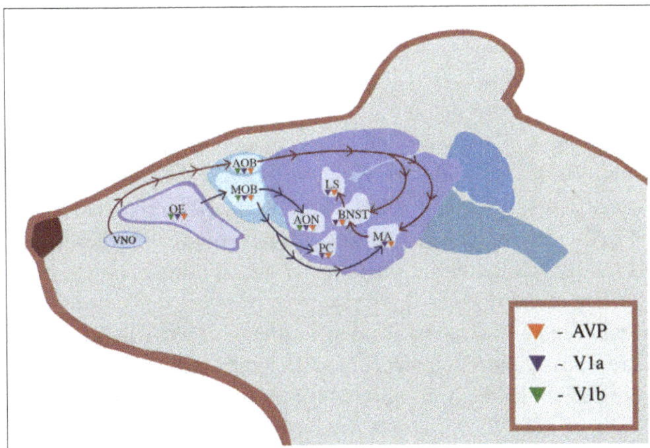

FIGURE 1 | The distribution of AVP (red triangles), V1a receptors (blue triangles), and V1b receptors (green triangles) in olfactory regions of the rodent brain. Information in the main olfactory system travels from the OE to the MOB and then is processed in the accessory olfactory nucleus, PC, and MA. Information in the accessory olfactory system travels from the VNO to the AOB and then to the MA, BNST, and LS.

This redundancy allows olfactory input to be processed simultaneously by non-dimorphic brain areas and by sexually dimorphic, AVP-rich areas such as the BNST, amygdala, and LS. For example, in male rats, exposure to the odors of a receptive female held behind a perforated plastic partition leads to Fos expression in the AVP neurons of the MA (53). The presence of this neuronal marker of gene activation in the MA indicates that the odor of the estrous female is driving activation of the MA and the interconnected hypothalamic brain areas that are associated with reproductive behavior. A different pattern of neural activation occurs in the brain of a female exposed to the odor of an estrous female. Similarly, female rough skin newts (*T. granulosa*) that have been treated with testosterone and AVT show male-typical responses to female odors, suggesting that manipulations of AVP and its homologs can alter olfactory processing of social cues. The ability of AVP to lead to differentiated responses to complex social odors would be favored by natural selection because these differentiated responses allow mammals to target their behavioral responses toward other individuals in a way that maximizes individual fitness. However, the specific role of AVP in driving complex behavioral responses to social odors has yet to be elucidated.

Arginine vasopressin alters olfactory processing in rats from the moment that olfactory information enters the brain via the MOB or the AOB, but this processing occurs in a variety of complex ways. In rats, the olfactory bulb contains a population of AVP neurons with V1b receptors that does not project outside of the olfactory bulb and that may regulate their own activity (54). This modulation within the bulb could decrease or increase sensitivity to social odors. Social odors also activate OR37 receptors in the main olfactory system, which provide direct, monosynaptic input into both the magnocellular and parvocellular AVP neurons of the PVN and the SON (55). It is not clear, however, whether activation of these receptors leads to release of AVP into the bloodstream, activation of brain areas associated with social behavior, or both. V1a and V1b receptors within the olfactory bulb are also associated with neurons that transmit information outside of the olfactory bulb, and additional V1a and V1b receptors have been localized in the olfactory epithelium (OE) and targets of the olfactory pathways such as the PC (56–58). The presence of AVP and its receptors in so many olfactory processing areas indicates that AVP is able to modulate olfactory information, as the information is evaluated by areas of the brain that direct behavioral responses.

Olfactory brain circuitry: interactions between olfactory pathways

Arginine vasopressin's influence on olfactory processing extends beyond the main and accessory olfactory systems. Although some processing of social odors appears to occur in a sexually dimorphic way to allow males and females to respond differentially to sexual cues, other processing of social odors follows similar neural pathways in both sexes. In mice, anatomical evidence suggests that olfactory cues may stimulate the non-dimorphic cells of the MA and activate the magnocellular cells of the SON (14). SON or PVN activation has the potential to lead to release of AVP in the bloodstream where it may alter the behavior of the animal by affecting the arousal level of the animal due to changes in blood pressure or autonomic activation. However, even though this pathway is not sexually dimorphic, modulation of the activity of this pathway might occur in a sexually dimorphic way through interactions with other neurotransmitter systems or with AVP in other neural pathways that are sexually dimorphic.

Our understanding of how AVP alters olfactory processing has been extended by the use of functional magnetic resonance imaging (fMRI) in addition to traditional neuroanatomical techniques. In this paradigm, fMRI BOLD responses are used to monitor changes in neural activation. Central administration of a V1a receptor antagonist in conjunction with the presentation of a male intruder increases BOLD responses in the anterior olfactory nucleus and in the infralimbic prefrontal cortex and decreases BOLD responses in the cortical amygdala in dams (27). The finding indicates that blocking AVP receptor binding during a threatening situation alters how olfactory cues are processed within the brain. In addition, the alteration in infralimbic prefrontal cortex activation is intriguing because this brain area has been implicated in the regulation of fear and autonomic responses to olfactory stimuli and projects to the BNST and LS (59). Because the BNST and LS have been associated with maternal aggression in rodents (22, 23), this pattern of neuronal activation may indicate readiness to attack an intruder. Although we are only beginning to understand how complex behavioral responses are integrated across the entire brain during social situations, these findings suggest that AVP's modulation of olfactory systems may have important implications for an animal's fitness. When AVP receptors are blocked, the typical fear response to an olfactory threat is diminished.

AVP and olfactory processing in Syrian hamsters

Arginine vasopressin also has been demonstrated to play a critical behavioral role in the interpretation of chemical signals during social interactions in Syrian hamsters (*Mesocricetus auratus*). In both male and female Syrian hamsters, infusions of AVP into the BNST, LS, or anterior hypothalamus increase the frequency of flank marking (60–62). V1a receptor binding in targets of this pathway, such as the ventromedial hypothalamus, is downregulated in response to social cues. Male Syrian hamsters who win repeated aggressive encounters show less submissive behavior and greater V1a receptor binding in the ventromedial hypothalamus than socially subjugated males (6). Therefore, social experience during development in Syrian hamsters leads to plasticity in AVP receptor distribution that shapes the production of olfactory signals. Although it is not known whether AVP also alters the interpretation of olfactory signals in this species, social odor preferences in both females and males are eliminated with lesions in brain areas that contain AVP and its receptors (63, 64). This plasticity indicates that social experiences that alter the distribution of AVP or its receptors within the brain may also shape a mammal's ability to produce and respond to olfactory signals.

Despite parallels between the role of AVP in regulating scent-marking behavior in male and female Syrian hamsters, the social context of AVP release may constrain scent mark production differently in males and females. For example, infusions of AVP or a V1a receptor antagonist into the anterior hypothalamus produce opposite effects in males and females. In female, but not male Syrian hamsters, AVP infusions decrease aggression whereas the V1a receptor antagonist infusions increase aggression (65). Together these results indicate that although AVP may shape the production of olfactory signals like flank marking, the social context of these signals determines how this peptide will influence social behavior. Selection pressures, therefore, can lead to sex differences in how AVP influences the processing of olfactory signals.

AVP and social recognition

The role of AVP in regulating the interpretation of olfactory signals has also been investigated in other rodents using various social recognition paradigms [reviewed in Ref. (50, 52, 66–69)]. A typical protocol involves the exposure of a rodent to an unfamiliar juvenile conspecific. After a delay of 30-120 min and infusion of AVP or one of its antagonists, the animal then is returned to a testing arena that contains either the same conspecific, a novel animal, or both [e.g., Ref. (70, 71)]. Exposure to the odor of a familiar animal typically leads to less olfactory exploration than exposure to the odor of a novel animal.

Arginine vasopressin influences social recognition via two separate pathways: one pathway that is contained entirely within the olfactory bulb and a second pathway that is sexually dimorphic and leads to the LS. Infusion of AVP into the olfactory bulb enhances social recognition in male rats (72). Although infusions of a commonly used V1a receptor antagonist in the olfactory bulb does not eliminate social recognition, performance in a social recognition test is impaired in male rats after infusions of OPC-21268, a non-peptide V1 receptor antagonist that diffuses more widely (54, 72). In both sexes, infusion of a V1a receptor antagonist into the LS decreases olfactory exploration of a novel same-sex juvenile rat (73). Although this finding is somewhat surprising because AVP immunoreactivity is lower in the LS in female rats, V1a receptors are more abundant in females (73). Therefore, the lower AVP content of the LS in females may be counteracted by the presence of additional receptors in this brain area. These findings also indicate that activation of AVP neural pathways may be important for social recognition in both sexes despite anatomical differences between the sexes.

Although initial processing of the olfactory cues used in social recognition occurs within the olfactory bulb, more complex processing occurs in sexually dimorphic AVP pathways. Innate variation in the production of AVP and its receptors within these areas leads to individual variation in social recognition. Female mice who were categorized as "high recognizers" because of strong performance in a social recognition test expressed less mRNA for AVP, V1a receptors, and V1b receptors in the lateral amygdala than "low recognizers," although no differences were identified in the BNST or MA (74). The ability to perform well during a social recognition task appears to result from downregulation of AVP in the lateral amygdala even if AVP in other brain areas like the LS is essential for processing the olfactory cues related to the social recognition task. In addition, in some rodent species, AVP pathways used in social recognition are responsive to changes in the environment that alter gene expression through epigenetic mechanisms that change the packaging of DNA and histones within the nucleus of a cell. For example, environmental influences such as maternal separation have been shown to alter methylation of DNA and to alter AVP gene expression (75). Similarly, administration of a histone deacetylase inhibitor like valproic acid creates epigenetic modifications that can alter olfactory processing. In female mice, valproic acid masculinizes AVP fiber density in the LS and increases the attraction of a female toward same-sex odors (76). This finding suggests that epigenetic mechanisms that are shaped by the prenatal and postnatal environment can alter AVP distribution within the brain and modify an animal's social behavior by modulating responses to olfactory stimuli.

The effects of central release of AVP on social recognition may be amplified by the simultaneous release of AVP into the bloodstream. During a social recognition test in mice using an intact male mouse as a stimulus animal, AVP is released in the SON as measured by microdialysis (77). Because AVP release from the SON leads to elevation of plasma AVP, this indicates that central activation and peripheral activation of AVP pathways may be linked. Lesions of the MA also disrupt the release of AVP from the SON, suggesting that olfactory processing by the pathway projecting from the MA to the LS may activate release of AVP from the SON (77). This connection between the MA and the magnocellular cells of the SON may modulate aggressive responses while elevating levels of AVP in the bloodstream (14).

Despite compelling data indicating that AVP regulates social recognition in both sexes, elimination of one type of AVP receptor does not block social recognition consistently. In male mice, a null mutation in the V1a or the V1b receptor leads to impairments in social recognition [V1a: (78) and V1b: (79)]. Deficits caused by a null mutation in the V1a receptor can be reversed by re-introducing the V1a receptor into the LS using a viral vector (80). However, other studies have failed to identify any impairment in social recognition in male V1a receptor knockout mice despite mild olfactory impairments (81). Female mice with a null mutation of the V1a receptor also display a normal Bruce effect, which is the loss of a pregnancy after the odor of urine of an unfamiliar male activates the vomeronasal system (82). In contrast, female mice with a null mutation in the V1b receptor do not show a normal Bruce effect, indicating that the V1b receptor may be more critical for this response in females (82). Inconsistencies between studies may result from the involvement of multiple receptor types and neurotransmitter systems in processing socially relevant olfactory signals.

Evolutionary significance of olfactory processing

The ability to discriminate between the odors of a mate, offspring, and an unfamiliar individual is important for individuals from social species. The evolutionary significance of olfactory investigation, however, may be compounded by the ability to extract additional complex information from odors. Male rats not only can discriminate between individuals but also avoid the odors of ill conspecifics. This avoidance response requires intact AVP neural pathways because exposure to these odors upregulates mRNA for V1a and V1b receptors in the MA, but does not occur if a rat receives a microinfusion of a V1a or V1b receptor antagonist into the MA (83). Although an increase in c-fos mRNA in the olfactory bulb and BNST indicated that those brain areas were activated by exposure to illness-related odors, V1a or V1b receptor binding was not elevated in these brain areas. Therefore, processing of illness-related odors in the AVP system occurs specifically in the MA, a brain area associated with fear. This example illustrates the idea that AVP pathways may assist with creating a complex emotional and behavioral response to the odor of a conspecific that varies depending on the conspecific's familiarity, sex, health, age, and other individual characteristics.

AVP AND AUDITORY PROCESSING

Neural processing of auditory signals in birds, fish, and frogs

Although AVP has most commonly been associated with processing of olfactory signals, AVP also assists with processing of auditory signals. A clear link between auditory processing and a non-mammalian AVP homolog, AVT, has been established in birds, frogs, and fish. For example, pairing male and female zebra finches (*Taeniopygia guttata*) increases AVT mRNA in the PVN and BNST of both sexes, and the magnitude of the increase in mRNA production in males is associated with the quantity of singing behaviors (84). Male zebra fiches that choose to sing to a female behind a wire barrier also have more AVT-immunoreactive neurons in the BNST than non-singers, again indicating a linkage between auditory signal production and social behavior in this species (85). In addition to these correlational linkages between AVT and singing behavior, direct manipulations of AVT using intraventricular infusions also increase singing behavior in female sparrows (*Zonotrichia leucophrys gambelii*; 86). Even though these studies do not indicate whether AVT influences auditory processing, an additional study in Lincoln's sparrows (*Melospiza lincolnii*) demonstrates that sparrows alter the effort used in song production and show changes in AVT-immunoreactivity depending on the quality of songs to which they are exposed (87).

Evidence linking AVT to auditory processing also has been found in fish and frogs. AVT is present in brain areas responsible for auditory integration in the plainfin midshipman fish (*Porichthys notatus*), a species where males vocalize to attract mates and during nest defense (88, 89). Similarly, AVT is more abundant in auditory processing areas of male bullfrogs (*Rana catesbeiana*) in comparison to female bullfrogs (90). Because calls are only produced by males in this species, this sexual dimorphism may indicate that AVT plays a key role in assessing the salience of auditory signals that are being produced by conspecifics. Manipulations of the AVT system support this idea because AVT infusions change call properties of túngara frogs (*Physalaemus pustulosus*), possibly interfering with communication between the sender and the recipient (91, 92). Similarly, in the gray tree frog (*Hyla versicolor*), auditory cues shape the effects of AVT on calling behavior because AVT only alters call quality when a male is in close proximity to another male (93). Together, these results indicate that AVT modulates calling behavior in response to auditory cues and allows animals to produce calls that are appropriate for a particular social context.

Neural processing of auditory signals in mammals

The distribution of AVP and its receptors within brain areas associated with auditory processing has been studied in less detail in mammals, possibly because much of the AVP research has focused on rodents that use olfaction as the primary sense for social assessments. Although it is known that female, but not male, guinea pigs (*Cavia porcellus*) display AVP-ir staining in the auditory brainstem, the function of this sexual dimorphism is unknown (94). In the few rodent species where the functional importance of AVP on vocalization has been studied, a role for both V1a and V1b receptors has been identified. Female mice with a null mutation in the V1b receptor show decreased ultrasonic vocalizations during resident-intruder aggressive encounters (95). Although vocal production is affected, it is not known whether auditory processing also differs between control mice and mice with a null mutation in the V1b receptor. Anatomical studies using singing mice (*Scotinomys teguina* and *Scotinomys xerampelinus*) that vocalize in social contexts have identified the presence of V1a receptors in brain areas used for vocal production and auditory responses (49). In both species of singing mice, V1a receptors are expressed in the medial geniculate nucleus, which is the region of the thalamus that processes auditory information (49). In addition, both species display V1a receptor binding in two brain areas associated with vocalization, the periaqueductal gray and anterior hypothalamus, with more extensive binding in the more vocal species, *S. teguina* (49). These findings are intriguing because they implicate AVP in the give-and-take of information that occurs during social communication. In mammalian species where vocalizations are used in social situations, selection may favor a role for AVP in modulating these signals.

Although the effects of central AVP on auditory processing have not been studied in humans due to methodological limitations, human genetic variation in V1a receptor haplotypes has been linked with auditory processing and communication. The number of repeats in the RS3 microsatellite marker for the V1a receptor has been positively linked with prepulse inhibition, a startle response that is suppressed in individuals with schizophrenia and other disorders of social communication (96, 97). This phenotype has been linked more closely to auditory communication in studies examining the relationship between V1a receptor variation and an individual's musical aptitude. In families containing either a professional or active amateur musician, the ability to detect structural changes in abstract sounds is linked with RS1 and RS3 microsatellite markers for the V1a receptor (98). Interest in music, another marker of interest in listening to auditory cues, is also associated with V1a receptor distribution in humans: the RS1 haplotype is most strongly associated with listening to music regularly at the present time and the RS3 haplotype is most prominently associated with listening to music regularly throughout the lifespan (99). Although studies using viral vectors to manipulate V1a receptor activity cannot be performed in humans, these correlational results indicate that central processing of auditory signals in humans is modulated by AVP and its receptors.

AVP as a hormone and acoustic processing in the ear

In addition to affecting neural processing of auditory signals, AVP in the bloodstream also affects hearing. Peripheral injections of AVP in rats create short-term hearing impairment as measured by evoked auditory brainstem responses to sound (100). In the inner ear, AVP also alters hearing by binding to V2 receptors and reducing the number of aquaporin-2 membrane channels, channels that increase water permeability (101). AVP binding to V2 receptors thus leads to hearing impairment through the accumulation of excess water in the membrane of the endolymphatic sac (102, 103). Because insulin interacts with the signaling pathway that regulates V2 receptors, disruption in this pathway in diabetic patients has been linked to hearing loss in humans (103). Similarly, excess endolymphatic fluid due to excess plasma AVP levels or V2 receptors in the inner ear produces the symptoms of Menière's disease, a disorder in humans that results in intermittent hearing loss, vertigo, and tinnitus (104–106). Therefore, release of AVP into the bloodstream in response to social or stressful stimuli may have a secondary effect of reducing sensitivity to sound cues.

Although excess AVP in the bloodstream may hamper the ability to detect auditory cues, smaller elevations in plasma AVP may increase recall of auditory information due to increased arousal. Peripheral administration of AVP can enhance performance in learning tasks due to elevation of heart rate, blood pressure, and other sympathetic nervous system activity [reviewed in Ref. (107)]. Administration of AVP via intranasal infusions in healthy, non-depressed elderly humans increases recall of auditory information, possibly due to this increase in arousal (108). Natural variation in AVP in humans also is correlated with performance on auditory learning tasks. In humans with major depression, plasma concentrations of AVP correlate positively with auditory memory as measured by a 10-WLLA test for audio recall (109). Diabetes insipidus, a disorder characterized by a mutation in the vasopressin prohormone that leads to lower plasma levels of AVP, is associated with decreased performance on a test of verbal memory in humans (110). Although elevations of AVP in the bloodstream can lower detection of auditory signals, once those signals are detected, AVP can enhance recall of information provided in those signals.

AVP AND PROCESSING OF TASTE INFORMATION

AVP and conditioned taste avoidance

A key to understanding the evolution of taste aversion in mammals and its link to social behavior has been provided by studies of gustatory learning in *Caenorhabditis elegans*, a nematode that utilizes chemoattraction to locate low salt environments (111). Modulation of this ability occurs through the action of a vasopressin/oxytocin-like neuropeptide, nematocin. When exposed to preferred low salt environments in the absence of food, worms with a null mutation for nematocin or its receptor are not able to learn to avoid these environments (111). Individuals lacking nematocin or its receptors also exhibit deficiencies in male mating behavior and other forms of social behavior due to altered activity of mechanosensory neurons (112). These findings implicate the ancient neuropeptide, nematocin, in the integration of sensory input into complex motor output in the model organism *C. elegans*. This link between AVP, taste, and social behavior seems to be preserved in more complex organisms like birds and mammals. In the zebra finch (*Taenioypygia guttata*), intraseptal infusion of a V1 antagonist reduces gregariousness and increases the latency to feed in the presence of a novel stimulus (113). However, in mammals, it is unclear whether the effects of AVP on taste also modify social behaviors.

Arginine vasopressin within the bloodstream may alter the processing of taste in mammals through a mechanism similar to the one described above for auditory learning. By altering arousal through activation of the sympathetic nervous system, AVP improves an animal's ability to learn to avoid an aversive stimulus. In rats, taste aversion to saccharine lasts longer if administration of desglycinamide-lysine vasopressin occurs prior to pairing of the taste of saccharine with nausea induced by injections of LiCl (114). Other studies, however, have demonstrated the opposite relationship with AVP injections leading to faster extinction of learned responses. The timing of AVP administration appears to be critical because the learned association disappears more rapidly if AVP is administered after the acquisition process, regardless of whether the AVP is administered peripherally or centrally (115–117). However, dosage of AVP does play a critical role because high doses are capable of inducing taste aversion without administration of LiCl following consumption of a sucrose solution (117). Although peripheral AVP injections produce similar effects as central AVP infusions, this effect still seems to result in part from the release of AVP from the neurons of the PVN. AVP is released in the PVN during extinction of taste avoidance responses in rats that have not been deprived of water as part of the testing protocol (118). Because radioimmunoassay shows no changes in AVP content in brain areas that have been associated with conditioned taste avoidance such as the medial septum, LS, insular cortex, or MA, this increase in AVP content in the PVN is most likely related to the osmoregulatory properties of AVP in the PVN (118). However, future studies may clarify the role of neural AVP in regulating taste aversion. Taken together, these data indicate that AVP can either improve sensory learning or hasten extinction of learned responses depending on the timing of AVP release.

AVP and modulation of taste

One molecular mechanism that AVP may use to modify taste is through modulation of the activity of epithelial sodium ion channels (ENaCs) that regulate salty and sour tastes [**Figure 2**; (119)]. ENaCs are found in the renal collecting duct, urinary

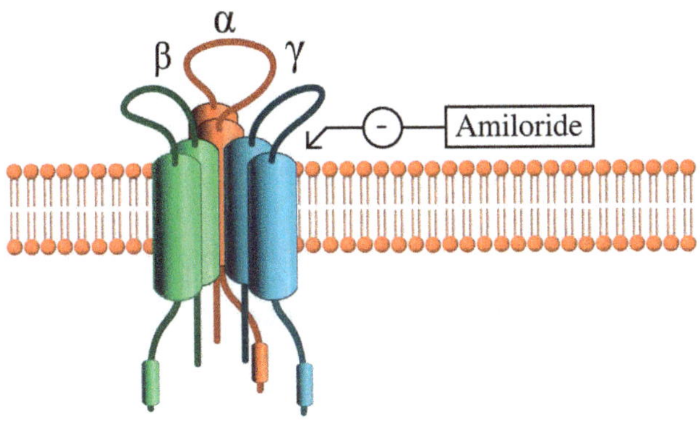

FIGURE 2 | Epithelial Na+ channel structure. ENaCs are composed of three subunits: α, β, and γ, and transport salt in a variety of epithelial tissues in the body. The α subunit alone is capable of functioning as a sodium transporter, but the addition of β and γ subunits increase the efficiency of this process. Sodium transport activity of ENaCs can be blocked with amiloride or enhanced with AVP.

bladder, lung, and taste buds and consist of three subunits that form a pore that selectively permits sodium to cross the membrane [reviewed in Ref. (120)]. In fungiform taste cells of hamsters, AVP increases sodium ion currents in ENaCs, indicating that the threshold for stimulation of these cells is being lowered (121). Therefore, AVP in the bloodstream may increase sensitivity to salty or sour tastes through its action on the ENaCs in taste cells. Under conditions where blood volume is low, this response may be part of a homeostatic mechanism to increase water retention in the blood by enhancing the palatability and consumption of salty food (121, 122). Although high doses of AVP appear to inhibit salt intake by making animals feel ill, central administration of lower doses of AVP stimulate salt intake whereas V_1 receptor antagonists inhibit salt intake (123). At the neural level, ENaCs also appear to be involved in regulating salt intake because they are co-localized with AVP in the magnocellular neurons of the SON and PVN, cells that assist with osmoregulation (124). Interestingly, these neural sodium channels are similar to ENaCs of the tongue in that both exhibit sensitivity to amiloride, a potassium-sparing diuretic that inhibits taste responses (124). In the brain, ENaCs may act as sensors of salt concentrations on the cells of the PVN and SON and lead to alterations in neural firing rates in response to fluctuations in salt concentration in the cerebrospinal fluid (124). Although it is unknown how ENaC activation by AVP may alter complex social behavior in mammals, these data indicate that behavioral responses that lead to release of AVP from the PVN and SON may also increase sensitivity to taste.

Disruption of taste sensitivity may be an important clue in diagnosing diseases that are accompanied by AVP dysregulation, such as syndrome of inappropriate ADH secretion (SIADH) (81, 125). In patients with SIADH related to lung cancer, the excess AVP alters taste perception (81, 126, 127). In patients with low serum sodium levels due to the effects of AVP on blood osmolality, correction of these levels led to improvement of taste function (81, 126, 127).

AVP AND VISUAL PROCESSING

Although visual information feeds into many brain areas that contain AVP, such as the BNST and LS (128, 129), the effect of AVP on processing of visual information has received little attention. Comparative analysis of visual opsin sequences in a variety of vertebrate species indicates that the visual opsins and AVP receptors are found in a shared genomic region that was duplicated twice during vertebrate evolution (130). However, the behavioral significance of the linkage between these sequences has not been examined. In chickens, a visual opsin has been co-localized with AVT in the neurons of the PVN, SON, and BNST (131). Although the function of opsins outside of the eye is unknown, these pigments may allow these neurons to respond to light and assist with coordination of circadian rhythmicity in behavior (131).

Connections between AVP and visual processing have been made in studies of visual learning, although these studies have focused more on AVP enhancement of sensory learning instead of AVP alteration of visual processing [e.g., Ref. (132, 133)]. In non-mammalian species, however, it has been demonstrated that AVT, a homolog of AVP, stimulates interest in visual cues associated with reproduction in rough skin newts (134). Additional studies in mammalian species that rely on visual cues during social interactions will help to clarify the role of AVP in visual processing.

CONCLUSION AND FUTURE DIRECTIONS

A social animal is bombarded with sensory cues throughout his or her lifetime. Even at birth, animals are usually attracted to the odors of their mothers but avoid unfamiliar odors. These and similar sensory cues are channeled through the central nervous system of the animal leading to output in the form of the social behaviors that are necessary for that individual's survival. In social rodents who heavily utilize their olfactory senses to distinguish threat from other environmental stimuli, AVP has been localized within the olfactory bulb itself and within the targets of the olfactory pathways. Therefore, as AVP neurons of the main and accessory olfactory systems are activated, they may modulate this olfactory input and direct it to the appropriate sites in the brain that regulate behavioral output. In addition, olfactory pathways also send information to the magnocellular neurons of the PVN and SON, which release AVP into the bloodstream. Additional research may clarify the degree of interplay between these two systems. The relationships between AVP in the olfactory system and other neurotransmitter systems and other sensory systems also should be explored in greater detail.

Although evidence also indicates that a relationship exists between AVP and other sensory modalities, these relationships have not been studied as extensively as the relationship between AVP and olfactory processing. Because most studies examining the role of AVP in sensory processing have been performed in rodents that use olfaction as the primary sense, other sensory modalities have received less attention. At this time, it is not known whether AVP in brain areas associated with mammalian visual, taste, or auditory processing shows the same level of plasticity in response to social or hormonal cues that shape behavior. It is also unknown whether manipulations of AVP can produce broad alterations in sensory processing in a variety of modalities in mammalian species with different social systems. How an animal is able to filter these social cues and make complex behavioral decisions needs to be explored in additional detail. However, it is clear that AVP modulates sensory processing through a variety of neural and hormonal pathways that are critical for the expression of species-typical social behavior.

Arginine vasopressin may be essential for integration of sensory input during complex forms of social behavior in mammals. As described earlier in this paper, fMRI has been used to assess neural activation in maternal rats presented with the threat of a male intruder (27). When a V1a antagonist is administered prior to exposure to the intruder, the gustatory cortex and olfactory areas of the brain show enhanced BOLD responses in females (27). This finding indicates that AVP is involved in regulating multiple sensory responses during complex social interactions, but should be explored under other social contexts and in additional species.

Studies using peripheral and central injections of AVP have demonstrated that the hormonal effects of AVP can shape gustatory, visual, and auditory learning through its effects on general levels of arousal. In addition, levels of AVP within the bloodstream can influence sensory processing in the ear and tongue through modulation of sodium channels. Within the ear, excess AVP has been associated with impaired hearing due to excess endolymph accumulation. In the tongue, AVP appears to modulate the activity of sodium channels known as ENaCs. Whether AVP shows similar ability to regulate visual signal transduction in a similar way has yet to be explored.

The apparent consequence of this fine-tuning of sensory input is that an animal is able to display appropriate social behavior in response to particular environmental stimuli. Animals with null mutations in vasopressin or its receptors demonstrate sensory deficits that appear to be potentially correlated with deficits in social behavior. In addition, the plasticity in AVP pathways during development that has been demonstrated in a variety of rodent species (2–4, 8, 135–137) may affect social behavior through alterations in the processing of sensory signals. However, the impact of developmental plasticity in AVP on sensory processing in multiple modalities has not yet been explored.

In humans, attempts have been made to link AVP with disorders that affect social behavior and involve sensory processing issues such as autism and schizophrenia [reviewed in Ref. (138)]. Because it is impossible to directly manipulate AVP or its receptors within specific brain areas in humans, the relationship between AVP and behavioral disorders has been assessed by correlating plasma AVP levels or V1a receptor promoter polymorphisms with behaviors associated with these disorders. Although the relationship between AVP and social behavior disorders has been difficult to establish in males, plasma levels of AVP have been linked to severity of psychosis in women with schizophrenia (139). Similarly, in girls with autism, plasma levels of AVP have been linked to the intensity of repetitive behaviors (140). Genetic linkages between AVP and the likelihood of developing a disorder of social behavior have also been identified in humans. A specific genetic polymorphism in the V1a receptor promoter was associated with increased susceptibility of psychopathology in children that had been exposed to war (141). The latter finding suggests that although certain V1a genotypes may predispose an individual to developing a disorder related to social behavior, exposure to environmental stressors also plays a role in the manifestation of the disorder. Therefore, it is possible that early social experiences may create life-long changes in the way that an individual perceives sensory cues in the surrounding world.

ACKNOWLEDGMENTS

We would like to thank C. Meredith, B. Craft, and two anonymous reviewers for their critical reading of an earlier draft of this manuscript. We also thank Jeremy Fancher for production of the figures. Funding for this work was provided by MJ Murdock Charitable Trust grants #2010181:JVZ:2/24/2011 and 2012224:JVZ:2/28/2013 to Janet K. Bester-Meredith.

REFERENCES

Caldwell HK, Lee H, Macbeth AH, Young WS III. Vasopressin: behav- ioral roles of an "original" neuropeptide. *Prog Neurobiol* (2008) 84(1):1–24. doi:10.1016/j.pneurobio.2007.10.007

Francis D, Young L, Meaney M, Insel T. Naturally occurring differences in maternal care are associated with the expression of oxytocin and vasopressin (V1a) receptors: gender differences. *J Neuroendocrinol* (2002) 14(5):349–53. doi:10.1046/j.0007-1331.2002.00776.x

Bester-Meredith J, Marler C. Vasopressin and the transmission of paternal behavior across generations in mated, cross-fostered *Peromyscus* mice. *Behav Neurosci* (2003) 117(3):455–63. doi:10.1037/0735-7044.117.3.455

Bester-Meredith J, Marler C. The association between male offspring aggres- sion and paternal and maternal behavior of *Peromyscus* mice. *Ethology* (2003) 109(10):797–808. doi:10.1046/j.0179-1613.2003.00917.x

Marler C, Bester-Meredith J, Trainor B. Paternal behavior and aggression: endocrine mechanisms and nongenomic transmission of behavior. *Adv Study Behav* (2003) 32:263–323. doi:10.1016/S0065-3454(03)01006-4

Cooper M, Karom M, Huhman K, Albers H. Repeated agonistic encoun- ters in hamsters modulate AVP V1a receptor binding. *Horm Behav* (2005) 48(5):545–51. doi:10.1016/j.yhbeh.2005.04.012

Frazier CRM, Trainor BC, Cravens CJ, Whitney TK, Marler CA. Paternal behavior influences development of aggression and vasopressin expression in male California mouse offspring. *Horm Behav* (2006) 50(5):699–707. doi:10.1016/j.yhbeh.2006.06.035

Bester-Meredith JK, Marler CA. Social experience during development and female offspring aggression in *Peromyscus* mice. *Ethology* (2007) 113(9):889–900. doi:10.1111/j.1439-0310.2007.01393.x

Bester-Meredith JK, Marler CA. Naturally occurring variation in vasopressin immunoreactivity is associated with maternal behavior in female *Peromyscus* mice. *Brain Behav Evol* (2012) 80(4):244–53. doi:10.1159/000341899

Haller J, Harold G, Sandi C, Neumann ID. Effects of adverse early-life events on aggression and anti-social behaviours in animals and humans. *J Neuroendocrinol* (2014) 26(10):724–38. doi:10.1111/jne.12182

Zhou L, Blaustein J, Devries G. Distribution of androgen receptor immunore- activity in vasopressin-immunoreactive and oxytocin-immunoreactive neu- rons in the male-rat brain. *Endocrinology* (1994) 134(6):2622–7. doi:10.1210/ en.134.6.2622

Devries G, Buijs R, Swaab D. Ontogeny of the vasopressinergic neurons of the suprachiasmatic nucleus and their extrahypothalamic projections in the rat- brain – presence of a sex difference in the lateral septum. *Brain Res* (1981) 218(1–2):67–78. doi:10.1016/0006-8993(81)90989-6

Wang Z. Species-differences in the vasopressin-immunoreactive pathways in the bed nucleus of the stria terminalis and medial amygdaloid nucleus in Prairie voles (*Microtus ochrogaster*) and Meadow voles (*Micro- tus pennsylvanicus*). *Behav Neurosci* (1995) 109(2):305–11. doi:10.1037/0735- 7044.109.2.305

Otero-Garcia M, Martin-Sanchez A, Fortes-Marco L, Martinez-Ricos J, Agustin-Pavon C, Lanuza E, et al. Extending the socio-sexual brain: arginine- vasopressin immunoreactive circuits in the telencephalon of mice. *Brain Struct Funct* (2014) 219(3):1055–81. doi:10.1007/s00429-013-0553-3

Devries G, Buijs R, Vanleeuwen F, Caffe A, Swaab D. The vasopressinergic innervation of the brain in normal and castrated rats. *J Comp Neurol* (1985) 233(2):236–54. doi:10.1002/cne.902330206

Devries G, Duetz W, Buijs R, Vanheerikhuize J, Vreeburg J. Effects of andro- gens and estrogens on the vasopressin and oxytocin innervation of the adult-rat brain. *Brain Res* (1986) 399(2):296–302. doi:10.1016/0006-8993(86)91519-2

Vanleeuwen F, Caffe A, Devries G. Vasopressin cells in the bed nucleus of the stria terminalis of the rat – sex-differences and the influence of androgens. *Brain Res* (1985) 325(1-2):391–4. doi:10.1016/0006-8993(85)90348-8

Kelly AM, Goodson JL. Functional significance of a phylogenetically wide- spread sexual dimorphism in vasotocin/vasopressin production. *Horm Behav* (2013) 64(5):840–6. doi:10.1016/j.yhbeh.2013.09.006

Rose J, Moore F. Behavioral neuroendocrinology of vasotocin and vasopressin and the sensorimotor processing hypothesis. *Front Neuroendocrinol* (2002) 23(4):317–41. doi:10.1016/S0091-3022(02)00004-3

Lukas M, Neumann ID. Social preference and maternal defeat-induced social avoidance in virgin female rats: sex differences in involvement of brain oxy- tocin and vasopressin. *J Neurosci Methods* (2014) 234:101–7. doi:10.1016/j.jneumeth.2014.03.013

Starr-Phillips EJ, Beery AK. Natural variation in maternal care shapes adult social behavior in rats. *Dev Psychobiol* (2014) 56(5):1017–26. doi:10.1002/dev. 21182

Bosch OJ. Maternal aggression in rodents: brain oxytocin and vasopressin mediate pup defence. *Philos Trans R Soc B Biol Sci* (2013) 368(1631):20130085. doi:10.1098/rstb.2013.0085

Bosch OJ, Neumann ID. Both oxytocin and vasopressin are mediators of mater- nal care and aggression in rodents: from central release to sites of action. *Horm Behav* (2012) 61(3):293–303. doi:10.1016/j.yhbeh.2011.11.002

Kessler MS, Bosch OJ, Bunck M, Landgraf R, Neumann ID. Maternal care dif- fers in mice bred for high vs. low trait anxiety: impact of brain vasopressin and cross-fostering. *Soc Neurosci* (2011) 6(2):156–68. doi:10.1080/17470919.2010.495567

Bosch OJ, Pfoertsch J, Beiderbeck DI, Landgraf R, Neumann ID. Maternal behaviour is associated with vasopressin release in the medial preoptic area and bed nucleus of the stria terminalis in the rat. *J Neuroendocrinol* (2010) 22(5):420–9. doi:10.1111/j.1365-2826.2010.01984.x

Bosch OJ, Neumann ID. Vasopressin released within the central amygdala pro- motes maternal aggression. *Eur J Neurosci* (2010) 31(5):883–91. doi:10.1111/j.1460-9568.2010.07115.x

Caffrey MK, Nephew BC, Febo M. Central vasopressin V1a receptors modulate neural processing in mothers facing intruder threat to pups. *Neuropharmacol- ogy* (2010) 58(1):107–16. doi:10.1016/j.neuropharm.2009.06.023

Nephew BC, Bridges RS, Lovelock DF, Byrnes EM. Enhanced maternal aggres- sion and associated changes in neuropeptide gene expression in multiparous rats. *Behav Neurosci* (2009) 123(5):949–57. doi:10.1037/a0016734

Bosch OJ, Neumann ID. Brain vasopressin is an important regulator of mater- nal behavior independent of dams' trait anxiety. *Proc Natl Acad Sci U S A* (2008) 105(44):17139–44. doi:10.1073/pnas.0807412105

Nephew BC, Bridges RS. Central actions of arginine vasopressin and a V1a receptor antagonist on maternal aggression, maternal behavior, and grooming in lactating rats. *Pharmacol Biochem Behav* (2008) 91(1):77–83. doi:10.1016/j.pbb.2008.06.013

Luther J, Tasker J. Voltage-gated currents distinguish parvocellular from mag- nocellular neurones in the rat hypothalamic paraventricular nucleus. *J Physiol* (2000) 523(1):193–209. doi:10.1111/j.1469-7793.2000.t01-1-00193.x

Raggenbass M. Overview of cellular electrophysiological actions of vasopressin. *Eur J Pharmacol* (2008) 583(2–3):243–54. doi:10.1016/j.ejphar.2007.11.074

Nakamura K, Ono T, Fukuda M, Uwano T. Paraventricular neuron chemosen- sitivity and activity related to blood-pressure control in emotional behavior. *J Neurophysiol* (1992) 67(2):255–64.

Roper JA, O'Carroll A, Young WS III, Lolait SJ. The vasopressin Avpr1b receptor: molecular and pharmacological studies. *Stress* (2011) 14(1):98–115. doi:10.3109/10253890.2010.512376

Stevenson EL, Caldwell HK. The vasopressin 1b receptor and the neural reg- ulation of social behavior. *Horm Behav* (2012) 61(3):277–82. doi:10.1016/j. yhbeh.2011.11.009

Donaldson ZR, Young LJ. Oxytocin, vasopressin, and the neurogenetics of sociality. *Science* (2008) 322(5903):900–4. doi:10.1126/science.1158668

Keverne E, Curley J. Vasopressin, oxytocin and social behaviour. *Curr Opin Neurobiol* (2004) 14(6):777–83. doi:10.1016/j.conb.2004.10.006

Phelps SM. From endophenotypes to evolution: social attachment, sexual fidelity and the avpr1a locus. *Curr Opin Neurobiol* (2010) 20(6):795–802. doi:10.1016/j.conb.2010.09.002

Slusarz M, Gieldon A, Slusarz R, Ciarkowski J. Analysis of interactions responsi- ble for vasopressin binding to human neurohypophyseal hormone receptors – molecular dynamics study of the activated receptor-vasopressin-G(alpha) sys- tems. *J Pept Sci* (2006) 12(3):180–9. doi:10.1002/psc.714

Chini B, Manning M. Agonist selectivity in the oxytocin/vasopressin recep- tor family: new insights and challenges. *Biochem Soc Trans* (2007) 35:737–41. doi:10.1042/BST0350737

Bamshad M, Novak M, Devries G. Sex and species-differences in the vaso- pressin innervation of sexually naive and parental Prairie voles, *Microtus ochrogaster* and Meadow voles, *Microtus pennsylvanicus*. *J Neuroendocrinol* (1993) 5(3):247–55. doi:10.1111/j.1365-2826.1993.tb00480.x

Bester-Meredith J, Young L, Marler C. Species differences in paternal behav- ior and aggression in *Peromyscus* and their associations with vasopressin immunoreactivity and receptors. *Horm Behav* (1999) 36(1):25–38. doi:10. 1006/hbeh.1999.1522

Fink S, Excoffier L, Heckel G. Mammalian monogamy is not controlled by a single gene. *Proc Natl Acad Sci U S A* (2006) 103(29):10956–60. doi:10.1073/pnas.0602380103

Turner LM, Young AR, Roempler H, Schoeneberg T, Phelps SM, Hoekstra HE. Monogamy evolves through multiple mechanisms: evidence from V1aR in deer mice. *Mol Biol Evol* (2010) 27(6):1269–78. doi:10.1093/molbev/msq013

Insel T, Wang Z, Ferris C. Patterns of brain vasopressin receptor distribution associated with social-organization in microtine rodents. *J Neurosci* (1994) 14(9):5381–92.

Young LJ, Winslow JT, Nilsen R, Insel TR. Species differences in V(1)a recep- tor gene expression in monogamous and nonmonogamous voles: behavioral consequences. *Behav Neurosci* (1997) 111(3):599–605. doi:10.1037/0735-7044. 111.3.599

Barrett CE, Keebaugh AC, Ahern TH, Bass CE, Terwilliger EF, Young LJ. Vari- ation in vasopressin receptor (Avpr1 a) expression creates diversity in behav- iors related to monogamy in prairie voles. *Horm Behav* (2013) 63(3):518–26. doi:10.1016/j.yhbeh.2013.01.005

Beery AK, Lacey EA, Francis DD. Oxytocin and vasopressin receptor distributions in a solitary and a social species of tuco-tuco (*Ctenomys haigi* and *Ctenomys sociabilis*). *J Comp Neurol* (2008) 507(6):1847–59. doi:10.1002/cne.21638

Campbell P, Ophir AG, Phelps SM. Central vasopressin and oxytocin recep- tor distributions in two species of singing mice. *J Comp Neurol* (2009) 516(4):321–33. doi:10.1002/cne.22116

Wacker DW, Engelmann M, Tobin VA, Meddle SL, Ludwig M. Vasopressin and social odor processing in the olfactory bulb and anterior olfactory nucleus. *Ann N Y Acad Sci* (2011) 1220:106–16. doi:10.1111/j.1749-6632.2010.05885.x

Wacker DW, Tobin VA, Noack J, Bishop VR, Duszkiewicz AJ, Engelmann M, et al. Expression of early growth response protein 1 in vasopressin neurones of the rat anterior olfactory nucleus following social odour exposure. *J Physiol* (2010) 588(23):4705–17. doi:10.1113/jphysiol.2010.196139

Wacker DW, Ludwig M. Vasopressin, oxytocin, and social odor recognition. *Horm Behav* (2012) 61(3):259–65. doi:10.1016/j.yhbeh.2011.08.014

Dass SAH, Vyas A. Copulation or sensory cues from the female augment Fos expression in arginine vasopressin neurons of the posterodorsal medial amyg- dala of male rats. *Front Zool* (2014) 11:42. doi:10.1186/1742-9994-11-42

Tobin VA, Hashimoto H, Wacker DW, Takayanagi Y, Langnaese K, Caquineau C, et al. An intrinsic vasopressin system in the olfactory bulb is involved in social recognition. *Nature* (2010) 464(7287):413–U110. doi:10.1038/nature08826

Bader A, Klein B, Breer H, Strotmann J. Connectivity from OR37 expressing olfactory sensory neurons to distinct cell types in the hypothalamus. *Front Neural Circuits* (2012) 6:84. doi:10.3389/fncir.2012.00084

Vaccari C, Lolait S, Ostrowski N. Comparative distribution of vasopressin V1b and oxytocin receptor messenger ribonucleic acids in brain. *Endocrinology* (1998) 139(12):5015–33. doi:10.1210/en.139.12.5015

Hernando F, Schoots O, Lolait S, Burbach J. Immunohistochemical localization of the vasopressin V1b receptor in the rat brain and pituitary gland: anatomical support for its involvement in the central effects of vasopressin. *Endocrinology* (2001) 142(4):1659–68. doi:10.1210/endo.142.4.8067

Levasseur G, Baly C, Grebert D, Durieux D, Salesse R, Caillol M. Anatomical and functional evidence for a role of arginine-vasopressin (AVP) in rat olfac- tory epithelium cells. *Eur J Neurosci* (2004) 20(3):658–70. doi:10.1111/j.1460-9568.2004.03516.x

Vertes R. Differential projections of the infralimbic and prelimbic cortex in the rat. *Synapse* (2004) 51(1):32–58. doi:10.1002/syn.10279

Irvin R, Szot P, Dorsa D, Potegal M, Ferris C. Vasopressin in the septal area of the golden-hamster controls scent marking and grooming. *Physiol Behav* (1990) 48(5):693–9. doi:10.1016/0031-9384(90)90213-N

Albers H, Ferris C. Role of the flank gland in vasopressin induced scent mark- ing behavior in the hamster. *Brain Res Bull* (1986) 17(3):387–9. doi:10.1016/ 0361-9230(86)90242-X

Huhman K, Albers H. Estradiol increases the behavioral-response to arginine- vasopressin (Avp) in the medial preoptic-anterior hypothalamus. *Peptides* (1993) 14(5):1049–54. doi:10.1016/0196-9781(93)90085-U

Been LE, Petrulis A. Lesions of the posterior bed nucleus of the stria terminalis eliminate opposite-sex odor preference and delay copulation in male Syrian hamsters: role of odor volatility and sexual experience. *Eur J Neurosci* (2010) 32(3):483–93. doi:10.1111/j.1460-9568.2010.07277.x

Martinez LA, Petrulis A. The medial preoptic area is necessary for sexual odor preference, but not sexual solicitation, in female Syrian hamsters. *Horm Behav* (2013) 63(4):606–14. doi:10.1016/j.yhbeh.2013.02.003

Gutzler SJ, Karom M, Erwin WD, Albers HE. Arginine-vasopressin and the regulation of aggression in female Syrian hamsters (*Mesocricetus auratus*). *Eur J Neurosci* (2010) 31(9):1655–63. doi:10.1111/j.1460-9568.2010.07190.x

Bielsky I, Young L. Oxytocin, vasopressin, and social recognition in mammals. *Peptides* (2004) 25(9):1565–74. doi:10.1016/j.peptides.2004.05.019

Ferguson J, Young L, Insel T. The neuroendocrine basis of social recognition. *Front Neuroendocrinol* (2002) 23(2):200–24. doi:10.1006/frne.2002.0229

Albers HE. The regulation of social recognition, social communication and aggression: vasopressin in the social behavior neural network. *Horm Behav* (2012) 61(3):283–92. doi:10.1016/j.yhbeh.2011.10.007

Winslow J, Insel T. Neuroendocrine basis of social recognition. *Curr Opin Neu- robiol* (2004) 14(2):248–53. doi:10.1016/j.conb.2004.03.009

Dantzer R, Koob G, Bluthe R, Lemoal M. Septal vasopressin modulates social memory in male-rats. *Brain Res* (1988) 457(1):143–7. doi:10.1016/0006-8993(88)90066-2

Popik P, Wolterink G, Debrabander H, Vanree J. Neuropeptides related to [Arg8]vasopressin facilitates social recognition in rats. *Physiol Behav* (1991) 49(6):1031–5. doi:10.1016/0031-9384(91)90327-K

Dluzen D, Muraoka S, Engelmann M, Landgraf R. The effects of infusion of arginine vasopressin, oxytocin, or their antagonists into the olfactory bulb upon social recognition responses in male rats. *Peptides* (1998) 19(6):999–1005. doi:10.1016/S0196-9781(98)00047-3

Veenema AH, Bredewold R, De Vries GJ. Vasopressin regulates social recogni- tion in juvenile and adult rats of both sexes, but in sex- and age-specific ways. *Horm Behav* (2012) 61(1):50–6. doi:10.1016/j.yhbeh.2011.10.002

Clipperton-Allen AE, Lee AW, Reyes A, Devidze N, Phan A, Pfaff DW, et al. Oxytocin, vasopressin and estrogen receptor gene expression in relation to social recognition in female mice. *Physiol Behav* (2012) 105(4):915–24. doi:10.1016/j.physbeh.2011.10.025

Murgatroyd C. Epigenetic programming of neuroendocrine systems during early life. *Exp Physiol* (2014) 99(1):62–5. doi:10.1113/expphysiol.2013. 076141

Murray EK, Varnum MM, Fernandez JL, de Vries GJ, Forger NG. Effects of neonatal treatment with valproic acid on vasopressin immunoreactivity and olfactory behaviour in mice. *J Neuroendocrinol* (2011) 23(10):906–14. doi:10.1111/j.1365-2826.2011.02196.x

Wang Y, Li X, Li L, Fu Q. Vasopres sin in the medial amygdala is essential for social recognition in the mouse. *J Neurol Sci* (2013) 30(1):81–7.

Bielsky I, Hu S, Szegda K, Westphal H, Young L. Profound impairment in social recognition and reduction in anxiety-like behavior in vasopressin V1a receptor knockout mice. *Neuropsychopharmacology* (2004) 29(3):483–93. doi:10.1038/sj.npp.1300360

DeVito LM, Konigsberg R, Lykken C, Sauvage M, Young WS III, Eichen- baum H. Vasopressin 1b receptor knock-out impairs memory for temporal order. *J Neurosci* (2009) 29(9):2676–83. doi:10.1523/JNEUROSCI.5488-08. 2009

Bielsky I, Hu S, Ren X, Terwilliger E, Young L. The V1a vasopressin receptor is necessary and sufficient for normal social recognition: a gene replacement study. *Neuron* (2005) 47(4):503–13. doi:10.1016/j.neuron.2005.06.031

Wersinger SR, Caldwell HK, Martinez L, Gold P, Hu S, Young WS III. Vaso- pressin 1a receptor knockout mice have a subtle olfactory deficit but normal aggression. *Genes Brain Behav* (2007) 6(6):540–51. doi:10.1111/j.1601-183X. 2006.00281.x

Wersinger SR, Temple JL, Caldwell HK, Young WS III. Inactivation of the oxy- tocin and the vasopressin (Avp) 1b receptor genes, but not the Avp 1a receptor gene, differentially impairs the Bruce effect in laboratory mice (*Mus musculus*). *Endocrinology* (2008) 149(1):116–21. doi:10.1210/en.2007-1056

Arakawa H, Arakawa K, Deak T. Oxytocin and vasopressin in the medial amygdala differentially modulate approach and avoidance behavior toward illness-related social odor. *Neuroscience* (2010) 171(4):1141–51. doi:10.1016/j.neuroscience.2010.10.013

Lowrey EM, Tomaszycki ML. The formation and maintenance of social rela- tionships increases nonapeptide mRNA in zebra finches of both sexes. *Behav Neurosci* (2014) 128(1):61–70. doi:10.1037/a0035416

Goodson JL, Rinaldi J, Kelly AM. Vasotocin neurons in the bed nucleus of the stria terminalis preferentially process social information and exhibit properties that dichotomize courting and non-courting phenotypes. *Horm Behav* (2009) 55(1):197–202. doi:10.1016/j.yhbeh.2008.10.007

Maney DL, Goode CT, Wingfield JC. Intraventricular infusion of arginine vasotocin induces singing in a female songbird. *J Neuroendocrinol* (1997) 9(7):487–91. doi:10.1046/j.1365-2826.1997.00635.x

Sewall KB, Dankoski EC, Sockman KW. Song environment affects singing effort and vasotocin immunoreactivity in the forebrain of male Lincoln's sparrows. *Horm Behav* (2010) 58(3):544–53. doi:10.1016/j.yhbeh.2010.04.002

Goodson J, Bass A. Vasotocin innervation and modulation of vocal-acoustic circuitry in the teleost *Porichthys notatus*. *J Comp Neurol* (2000) 422(3):363–79. doi:10.1002/1096-9861(20000703)422:3<363::AID-CNE4>3.0.CO;2-8

Goodson J, Evans A, Bass A. Putative isotocin distributions in sonic fish: relation to vasotocin and vocal-acoustic circuitry. *J Comp Neurol* (2003) 462(1):1–14. doi:10.1002/cne.10679

Caruana DA, Alexander GM, Dudek SM. New insights into the regulation of synaptic plasticity from an unexpected place: hippocampal area CA2. *Learn Mem* (2012) 19(9):391–400. doi:10.1101/lm.025304.111

Kime NM, Whitney TK, Davis ES, Marler CA. Arginine vasotocin promotes calling behavior and call changes in male tungara frogs. *Brain Behav Evol* (2007) 69(4):254–65. doi:10.1159/000099613

Kime NM, Whitney TK, Ryan MJ, Rand AS, Marler CA. Treatment with arginine vasotocin alters mating calls and decreases call attractiveness in male tungara frogs. *Gen Comp Endocrinol* (2010) 165(2):221–8. doi:10.1016/j.ygcen.2009. 06.023

Trainor BC, Rouse KL, Marler CA. Arginine vasotocin interacts with the social environment to regulate advertisement calling in the gray treefrog (*Hyla versi- color*). *Brain Behav Evol* (2003) 61(4):165–71. doi:10.1159/000070700

Duboisdauphin M, Tribollet E, Dreifuss J. A sexually dimorphic vasopressin innervation of auditory pathways in the Guinea-Pig brain. *Brain Res* (1987) 437(1):151–6. doi:10.1016/0006-8993(87)91536-8

Scattoni ML, McFarlane HG, Zhodzishsky V, Caldwell HK, Young WS, Ricceri L, et al. Reduced ultrasonic vocalizations in vasopressin 1b knockout mice. *Behav Brain Res* (2008) 187(2):371–8. doi:10.1016/j.bbr.2007.09.034

Degerman E, Rauch U, Lindberg S,

Caye-Thomasen P, Hultgardh A, Magnusson M. Expression of insulin signalling components in the sensory epithelium of the human saccule. *Cell Tissue Res* (2013) 352(3):469–78. doi:10.1007/s00441- 013-1614-x

Parker JT, Rodriguez N, Lawal B, Delevan CJ, Bamshad M. Mating increases male's interest in other females: a cognitive study in socially monogamous prairie voles (*Microtus ochrogaster*). *Behav Processes* (2011) 88(2):127–34. doi:10.1016/j.beproc.2011.08.010

Lechner SG, Markworth S, Poole K, Smith ESJ, Lapatsina L, Frahm S, et al. The molecular and cellular identity of peripheral osmoreceptors. *Neuron* (2011) 69(2):332–44. doi:10.1016/j.neuron.2010.12.028

Jager M, Chiori R, Alie A, Dayraud C, Queinnec E, Manuel M. New insights on ctenophore neural anatomy: immunofluorescence study in *Pleurobrachia pileus* (Muller, 1776). *J Exp Zool B Mol Dev Evol* (2011) 316B(3):171–87. doi:10.1002/jez.b.21386

Naganuma H, Kawahara K, Tokumasu K, Satoh R, Okamoto M. Effects of arginine vasopressin on auditory brainstem response and cochlear morphol- ogy in rats. *Auris Nasus Larynx* (2014) 41(3):249–54. doi:10.1016/j.anl.2013. 12.004

Eckhard A, Gleiser C, Arnold H, Rask-Andersen H, Kumagami H, Mueller M, et al. Water channel proteins in the inner ear and their link to hear- ing impairment and deafness. *Mol Aspects Med* (2012) 33(5–6):612–37. doi:10.1016/j.mam.2012.06.004

Kumagami H, Loewenheim M, Beitz E, Wild K, Schwartz H, Yamashita K, et al. The effect of anti-diuretic hormone on the endolymphatic sac of the inner ear. *Pflugers Arch* (1998) 436(6):970–5. doi:10.1007/s004240050731

Takumida M, Kakigi A, Egami N, Nishioka R, Anniko M. Localization of aqua- porins 1, 2, and 3 and vasopressin type 2 receptor in the mouse inner ear. *Acta Otolaryngol* (2012) 132(8):807–13. doi:10.3109/00016489.2012.662718

Kitahara T, Doi K, Maekawa C, Kizawa K, Horii A, Kubo T, et al. Meniere's attacks occur in the inner ear with excessive vasopressin type-2 receptors. *J Neuroendocrinol* (2008) 20(12):1295–300. doi:10.1111/j.1365-2826.2008.01792.x

Aoki M, Hayashi H, Kuze B, Mizuta K, Ito Y. The association of the plasma vasopressin level during attacks wit h a prognosis of Meniere's disease. *Int J Audiol* (2010) 49(1):1–6. doi:10.3109/14992020903160850

Maekawa C, Kitahara T, Kizawa K, Okazaki S, Kamakura T, Horii A, et al. Expression and translocation of aquaporin-2 in the endolymphatic sac in patients with Meniere's disease. *J Neuroendocrinol* (2010) 22(11):1157–64. doi:10.1111/j.1365-2826.2010.02060.x

Croiset G, Nijsen M, Kamphuis P. Role of corticotropin-releasing factor, vaso- pressin and the autonomic nervous system in learning and memory. *Eur J Pharmacol* (2000) 405(1–3):225–34. doi:10.1016/S0014-2999(00)00556-2

Kline RJ, O'Connell LA, Hofmann HA, Holt GJ, Khan IA. The distribution of an AVT V1a receptor in the brain of a sex changing fish, Epinephelus adscensionis. *J Chem Neuroanat* (2011) 42(1):72–88. doi:10.1016/j.jchemneu.2011.06.005

Stern JE, Filosa JA. Bidirectional neuro-glial signaling modalities in the hypo- thalamus: role in neurohumoral regulation. *Auton Neurosci* (2013) 175(1- 2):51–60. doi:10.1016/j.autneu.2012.12.009

Zubrzycka M, Janecka A. Effect of tooth pulp and periaqueductal central gray electrical stimulation on beta-endorphin release into the fluid perfusing the cerebral ventricles in rats. *Brain Res* (2011) 1405:15–22. doi:10.1016/j.brainres. 2011.06.030

Beets I, Janssen T, Meelkop E, Temmerman L, Suetens N, Rademakers S, et al. Vasopressin/oxytocin-related signaling regulates gustatory associative learning in *C. elegans*. *Science* (2012) 338(6106):543–5. doi:10.1126/science. 1226860

Garrison JL, Macosko EZ, Bernstein S, Pokala N, Albrecht DR, Bargmann CI. Oxytocin/vasopressin-related peptides have an ancient role in reproductive behavior. *Science* (2012) 338(6106):540–3. doi:10.1126/science.1226201

Kelly AM, Kingsbury MA, Hoffbuhr K, Schrock SE, Waxman B, Kabelik D, et al. Vasotocin neurons and septal V-1a-like receptors potently modulate songbird flocking and responses to novelty. *Horm Behav* (2011) 60(1):12–21. doi:10.1016/j.yhbeh.2011.01.012

Vawter M, Green K. Effects of desglycinamide-lysine vasopressin on a condi- tioned taste-aversion in rats. *Physiol Behav* (1980) 25(6):851–4. doi:10.1016/ 0031-9384(80)90303-0

Hayes U, Chambers K. Central infusion of vasopressin in male rats acceler- ates extinction of conditioned taste avoidance induced by LiCl. *Brain Res Bull* (2002) 57(5):727–33. doi:10.1016/S0361-9230(02)00747-5

Hayes U, Chambers K. Peripheral vasopressin accelerates extinction of con- ditioned taste avoidance. *Physiol Behav* (2005) 84(1):147–56. doi:10.1016/j. physbeh.2004.11.001

Hayes U, Chambers K. High doses of vasopressin delay the onset of extinc- tion and strengthen acquisition of LiCl-induced conditioned taste avoidance. *Physiol Behav* (2005) 84(4):625–33. doi:10.1016/j.physbeh.2005.02.012

Brownson E, Brinton R, Chambers K. Vasopressin content in select brain regions during extinction of a conditioned taste aversion. *Brain Res Bull* (2002) 59(2):125–34. doi:10.1016/S0361-9230(02)00861-4

Okada Y, Miyamoto T, Sato T. Vasopressin increases frog gustatory neural responses elicited by NaCl and HCl. *Comp Biochem Physiol A Physiol* (1991) 100(3):693–6. doi:10.1016/0300-9629(91)90391-O

Snyder P. Minireview: regulation of epithelial Na+ channel trafficking. *Endocrinology* (2005) 146(12):5079–85. doi:10.1210/en.2005-0894

Gilbertson T, Roper S, Kinnamon S. Proton currents through amiloride- sensitive Na+ channels in isolated hamster taste cells - enhancement by vaso- pressin and camp. *Neuron* (1993) 10(5):931–42. doi:10.1016/0896-6273(93)90208-9

Greenwood MP, Greenwood M, Paton JFR, Murphy D. Salt appetite is reduced by a single experience of drinking hypertonic saline in the adult rat. *PLoS One* (2014) 9(8):e104802. doi:10.1371/journal.pone.0104802

Flynn F, Kirchner T, Clinton M. Brain vasopressin and sodium appetite. *Am J Physiol Regul Integr Comp Physiol* (2002) 282(4):R1236–44. doi:10.1152/ ajpregu.00181.2001

Teruyama R, Sakuraba M, Wilson LL, Wandrey NEJ, Armstrong WE. Epithelial Na+ sodium channels in magnocellular cells of the rat supraoptic and par- aventricular nuclei. *Am J Physiol Endocrinol Metab* (2012) 302(3):E273–85. doi:10.1152/ajpendo.00407.2011

Gewirtz JR, Bisognano JD. Catheter-based renal sympathetic denervation: a targeted approach to resistant hypertension. *Cardiol J* (2011) 18(1):97–102.

Pirodda A, Ferri GG, Raimondi MC, Borghi C. Diuretics in Meniere disease: a therapy or a potential cause of harm? *Med Hypotheses* (2011) 77(5):869–71. doi:10.1016/j.mehy.2011.07.060

Borraccia V, Sblano S, Carabellese F, De Sario R, Zefferino R, Vinci F. Stress-related temporary hearing loss-evaluation of bio-humoral parameters: forensic and criminological applications. *J Forensic Sci* (2012) 57(4):946–51. doi:10.1111/j.1556-4029.2012.02161.x

Ohkura S, FabreNys C, Broad K, Kendrick K. Sex hormones enhance the impact of male sensory cues on both primary and association cortical com- ponents of visual and olfactory processing pathways as well as in limbic and hypothalamic regions in female sheep. *Neuroscience* (1997) 80(1):285–97. doi:10.1016/S0306-4522(97)00103-6

Morin L, Blanchard J. Forebrain connections of the hamster intergeniculate leaflet: comparison with those of ventral lateral geniculate nucleus and retina. *Vis Neurosci* (1999) 16(6):1037–54. doi:10.1017/S0952523899166069

Lagman D, Daza DO, Widmark J, Abalo XM, Sundstrom G, Larhammar D. The vertebrate ancestral repertoire of visual opsins, transducin alpha subunits and oxytocin/vasopressin receptors was established by duplication of their shared genomic region in the two rounds of early vertebrate genome duplications. *BMC Evol Biol* (2013) 13:238. doi:10.1186/1471-2148-13-238

Ohuchi H, Yamashita T, Tomonari S, Fujita-Yanagibayashi S, Sakai K, Noji S, et al. A non-mammalian type opsin 5 functions dually in the photorecep- tive and non-photoreceptive organs of birds. *PLoS One* (2012) 7(2):e31534. doi:10.1371/journal.pone.0031534

Paban V, AlescioLautier B, Devigne C, SoumireuMourat B. Effects of arginine(8)-vasopressin administered at different times in the learning of an appetitive visual discriminative task in mice. *Behav Brain Res* (1997) 87(2):149–57. doi:10.1016/S0166-4328(96)02275-9

Jentsch J, Arguello P, Anzivino L. Null mutation of the arginine-vasopressin gene in rats slows attentional engagement and facilitates response accu- racy in a lateralized reaction time task. *Neuropsychopharmacology* (2003) 28(9):1597–605. doi:10.1038/sj.npp.1300194

Thompson R, Moore F. The effects of sex steroids and vasotocin on behav- ioral responses to visual and olfactory sexual stimuli in ovariectomized female roughskin newts. *Horm Behav* (2003) 44(4):311–8. doi:10.1016/S0018-506X(03)00161-2

Ferris C. Adolescent stress and neural plasticity in hamsters: a vasopressin- serotonin model of inappropriate aggressive behaviour. *Exp Physiol* (2000) 85:85S–90S. doi:10.1111/j.1469-445X.2000.tb00011.x

Bester-Meredith J, Marler C. Vasopressin and aggression in cross-fostered Cal- ifornia mice (*Peromyscus californicus*) and white-footed mice (*Peromyscus leu- copus*). *Horm Behav* (2001) 40(1):51–64. doi:10.1006/hbeh.2001.1666

Curley JP, Davidson S, Bateson P, Champagne FA. Social enrichment during postnatal development induces transgenerational effects on emotional and reproductive behavior in mice. *Front Behav Neurosci* (2009) 3:25. doi:10.3389/ neuro.08.025.2009

Francis SM, Sagar A, Levin-Decanini T, Liu W, Carter CS, Jacob S. Oxytocin and vasopressin systems in genetic syndromes and neurodevelopmental disorders. *Brain Res* (2014) 1580:199–218. doi:10.1016/j.brainres.2014.01.021

Rubin LH, Carter CS, Bishop JR, Pournajafi-Nazarloo H, Harris MSH, Hill SK, et al. Peripheral vasopressin but not oxytocin relates to severity of acute psychosis in women with acutely-ill untreated first-episode psychosis. *Schizophr Res* (2013) 146(1–3):138–43. doi:10.1016/j.schres.2013.01.019

Miller M, Bales KL, Taylor SL, Yoon J, Hostetler CM, Carter CS, et al. Oxy- tocin and vasopressin in children and adolescents with autism spectrum dis- orders: sex differences and associations with symptoms. *Autism Res* (2013) 6(2):91–102. doi:10.1002/aur.1270

Feldman R, Vengrober A, Ebstein RP. Affiliation buffers stress: cumulative genetic risk in oxytocin-vasopressin genes combines with early caregiving to predict PTSD in war-exposed young children. *Transl Psychiatry* (2014) 4:e370. doi:10.1038/tp.2014.6

15

Membrane-initiated non-genomic signaling by estrogens in the hypothalamus: cross-talk with glucocorticoids with implications for behavior

Jennifer Rainville[1], Kevin Pollard[2] and Nandini Vasudevan[1,2]*

[1] Department of Cell and Molecular Biology, Tulane University, New Orleans, LA, USA
[2] Neuroscience Program, Tulane University, New Orleans, LA, USA

Edited by:
Hubert Vaudry, University of Rouen, France

Reviewed by:
Aldo Lucion, Universidade Federal do Rio Grande do Sul, Brazil
Denise D. Belsham, University of Toronto, Canada

***Correspondence:**
Nandini Vasudevan, Department of Cell and Molecular Biology, Tulane University, 2000 Percival Stern Hall, New Orleans, LA 70118, USA
e-mail: nandini@tulane.edu

The estrogen receptor and glucocorticoid receptor are members of the nuclear receptor superfamily that can signal using both non-genomic and genomic transcriptional modes. Though genomic modes of signaling have been well characterized and several behaviors attributed to this signaling mechanism, the physiological significance of non-genomic modes of signaling has not been well understood. This has partly been due to the controversy regarding the identity of the membrane ER (mER) or membrane GR (mGR) that may mediate rapid, non-genomic signaling and the downstream signaling cascades that may result as a consequence of steroid ligands binding the mER or the mGR. Both estrogens and glucocorticoids exert a number of actions on the hypothalamus, including feedback. This review focuses on the various candidates for the mER or mGR in the hypothalamus and the contribution of non-genomic signaling to classical hypothalamically driven behaviors and changes in neuronal morphology. It also attempts to categorize some of the possible functions of non-genomic signaling at both the cellular level and at the organismal level that are relevant for behavior, including some behaviors that are regulated by both estrogens and glucocorticoids in a potentially synergistic manner. Lastly, it attempts to show that steroid signaling via non-genomic modes may provide the organism with rapid behavioral responses to stimuli.

Keywords: hypothalamus, spine density, membrane-initiated signaling, GPCR, estrogen receptor variants, aggression, lordosis, glucocorticoid receptor

GENOMIC AND NON-GENOMIC SIGNALING BY NUCLEAR RECEPTORS

Nuclear receptor ligands such as estrogen and glucocorticoids signal via both non-genomic and genomic pathways within cells. The genomic or transcriptional pathway is the best elucidated primarily due to the well-characterized nature of the estrogen receptor (ER)α and β and the glucocorticoid receptor (GR), all of which are members of the nuclear receptor superfamily. Once bound to their cognate ligands, these receptors act as ligand-activated transcription factors in the nucleus by binding to specific enhancer elements such as the estrogen response element (ERE) (1) and glucocorticoid response element (GRE) (2) in the promoters of genes. Both receptors have a modular structure, with a conserved DNA-binding domain, multiple transactivation domains, and a C-terminal ligand-binding domain (3, 4).

On the other hand, non-genomic signaling, first described by Szego and Davis in 1967, as the rapid increase in cAMP in the uterus occurred within 15 min of 17β-estradiol (17β-E) administration to ovariectomized mice (5). In the central nervous system (CNS), 17β-E was shown to rapidly depolarize pro-opiomelanocortin (POMC) hypothalamic neurons via Akt or protein kinase (PK) B, extracellular regulated kinase (ERK/MAPK), PKA, and PKC pathways (6, 7). In other tissues such as rat hippocampal neurons, phospho-cAMP response element binding protein (pCREB) increased within 1 h of 17β-E addition and this increase was blocked by inhibitors to both calmodulin kinase II (CamKII) and ERK pathways (8). In the case of corticosterone-mediated rapid actions, treatment of neurons with dexamethasone, a synthetic glucocorticoid, rapidly induced the nuclear localization of the GR (9, 10), an effect potentiated by the inhibition of p38MAPK (11). Extracts from rat hippocampal synaptoneurosomes showed a reduction in Akt and ERK phosphorylation within 30 min in response to pharmacological inhibition of the GR by RU-486 (12), suggesting that the classical nuclear receptor was required for non-genomic signaling in the hippocampus. Apart from kinase activation, dexamethasone-mediated negative feedback at the corticotropin releasing hormone (CRH) neuron was also rapid, consisting of suppression of the excitatory drive to the CRH neuron, mediated by endocannabinoids acting as a retrograde messenger to the presynaptic glutamatergic neuron (13), an effect mimicked with a membrane-limited dexamethasone conjugated to bovine serum albumin (Dex-BSA) (13). Hence, non-genomic signaling by steroid hormones is extra-nuclear signaling that is initiated by the endogenous ligand within minutes, in contrast to the hours required to detect transcriptionally regulated proteins.

Central to this concept of non-genomic signaling that is typically demonstrated by the use of membrane-limited conjugates

(14), is the idea of a receptor that initiates such signaling from the plasma membrane. However, with the exception of the membrane progesterone receptors (mPRs) that belong to the progestin and adipoQ receptor (PAQR) family, the identity of the membrane ER (mER) and membrane GR (mGR) has remained elusive (15). This review aims to describe the current candidates for the mER and the mGR that mediate rapid non-genomic signaling from the plasma cell membrane as well as focus on rapid actions that are relevant for hypothalamically driven behaviors that are dependent on estrogens but that have a glucocorticoid-regulated component. We concentrate on the hypothalamus since this is a classically steroid-responsive area of the brain and is critical for several estrogen-dependent behaviors (16). For more general reviews on rapid actions of estrogens and glucocorticoids in the CNS, including tools that are typically used to elucidate membrane-initiated non-genomic effects, the reader is referred to (7, 14, 17–19).

THE MEMBRANE ER AND GR

In the CNS, both ^{3}H-labeled 17β-E (20) and a ^{125}I-labeled membrane-impermeant conjugate where 17β-E is attached to bovine serum albumin (E2-BSA) (21) showed relatively high affinity binding to rat plasma membranes, suggesting the presence of a mER. What is a good definition for a mER or mGR? Previously, Micevych et al. (22) have suggested that ICI 182,780 antagonism, stereospecific 17β-E binding and sequence homology to the ERα and ERβ should be considered pre-requisites for a protein to be termed a mER. We propose, given the off-target effects of ICI 182,780 (23) that the definition of the mER or mGR be modified slightly to consider proteins capable of specific binding to 17β-E or to dexamethasone (in the case of the mGR), presence at/near the plasma membrane and signaling from the membrane. It should be noted that this definition would exclude the binding of proteins to 17α-E, an estrogen often used in studies of as an inactive isomer of 17β-estradiol, but that recently has been shown to increase neurogenesis and to mediate neuroprotection (24). Most studies described below show evidence of the candidate mER at the plasma membrane and its ability to rapidly within minutes modulate rapid signaling pathways such as kinase regulation or calcium flux. A few studies also demonstrate the regulation of the candidate ER at the membrane.

ERα AS THE mER

As we will focus on outputs dependent on the hypothalamus in this review, we will initially discuss the nuclear classical ERα as a candidate mER because (a) this is the most abundant ER isoform in the medial preoptic area (mPOA), ventromedial hypothalamus (VMH), and arcuate nucleus (ARH) (25–27) and (b) loss of ERα in the hypothalamus abrogated hypothalamically driven lordosis behavior in females (28) and aggressive behavior in males (29). A number of studies using 17β-E binding, electron microscopy, immunocytochemistry, and western blotting have examined the idea that a small percentage (3–5%) of the total pool of the classical ERα is present on the plasma membrane (30). Consistent with this idea, immunocytochemistry using minimal fixation in both the breast cancer MCF-7 cell line (31) and anterior pituitary GH3 cell line (32), revealed ERα at the membrane in caveolae in some, but not all cells. MCF-7 cells with ERα at the plasma membrane showed increased phospho-ERK (pERK) within 10 min of application of either 17β-E or a membrane-limited E2-peroxidase conjugate (33). In the CNS, ERα was localized to the dendrites and axon terminals in the guinea pig hypothalamus (34), while ERα was detected in axon terminals, dendritic spines, as well as in astrocytes in the CA1 using immuno-electron microscopy in the proestrous female rat (35). In the dorsal CA1 from the female rat, ERα was present in synaptic vesicles in the axon of some GABAergic basket cells; 17β-E moved these ERα-containing vesicles toward synapses within 24 h (36). In addition, some proportion of this extra-nuclear ERα at synaptosomes and vesicles was phosphorylated though the function of phosphorylation in localization of the ERα remains unknown (37). In hypothalamic neurons and astrocytes obtained from both male and female rats, a full-length 66 kDa form of the ERα and a 52 kDa variant has been detected using surface biotinylation and immunocytochemistry (38, 39). These studies demonstrate that the nuclear ERα is present at the plasma membrane in many cell types, including the hypothalamus.

TARGETING OF ERα TO THE PLASMA MEMBRANE

Though hydropathicity analysis shows that ERα may have a potential trans-membrane domain (38), the idea that ERα requires a membrane protein to tether it to the plasma membrane has been cemented primarily by the discovery of caveolin proteins that can anchor the ERα in lipid rafts and caveolae. Caveolin proteins are highly conserved structural proteins that are necessary and sufficient for the existence of caveolae, a subset of lipid rafts (40) that comprise a restricted compartment for signaling molecules associated with the plasma membrane. Initially, ERα was reported to interact with caveolin 1 (Cav-1) in MCF-7 and vascular smooth muscle cells (VSMC) (41). The caveolins in turn act as adaptor proteins to couple ERα selectively to either other proteins such as the metabotrophic glutamate receptors (mGluR) or to processes such as palmitoylation. In the hippocampus of the female rat, Cav-1 interacted with mGluR1a so that 17β-E activated downstream $G\alpha_q$ and ERK signaling. This, in turn, increased pCREB activation within 5 min of 17β-E application (42). Hence, inhibitors to phospholipase C (PLC) and ERK and mGluR1a as well as a dominant negative Cav-1 mutant decreased pCREB activation (42). On the other hand, Cav-3 tethered ERα in hippocampal neurons to mGluR2/3; this pathway activated $G\alpha_i$ signaling, leading to the inhibition of PKA and the subsequent downregulation of pCREB (42). Hence, the type of caveolin dictated the final divergent pCREB response though the physiological conditions wherein ERα may bind to Cav-1 versus Cav-3 are unknown. In hypothalamic astrocytes, the coupling of ERα to mGluR1a resulted in an increase of calcium within 2 min of 17β-E application; this was blocked both by the ERα and ERβ antagonist, ICI 182,780 and by the mGluR1a antagonist LY 367385 (43). In striatal neurons, Cav-1 facilitated the tethering of ERα to mGluR5 and subsequent $G\alpha_q$ signaling (44). Hence, caveolins may not only tether ERs into caveolae in the plasma membrane in different cell types but also subserve tissue-specific signaling to specific Gα subunits by co-opting different mGluR partners. The coupling of ERα to mGluRs may allow downstream signaling to be potentiated by rendering it sensitive to two ligands, i.e., 17β-E for the ER and glutamate for the mGluR. This is supported by the data that in hypothalamic astrocytes, glutamate, and 17β-E combined elicited greater Ca^{+2} increases than either ligand alone (43).

In addition to the role that mGluRs play in linking ERα to Gα proteins, ERα can also directly bind Gα subunits. 17β-E inhibited cAMP production within 5 min of addition to GT1–7 immortalized GnRH neurons via ERα that is physically tethered to $G\alpha_{i3}$ (45) protein that can be detected in co-immunoprecipitation experiments. Interestingly, addition of 17β-E decreased the amount of membrane-associated $G\alpha_{i3}$ and this decrease was blocked by the ER antagonist ICI 182,780 suggesting control of the signaling cascade by the ligand, similar to classical G-protein coupled receptors (GPCRs) (45). Though ERα has been demonstrated to tether to $G\alpha_i$ in the caveolae of endothelial cells to increase the activity of nitric oxide synthase (46), this mode of regulation of nitric oxide synthase by 17β-E has not been shown in the CNS.

Apart from serving as adaptors, the binding of caveolins to the ER also increases palmitoylation of the ER, a process by which palmitate, a C16 fatty acid is added to an internal cysteine via a thioester bond. In the human ERα, a canonical palmitoylation site exists at the cysteine amino acid residue at position 447 (C447); the corresponding site in the mouse ERα is the C451 (31). Mutant ERα where the C447 site was mutated to alanine (C447A) did not bind Cav-1, was not localized at the membrane in HeLa cells and showed decreased pERK activation in response to a 10-min application of 17β-E (47). Additionally, when a non-classical palmitoylation site, S522, in the ERα was mutated, localization at the plasma membrane and Cav-1 binding to ERα was decreased (48) in Chinese hamster ovary (CHO) cells. This mutant also decreased the ability of 17β-E to increase pCREB in hippocampal neurons from the female rat (42). Other binding partners for the ERα also lead to increases in palmitoylation and subsequent membrane localization. For example, the amino acid residue cysteine at position 451 of the mouse ERα also binds the heat-shock protein 27 (hsp27), which increased the rate of palmitoylation at this site. Therefore, siRNA to hsp27 decreased palmitoylation with subsequent decrease of ERα at the plasma membrane and decreased phospho-Akt (pAkt) normally induced by a 10 min application of 17β-E (49). The C-terminal of mouse ERα (Leu512–514) is important in ERα dimerization at the plasma membrane; mutation of these residues decreased pAkt and cAMP generation within 5 min of 17β-E addition and decreased the activation of both $G\alpha_s$ and $G\alpha_q$ subunits in the CHO cell line (50) (**Figure 1**). In the CNS, it is unknown if the ERα at the membrane exists as dimers and if these dimers use caveolin proteins as adaptors. It is also unclear if caveolin binding to the ERα precedes greater palmitoylation since ERα mutations that destroy the interaction with caveolin also destroy palmitoylation. Recently, E2-BSA has been shown to transcriptionally upregulate Cav-1 via a PI3K and ERK pathway within 12 h in endothelial cells (51). Hence, 17β-E may increase non-genomic signaling both by increasing the palmitoylation of ERα within rapid time frames and within longer time frames via the transcriptional upregulation of Cav-1.

REGULATION OF ERα AT THE MEMBRANE BY 17β-E

Similar to the tissue specificity shown by ERα-mediated rapid, non-genomic signaling, ERα at the membrane is also regulated by 17β-E in both temporal and tissue-specific manner. In hypothalamic astrocytes (38) and neurons (39) and in a hypothalamic cell line, mHypoE-38 (52), 17β-E increased the amount of both the 52 and 66 kDa mER in the cell membrane within 30 min. This increase of mERα at the plasma membrane can be blocked by ICI 182,780 and the mGluR1a antagonist LY 367385 but does not occur with E2-BSA, suggesting that this is an internal, non-membrane-initiated rapid effect that is dependent on the mGluR1a receptor. In contrast, in MCF-7 cells, 17β-E decreased Cav-1 within 8 h, thus decreasing the amount of ERα at the membrane. Similarly, 17β-E

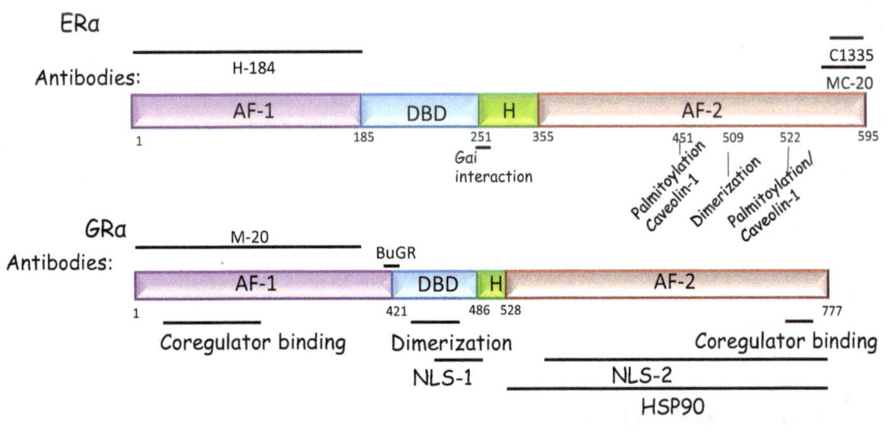

FIGURE 1 | Domain structure of the ERα and the GRα. ERα and GRα are classical intracellular nuclear receptors but may also be present on the plasma membrane. Both receptors have a N-terminal AF-1 domain, a central DNA binding domain, a hinge domain (H), and a C-terminal AF-2 domain, required to bind ligand. ERα: the antibodies most commonly used to detect ERα are the H184 (Santa Cruz Biotechnology, TX, USA) antibody raised to the N-terminal domain and the MC-20 (Santa Cruz Biotechnology, TX, USA) and C1335 (Upstate Biotechnology, NY, USA) raised to the C-terminal domain. In addition, the sites that may tether the ERα to the plasma membrane are marked. These are residues required for caveolin or $G\alpha_i$ binding or residues that are palmitoylated or required for dimerization at the membrane. GRα: the antibodies most commonly used to detect GRα are the BuGR antibody (Abcam Inc., MA, USA) and the M-20 (Santa Cruz Biotechnology, TX, USA) antibody, directed to the N-terminal domain. The NLS refers to the nuclear localization signal since nuclear localization of this receptor can occur rapidly and is a non-genomic effect.

treatment of hippocampal slices from female rats removed ERα from the synaptosomal plasma membrane by depalmitoylation within 20 min (37). In CHO cells, palmitate incorporation into ERα and association with Cav-1 decreased within 60 min of 17β-E administration, suggesting that ERα at the plasma membrane was lowered, consistent with this idea, ERK activation also decreased (47). Decreasing ERα at the membrane in these cells may allow for a decrease in non-genomic signaling and may mark a shift toward genomic transcription. In contrast, in the VSMC, 17β-E increased both Cav-1 and Cav-2 and increased ERα localization at the plasma membrane (41). Such increased ERα localization in response to the endogenous ligand may be a mechanism to sustain non-genomic signaling in some cell types.

Similar to other trans-membrane GPCRs, which may undergo desensitization via internalization in a G-protein receptor kinase 2 (GRK2)-β-arrestin-dependent manner (18), 17β-E application to cortical neuronal cultures rapidly induced GRK2 phosphorylation within 5 min and β-arrestin1 and c-Src recruitment to the ERα within 60 min. Predictably, since β-arrestin1 tagging of trans-membrane GPCRs provides a scaffold for c-Src attachment and subsequent ERK activation (53), siRNA to β-arrestin1 abrogated the 17β-E induction of pERK in these neurons (54). Though the exact partners of the ERα in this internalized signalosome are unknown, ERα internalization is initiated from the membrane since E2-BSA also promotes internalization (54). Internalization of the ERα has also been tested more directly by using a surface biotinylation technique followed by stripping the surface biotin with glutathione after 17β-E addition to cells. Hence, the continued presence of biotin in this preparation would argue that the receptor was internalized and protected against glutathione action. In hypothalamic neurons, addition of 17β-E caused internalization of both the 52 and 66 kDa forms within 30 min, with internalization of the 52 kDa form persisting for 2 h (54), demonstrating that recycling and internalization of the classical ERα as well as the 52 kDa variant occurs in a rapid time frame. An unresolved issue is the rapid decrease in total ERα protein and mRNA in the hypothalamus on 17β-E application that has been shown by several investigators (55, 56). However, it is difficult to reconcile this with the increase in plasma mERα that is seen in the hypothalamic primary neuronal and astrocytic cultures (38, 39) and in the hypothalamic cell line mHypoE-38 (52) unless ERα from other non-membrane locations decrease to a large extent; this could be a parameter to be investigated in future studies. This could also be due to the recent studies that show an increase ERα at the plasma membrane being carried out in primary cultures versus hypothalamic tissue that retain neuronal connectivity in the older studies.

DEPENDENCE OF RAPID SIGNALING ON ERα AND ERβ

In addition to direct demonstration of the ERα either at the membrane or tethering to an intrinsic membrane protein, the ER dependence of kinase activation has also been investigated. Several studies, described in this review, have used the ERα and ERβ antagonist ICI 182,780 to antagonize a rapid signaling pathway or a genetic approach that deletes either ERα or ERβ specifically in the whole animal. The availability of ERα and ERβ knockout animals, i.e., ERαKO and ERβKO, has been useful to understand the ER dependence of 17β-E-mediated non-genomic signaling *in vivo*, particularly in light of an absence of a specific antibody to the ERβ (57). In wild-type female mice, subcutaneous administration of 17β-E caused the activation of CREB and ERK within an hour, as measured by immunohistochemistry for the phosphorylated forms of these molecules. When either ERα or ERβ or both were deleted, a complex brain nuclei-specific and isoform-specific ER dependence was revealed, which may in part be due to the tissue distribution of the ER isoforms in the brain (**Table 1** below) (58). For example, in the ventrolateral VMH (vl-VMH), the loss of ERα results in the reduction of pCREB on 17β-E administration and this could be because the predominant ER isoform is the ERα and it is possible that the loss of ERα cannot be compensated by smaller amounts of ERβ (58). The use of ERαKO, ERβKO, and ERαβKO mice in this study showed that ERα is hence both necessary and sufficient for the induction of pCREB. In the mPOA, 17β-E could induce pCREB via either ERα or ERβ but required both ERα and ERβ to act in conjunction in order to induce pERK (58), demonstrating that ER isoforms can regulate rapid signaling differentially in the same tissue. The regulation in male mice is unknown and is under investigation in our laboratory.

ERα VARIANTS

In both hypothalamic neurons and astrocytes (38), a variant 52 kDa ERα (ERα-52), detected with a C-terminal antibody that also detects the full-length 66 kDa, was expressed in much higher amounts than the ERα-66 kDa form. Based on RT-PCR analysis using flanking primers to this exon in the mouse hypothalamic cell line mHypoE-38, this is believed to be an ERα that lacks exon 4 (ERαΔ4) (52). In astrocytes, only the 66 kDa form is thought to be interact with mGluR1 (43) and the interaction, signaling properties, and function, if unique, of the 52 kDa variant remain unknown. A 36 kDa variant lacking the AF-1 and AF-2 domains with a unique C-terminus was detected in human breast

Table 1 | Comparison of CREB and ERK between wild-type (WT), ERα knockout (ERαKO), ERβ knockout (ERβKO), and double ERα ERβ knockout (ERαβKO) female mouse brain.

Genotype	vlVMH		mPOA		Medial septum	
	pCREB	pERK	pCREB	pERK	pCREB	pERK
WT	++	NR	++	++	++	NR
ERαKO	–	NR	++	–	++	NR
ERβKO	++	NR	++	–	–	NR
ERαβKO	–	NR	–	–	–	NR

pCREB and pERK in 17β-E injected mice was quantitated by immunohistochemistry and compared to the levels of pCREB and pERK present in mice injected with the vehicle, in the ventrolateral VMH (vl-VMH), the medial preoptic area (mPOA) and the medial septum in female ovariectomized mice injected with 10 μg 17β-E and sacrificed an hour after injection. In WT mice, 17β-E increased pCREB in the vl-VMH and pERK and pCREB in the mPOA. ER isoform dependence varies according to the output (pCREB or pERK) measured and the nuclei. ++: upregulation compared to vehicle-treated mice. –: no upregulation compared to vehicle-treated mice. NR= data not recorded. Data are from Ref. (58).

cancer cells, coded for by a unique promoter located in intron 1 of the *Esr1*gene (59) and can be detected by a specific antibody. ERα-36 was localized to the plasma membrane, mediated rapid ERK signaling, and is induced by the selective activation of the GPR30 (discussed in Section "GPR30") by the agonist, G-1 (60). Importantly, this GPR30-selective activator, G-1, has also been demonstrated to bind and activate ERα-36 (60), suggesting that some of the responses attributed to the GPR30 might be via ERα-36. A 46 kDa variant observed in endothelial cells is also localized to the plasma membrane (61) and is composed of a splice variant missing the first 173 amino acids of ERα-66 (62). ERα-46 cannot be detected with an N-terminus antibody raised to ERα-66 such as H-184 (**Figure 1**), but should be identifiable with a C-terminus ERα antibody. A novel ER is the ER-X, an ER of 63 kDa that is expressed in the neocortex in the caveolae membrane fraction, can be identified with ERα and ERβ antibodies and is present in the ERα knockout animal (63). This ER, whose structure remains unidentified, mediated ERK signaling by both 17α-estradiol and 17β-estradiol and would not meet the criteria for a mER, based on our previous definition. The function and expression pattern of the ER-X is unknown though it was upregulated after ischemic injury (63) in the adult. If it is not present in the adult hypothalamus, it is unlikely to be a receptor that mediates normal behavior that is dependent on the hypothalamus (63). So far, neither ERα-36 nor ERα-46 has been demonstrated in the CNS, though it is possible that some antibodies directed toward the DNA-binding domain or, in the case of the 46 kDa variant, the C-terminal domain of the full-length 66 kDa ERα such as MC-20 or C1335 (**Figure 1**) may detect these forms in studies that use solely immunocytochemistry.

Gα-COUPLED mERs

The idea that the mER is a $G\alpha_q$-coupled receptor has been explored in the POMC neuron in the ARH, primarily by the laboratories of Kelly and Ronnekliev (7, 64, 65). In POMC neurons, 17β-E and E2-BSA uncoupled the inhibitory μ-opioid receptor from the G-protein coupled inward rectifying K^+ (GIRK) channel, in a PLC-, PKC-, and PKA-dependent manner (66, 67), thus decreasing hyperpolarization of these neurons and increasing neuronal excitability. Pharmacological characterization revealed that a $G\alpha_q$ receptor upregulated PLC and calcium release, which in turn activated PKC and PKA. Subsequent PKA phosphorylation of the GIRK channel uncoupled the μ-opioid receptor (7, 68) from GIRK. Though this response was specific for 17β-E versus 17α-E and was blocked by the ERα and ERβ antagonist ICI 182,780, it also occurred in ERαKO, ERβKO, and GPR30 KO mice (69), suggesting that a novel mER is coupled to $G\alpha_q$. This signaling pathway can be activated by a selective ligand, STX, which does not bind ERα, ERβ, or GPR30. Both STX and 17β-E also reduced post-ovariectomy weight gain, suggesting that this novel $G\alpha_q$-coupled mER is important in energy homeostasis. Leptin receptors on POMC neurons caused depolarization rapidly via the JAK/STAT and PI3K pathways that open calcium-dependent TRPC channels (70); 17β-E signaling may synergize with leptin action by increasing calcium rapidly in these neurons via this $G\alpha_q$-mER. Several reviews (7, 68, 69, 71–74) detail the studies on this STX-activated receptor.

GPR30

The GPR30, also known as GPER1, is a former orphan GPCR that was shown to bind 17β-E and increase cAMP in breast cancer SKBR3 cells via an increase in adenylyl cyclase activity (75). In the rat hypothalamus, GPR30 expression is particularly high in the PVN and SON (76) with low expression in the VMH. Cell fractionation and immunocytochemistry revealed GPR30 to be localized at the plasma membrane in both the SKBR3 ($GPR30^+$, $ER\alpha^-$, $ER\beta^-$) and MDA-MB-231 ($GPR30^-$, $ER\alpha^-$, $ER\beta^+$; GPR30 overexpression) breast cancer cell lines (77). Though GPR30 was not detected at the plasma membrane using surface biotinylation in hypothalamic astrocytes (38), GPR30 was localized to the post-synaptic density in the hippocampus and associates with PSD-95 through its C-terminal tail (78). This association with PSD-95 can localize GPR30 to the plasma membrane, independent of 17β-E. Immuno-electron microscopy analysis of rat hippocampi also revealed membrane localization with no intracellular staining (79). However, it can be detected intracellularly in normal mammary gland epithelial cells (80) and colocalized with a marker of the Golgi apparatus in primary cultures of the hippocampus (81). Also, overexpressed GPR30 in COS7 cells exhibits localization at the endoplasmic reticulum and the Golgi (82), suggesting that cell type can determine localization. In addition, HeLa cells transfected with FLAG-GPR30 show mostly staining at the membrane while cells transfected with GFP-GPR30 show staining mainly in the endoplasmic reticulum [(79) #6908], suggesting that inclusion of molecular tags may interfere with proper intracellular trafficking, possibly confounding the interpretation of experiments relying on ectopic expression of GPR30.

Studies describing the regulation of internalization of GPR30 have also yielded conflicting results. When FLAG-GPR30 was ectopically expressed in HeLa cells, receptor endocytosis was ligand dependent and internalized GPR30 occupied a diffuse cytoplasmic localization consistent with classical receptor recycling or proteasomal degradation pathways (79). In human embryonic kidney (HEK)-293 cells, GPR30 internalization was not only ligand-dependent but also occurs constitutively (83). While most GPCRs are either recycled to the plasma membrane via endosomes or degraded in lysosomes to limit excessive signaling, GPR30 rapidly accumulates in the perinuclear compartment via clathrin-coated vesicles (83). It is thought that this Rab 11-dependent accumulation is in the trans-Golgi network and degradation occurs via an ubiquitin-proteasome-mediated pathway, unlike the endosomal degradation or recycling to the surface that is typical for other GPCRs (83). Since this pathway for internalization and degradation is rapid and constitutive, Cheng et al. propose this as the reason for the difficulty in detecting GPR30 at the plasma membrane in some cell lines (83).

GPR30 can signal via both the $G\alpha_s$ and the $G_{\beta\gamma}$ subunits that are associated with the receptor upon activation. The Gβγ subunit transactivated the EGFR receptor leading to downstream activation ERK protein, while simultaneous activation of the $G\alpha_s$ subunit by 17β-E inactivated ERK signaling through activation of adenylyl cyclase and PKA, thus limiting cAMP signaling to a short time frame (23). Furthermore, although GPR30 protein was readily detectable in both the microsomal and plasma membrane subcellular fractions of breast cancer cell lines, only GPR30 in the plasma membrane fraction bound ligand and activated G-protein signaling, suggesting that only membrane-associated GPR30 protein is functional (77). However, GPR30 activation in COS7 cells initiated intracellular calcium mobilization and nuclear accumulation of PIP3 via EGFR transactivation (82) via a non-membrane-initiated signaling mechanism since calcium flux was not replicated by membrane restricted estradiol derivatives (84). These discrepant results have yet to be reconciled. A recent study reported that GPR30 could decrease cAMP that was elevated by heterologous ligands, such as forskolin, via the C-terminal PDZ domain (85). This domain could bind membrane-activated guanylate cyclases (MAGUKs), which act as adaptors for AKAP5 (PKA anchoring protein) that in turn decreased adenylate cyclase activity. This would decrease the cAMP that is elevated by 17β-E binding of the GPR30 and may serve to limit the time frame of GPR30 signaling (85). Hence, both ERK and cAMP signaling downstream of the GPR30 may be restricted to very short time frames.

THE iGR AS THE mGR

Similar to the ERα being considered a possible mER, the intracellular GR (iGR) that exists as a complex with heat-shock protein 90 (HSP90), p23, and a tetratricopeptide protein (86) in the cytoplasm has been proposed as a candidate mGR (87). Stable reduction of mGR levels in CD14^{+} monocytes using stably transfected siRNA to iGRα suggested that both mGR and iGR were derived from the same transcript (88). GR exists in two isoforms, GRα and GRβ. GRβ, generated by alternative splicing, lacks the last 50 amino acids of the GRα carboxy terminus, and instead possesses a unique 15 amino acid sequence at its C-terminus (89). GRβ neither binds glucocorticoids nor has intrinsic transcriptional activity, but has been implicated as a dominant negative inhibitor of GRα activity through formation of a non-functional heterodimer (90). Higher concentrations of GRβ relative to GRα, therefore, result in decreased glucocorticoid sensitivity. However, levels of GRβ protein in the brain are extremely low (89) and this is not thought to be a regulator of GRα in the brain. The presence of mGRα was detected at very low levels in human lymphocytes and leukocytes using membrane-impermeable fluorescent liposomes and GR-specific antibodies (91) such as M-20 (**Figure 1**). Similar to the tethering of ERα to the plasma membrane, mGRα has been associated with Cav-1 in MCF-7 cells (92). However, while plasma membrane association of other steroid hormone receptors, including ER, is dependent on palmitoylation, mutation of the homologous sequence in GR did not affect membrane localization (93), suggesting that other mechanisms must tether mGR to the plasma membrane. In the brain, most of the rapid effects of glucocorticoids have been confined to the hippocampus and to the hypothalamus. Membrane glucocorticoid receptors were first observed in the synaptic plasma membrane fractions (SPM) of rat brain via [3H]-corticosterone binding assays (20). Hypothalamic SPM had a higher binding capacity than hippocampal or cortical SPM, which is in contrast to corticosterone binding of the iGR, which is lower in the hypothalamus and much higher in cerebral cortex and hippocampus (94). Synaptosomal fractions from rat hippocampus contained plasma membrane-associated GR (95) and GR immunoreactivity was observed at the plasma membranes and vesicle membranes of the hypothalamus (96) while in the CA1, GR was shown in the spine (97). Functionally, JNK and p38 MAPK were activated within 10 min of glucocorticoid administration in primary hippocampal neurons (98). The hypothalamo–pituitary–adrenal (HPA) axis is also subject to rapid negative feedback at the level of the hypothalamus (99). Bath application of glucocorticoids to rat hypothalamic slices caused a rapid suppression of glutamate-mediated excitatory synaptic currents onto CRH neurons that was decreased by a CB1 receptor antagonist (13). The release of endocannabinoids that bind to the CB1 receptor is dependent on corticosterone rapidly acting on the CRH neuron and is dependent on $G\alpha_s$-driven PKA activation in the CRH neuron (100). However, the release of nitric oxide (NO) that increased GABAergic inhibition (101) onto the CRH neuron was dependent on Gβγ signaling (100). Hence, in the PVN, rapid negative feedback by glucocorticoids on post-synaptic CRH neurons is exerted by a combination of suppression of presynaptic glutamatergic neurons and excitation of presynaptic GABAergic neurons. The identity of the mGR that can signal via both $G\alpha_s$ and Gβγ subunits in the CRH neuron remains unknown.

UNRESOLVED QUESTIONS: mER AND mGR

As is evident in the preceding sections, several questions about the identity of the mER and mGR remain. Though the strongest evidence exists for a post-translationally modified classical ER, there are other viable candidates for the ER (102) based both on evidence of proteins that interact with antibodies raised to the classical ER or to the continued existence of non-genomic effects in ERαKO and ERβKO mice (63). Different ER proteins might be mERs in different tissues (14) or different proteins might be mERs in the same tissue at different times to generate divergent rapid signaling outcomes within the same cell or different tissues that is congruent with incoming stimuli. It is also possible that the time frame of non-genomic signaling might be different when there are different mERs present – a GPCR such as GPR30 may activate the ERK and PKA pathways very transiently whereas ERα or ERβ at the membrane may be capable of more sustained activation. Again, this would change the response of the cell to stimuli, depending on the mER present. Second, if the mER is the ERα, the mechanism by which only a small proportion of the total ERα is targeted to the membrane is not known and strengthens the idea that different pools of ERα may exist within cells (30) with different functions. The rationale for the variable amount of ERα at the membrane in some cells versus others in cell lines is also unclear but could allow for 17β-E to employ non-genomic versus genomic signaling to different extents in different cells, which maybe at different physiological states. Third, apart from the difficulty in studying ERβ localization or interaction with other proteins due to the unavailability of a reliable antibody (57), the localization of the ERα variants is also particularly understudied, but the predominance of the 52 kDa form as opposed to the full-length 66 kDa form in the CNS (39, 52) argues for an important role of these variants in estrogen signaling in the brain, as opposed to other classical estrogen-responsive tissues such as the uterus. The rapid actions of these different ERα variants may also oppose each other in some cases (39). It is, therefore, likely that the ratio of different ERs, including mERs expressed in each cell that determines the cellular response to 17β-E exposure. The significance of these spatially separated and functionally opposing ER populations may be to modulate the hypothalamic and hippocampal neuron response to estrogen and prevent runaway signaling. Fourth, though the GPR30 has a role to play in estrogen-mediated physiology, the acceptance of GPR30 as a mER has not been universal (103) with some investigators preferring to term it as a "collaborator" to the ERα, which is deemed to be the primary mER that signals from the membrane (30). If GPR30 or $G\alpha_q$-coupled novel proteins are the mERs in some tissues, it is also possible that they crosstalk with classical ERα or ERβ, accounting in some studies for the ICI-mediated antagonism of the effect. Though this cooperation between GPR30 and ERα has been shown to have a proliferative effect on ovarian cancer cells (104), a functional effect has not been demonstrated in the hypothalamus. In the ventral hippocampus in male mice, Hart et al. showed an injection of G-1 could increase the phosphorylation of an ERK-sensitive serine site on the ERα at position 118 within 30 min, suggesting that these two receptors could interact with each in the CNS (105). Future studies on the colocalization and the functional interaction between ERα and GPR30 in the hypothalamus will prove useful in this regard. There are far fewer studies on the mGR, when compared to the mER, and most studies investigate the possibility of the mGR being equivalent to the iGR. Surprisingly, the idea that different G-protein subunits, particularly that the Gβγ subunit can support signaling from the unidentified mGR in the CRH neuron and from the $G\alpha_q$-coupled, STX-activated mER in the POMC neuron is also seen with a traditional GPCR such as GPR30. Whether signaling from both G-protein subunits is concomitant or if one signaling pathway predominates, under certain physiological conditions, is not known.

Lastly, the model generated by the existing literature is that the mER or mGR is at the inner leaflet of the membrane, associated with intrinsic membrane proteins or scaffolds such as caveolin. However, surface biotinylation experiments imply that some part of the mER or mGR is exposed to the extracellular mileu (18). Though an abundance of hydrophobic amino acids in the ligand-binding domain of the mER predicts that this domain might insert into the plasma membrane (106), no study has demonstrated this in the CNS. While recycling of this receptor from the membrane is to be expected, the pathways (Rab-mediated or β-arrestin mediated) are possibly cell-specific and are worthy of more attention since non-genomic signaling is possibly terminated during internalization.

MORPHOLOGICAL AND BEHAVIORAL OUTPUTS IN THE CNS DEPENDENT ON NON-GENOMIC SIGNALING BY ESTROGENS AND GLUCOCORTICOIDS

Though kinase regulation and calcium flux has been shown to occur rapidly when cells are exposed to the hormone in a number of tissues and the idea of non-genomic signaling more accepted than ever before, the relevance of non-genomic signaling for behavior has remained murky. Here, we shall confine ourselves to primarily hypothalamically driven behaviors or possible neural correlates that are either rapidly induced by 17β-E or E2-BSA or that may have a non-genomic component. Finally, we will discuss the intersection of glucocorticoid rapid signaling in a 17β-E-mediated behavior.

SPINOGENESIS

Estrogen is critical in the display of female sex behavior in rodents by acting on the hypothalamus; retrograde tract tracing using the pseudorabies virus (PRV) injected into the lumbar muscles labeled the lordosis circuit, in particular, the plexus of oxytocin fibers in the vl-VMH (107). In the hypothalamus, estradiol benzoate (EB) injections to ovariectomized rats increased spine density by 48% in the vl-VMH as compared to oil injections (108). Surprisingly, only 3% of PRV-labeled neurons were $ER\alpha^+$ and these were not the neurons that showed an increase in spine density (109) upon EB administration. These data argue that the increase in spine density in the VMH may be only indirectly dependent on ERα signaling or could be due to another ER while the longer time frames used in the study do not allow us to conclude if there is a non-genomic component. A candidate could be the GPR30 receptor, which is expressed in the vl-VMH; the role of this receptor in spinogenesis in the hypothalamus is not known. Rapid effects on spinogenesis and spine morphology following GR activation have been observed in the hippocampus, but not in the hypothalamus. CA1 neurons from male rat hippocampal slices treated with dexamethasone for 1 h demonstrated a translation-independent increase in spine density, which was lost with co-application of dexamethasone with either the GR antagonist RU-486 or the NMDA receptor blocker MK-801 (95). The proportion of mushroom-shaped and thin-type spines was also increased following GR activation (95).

Does non-genomic signaling play a role in the increase in spine density by estrogens or by glucorticoids? The mGluR1a antagonist, LY367385 in the ARH decreased phosphorylated cofilin levels that are induced within an hour of EB injection and that are required for actin reorganization and spinogenesis, suggesting that at least some of the initial aspects of spinogenesis are mediated via non-genomic signaling from the ERα-mGluR1a complex at the membrane (110). Though EB can increase filopodial spines in the ARH within 4 h of treatment, mushroom shaped, more stable spines require time frames in excess of 20 h and parallels the time frames required for the full display of lordosis behavior, suggesting that rapid non-genomic signaling is insufficient for formation of stable spines (110). Stabilization of the PSD-95 protein, a scaffolding protein enriched in mushroom-shaped dendritic spines, was dependent on pAkt and also required 48 h of 17β-E treatment in differentiated NG-108 cells (111). Another model for the increase in 17β-E-mediated increase in spine density in the hypothalamus is that 17β-E stimulates PI3K activation pre-synaptically, inducing glutamate release, followed by NMDA receptor activation and ERK signaling post-synaptically, with a subsequent increase in spinophilin protein that was correlated with an increase in stable dendritic spines (112) on the post-synaptic neuron. Both ERK and PI3K signaling are implicated in the increase in spine density, though the formation of mature mushroom spines also appears to require transcription (113). Though there are no reports of glucocorticoid-mediated regulation of spine density in the hypothalamus, suppression of PKA, PKC, MAPK, or PI3K signaling completely blocked GR-mediated spinogenesis in CA1 neurons, suggesting that GR signals through convergent kinase pathways to increase actin polymerization, which would allow for spine changes (114). In CA1 neurons, treatment with the synthetic glucocorticoid dexamethasone increased p-cofilin levels within 30 min, similar to the rapid induction seen in the ARH by EB (97).

Consistent with the idea that 17β-E-mediated spinogenesis in the VMH has a functional consequence, cytochalasin D, an actin polymerization inhibitor, blocked the formation of spines in the ARH and reduced lordosis (110) though the relevance of such spinogenesis to sex behavior in rodents (see Sex Behavior or Lordosis in Females) is unknown. The consequences of spine disruption for other behaviors such as aggressive behavior or male sex behavior (see Male Sex Behavior) are also unknown. Though most of the studies have shown effects on spine density or morphology in longer time frames that do not allow one to parse non-genomic actions from transcription, spine density on the apical dendrite in the stratum radiatum and in the stratum lacunosum moleculare of the CA1 neuron was increased within 40 min by the ERα selective agonist, propyl pyrazole triol (PPT); however, these were at high doses that were not correlated with doses of PPT that led to an improvement in social memory within 40 min of administration (115). In mature rat cortical neurons, 17β-E rapidly increased ERK and p21-activated kinase to increase dendritic spine density (116) within 30 min. Though this suggests that non-genomic signaling may be sufficient for an increase in spine density at least in the hippocampus and cortex, this has to be confirmed with experiments that utilize a transcription inhibitor. A similar rapid effect of estrogen on spine density in the hypothalamus has not been demonstrated.

SEX BEHAVIOR OR LORDOSIS IN FEMALES

Lordosis in rodents is a 17β-E-driven behavior where integration of sensory information within the limbic-hypothalamic circuit culminates in VMH projections onto neurons of the periaqueductal gray (PAG) and spinal cord motor neurons, resulting in the classical lordosis posture (16). A series of elegant experiments from the laboratory of Micevych delineated a microcircuit consisting of neuronal afferents from the ARH to the mPOA (113). In this circuit, the initial membrane-initiated signaling by 17β-E in the ARH neurons increased PKCθ (117) and released neuropeptide Y that activates β-endorphin expressing ARH neurons that project into the mPOA (118). In the mPOA, β-endorphin released from the ARH caused the internalization of μ-opioid receptors (MOR) within 30 min of E2-BSA (119) administration into the ARH, suggesting that this is a membrane-initiated non-transcriptional event. This transient inhibition of lordosis initiated by MOR internalization is removed 30 h later by progesterone (120). A number of different receptors, including ERα and mGluR1a, play a role in this membrane-initiated signaling to influence lordosis behavior. Not only does ERα and mGluR1a colocalize in about 23% of ERα-expressing neurons but deletion of ERα also blocked MOR internalization in the mPOA (121) and abolishes lordosis (122). Blocking of MOR internalization with application of an mGluR1 antagonist or Cav-1 siRNA into the ARH also, in turn, reduced lordosis (119, 123). Though this suggests that ERα and mGluR1 signal together as in the hippocampus (124), the selective mER agonist, STX in the ARH also induced MOR internalization and lordosis (125), an effect blocked by the mGluR1a antagonist. This suggests that in the ARH, both ERα and the $G\alpha_q$-mER may couple to mGluR1a and facilitate lordosis, though the mechanisms by which this occurs are unclear. Apart from these receptors, the localization of the GPR30 in the hypothalamus (126) and the ability of G-1, an agonist at the GPR30 to facilitate lordosis in female ovariectoimized mice (127) argues that GPR30 signaling is also important, at least in mice. It is unknown if the ERα, the $G\alpha_q$-mER, and the GPR30 interact or signal to each other or represent independent parallel signaling pathways that drive lordosis in estrogen primed ovariectomized female rodents, though any model must take into account the necessity of ERα in the VMH for lordosis.

Since Kow et al. demonstrated that E2-BSA alone in the VMH does not induce lordosis (128), we can presume that non-genomic signaling is insufficient but may potentiate or prime lordosis that is in itself dependent on nuclear transcription (129) via a coupled signaling pathway (130). Consistent with this idea, a mouse that possesses an ERα that cannot bind an ERE ($ER\alpha^{-/AA}$) (131) did not display lordosis behavior (132), demonstrating the importance of 17β-E-bound ERα transcriptional action at an ERE for lordosis. Also, combined E2-BSA and 17β-E administrations into the VMH increase progesterone receptor (PR) protein levels higher than either hormone alone (133), demonstrating potentiation of transcription by a membrane-limited estrogen conjugate. The reduction of ERα in the VMH using adenovirus-associated shRNA viral vectors that abolished lordosis behavior (29) shows the absolute requirement for the ERα, which could be due to its participation both as a mER and as a nuclear transcription factor in the VMH. An additional role could be the signaling initiated by ERα acting as a mER in the ARH but as a transcription factor that upregulates the PR in the VMH (134), both processes that are required for lordosis. In this scenario, membrane-initiated signaling in the ARH results in transient inhibition of lordosis so that 17β-E can transcriptionally activate genes such as the PR in the VMH that are important for the full display of lordosis that occurs 30 h later (113).

MALE SEX BEHAVIOR

In males, 17β-E given intraperitoneally at high concentrations to castrated adult rats increased some aspects of male sex behavior, i.e., genital sniffs and mounting within 15 min, a time frame commensurate with non-genomic actions (135). However, since protein synthesis inhibitors (136) and the presence of the ERE-binding mutant, the $ER\alpha^{-/AA}$ mouse abolished male sex behavior (131), it is reasonable to conclude that male sex behavior, similar to female sex behavior, has a non-genomic component that is not sufficient for the full display of the behavior. Though most of the studies investigate the role of testosterone in males (137, 138), testosterone can be converted to 17β-E by aromatase (139). In the castrated and testosterone supplemented quail that was treated with the aromatase inhibitor, vorozole, administration of 17β-E or E2-BSA intracerebroventricularly (icv) increased appetitive sexual behavior but not the final consummatory aspects of sexual behavior within 15 min (140). This appetitive sexual behavior was also blocked by vorozole, administered icv 15 min before behavioral testing (140). This implies that neuroestrogens that are rapidly generated in response to stimuli such as the sight of a female signal rapidly to initiate appetitive sexual behavior. Though ICI 182,780 antagonized the increase in appetitive sexual behavior seen rapidly with 17β-E administration (140), the exact mER that mediates the rapid regulation of sex behavior or aromatase in the quail or the mouse is unknown. In the male mouse, consistent with the interpretation that arises from the data in the quail, 17β-E administered to aromatase knockout male mice reversed the lack of sex behavior while vorozole decreased sex behavior in C57BL/6 mice within 15 min of administration (141). Stimuli-dependent rapid regulation of aromatase could represent a mechanism to locally elevate neuroestrogens, which then increase sex behavior in male quail or in the male rodent. However, contrary to this expectation, aromatase activity decreased rapidly when male quail were exposed to female stimuli but neuroestrogen concentrations itself increased in the mPOA (142), a nuclei important for male sex behavior. However, it is important to note that the acute action of 17β-E on appetitive sexual behavior in the male quail was always preceded by initial copulation with a receptive female to establish this learned response, wherein the sight of the same female would initiate appetitive sexual behavior (143). In this case, it is possible that prior sexual experience may initiate transcriptional signaling by 17β-E, which in turn primes rapid non-genomic signaling to achieve greater efficiency in subsequent sexual interactions and optimize reproduction; this remains to be tested. Similar to female sex behavior, the non-genomic component in male sex behavior is important for the initial approach and mounting aspects of male sex behavior.

AGGRESSION IN MALES

Castration in male rodents removes both testosterone and estrogens and results in loss of aggression in response to territorial intrusion (144, 145). The importance of estrogen in male aggressive behavior is shown by the deletion of aromatase, which abolished aggression by male mice in a resident-intruder paradigm, though this is possibly also due to organizational defects since 17β-E reinstated aggression only when administered before postnatal day 7 (146). In CD-1 outbred male mice, ERα concentrations in several areas of the circuit involved in aggression such as the bed nucleus of the stria terminalis (BNST), the lateral septum (LS), and the anterior hypothalamus (AH) was higher in more aggressive mice (147). Reduction of ERα in the VMH by adenovirus mediated transfer of siRNA to ERα abolished aggressive behavior in male mice, demonstrating that ERα expression in the VMH is necessary for aggression in adult male mice (29), just as it was important for sex behavior in male mice. In California, beach mice that were castrated and supplemented with testosterone and an aromatase inhibitor so that they possessed testosterone but not estrogen, aggression increased rapidly within 15 min of injection with cyclodextrin-conjugated 17β-E (148). This suggests that testosterone alone was not sufficient to elicit aggressive behavior in a resident-intruder paradigm and that 17β-E is necessary to activate aggression. The time frame and the inability of cycloheximide (149) to decrease this aggression in the beach mouse argue that 17β-E acts non-genomically, though most studies on aggression, with the exception of those cited in this paragraph, in the rat and mouse have used time frames that do not allow us to parse a non-genomic effect from a genomic/coupled signaling effect.

What is the source of 17β-E? In rodents, aromatase is expressed in axon terminals (150–152) particularly in the hypothalamus (153) and brain 17β-E concentrations in the male rat are equal to or higher (~8 nM) than in the plasma (154). Hence, 17β-E generated at the synapse has been envisioned to function as a neuromodulator in short time frames (155), in line with the data in male birds where neuroestrogens generated at axon terminals are important in learning in songbirds (156) and in sex behavior in the quail (157, 158). In the castrated male rat, EB synergized with dihydrotestosterone (DHT) to increase aromatase activity (159). In addition, 17β-E can transcriptionally induce the aromatase gene via ERα-c-jun complex binding to AP-1 elements in the brain-specific promoter of aromatase (160). Therefore, similar to spinogenesis, the regulation of aromatase by 17β-E itself may represent another correlate where both rapid, non-genomic and slower, transcriptional mechanisms converge. The areas of the brain wherein this may occur in the rodent are not clear and are being investigated in our laboratory.

Though 17β-E can rapidly increase aggression by modulating neurotransmitter release [(145) and references therein], it may also do via regulating the HPA axis. In the white-crowned sparrow, neither brain 17β-E concentrations nor aromatase activity in nuclei involved in aggression were correlated with aggressive behavior (161) though corticosterone did increase rapidly. What is the link between glucocorticoids and aggression? Though aggression itself is stressful and leads to secretion of glucocorticoids, dominance in an aggressive encounter typically leads to lowering of the corticosterone level (162). However, pre-fight corticosterone levels have been shown to be associated with aggressiveness in fish and acute treatment with adrenocorticotrophic hormone (ACTH) increased fighting behavior in male mice (163) while acute treatment with corticosterone 2 min before an encounter increased aggressiveness in male rats (164) and risk assessment in the open field and elevated plus maze tests (165). Supporting the idea that corticosterone is important in regulation the onset of aggressive behavior, acute treatment with GR antagonists (166, 167) or prevention of glucocorticoid synthesis (164) prevented aggression when presented with social challenge. Since acute central application of corticosterone increased aggression within 7 min and protein synthesis inhibitors did not decrease it, non-genomic signaling by glucocorticoids in the CNS is most likely required to increase aggression (164). Consistent with this idea, acute corticosterone injection also decreased the magnitude of electrical stimulation to the hypothalamus required to elicit attack (168). In addition, corticosterone administration to rats in established colonies did not change aggression, demonstrating that glucocorticoids promote aggression only in ethologically relevant situations such as territorial intrusion (169). However, chronic elevated levels of glucocorticoids, such as seen in stressed or socially defeated animals decrease aggression and increased submissiveness in hamsters (170, 171), mice (172), and rats (173, 174). This is thought to be due to genomic signaling by glucocorticoids though the molecular mechanisms by which glucocorticoids facilitate or inhibit aggression are unclear (175).

Gonadal status can modify the actions of glucocorticoids on the hypothalamus or can regulate corticosterone levels itself. For example, gonadal steroids can modify glucocorticoid-mediated

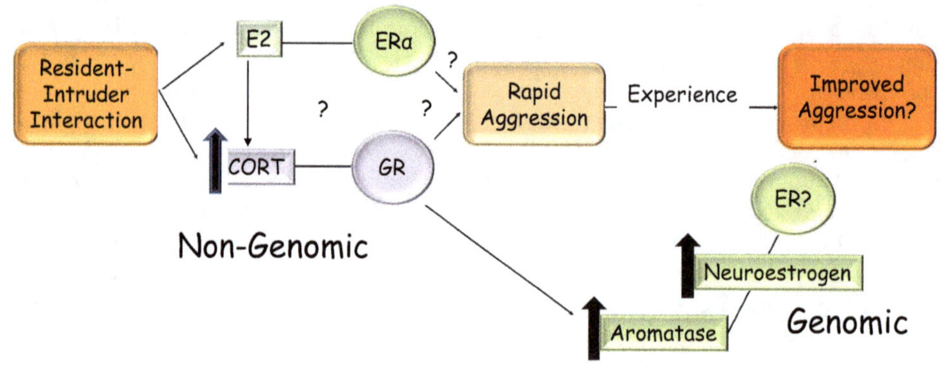

FIGURE 2 | Hypothetical model in the rodent for the rapid and sustained increase in aggression that is seen when an intruder enters a resident's home-cage. On visual and/or olfactory cues, 17β-E in the brain may increase corticosterone via an unknown mechanism. This increase in corticosterone may rapidly and non-genomically increase aggressive behavior. The mechanism by which corticosterone does so is not known but may involve the regulation of aromatase and could be GR mediated. It is not known if 17β-E's regulation of aggressive behavior is solely via corticosterone increase or these are two parallel pathways, which require ERα, as shown in the figure. Elevated corticosterone levels can increase transcription from the brain-specific aromatase promoter, which in turn increases neuroestrogens. This may contribute to shorter latencies of attack in successive bouts. The interaction of estrogen and corticosterone ensures that the resident rodent is aggressive only in the presence of a relevant external cue, i.e., intruder and a relevant internal cue, i.e., sufficient 17β-E.

negative feedback on CRH. 17β-E chronically administered to gonadectomized and adrenalectomized female rats treated with high doses of corticosterone increased CRH mRNA levels, thus counteracting negative feedback, while DHT treatment to male rats had an opposing effect and caused a further decrease in CRH levels (176). In female ovariectomized rats, icv, but not systemic, 17β-E injection increased corticosterone rapidly within 30 min, an effect mimicked with the ERα selective agonist, PPT, injected into the PVN (177). In gonadectomized male rats, CRH mRNA was higher when they were treated with EB but lower when treated with DHT, implying that estrogens can regulate the HPA axis in males also (178). A number of mechanisms may be involved in the rapid increase of aggression by glucocorticoids in response to social challenge, including the regulation of dopamine (179, 180) and serotonin (181, 182) neurotransmission. Here, we will focus on one such mechanism that is responsive to both estrogens and glucocorticoids in the hypothalamus, namely, the regulation of aromatase. Acute stressors, which increase glucocorticoids, increased neuroestrogen concentrations in the PVN and aromatase mRNA in the PVN within an hour in female rats, suggesting that corticosteroid release may also increase neuroestrogen in the hypothalamus (183). Similarly, in male quail, rapid increases in aromatase activity also occurred on restraint stress in the mPOA (184), demonstrating that corticosterone can affect aromatase using a non-genomic signaling mechanism that is yet unknown, in both birds and rodents. Furthermore, aromatase protein levels are increased in response to glucocorticoid treatment in a hypothalamic cell line via a transcriptional mechanism (185), leading to a possible increase in the amount of aromatase that may increase the efficiency of winning future bouts. These data demonstrate that 17β-E in the brain can increase plasma corticosterone, which in turn can increase aromatase activity and/or transcription in the hypothalamus leading to a positive feedback circuit that may be active under physiologically relevant stressful contexts such territorial intrusion. The relevance of this pathway

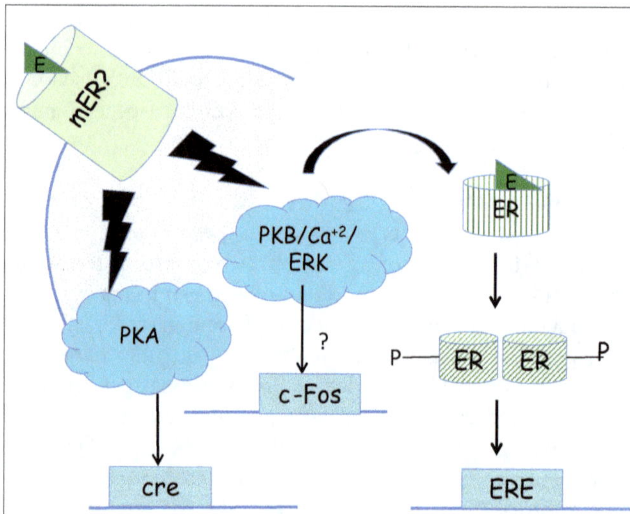

FIGURE 3 | Priming of transcription within neurons by non-genomic signaling. Non-genomic signaling, initiated at the plasma membrane by an unknown mER can activate ERK signaling, which in turn may cause phosphorylation of the ERα and increased transcription from promoters than contain EREs (130). Alternatively, ERK signaling may also lead via unknown mechanisms to increased transcription from the c-Fos promoter (190) while PKA signaling generated by the mER may lead to increased transcription from promoters that have a cAMP response element (CRE) enhancer (189).

(**Figure 2**) to aggression is under active investigation in our laboratory, with the idea that glucocorticoid control of aggressive behavior is dependent on neuroestrogen concentrations in the brain.

FUNCTIONS OF NON-GENOMIC SIGNALING

One function of non-genomic signaling within a cell could be to provide cells with another pathway by which they can respond differently to the same endogenous ligand. For example, acute signaling by glucocorticoids increases aggression in an ethologically relevant context but chronic signaling by glucocorticoids increases submission (186). A parallel is seen with the regulation of the CRH neuron by acute or chronic glucocorticoid exposure via the regulation of synaptic inputs in the opposite direction. In the acute phase, rapid signaling by glucocorticoids increases negative feedback on the CRH neuron decreasing the firing of the neuron (187), while chronic exposure to glucocorticoids decreases negative feedback on the CRH and increases CRH mRNA, increasing HPA axis reactivity (188). A second function of membrane-initiated signaling might be to prime nuclear transcription via the phosphorylation of ERα, seen in a neuroblastoma cell line (130) (**Figure 3**), leading to greater transcription from genes with EREs in their promoters. In some cases, rapid signaling could also activate genes that do not have classical EREs in their promoters. For example, PKA signaling induced by 17β-E in the SK-N-SH neuronal cell line was required to induce the neurotensin/neuromedin gene (189), while E2-BSA in this cell line activated a reporter gene driven by a c-Fos promoter in an ERK-dependent manner (190). The idea that non-genomic signaling might prime later outputs such as behavior is also evident from the studies on sex behavior in female and male rodents. Apart from the potentiation of transcription by rapid signaling, non-genomic signaling could also decrease transcription if the decrease in transcription is ultimately important in leading to an optimal cellular response. For example, the increase in PI3K and MAPK activation that occurs within 30 min via ERα in the mHypoE-38 hypothalamic cell line is required for the long-term repression of neuropeptide Y by 17β-E (191). Third, non-genomic signaling via one pathway could also synergize with rapid signaling pathways initiated by other ligands. For instance, 17β-E-induced increases in calcium in POMC neurons augmented the activation of the calcium-sensitive TRPC channels (192) already upregulated by leptin (65). Additionally, 17β-E also transcriptionally induced PI3K p85 subunit in the hypothalamus (193, 194) and this combined with the non-genomic signaling-mediated increase in calcium potentiates the PI3K and calcium-mediated TRPC channel opening activated by leptin (70). In this case, 17β-E utilized both non-genomic, i.e., calcium increase and genomic signaling, i.e., PI3K transcriptional upregulation to synergize with the rapid signaling initiated by the leptin receptor to converge onto neuronal depolarization. Fourth, non-genomic signaling pathways may also synergize with a parallel, independent transcriptional pathway, in response to the same ligand. The rapid action of glucocorticoids in decreasing glutamatergic inputs to the CRH neuron combined with slower transcriptional downregulation of the CRH and vasopressin gene are dual pathways that achieve negative feedback

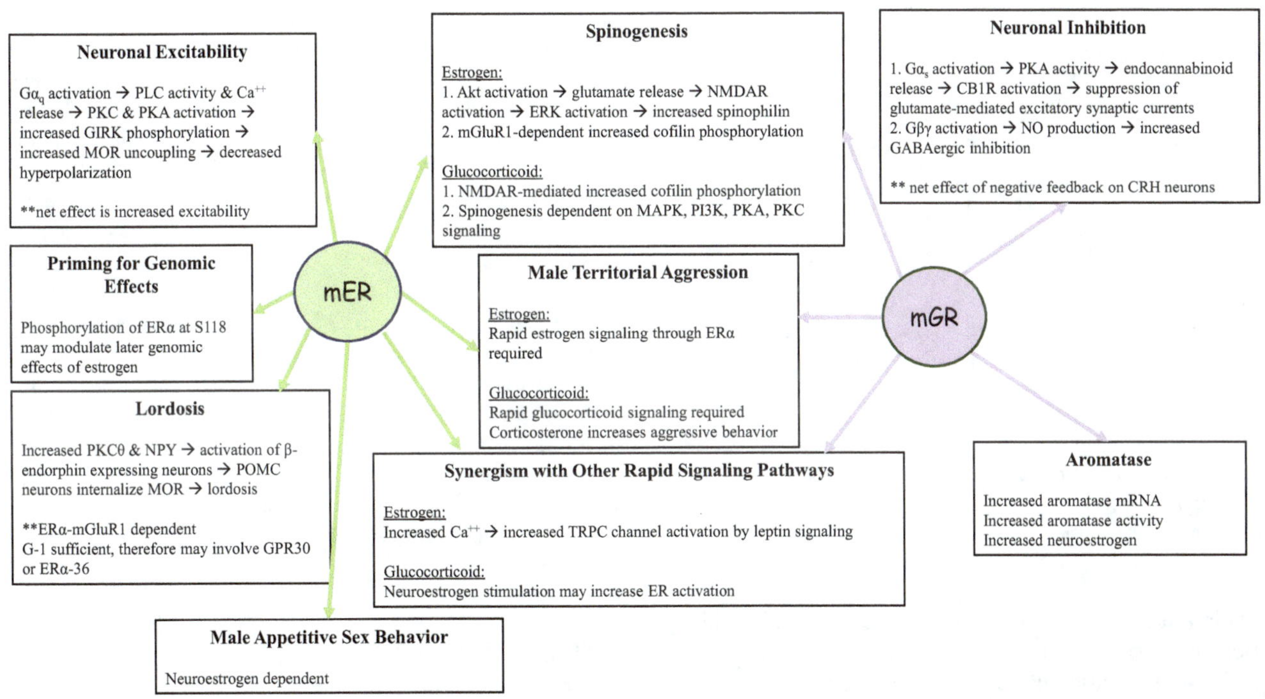

FIGURE 4 | Functions of non-genomic signaling initiated by the mER or the mGR in the CNS. Both mER and mGR contribute to the regulation of male territorial aggression and spinogenesis in neurons, as well as synergizing with other rapid signaling pathways. In the pre-opiomelanocortin (POMC) neuron shown on the left, non-genomic signaling by the mER increases neuronal excitability while rapid negative feedback by the mGR in corticotropin releasing hormone (CRH) neurons decreases neuronal excitability (shown on the right). In addition, the mER plays a role in male sexual behavior and may interact with GPR30 regulates lordosis behavior in female rodents. Glucocorticoids via the mGR also increase neuroestrogen concentrations, via aromatase activity and the increase in aromatase protein, thus providing a route by which the actions of estrogens and glucocorticoids can converge in the brain.

Table 2 | Receptors that are activated or inhibited by the natural estrogen 17β-estradiol, the natural glucocorticoid, corticosterone, a membrane-limited estrogen conjugate (E2-BSA) or glucocorticoid-conjugate (Dex-BSA), or selective agonists or antagonists.

Hormone/drug	Receptor activation	Receptor antagonism	Reference
17β-estradiol	All ERs	None	
E2-BSA	All mERs	None	
Propyl pyrazole triol (PPT)	ERα; 410-fold selectivity over ERβ. Also binds GPR30	None reported	(199)
R,R(THC)	ERα	ERβ	(200)
Diarylpropionitrile (DPN)	ERβ; 70-fold selectivity over ERα	None reported	(201)
ICI 182,780	GPR30	ERα/ERβ	(202)
G-1	GPR30 and ERα-36	None reported	(60)
G-15	ERα or ERβ; activates ERE	GPR30	(203)
G-36	None reported	GPR30	(203)
Corticosterone	All GRs Mineralocorticoid receptor	None reported	(204)
Dexamethasone	All GRs MR (30% of affinity to GR)	None reported	(204)
Dex-BSA	All mGRs	None reported	
RU-486 (mifepristone)	None reported	GR, progesterone receptor	(205)

As can be seen, several selective agonists or antagonists show cross-reactivity to other receptors for estrogens and to other receptors for mineralocorticoids and progestins, in the case of the glucorticoids. Hence, results obtained using these compounds must be carefully interpreted.
MR, mineralocorticoid receptor.

regulation in the PVN (19). Glucocorticoid-mediated rapid regulation of aromatase combined with the slower transcriptional increase or aromatase mRNA and protein is yet another example where both modes would finally increase neuroestrogens in the hypothalamus. Lastly, non-genomic signaling in one cell type may also synergize with genomic signaling in another cell type to converge onto behavioral outputs. This is demonstrated by the ability of 17β-E to elicit a rapid calcium increase in hypothalamic astrocytes that is required for the increased synthesis of neuroprogesterone (195). This release of progesterone that binds to the PR that is transcriptionally induced by the liganded ERα in hypothalamic neurons is required for lordosis behavior in rodents (195). Some of these functions of non-genomic signaling are shown in **Figure 4.**

FUTURE DIRECTIONS

Understanding the many facets of non-genomic signaling would also spotlight the role and source of the ligand. The idea that local estrogen synthesis in the brain, i.e., neuroestrogens is important in transducing environmental stimuli to behavior is fairly recent and has mostly been explored in birds (155, 156, 196). In addition, this would bring into focus the role of estrogens in males; traditionally, classical female-typical behaviors such as lordosis have received far more attention in the estrogen field. Second, many of the studies described above were done in rats whereas there are hints that there may be subtle differences in the mouse. For example, though there is very little GPR30 protein reported in the rat amygdala (76), there is high expression of GPR30 in the mouse basolateral amygdala and intra-amygdalar injection of G-1 attenuates behaviors that denote anxiety in the mouse (197). Similarly, though G-1 failed to regulate sex behavior in the female rat (198), it could do so in the female mouse (127). Though studies on rapid non-genomic signaling have become more mainstream, a number of mechanistic aspects of non-genomic signaling and coupled signaling remain unknown including the temporal nature of the shift from non-genomic signaling to genomic signaling. The role of the ERα variants and GR variants in any of these hypothalamically driven behaviors or in spinogenesis is unclear, with almost no studies on the subject. In this regard, it is worth nothing that studies using agonists or antagonists should be careful to verify if the effects are specific – for example, some of the G-1 mediated effects could be via ERα-36 and some of the ICI-mediated effects could be via GPR30 (**Table 2**).

Complementary studies using deletions of the genes in animals or preferably using site-specific or temporally specific deletion would prove useful to establish specificity. The detailed molecular pathways by which 17β-E regulates spinogenesis or behaviors in the VMH are also not well worked out, though there has been considerable progress in the last decade on the receptors that might be involved. Lastly, understanding non-genomic signaling is possibly a mechanism to convey information about external physiologically relevant stimuli rapidly to the animal to generate both acute and chronic outcomes.

ACKNOWLEDGMENTS

We gratefully acknowledge discussions with Dr. Jeffrey Tasker, Department of Cell and Molecular Biology, Tulane University, particularly on the GR, during the preparation of this manuscript and thank Dr. Sara Clark for proofreading of the manuscript. This work is supported by the NSF CAREER IOS 1053716 grant, awarded to NV and the Louisiana Board of Regents Fellowship awarded to KP.

REFERENCES

Nilsson S, Makela S, Treuter E, Tujague M, Thomsen J, Andersson G, et al. Mechanisms of estrogen action. *Physiol Rev* (2001) 81:1535–65.

Hamilton KJ, Arao Y, Korach KS. Estrogen hormone physiology: reproduc- tive findings from estrogen receptor mutant mice. *Reprod Biol* (2014) 14:3–8. doi:10.1016/j.repbio.2013.12.002

Aranda A, Pascual A. Nuclear hormone receptors and gene expression. *Physiol Rev* (2001) 81:1269–304.

Huang P, Chandra V, Rastinejad F. Structural overview of the nuclear recep- tor superfamily: insights into physiology and therapeutics. *Annu Rev Physiol* (2010) 72:247–72. doi:10.1146/annurev-physiol-021909-135917

Szego CM, Davis JS. Adenosine 3',5'-monophosphate in rat uterus: acute ele- vation by estrogen. *Proc Natl Acad Sci U S A* (1967) 58:1711–8. doi:10.1073/pnas.58.4.1711

Malyala A, Kelly MJ, Ronnekleiv OK. Estrogen modulation of hypothala- mic neurons: activation of multiple signaling pathways and gene expression changes. *Steroids* (2005) 70:397–406. doi:10.1016/j.steroids.2005.03.004

Kelly MJ, Ronnekleiv OK. Membrane-initiated estrogen signaling in hypothal- amic neurons. *Mol Cell Endocrinol* (2008) 290:14–23. doi:10.1016/j.mce.2008. 04.014

Segal M, Murphy DD. CREB activation mediates plasticity in cultured hip- pocampal neurons. *Neural Plast* (1998) 6:1–7. doi:10.1155/NP.1998.1

Htun H, Barsony J, Renyi I, Gould DL, Hager GL. Visualization of glucocorti- coid receptor translocation and intranuclear organization in living cells with a green fluorescent protein chimera. *Proc Natl Acad Sci U S A* (1996) 93:4845–50. doi:10.1073/pnas.93.10.4845

Hache RJ, Tse R, Reich T, Savory JG, Lefebvre YA. Nucleocytoplasmic traffick- ing of steroid-free glucocorticoid receptor. *J Biol Chem* (1999) 274:1432–9. doi:10.1074/jbc.274.3.1432

Bouazza B, Debba-Pavard M, Amrani Y, Isaacs L, O'connell D, Ahamed S, et al. Basal p38 mitogen-activated protein kinase regulates unliganded glucocorti- coid receptor function in airway smooth muscle cells. *Am J Respir Cell Mol Biol* (2014) 50:301–15. doi:10.1165/rcmb.2012-0522OC

Chen DY, Bambah-Mukku D, Pollonini G, Alberini CM. Glucocorticoid recep- tors recruit the CaMKIIalpha-BDNF-CREB pathways to mediate memory consolidation. *Nat Neurosci* (2012) 15:1707–14. doi:10.1038/nn.3266

Di S, Malcher-Lopes R, Halmos KC, Tasker JG. Nongenomic glucocorticoid inhibition via endocannabinoid release in the hypothalamus: a fast feedback mechanism. *J Neurosci* (2003) 23:4850–7.

Vasudevan N, Pfaff DW. Membrane-initiated actions of estrogens in neuroen- docrinology: emerging principles. *Endocr Rev* (2007) 28:1–19. doi:10.1210/er.2005-0021

Warner M, Gustafsson JA. Nongenomic effects of estrogen: why all the uncer- tainty? *Steroids* (2006) 71:91–5. doi:10.1016/j.steroids.2005.09.001

Pfaff DW, McCarthy M, Schwartz-Giblin S, Kow LM. Female reproductive behavior. In: Knobil E, Neill J, editors. *The Physiology of Reproduction*. New York, NY: Raven (1994). p. 107–220.

Dallman MF. Fast glucocorticoid actions on brain: back to the future. *Front Neuroendocrinol* (2005) 26:103–8. doi:10.1016/j.yfrne.2005.08.001

Micevych P, Dominguez R. Membrane estradiol signaling in the brain. *Front Neuroendocrinol* (2009) 30:315–27. doi:10.1016/j.yfrne.2009.04.011

Hill MN, Tasker JG. Endocannabinoid signaling, glucocorticoid-mediated neg- ative feedback, and regulation of the hypothalamic-pituitary-adrenal axis. *Neu- roscience* (2012) 204:5–16. doi:10.1016/j.neuroscience.2011.12.030

Towle AC, Sze PY. Steroid binding to synaptic plasma membrane: differen- tial binding of glucocorticoids and gonadal steroids. *J Steroid Biochem* (1983) 18:135–43. doi:10.1016/0022-4731(83)90079-1

Zheng J, Ali A, Ramirez VD. Steroids conjugated to bovine serum albumin as tools to demonstrate specific steroid neuronal membrane binding sites. *J Psychiatry Neurosci* (1996) 21:187–97.

Micevych P, Kuo J, Christensen A. Physiology of membrane oestrogen receptor signalling in reproduction. *J Neuroendocrinol* (2009) 21:249–56. doi:10.1111/ j.1365-2826.2009.01833.x

Filardo EJ. Epidermal growth factor receptor (EGFR) transactivation by estro- gen via the G-protein-coupled receptor, GPR30: a novel signaling pathway with potential significance for breast cancer. *J Steroid Biochem Mol Biol* (2002) 80:231–8. doi:10.1016/S0960-0760(01)00190-X

Pietranera L, Brocca ME, Roig P, Lima A, Garcia-Segura LM, De Nicola AF. 17alpha-Oestradiol-induced neuroprotection in the brain of spontaneously hypertensive rats. *J Neuroendocrinol* (2014) 26:310–20. doi:10.1111/jne.12151

Shughrue PJ, Lane MV, Merchenthaler I. Comparative distribution of estrogen receptor-alpha and -beta mRNA in the rat central nervous system. *J Comp Neu- rol* (1997) 388:507–25. doi:10.1002/(SICI)1096-9861(19971201)388:4<507::AID-CNE1>3.0.CO;2-6

Laflamme N, Nappi RE, Drolet G, Labrie C, Rivest S. Expression and neu- ropeptidergic characterization of estrogen receptors (ERalpha and ERbeta) throughout the rat brain: anatomical evidence of distinct roles of each sub- type. *J Neurobiol* (1998) 36:357–78. doi:10.1002/(SICI)1097-4695(19980905) 36:3<357::AID-NEU5>3.0.CO;2-V

Mitra SW, Hoskin E, Yudkovitz J, Pear L, Wilkinson HA, Hayashi S, et al. Immunolocalization of estrogen receptor beta in the mouse brain: com- parison with estrogen receptor alpha. *Endocrinology* (2003) 144:2055–67. doi:10.1210/en.2002-221069

Musatov S, Chen W, Pfaff DW, Kaplitt MG, Ogawa S. RNAi-mediated silencing of estrogen receptor {alpha} in the ventromedial nucleus of hypothalamus abol- ishes female sexual behaviors. *Proc Natl Acad Sci U S A* (2006) 103:10456–60. doi:10.1073/pnas.0603045103

Sano K, Tsuda MC, Musatov S, Sakamoto T, Ogawa S. Differential effects of site-specific knockdown of estrogen receptor alpha in the medial amygdala, medial pre-optic area, and ventromedial nucleus of the hypothalamus on sex- ual and aggressive behavior of male mice. *Eur J Neurosci* (2013) 37:1308–19. doi:10.1111/ejn.12131

Levin ER. Membrane oestrogen receptor alpha signalling to cell functions. *J Physiol* (2009) 587:5019–23. doi:10.1113/jphysiol.2009.177097

Zivadinovic D, Gametchu B, Watson CS. Membrane estrogen receptor-alpha levels in MCF-7 breast cancer cells predict cAMP and proliferation responses. *Breast Cancer Res* (2005) 7:R101–12. doi:10.1186/bcr959

Bulayeva NN, Wozniak AL, Lash LL, Watson CS. Mechanisms of membrane estrogen receptor-alpha-mediated rapid stimulation of Ca2+ levels and pro- lactin release in a pituitary cell line. *Am J Physiol Endocrinol Metab* (2005) 288:E388–97. doi:10.1152/ajpendo.00349.2004

Zivadinovic D, Watson CS. Membrane estrogen receptor-alpha levels predict estrogen-induced ERK1/2 activation in MCF-7 cells. *Breast Cancer Res* (2005) 7:R130–44. doi:10.1186/bcr959

Blaustein JD, Lehman MN, Turcotte JC, Greene G. Estrogen receptors in den- drites and axon terminals in the guinea pig hypothalamus. *Endocrinology* (1992) 131:281–90. doi:10.1210/endo.131.1.1612006

Milner TA, McEwen BS, Hayashi S, Li CJ, Reagan LP, Alves SE. Ultrastructural evidence that hippocampal alpha estrogen receptors are located at extranuclear sites. *J Comp Neurol* (2001) 429:355–71. doi:10.1002/1096-9861(20010115)429:3<355::AID-CNE1>3.0.CO;2-\#

Hart SA, Snyder MA, Smejkalova T, Woolley CS. Estrogen mobilizes a subset of estrogen receptor-alpha-immunoreactive vesicles in inhibitory presynap- tic boutons in hippocampal CA1. *J Neurosci* (2007) 27:2102–11. doi:10.1523/JNEUROSCI.5436-06.2007

Tabatadze N, Smejkalova T, Woolley CS. Distribution and posttranslational modification of synaptic ERalpha in the adult female rat hippocampus. *Endocrinology* (2013) 154:819–30. doi:10.1210/en.2012-1870

Bondar G, Kuo J, Hamid N, Micevych P. Estradiol-induced estrogen receptor- alpha trafficking. *J Neurosci* (2009) 29:15323–30. doi:10.1523/JNEUROSCI. 2107-09.2009

Dominguez R, Micevych P. Estradiol rapidly regulates membrane estrogen receptor alpha levels in hypothalamic neurons. *J Neurosci* (2010) 30:12589–96. doi:10.1523/JNEUROSCI.1038-10.2010

Patel HH, Insel PA. Lipid rafts and caveolae and their role in compart- mentation of redox signaling. *Antioxid Redox Signal* (2009) 11:1357–72. doi:10.1089/ARS.2008.2365

Razandi M, Oh P, Pedram A, Schnitzer J, Levin ER. ERs associate with and regu- late the production of caveolin: implications for signaling and cellular actions. *Mol Endocrinol* (2002) 16:100–15. doi:10.1210/mend.16.1.0757

Boulware MI, Weick JP, Becklund BR, Kuo SP, Groth RD, Mermelstein PG. Estradiol activates group I and II metabotropic glutamate receptor signaling, leading to opposing influences on cAMP response element-binding protein. *J Neurosci* (2005) 25:5066–78. doi:10.1523/JNEUROSCI.1427-05.2005

Kuo J, Hariri OR, Bondar G, Ogi J, Micevych P. Membrane estrogen receptor- alpha interacts with metabotropic glutamate receptor type 1a to mobi- lize intracellular calcium in hypothalamic astrocytes. *Endocrinology* (2009) 150:1369–76. doi:10.1210/en.2008-0994

Meitzen J, Mermelstein PG. Estrogen receptors stimulate brain region specific metabotropic glutamate receptors to rapidly initiate signal transduction path- ways. *J Chem Neuroanat* (2011) 42:236–41. doi:10.1016/j.jchemneu.2011.02.002

Navarro CE, Abdul Saeed S, Murdock C, Martinez-Fuentes AJ, Arora KK, Krs- manovic LZ, et al. Regulation of cyclic adenosine 3',5'-monophosphate sig- naling and pulsatile neurosecretion by Gi-coupled plasma membrane estro- gen receptors in immortalized gonadotropin-releasing hormone neurons. *Mol Endocrinol* (2003) 17:1792–804. doi:10.1210/me.2003-0040

Chambliss KL, Shaul PW. Estrogen modulation of endothelial nitric oxide syn- thase. *Endocr Rev* (2002) 23:665–86. doi:10.1210/er.2001-0045

Acconcia F, Ascenzi P, Bocedi A, Spisni E, Tomasi V, Trentalance A, et al. Palmitoylation-dependent estrogen receptor alpha membrane localization: regulation by 17beta-estradiol. *Mol Biol Cell* (2005) 16:231–7. doi:10.1091/mbc.E04-07-0547

Razandi M, Alton G, Pedram A, Ghonshani S, Webb P, Levin ER. Identification of a structural determinant necessary for the localization and function of estro- gen receptor alpha at the plasma membrane. *Mol Cell Biol* (2003) 23:1633–46. doi:10.1128/MCB.23.5.1633-1646.2003

Razandi M, Pedram A, Levin ER. Heat shock protein 27 is required for sex steroid receptor trafficking to and functioning at the plasma membrane. *Mol Cell Biol* (2010) 30:3249–61. doi:10.1128/MCB.01354-09

Razandi M, Pedram A, Merchenthaler I, Greene GL, Levin ER. Plasma mem- brane estrogen receptors exist and functions as dimers. *Mol Endocrinol* (2004) 18:2854–65. doi:10.1210/me.2004-0115

Tan Z, Zhou LJ, Li Y, Cui YH, Xiang QL, Lin GP, et al. E(2)-BSA activates caveolin-1 via PI(3)K/ERK1/2 and lysosomal degradation pathway and con- tributes to EPC proliferation. *Int J Cardiol* (2012) 158:46–53. doi:10.1016/j.ijcard.2010.12.106

Dominguez R, Dewing P, Kuo J, Micevych P. Membrane-initiated estra- diol signaling in immortalized hypothalamic N-38 neurons. *Steroids* (2013) 78:607–13. doi:10.1016/j.steroids.2012.12.008

Dewire SM, Ahn S, Lefkowitz RJ, Shenoy SK. Beta-arrestins and cell signal- ing. *Annu Rev Physiol* (2007) 69:483–510. doi:10.1146/annurev.ph.69.013107. 100021

Dominguez R, Hu E, Zhou M, Baudry M. 17beta-estradiol-mediated neu- roprotection and ERK activation require a pertussis toxin-sensitive mech- anism involving GRK2 and beta-arrestin-1. *J Neurosci* (2009) 29:4228–38. doi:10.1523/JNEUROSCI.0550-09.2009

Blaustein JD. Cytoplasmic estrogen receptors in rat brain: immunocytochemi- cal evidence using three antibodies with distinct epitopes. *Endocrinology* (1992) 131:1336–42. doi:10.1210/endo.131.3.1380440

Meredith JM, Auger CJ, Blaustein JD. Down-regulation of estrogen receptor immunoreactivity by 17 beta-estradiol in the guinea pig forebrain. *J Neuroen- docrinol* (1994) 6:639–48. doi:10.1111/j.1365-2826.1994.tb00630.x

Snyder MA, Smejkalova T, Forlano PM, Woolley CS. Multiple ERbeta antisera label in ERbeta knockout and null mouse tissues. *J Neurosci Methods* (2010) 188:226–34. doi:10.1016/j.jneumeth.2010.02.012

Abraham IM, Todman MG, Korach KS, Herbison AE. Critical in vivo roles for classical estrogen receptors in rapid estrogen actions on intracellular signaling in mouse brain. *Endocrinology* (2004) 145:3055–61. doi:10.1210/en.2003-1676

Wang Z, Zhang X, Shen P, Loggie BW, Chang Y, Deuel TF. A variant of estrogen receptor-{alpha}, hER-{alpha}36: transduction of estrogen- and antiestrogen- dependent membrane-initiated mitogenic signaling. *Proc Natl Acad Sci U S A* (2006) 103:9063–8. doi:10.1073/pnas.0603339103

Kang L, Zhang X, Xie Y, Tu Y, Wang D, Liu Z, et al. Involvement of estrogen receptor variant ER-alpha36, not GPR30, in nongenomic estrogen signaling. *Mol Endocrinol* (2010) 24:709–21. doi:10.1210/me.2009-0317

Li L, Haynes MP, Bender JR. Plasma membrane localization and function of the estrogen receptor alpha variant (ER46) in human endothelial cells. *Proc Natl Acad Sci U S A* (2003) 100:4807–12. doi:10.1073/pnas.0831079100

Flouriot G, Brand H, Denger S, Metivier R, Kos M, Reid G, et al. Identification of a new isoform of the human estrogen receptor-alpha (hER-alpha) that is encoded by distinct transcripts and that is able to repress hER-alpha activation function 1. *EMBO J* (2000) 19:4688–700. doi:10.1093/emboj/19.17.4688

Toran-Allerand CD, Guan X, Maclusky NJ, Horvath TL, Diano S, Singh M, et al. ER-X: a novel, plasma membrane-associated, putative estrogen receptor that is regulated during development and after ischemic brain injury. *J Neurosci* (2002) 22:8391–401.

Kelly MJ, Qiu J, Ronnekleiv OK. Estrogen signaling in the hypothalamus. *Vitam Horm* (2005) 71:123–45. doi:10.1016/S0083-6729(05)71005-0

Kelly MJ, Ronnekleiv OK. Membrane-initiated actions of estradiol that regulate reproduction, energy balance and body temperature. *Front Neuroendocrinol* (2012) 33:376–87. doi:10.1016/j.yfrne.2012.07.002

Kelly MJ, Lagrange AH, Wagner EJ, Ronnekleiv OK. Rapid effects of estrogen to modulate G protein-coupled receptors via activation of protein kinase A and protein kinase C pathways. *Steroids* (1999) 64:64–75. doi:10.1016/S0039- 128X(98)00095-6

Kelly MJ, Ronnekleiv OK, Ibrahim N, Lagrange AH, Wagner EJ. Estrogen mod- ulation of K(+) channel activity in hypothalamic neurons involved in the con- trol of the reproductive axis. *Steroids* (2002) 67:447–56. doi:10.1016/S0039-128X(01)00181-7

Roepke TA, Qiu J, Bosch MA, Ronnekleiv OK, Kelly MJ. Cross-talk between membrane-initiated and nuclear-initiated oestrogen signalling in the hypo- thalamus. *J Neuroendocrinol* (2009) 21:263–70. doi:10.1111/j.1365-2826.2009.01846.x

Qiu J, Ronnekleiv OK, Kelly MJ. Modulation of hypothalamic neuronal activ- ity through a novel G-protein-coupled estrogen membrane receptor. *Steroids* (2008) 73:985–91. doi:10.1016/j.steroids.2007.11.008

Qiu J, Fang Y, Ronnekleiv OK, Kelly MJ. Leptin excites proopiomelanocortin neurons via activation of TRPC channels. *J Neurosci* (2010) 30:1560–5. doi:10.1523/JNEUROSCI.4816-09.2010

Kelly MJ, Ronnekleiv OK. A selective membrane estrogen receptor agonist maintains autonomic functions in hypoestrogenic states. *Brain Res* (2013) 1514:75–82. doi:10.1016/j.brainres.2013.03.020

Smith AW, Bosch MA, Wagner EJ, Ronnekleiv OK, Kelly MJ. The mem- brane estrogen receptor ligand STX rapidly enhances GABAergic signaling in NPY/AgRP neurons: role in mediating the anorexigenic effects of 17beta-estradiol. *Am J Physiol Endocrinol Metab* (2013) 305:E632–40. doi:10.1152/ ajpendo.00281.2013

Nestor CC, Kelly MJ, Ronnekleiv OK. Cross-talk between reproduction and energy homeostasis: central impact of estrogens, leptin and kisspeptin signal- ing. *Horm Mol Biol Clin Investig* (2014) 17:109–28. doi:10.1515/hmbci-2013-0050

Smith AW, Ronnekleiv OK, Kelly MJ. Gq-mER signaling has opposite effects on hypothalamic orexigenic and anorexigenic neurons. *Steroids* (2014) 81:31–5. doi:10.1016/j.steroids.2013.11.007

Thomas P, Pang Y, Filardo EJ, Dong J. Identity of an estrogen membrane recep- tor coupled to a G protein in human breast cancer cells. *Endocrinology* (2005) 146:624–32. doi:10.1210/en.2004-1064

Brailoiu E, Dun SL, Brailoiu GC, Mizuo K, Sklar LA, Oprea TI, et al. Distri- bution and characterization of estrogen receptor G protein-coupled recep- tor 30 in the rat central nervous system. *J Endocrinol* (2007) 193:311–21. doi:10.1677/JOE-07-0017

Filardo E, Quinn J, Pang Y, Graeber C, Shaw S, Dong J, et al. Activation of the novel estrogen receptor G protein-coupled receptor 30 (GPR30) at the plasma membrane. *Endocrinology* (2007) 148:3236–45. doi:10.1210/en.2006- 1605

Akama KT, Thompson LI, Milner TA, McEwen BS. Post-synaptic density-95 (PSD-95) binding capacity of G-protein-coupled receptor 30 (GPR30), an estrogen receptor that can be identified in hippocampal dendritic spines. *J Biol Chem* (2013) 288:6438–50. doi:10.1074/jbc.M112.412478

Funakoshi T, Yanai A, Shinoda K, Kawano MM, Mizukami Y. G protein-coupled receptor 30 is an estrogen receptor in the plasma membrane. *Biochem Biophys Res Commun* (2006) 346:904–10. doi:10.1016/j.bbrc.2006.05.191

Cheng SB, Graeber CT, Quinn JA, Filardo EJ. Retrograde transport of the trans- membrane estrogen receptor, G-protein-coupled-receptor-30 (GPR30/GPER) from the plasma membrane towards the nucleus. *Steroids* (2011) 76:892–6. doi:10.1016/j.steroids.2011.02.018

Matsuda K, Sakamoto H, Mori H, Hosokawa K, Kawamura A, Itose M, et al. Expression and intracellular distribution of the G protein-coupled receptor 30 in rat hippocampal formation. *Neurosci Lett* (2008) 441:94–9. doi:10.1016/j.neulet.2008.05.108

Revankar CM, Cimino DF, Sklar LA, Arterburn JB, Prossnitz ER. A trans- membrane intracellular estrogen receptor mediates rapid cell signaling. *Science* (2005) 307:1625–30. doi:10.1126/science.1106943

Cheng SB, Quinn JA, Graeber CT, Filardo EJ. Down-modulation of the G-protein-coupled estrogen receptor, GPER, from the cell surface occurs via a trans-Golgi-proteasome pathway. *J Biol Chem* (2011) 286:22441–55. doi:10.1074/jbc.M111.224071

Revankar CM, Mitchell HD, Field AS, Burai R, Corona C, Ramesh C, et al. Synthetic estrogen derivatives demonstrate the functionality of intracellular GPR30. *ACS Chem Biol* (2007) 2:536–44. doi:10.1021/cb700072n

Broselid S, Berg KA, Chavera TA, Kahn R, Clarke WP, Olde B, et al. G protein-coupled receptor 30 (GPR30) forms a plasma membrane complex with membrane-associated guanylate kinases (MAGUKs) and protein kinase A-anchoring protein 5 (AKAP5) that constitutively inhibits cAMP production. *J Biol Chem* (2014) 289:22117–27. doi:10.1074/jbc.M114.566893

Heitzer MD, Wolf IM, Sanchez ER, Witchel SF, Defranco DB. Glucocorticoid receptor physiology. *Rev Endocr Metab Disord* (2007) 8:321–30. doi:10.1007/ s11154-007-9059-8

Stahn C, Buttgereit F. Genomic and nongenomic effects of glucocorticoids. *Nat Clin Pract Rheumatol* (2008) 4:525–33. doi:10.1038/ncprheum0898

Strehl C, Gaber T, Lowenberg M, Hommes DW, Verhaar AP, Schellmann S, et al. Origin and functional activity of the membrane-bound glucocorticoid receptor. *Arthritis Rheum* (2011) 63:3779–88. doi:10.1002/art.30637

Pujols L, Mullol J, Roca-Ferrer J, Torrego A, Xaubet A, Cidlowski JA, et al. Expression of glucocorticoid receptor alpha- and beta-isoforms in human cells and tissues. *Am J Physiol Cell Physiol* (2002) 283:C1324–31. doi:10.1152/ajpcell. 00363.2001

Oakley RH, Cidlowski JA. The biology of the glucocorticoid receptor: new signaling mechanisms in health and disease. *J Allergy Clin Immunol* (2013) 132:1033–44. doi:10.1016/j.jaci.2013.09.007

Bartholome B, Spies CM, Gaber T, Schuchmann S, Berki T, Kunkel D, et al. Membrane glucocorticoid receptors (mGCR) are expressed in normal human peripheral blood mononuclear cells and up-regulated after in vitro stimu- lation and in patients with rheumatoid arthritis. *FASEB J* (2004) 18:70–80. doi:10.1096/fj.03-0328com

Vernocchi S, Battello N, Schmitz S, Revets D, Billing AM, Turner JD, et al. Mem- brane glucocorticoid receptor activation induces proteomic changes aligning with classical glucocorticoid effects. *Mol Cell Proteomics* (2013) 12:1764–79. doi:10.1074/mcp.M112.022947

Samarasinghe RA, Di Maio R, Volonte D, Galbiati F, Lewis M, Romero G, et al. Nongenomic glucocorticoid receptor action regulates gap junction intercellu- lar communication and neural progenitor cell proliferation. *Proc Natl Acad Sci U S A* (2011) 108:16657–62. doi:10.1073/pnas.1102821108

McEwen BS, De Kloet R, Wallach G. Interactions in vivo and in vitro of corti- coids and progesterone with cell nuclei and soluble macromolecules from rat brain regions and pituitary. *Brain Res* (1976) 105:129–36. doi:10.1016/0006-8993(76)90928-8

Komatsuzaki Y, Murakami G, Tsurugizawa T, Mukai H, Tanabe N, Mitsuhashi K, et al. Rapid spinogenesis of pyramidal neurons induced by activation of glucocorticoid receptors in adult male rat hippocampus. *Biochem Biophys Res Commun* (2005) 335:1002–7. doi:10.1016/j.bbrc.2005.07.173

Liposits Z, Bohn MC. Association of glucocorticoid receptor immunoreactivity with cell membrane and transport vesicles in hippocampal and hypothalamic neurons of the rat. *J Neurosci Res* (1993) 35:14–9. doi:10.1002/jnr.490350103

Jafari M, Seese RR, Babayan AH, Gall CM, Lauterborn JC. Glucocorticoid receptors are localized to dendritic spines and influence local actin signaling. *Mol Neurobiol* (2012) 46:304–15. doi:10.1007/s12035-012-8288-3

Qi AQ, Qiu J, Xiao L, Chen YZ. Rapid activation of JNK and p38 by glucocor- ticoids in primary cultured hippocampal cells. *J Neurosci Res* (2005) 80:510–7. doi:10.1002/jnr.20491

Evanson NK, Tasker JG, Hill MN, Hillard CJ, Herman JP. Fast feedback inhi- bition of the HPA axis by glucocorticoids is mediated by endocannabinoid signaling. *Endocrinology* (2010) 151:4811–9. doi:10.1210/en.2010-0285

Di S, Maxson MM, Franco A, Tasker JG. Glucocorticoids regulate glutamate and GABA synapse-specific retrograde transmission via divergent nongenomic signaling pathways. *J Neurosci* (2009) 29:393–401. doi:10.1523/JNEUROSCI. 4546-08.2009

Di S, Malcher-Lopes R, Marcheselli VL, Bazan NG, Tasker JG. Rapid glucocorticoid-mediated endocannabinoid release and opposing regulation of glutamate and gamma-aminobutyric acid inputs to hypothalamic magnocel- lular neurons. *Endocrinology* (2005) 146:4292–301. doi:10.1210/en.2005-0610

Toran-Allerand CD. Minireview: a plethora of estrogen receptors in the brain: where will it end? *Endocrinology* (2004) 145:1069–74. doi:10.1210/en.2003- 1462

Otto C, Rohde-Schulz B, Schwarz G, Fuchs I, Klewer M, Brittain D, et al. G protein-coupled receptor 30 localizes to the endoplasmic reticulum and is not activated by estradiol. *Endocrinology* (2008) 149:4846–56. doi:10.1210/en.2008-0269

Albanito L, Lappano R, Madeo A, Chimento A, Prossnitz ER, Cappello AR, et al. G-protein-coupled receptor 30 and estrogen receptor-alpha are involved in the proliferative effects induced by atrazine in ovarian cancer cells. *Environ Health Perspect* (2008) 116:1648–55. doi:10.1289/ehp.11297

Hart D, Nilges M, Pollard K, Lynn T, Patsos O, Shiel C, et al. Activation of the G-protein coupled receptor 30 (GPR30) has different effects on anxiety in male and female mice. *Steroids* (2014) 81:49–56. doi:10.1016/j.steroids.2013.11.004

Kumar V, Green S, Staub A, Chambon P. Localisation of the oestradiol-binding and putative DNA-binding domains of the human oestrogen receptor. *EMBO J* (1986) 5:2231–6.

Daniels D, Miselis RR, Flanagan-Cato LM. Central neuronal circuit inner- vating the lordosis-producing muscles defined by transneuronal transport of pseudorabies virus. *J Neurosci* (1999) 19:2823–33.

Calizo LH, Flanagan-Cato LM. Estrogen selectively regulates spine density within the dendritic arbor of rat ventromedial hypothalamic neurons. *J Neu- rosci* (2000) 20:1589–96.

Flanagan-Cato LM, Calizo LH, Daniels D. The synaptic organization of VMH neurons that mediate the effects of estrogen on sexual behavior. *Horm Behav* (2001) 40:178–82. doi:10.1006/hbeh.2001.1679

Christensen A, Dewing P, Micevych P. Membrane-initiated estradiol signaling induces spinogenesis required for female sexual receptivity. *J Neurosci* (2011) 31:17583–9. doi:10.1523/JNEUROSCI.3030-11.2011

Akama KT, McEwen BS. Estrogen stimulates postsynaptic density-95 rapid protein synthesis via the Akt/protein kinase B pathway. *J Neurosci* (2003) 23:2333–9.

Schwarz JM, Liang SL, Thompson SM, McCarthy MM. Estradiol induces hypo- thalamic dendritic spines by enhancing glutamate release: a mechanism for organizational sex differences. *Neuron* (2008) 58:584–98. doi:10.1016/j.neuron. 2008.03.008

Micevych P, Christensen A. Membrane-initiated estradiol actions medi- ate structural plasticity and reproduction. *Front Neuroendocrinol* (2012) 33:331–41. doi:10.1016/j.yfrne.2012.07.003

Komatsuzaki Y, Hatanaka Y, Murakami G, Mukai H, Hojo Y, Saito M, et al. Corticosterone induces rapid spinogenesis via synaptic glucocorticoid receptors and kinase networks in hippocampus. *PLoS One* (2012) 7:e34124. doi:10.1371/journal.pone.0034124

Phan A, Lancaster KE, Armstrong JN, Maclusky NJ, Choleris E. Rapid effects of estrogen receptor alpha and beta selective agonists on learning and den- dritic spines in female mice. *Endocrinology* (2011) 152:1492–502. doi:10.1210/ en.2010-1273

Srivastava DP, Woolfrey KM, Liu F, Brandon NJ, Penzes P. Estrogen receptor beta activity modulates synaptic signaling and structure. *J Neurosci* (2010) 30:13454–60. doi:10.1523/JNEUROSCI.3264-10.2010

Dewing P, Christensen A, Bondar G, Micevych P. Protein kinase C signaling in the hypothalamic arcuate nucleus regulates sexual receptivity in female rats. *Endocrinology* (2008) 149:5934–42. doi:10.1210/en.2008-0847

Sinchak K, Micevych P. Visualizing activation of opioid circuits by internal- ization of G protein-coupled receptors. *Mol Neurobiol* (2003) 27:197–222. doi:10.1385/MN:27:2:197

Dewing P, Boulware MI, Sinchak K, Christensen A, Mermelstein PG, Micevych P. Membrane estrogen receptor-alpha interactions with metabotropic gluta- mate receptor 1a modulate female sexual receptivity in rats. *J Neurosci* (2007) 27:9294–300. doi:10.1523/JNEUROSCI.0592-07.2007

Sinchak K, Micevych PE. Progesterone blockade of estrogen activation of mu- opioid receptors regulates reproductive behavior. *J Neurosci* (2001) 21:5723–9.

Micevych PE, Rissman EF, Gustafsson JA, Sinchak K. Estrogen receptor-alpha is required for estrogen-induced mu-opioid receptor internalization. *J Neurosci Res* (2003) 71:802–10. doi:10.1002/jnr.10526

Ogawa S, Eng V, Taylor J, Lubahn DB, Korach KS, Pfaff DW. Roles of estrogen receptor-alpha gene expression in reproduction-related behaviors in female mice. *Endocrinology* (1998) 139:5070–81. doi:10.1210/en.139.12.5070

Christensen A, Micevych P. CAV1 siRNA reduces membrane estrogen receptor-alpha levels and attenuates sexual receptivity. *Endocrinology* (2012) 153:3872–7. doi:10.1210/en.2012-1312

Mermelstein PG, Micevych PE. Nervous system physiology regulated by membrane estrogen receptors. *Rev Neurosci* (2008) 19:413–24. doi:10.1515/ REVNEURO.2008.19.6.413

Christensen A, Micevych P. A novel membrane estrogen receptor activated by STX induces female sexual receptivity through an interaction with mGluR1a. *Neuroendocrinology* (2013) 97:363–8. doi:10.1159/000351077

Hazell GG, Yao ST, Roper JA, Prossnitz ER, O'carroll AM, Lolait SJ. Localisa- tion of GPR30, a novel G protein-coupled oestrogen receptor, suggests mul- tiple functions in rodent brain and peripheral tissues. *J Endocrinol* (2009) 202:223–36. doi:10.1677/JOE-09-0066

Anchan D, Clark S, Pollard K, Vasudevan N. GPR30 activation decreases anxi- ety in the open field test but not in the elevated plus maze test in female mice. *Brain Behav* (2014) 4:51–9. doi:10.1002/brb3.197

Kow LM, Pfaff DW. The membrane actions of estrogens can potentiate their lordosis behavior-facilitating genomic actions. *Proc Natl Acad Sci U S A* (2004) 101:12354–7. doi:10.1073/pnas.0404889101

Pfaff DW, Ogawa S, Kia HK, Vasudevan N, Krebs C, Frohlich J, et al. Genetic mechanisms in neural and hormonal controls over female reproductive behav- iors. In: Pfaff DW, Arnold A, Etgen A, Fahrbach S, Rubin R, editors. *Hormones, Brain and Behavior.* San Diego, CA: Academic Press (2002). p. 441–60.

Clark S, Rainville J, Zhao X, Katzenellenbogen BS, Pfaff D, Vasudevan N. Estro- gen receptor-mediated transcription involves the activation of multiple kinase pathways in neuroblastoma cells. *J Steroid Biochem Mol Biol* (2014) 139:45–53. doi:10.1016/j.jsbmb.2013.09.010

McDevitt MA, Glidewell-Kenney C, Weiss J, Chambon P, Jameson JL, Levine JE. Estrogen response element-independent estrogen receptor (ER)-alpha signal- ing does not rescue sexual behavior but restores normal testoster- one secre- tion in male ERalpha knockout mice. *Endocrinology* (2007) 148:5288–94. doi:10.1210/en.2007-0673

McDevitt MA, Glidewell-Kenney C, Jimenez MA, Ahearn PC, Weiss J, Jame- son JL, et al. New insights into the classical and non-classical actions of estro- gen: evidence from estrogen receptor knockout and knock-in mice. *Mol Cell Endocrinol* (2008) 290:24–30. doi:10.1016/j.mce.2008.04.003

Sa SI, Pereira PA, Malikov V, Ferreira IM, Madeira MD. The role of plasma membrane estrogen receptors in mediating the estrogen induction of proges- terone receptors in hypothalamic ventromedial neurons. *J Comp Neurol* (2014) 522:298–307. doi:10.1002/cne.23396

Parsons B, McEwen B, Pfaff D. A discontinuous schedule of estradiol treatment is sufficient to activate progesterone-facilitated feminine sexual behavior and to increase cytosol receptors for progestins in the hypothalamus of the rat. *Endocrinology* (1982) 110:613–9. doi:10.1210/endo-110-2-613

Cross E, Roselli CE. 17beta-estradiol rapidly facilitates chemoinvestigation and mounting in castrated male rats. *Am J Physiol* (1999) 276:R1346–50.

McGinnis MY, Kahn DF. Inhibition of male sexual behavior by intra- cra- nial implants of the protein synthesis inhibitor anisomycin into the medial preoptic area of the rat. *Horm Behav* (1997) 31:15–23. doi:10.1006/hbeh.1997. 1367

Soma KK. Testosterone and aggression: Berthold, birds and beyond. *J Neuroen- docrinol* (2006) 18:543–51. doi:10.1111/j.1365-2826.2006.01440.x

Gleason ED, Fuxjager MJ, Oyegbile TO, Marler CA. Testosterone release and social context: when it occurs and why. *Front Neuroendocrinol* (2009) 30:460–9. doi:10.1016/j.yfrne.2009.04.009

Naftolin F, MacLusky NJ. Aromatase in the central nervous system. *Cancer Res* (1982) 42:3274s–6s.

Seredynski AL, Balthazart J, Christophe VJ, Ball GF, Cornil CA. Neuroestro- gens rapidly regulate sexual motivation but not performance. *J Neurosci* (2013) 33:164–74. doi:10.1523/JNEUROSCI.2557-12.2013

Taziaux M, Keller M, Bakker J, Balthazart J. Sexual behavior activity tracks rapid changes in brain estrogen concentrations. *J Neurosci* (2007) 27:6563–72. doi:10.1523/JNEUROSCI.1797-07.2007

Dickens MJ, De Bournonville C, Balthazart J, Cornil CA. Relationships between rapid changes in local aromatase activity and estradiol concentrations in male and female quail brain. *Horm Behav* (2014) 65:154–64. doi:10.1016/j.yhbeh. 2013.12.011

Cornil CA, Ball GF, Balthazart J. Rapid control of male typical behav- iors by brain-derived estrogens. *Front Neuroendocrinol* (2012) 33:425–46. doi:10.1016/j.yfrne.2012.08.003

Floody O, Pfaff D. Steroid hormones and aggressive behavior: approaches to the study of hormone-sensitive brain mechanisms for behavior. *Res Publ Assoc Res Nerv Ment Dis* (1974) 52:149–85.

Nelson RJ, Trainor BC. Neural mechanisms of aggression. *Nat Rev Neurosci* (2007) 8:536–46. doi:10.1038/nrn2174

Toda K, Saibara T, Okada T, Onishi S, Shizuta Y. A loss of aggressive behaviour and its reinstatement by oestrogen in mice lacking the aromatase gene (Cyp19). *J Endocrinol* (2001) 168:217–20. doi:10.1677/joe.0.1680217

Trainor BC, Greiwe KM, Nelson RJ. Individual differences in estrogen recep- tor alpha in select brain nuclei are associated with individual differences in aggression. *Horm Behav* (2006) 50:338–45. doi:10.1016/j.yhbeh.2006.04.002

Trainor BC, Lin S, Finy MS, Rowland MR, Nelson RJ. Photoperiod reverses the effects of estrogens on male aggression via genomic and nongenomic pathways. *Proc Natl Acad Sci U S A* (2007) 104:9840–5. doi:10.1073/pnas.0701819104

Laredo SA, Villalon Landeros R, Dooley JC, Steinman MQ, Orr V, Silva AL, et al. Nongenomic effects of estradiol on aggression under short day photoperiods. *Horm Behav* (2013) 64:557–65. doi:10.1016/j.yhbeh.2013.06.002

Naftolin F, Horvath TL, Jakab RL, Leranth C, Harada N, Balthazart J. Aromatase immunoreactivity in axon terminals of the vertebrate brain. An immunocyto- chemical study on quail, rat, monkey and human tissues. *Neuroendocrinology* (1996) 63:149–55. doi:10.1159/000126951

Horvath TL, Roa-Pena L, Jakab RL, Simpson ER, Naftolin F. Aromatase in axonal processes of early postnatal hypothalamic and limbic areas includ- ing the cingulate cortex. *J Steroid Biochem Mol Biol* (1997) 61:349–57. doi:10.1016/S0960-0760(97)80032-5

Naftolin F, Horvath TL, Balthazart J. Estrogen synthetase (aromatase) immuno- histochemistry reveals concordance between avian and rodent limbic systems and hypothalami. *Exp Biol Med (Maywood)* (2001) 226:717–25.

Wu MV, Manoli DS, Fraser EJ, Coats JK, Tollkuhn J, Honda S, et al. Estro- gen masculinizes neural pathways and sex-specific behaviors. *Cell* (2009) 139:61–72. doi:10.1016/j.cell.2009.07.036

Hojo Y, Murakami G, Mukai H, Higo S, Hatanaka Y, Ogiue-Ikeda M, et al. Estrogen synthesis in the brain – role in synaptic plasticity and memory. *Mol Cell Endocrinol* (2008) 290:31–43. doi:10.1016/j.mce.2008.04.017

Saldanha CJ, Remage-Healey L, Schlinger BA. Synaptocrine signaling: steroid synthesis and action at the synapse. *Endocr Rev* (2011) 32:532–49. doi:10.1210/ er.2011-0004

Remage-Healey L, Oyama RK, Schlinger BA. Elevated aromatase activity in forebrain synaptic terminals during song. *J Neuroendocrinol* (2009) 21:191–9. doi:10.1111/j.1365-2826.2009.01820.x

Balthazart J, Baillien M, Cornil CA, Ball GF. Preoptic aromatase modulates male sexual behavior: slow and fast mechanisms of action. *Physiol Behav* (2004) 83:247–70. doi:10.1016/j.physbeh.2004.08.025

Cornil CA, Seredynski AL, de Bournonville C, Dickens MJ, Charlier TD, Ball GF, et al. Rapid control of reproductive behaviour by locally synthe- sised oestrogens: focus on aromatase. *J Neuroendocrinol* (2013) 25:1070–8. doi:10.1111/jne.12062

Roselli CE. Synergistic induction of aromatase activity in the rat brain by estra- diol and 5 alpha-dihydrotestosterone. *Neuroendocrinology* (1991) 53:79–84. doi:10.1159/000125701

Yilmaz MB, Wolfe A, Cheng YH, Glidewell-Kenney C, Jameson JL, Bulun SE. Aromatase promoter I.f is regulated by estrogen receptor alpha (ESR1) in mouse hypothalamic neuronal cell lines. *Biol Reprod* (2009) 81:956–65. doi:10.1095/biolreprod.109.077206

Charlier TD, Newman AE, Heimovics SA, Po KW, Saldanha CJ, Soma KK. Rapid effects of aggressive interactions on aromatase activity and oestradiol in discrete brain regions of wild male white-crowned sparrows. *J Neuroendocrinol* (2011) 23:742–53. doi:10.1111/j.1365-2826.2011.02170.x

Bronson FH, Eleftheriou BE. Adrenal response to fighting in mice: separation of physical and psychological causes. *Science* (1965) 147:627–8. doi:10.1126/ science.147.3658.627

Mainardi M, Valenti G, Valsecchi P, Parmigiani S, Brain PF, Vescovi P. Acute effects of low doses of two ACTH preparations on fighting behavior in male mice. *Med Sci Res* (1987) 15:649–50.

Mikics E, Kruk MR, Haller J. Genomic and non-genomic effects of glucocor- ticoids on aggressive behavior in male rats. *Psychoneuroendocrinology* (2004) 29:618–35. doi:10.1016/S0306-4530(03)00090-8

Mikics E, Barsy B, Barsvari B, Haller J. Behavioral specificity of non-genomic glucocorticoid effects in rats: effects on risk assessment in the elevated plus- maze and the open-field. *Horm Behav* (2005) 48:152–62. doi:10.1016/j.yhbeh.2005.02.002

Schjolden J, Basic D, Winberg S. Aggression in rainbow trout is inhib- ited by both MR and GR antagonists. *Physiol Behav* (2009) 98:625–30. doi:10.1016/j.physbeh.2009.09.018

Chang C, Li CY, Earley RL, Hsu Y. Aggression and related behavioral traits: the impact of winning and losing and the role of hormones. *Integr Comp Biol* (2012) 52:801–13. doi:10.1093/icb/ics057

Kruk MR, Halasz J, Meelis W, Haller J. Fast positive feedback between the adrenocortical stress response and a brain mechanism involved in aggressive behavior. *Behav Neurosci* (2004) 118:1062–70. doi:10.1037/0735-7044.118.5. 1062

Mikics E, Barsy B, Haller J. The effect glucocorticoids on aggressiveness in established colonies of rats. *Psychoneuroendocrinology* (2007) 32:160–70. doi:10.1016/j.psyneuen.2006.12.002

Hayden-Hixson DM, Ferris CF. Cortisol exerts site-, context- and dose- dependent effects on agonistic responding in hamsters. *J Neuroendocrinol* (1991) 3:613–22. doi:10.1111/j.1365-2826.1991.tb00326.x

Hayden-Hixson DM, Ferris CF. Steroid-specific regulation of agonistic responding in the anterior hypothalamus of male hamsters. *Physiol Behav* (1991) 50:793–9. doi:10.1016/0031-9384(91)90020-O

Leshner AI, Korn SJ, Mixon JF, Rosenthal C, Besser AK. Effects of corticos- terone on submissiveness in mice: some temporal and theoretical considera- tions. *Physiol Behav* (1980) 24:283–8. doi:10.1016/0031-9384(80)90087-6

Blanchard DC, Spencer RL, Weiss SM, Blanchard RJ, McEwen B, Sakai RR. Visible burrow system as a model of chronic social stress: behavioral and neuroendocrine correlates. *Psychoneuroendocrinology* (1995) 20:117–34. doi:10.1016/0306-4530(94)E0045-B

Blanchard RJ, Dulloog L, Markham C, Nishimura O, Nikulina Compton J, Jun A, et al. Sexual and aggressive interactions in a visible burrow system with provi- sioned burrows. *Physiol Behav* (2001) 72:245–54. doi:10.1016/S0031-9384(00) 00403-0

Haller J. The glucocorticoid/aggression relationship in animals and humans: an analysis sensitive to behavioral characteristics, glucocorticoid secretion pat- terns, and neural mechanisms. *Curr Top Behav Neurosci* (2014) 17:73–109. doi:10.1007/7854_2014_284

Patchev VK, Almeida OF. Gonadal steroids exert facilitating and "buffering" effects on glucocorticoid-mediated transcriptional regulation of corticotropin- releasing hormone and corticosteroid receptor genes in rat brain. *J Neurosci* (1996) 16:7077–84.

Liu J, Bisschop PH, Eggels L, Foppen E, Fliers E, Zhou JN, et al. Intrahypo- thalamic estradiol modulates hypothalamus-pituitary-adrenal-axis activity in female rats. *Endocrinology* (2012) 153:3337–44. doi:10.1210/en.2011-2176

Lund TD, Munson DJ, Haldy ME, Handa RJ. Androgen inhibits, while oestrogen enhances, restraint-induced activation of neuropeptide neurones in the par- aventricular nucleus of the hypothalamus. *J Neuroendocrinol* (2004) 16:272–8. doi:10.1111/j.0953-8194.2004.01167.x

Anstrom KK, Miczek KA, Budygin EA. Increased phasic dopamine signaling in the mesolimbic pathway during social defeat in rats. *Neuroscience* (2009) 161:3–12. doi:10.1016/j.neuroscience.2009.03.023

Barik J, Marti F, Morel C, Fernandez SP, Lanteri C, Godeheu G, et al. Chronic stress triggers social aversion via glucocorticoid receptor in dopaminoceptive neurons. *Science* (2013) 339:332–5. doi:10.1126/science.1226767

Haller J, Halasz J, Makara GB, Kruk MR. Acute effects of glucocorticoids: behavioral and pharmacological perspectives. *Neurosci Biobehav Rev* (1998) 23:337–44. doi:10.1016/S0149-7634(98)00035-9

Summers CH, Winberg S. Interactions between the neural regulation of stress and aggression. *J Exp Biol* (2006) 209:4581–9. doi:10.1242/jeb.02565

Liu J, Hu P, Qi XR, Meng FT, Kalsbeek A, Zhou JN. Acute restraint stress increases intrahypothalamic oestradiol concentrations in conjunction with increased hypothalamic oestrogen receptor beta and aromatase mRNA expres- sion in female rats. *J Neuroendocrinol* (2011) 23:435–43. doi:10.1111/j.1365-2826.2011.02123.x

Dickens MJ, Cornil CA, Balthazart J. Neurochemical control of rapid stress- induced changes in brain aromatase activity. *J Neuroendocrinol* (2013) 25:329–39. doi:10.1111/jne.12012

Brooks DC, Zhao H, Yilmaz MB, Coon VJ, Bulun SE. Glucocorticoid-induction of hypothalamic aromatase via its brain-specific promoter. *Mol Cell Endocrinol* (2012) 362:85–90. doi:10.1016/j.mce.2012.05.012

Haller J, Mikics E, Makara GB. The effects of non-genomic glucocorticoid mechanisms on bodily functions and the central neural system. A critical eval- uation of findings. *Front Neuroendocrinol* (2008) 29:273–91. doi:10.1016/j.yfrne.2007.10.004

Hill MN, Patel S, Campolongo P, Tasker JG, Wotjak CT, Bains JS. Functional interactions between stress and the endocannabinoid system: from synaptic signaling to behavioral output. *J Neurosci* (2010) 30:14980–6. doi:10.1523/JNEUROSCI.4283-10.2010

Choi DC, Evanson NK, Furay AR, Ulrich-Lai YM, Ostrander MM, Herman JP. The anteroventral bed nucleus of the stria terminalis differentially regulates hypothalamic-pituitary-adrenocortical axis responses to acute and chronic stress. *Endocrinology* (2008) 149:818–26. doi:10.1210/en.2007-0883

Watters JJ, Dorsa DM. Transcriptional effects of estrogen on neuronal neu- rotensin gene expression involve cAMP/protein kinase A dependent mecha- nisms. *J Neurosci* (1998) 18:6672–80.

Watters JJ, Campbell JS, Cunningham MJ, Krebs EG, Dorsa DM. Rapid mem- brane effects of steroids in neuroblastoma cells: effects of estrogen on mito- gen activated protein kinase signalling cascade and c-fos immediate early gene transcription. *Endocrinology* (1997) 138:4030–3. doi:10.1210/endo.138.9.5489

Titolo D, Mayer CM, Dhillon SS, Cai F, Belsham DD. Estrogen facilitates both phosphatidylinositol 3-kinase/Akt and ERK1/2 mitogen-activated pro- tein kinase membrane signaling required for long-term neuropeptide Y transcriptional regulation in clonal, immortalized neurons. *J Neurosci* (2008) 28:6473–82. doi:10.1523/JNEUROSCI.0514-08.2008

Constantin S, Caligioni CS, Stojilkovic S, Wray S. Kisspeptin-10 facilitates a plasma membrane-driven calcium oscillator in gonadotropin-releasing hormone-1 neurons. *Endocrinology* (2009) 150:1400–12. doi:10.1210/en.2008- 0979

Malyala A, Pattee P, Nagalla SR, Kelly MJ, Ronnekleiv OK. Suppression subtrac- tive hybridization and microarray identification of estrogen-regulated hypo- thalamic genes. *Neurochem Res* (2004) 29:1189–200. doi:10.1023/B:NERE. 0000023606.13670.1d

Roepke TA, Malyala A, Bosch MA, Kelly MJ, Ronnekleiv OK. Estrogen reg- ulation of genes important for K+ channel signaling in the arcuate nucleus. *Endocrinology* (2007) 148:4937–51. doi:10.1210/en.2007-0605

Micevych PE, Chaban V, Ogi J, Dewing P, Lu JK, Sinchak K. Estradiol stimu- lates progesterone synthesis in hypothalamic astrocyte cultures. *Endocrinology* (2007) 148:782–9. doi:10.1210/en.2006-0774

Remage-Healey L, Saldanha CJ, Schlinger BA. Estradiol synthesis and action at the synapse: evidence for "synaptocrine" signaling. *Front Endocrinol* (2011) 2:28. doi:10.3389/fendo.2011.00028

Tian Z, Wang Y, Zhang N, Guo YY, Feng B, Liu SB, et al. Estrogen recep- tor GPR30 exerts anxiolytic effects by maintaining the balance between GABAergic and glutamatergic transmission in the basolateral amygdala of ovariectomized mice after stress. *Psychoneuroendocrinology* (2013) 38:2218–33. doi:10.1016/j.psyneuen.2013.04.011

Lebesgue D, Reyna-Neyra A, Huang X, Etgen AM. GPR30 differentially reg- ulates short latency responses of luteinising hormone and prolactin secretion to oestradiol. *J Neuroendocrinol* (2009) 21:743–52. doi:10.1111/j.1365-2826.2009.01893.x

Petrie WK, Dennis MK, Hu C, Dai D, Arterburn JB, Smith HO, et al. G protein- coupled estrogen receptor-selective ligands modulate endometrial tumor growth. *Obstet Gynecol Int* (2013) 2013:472720. doi:10.1155/2013/472720

Sun J, Meyers MJ, Fink BE, Rajendran R, Katzenellenbogen JA, Katzenellen- bogen BS. Novel ligands that function as selective estrogens or antiestrogens for estrogen receptor-alpha or estrogen receptor-beta. *Endocrinology* (1999) 140:800–4. doi:10.1210/endo.140.2.6480

Meyers MJ, Sun J, Carlson KE, Marriner GA, Katzenellenbogen BS, Katzenellen- bogen JA. Estrogen receptor-beta potency-selective ligands: structure-activity relationship studies of diarylpropionitriles and their acetylene and polar ana- logues. *J Med Chem* (2001) 44:4230–51. doi:10.1021/jm010254a

Filardo EJ, Quinn JA, Frackelton AR Jr, Bland KI. Estrogen action via the G protein-coupled receptor, GPR30: stimulation of adenylyl cyclase and cAMP- mediated attenuation of the epidermal growth factor receptor-to-MAPK sig- naling axis. *Mol Endocrinol* (2002) 16:70–84. doi:10.1210/mend.16.1.0758

Dennis MK, Field AS, Burai R, Ramesh C, Petrie WK, Bologa CG, et al. Identifi- cation of a GPER/GPR30 antagonist with improved estrogen receptor counter- selectivity. *J Steroid Biochem Mol Biol* (2011) 127:358–66. doi:10.1016/j.jsbmb. 2011.07.002

Lan NC, Graham B, Bartter FC, Baxter JD. Binding of steroids to mineralocor- ticoid receptors: implications for in vivo occupancy by glucocorticoids. *J Clin Endocrinol Metab* (1982) 54:332–42. doi:10.1210/jcem-54-2-332

16

Insulin, aging, and the brain: mechanisms and implications

Abimbola A. Akintola* and Diana van Heemst

Department of Gerontology and Geriatrics, Leiden University Medical Center, Leiden, Netherlands

Edited by:
Hubert Vaudry, University of Rouen, France

Reviewed by:
Catarina Oliveira, University of Coimbra, Portugal
Andrzej Bartke, Southern Illinois University School of Medicine, USA

****Correspondence:***
Abimbola A. Akintola, Department of Gerontology and Geriatrics, Leiden University Medical Center, C7-124, Albinusdreef 2, Leiden 2333 ZA, Netherlands
e-mail: a.a.akintola@lumc.nl

There is now an impressive body of literature implicating insulin and insulin signaling in successful aging and longevity. New information from *in vivo* and *in vitro* studies concerning insulin and insulin receptors has extended our understanding of the physiological role of insulin in the brain. However, the relevance of these to aging and longevity remains to be elucidated. Here, we review advances in our understanding of the physiological role of insulin in the brain, how insulin gets into the brain, and its relevance to aging and longevity. Furthermore, we examine possible future therapeutic applications and implications of insulin in the context of available models of delayed and accelerated aging.

Keywords: insulin, insulin receptors, brain, inflammation, delayed aging, accelerated aging, longevity

INTRODUCTION

Pathways that orchestrate the responses of the organism to changes in its environment have been implicated in the genetic regulation of lifespan across different species. One of the key pathways identified by genetic analysis of long-lived *Caenorhabditis elegans* (*C. elegans*) mutants is insulin/insulin-like growth factor-1 (IGF-1) signaling (IIS) (1, 2). In invertebrates, multiple insulin/IGF-1-like ligands signal via a common receptor, which shows homology to the mammalian insulin and IGF-1 receptors. Also in mammals, insulin/IGF-1 signaling has been linked to aging, lifespan, and longevity (3). Although in mammals, insulin and IGF-1 act predominantly via distinct receptors, there is extensive overlap and interaction in their downstream signaling cascades, making it difficult to separate effects of insulin signaling from those of IGF-1 signaling. The long-lived phenotype of FIRKO mice, which were made by selective disruption of the insulin receptor (IR) in adipose tissue, supports a role of insulin signaling in longevity (4). Moreover, many of the long-lived mouse mutants with disrupted GH/IGF-1 signaling display enhanced insulin sensitivity. In humans, a hallmark phenotype of healthy longevity is maintenance of insulin sensitivity (5, 6), which has been observed in familial human longevity (7, 8), as well as in centenarians (9–11). Insulin influences all aspects of human physiology (12, 13). Besides regulating peripheral glucose homeostasis, insulin is an important neuromodulator that contributes to neurobiological processes (14), with growing evidence that insulin supports behavioral, cellular, biochemical, and molecular functions (15). In literature, evidence linking aging and insulin signaling includes prolongation of life span in rodents via genetic mutations affecting insulin signaling pathways or via interventions that down-regulate nutrient sensing pathways such as caloric restriction. Further evidence includes data on the role of type 2 diabetes in accelerated aging syndromes, and the increased incidence of insulin resistance with age (16). In model organisms (nematodes and fruit flies), specific neural manipulations of insulin signaling have also been linked to aging and lifespan (17, 18). Insulin is produced in the brain of these organisms, making it undoubtedly a neuropeptide. In mammals and humans, IRs are highly abundant in many brain areas and nuclei, but it remains unclear if insulin is produced in the brain. Furthermore, the physiological and pathophysiological mechanisms of insulin action in the brain in relation to aging and longevity remain to be elucidated.

With the global population aging, there has been an astonishing increase in the prevalence of obesity (19), metabolic syndrome (20), type 2 diabetes (21), and neurodegenerative diseases (22). Insulin resistance is a shared feature in these diverse pathologies (13, 23–26). It therefore becomes critical to understand the role of insulin in healthy longevity, as this may be relevant to combatting age-related disorders that have been linked to disturbances in glucose metabolism. The aim of this article is to review advances in our knowledge about insulin, insulin signaling, and the brain, and to present these in the context of available models of delayed and accelerated aging. Furthermore, we will examine the links between inflammation, metabolic health, and brain health, and their effect on aging. Finally, we will review therapeutic options to enhance brain insulin action, including measures to enhance local brain insulin levels as well as measures to enhance the brain responses to insulin.

INSULIN AND THE BRAIN: A CENTURY OF DISCOVERIES

Insulin, after discovery in 1921, was initially considered a peripheral hormone and thus unable to cross the blood–brain barrier (BBB) (27). However, in 1967, Margolis and Altszuler demonstrated in dogs that the concentration of cerebrospinal fluid (CSF) insulin increased after an increase in plasma insulin (28), thus showing that insulin is able to cross the blood–CSF barrier. In 1978, Havrankova et al. demonstrated the widespread presence of IRs in the central nervous system (CNS) of the rat (29). Later that year, they further demonstrated that high levels of insulin were present in rat brain extracts, and found that the concentration of insulin in the CNS was considerably higher than its concentration in the circulation (30). They thus proposed a physiological role for insulin in the CNS. In the 1980s, further evidence that insulin from peripheral circulation crosses the BBB thus gaining access to the brain was provided. In 1983, Dorn et al. demonstrated that the human brain contains insulin in concentrations much higher than the blood, the highest being in the hypothalamus (31). Furthermore, they showed the presence of high concentrations of insulin in the brains and spinal cords of human cadavers, mice, and rats (32). Baskin et al. demonstrated uptake in the hypothalamus of [125I]iodoinsulin after the insulin had been stereotaxically injected into a lateral cerebral ventricle. Furthermore, they detected insulin-like immunoreactivity in the periventricular, supraoptic, suprachiasmatic, arcuate, and lateral hypothalamic nuclei of the rat hypothalamus (33, 34). In 1992, Schechter et al. delineated the ontogeny of rabbit brain insulin concentration and demonstrated that insulin availability is developmentally regulated (35). In the past decade, studies of the effects of insulin in the brain have been enhanced after development of non-invasive methods of selective delivery of insulin into the brain, via the intranasal route, circumventing peripheral effects of systemic hypoglycemia (36). This has advanced our understanding of potentially therapeutic effects of enhancing insulin concentrations in the brain. Furthermore, studies in recent years have brought forward the role of insulin signaling in the hypothalamus, as a key player in regulation of hepatic glucose production and food intake (37).

BRAIN INSULIN: IS INSULIN A NEUROPEPTIDE IN HUMANS?

In the rabbit, discordance was observed between insulin concentrations in serum and CSF (35). Insulin was found to be present in high concentrations in brain micro-vessels (38), brain extracts (39), and immature nerve cell bodies (35, 40), despite that only 0.046% of peripheral insulin crosses the BBB in mice (12, 41). Moreover, brain insulin concentrations were observed to vary according to developmental stages, with peak amounts being observed during the critical phases of brain growth and development (42). Taken together, these results suggest that brain insulin availability is strictly regulated and can reach high levels in the CNS. This raises the question as to the source of brain insulin, does all of brain insulin derive from the periphery or is insulin also synthesized in the brain (**Figure 1**)?

There is unequivocal evidence for selective, regulated, time dependent, temperature sensitive, carrier mediated, and saturable insulin transport to the brain (43–50). In mice, human insulin was shown to access the CNS after crossing the BBB (51). In rabbits, insulin infused into the carotid artery was shown to have crossed the BBB into the peri-capillary space and brain parenchyma with preservation of the peptide's integrity (45). In dogs, studies using a three component mathematical model (plasma, intermediate component, and CSF) have shown that insulin delivery to the CNS fits a receptor-mediated saturable process (43). In healthy humans, during hyperinsulinemic, euglycemic clamp studies, increase in circulating insulin was demonstrated to rapidly affect brain activity, alongside rapid cerebral insulin signal transduction, independent of the systemic effects of the insulin (48).

Apart from passage through the BBB, direct access of insulin to the CSF has also been demonstrated (**Figure 1**). This alternative

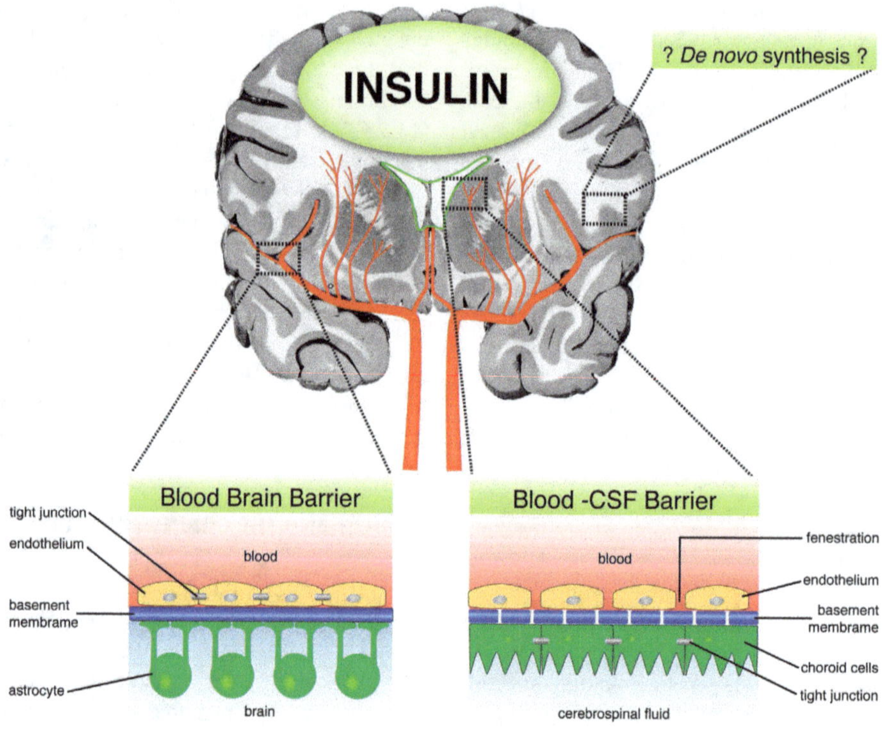

FIGURE 1 | Sources of brain insulin. Schematic diagram showing the possible sources of brain insulin. First, peripheral insulin can access the brain through the blood brain barrier (BBB) via a selective, carrier-mediated transport system. Second, insulin may diffuse through the blood–CSF barrier in circumventricular regions, which are lacking in BBB. Third, there is some limited evidence suggesting the possibility of *de novo* insulin synthesis in the brain.

route occurs through circumventricular regions, such as the area postrema, which lack a BBB (34, 52–54). Unlike the BBB that contains tight junctions, the capillaries in the circumventricular regions are porous, thereby allowing plasma solubles to diffuse freely and directly into these areas (55). The route through which insulin accesses the brain has implications for the rate of convection and diffusion in the brain, and distribution of the insulin into the brain parenchyma. Following intraventricular administration of insulin, insulin becomes distributed through the ventricular compartments and to the surface of the brain bathed by the subarachnoid space, with relatively slow rate of diffusion into the brain parenchyma, and is minimal at distances more than 1–2 mm removed from the CSF surface (55, 56). In addition, insulin delivered into the CSF undergoes relatively rapid bulk flow through the CSF flow tracks. For example, the entire CSF volume is turned over every 4–5 h following production at the choroid plexus in the human brain (55).

In model organisms, insulin is biosynthesized by neurons in the brain and it exerts both local and remote actions, including regulation of homeostasis; making it undoubtedly a neuropeptide. In humans, however, insulin is mainly produced in the pancreas, which raises the question as to whether insulin can be considered a neuropeptide in humans. Neuropeptides have been defined as "small proteinaceous substances produced and released by neurons through the regulated secretory route and acting on neural substrates" (57). Neuropeptides have been shown to have strict, cell specific expression patterns, on which the physiological or behavioral role of the peptides is based. Criteria for classification as a neuropeptide include gene expression and biosynthesis by neurons; storage, and regulated release upon demand and ability to modulate or mediate neural functioning directly through receptors (57). Although IRs are highly abundant in many brain areas and nuclei, it remains unclear if insulin is produced in the brain. Therefore, following the strict criteria for neuropeptide definition, it becomes debatable if mammalian insulin is a true neuropeptide.

Evidence in favor of insulin synthesis in the brain mostly derives from *in vitro* studies, including the study by Clarke et al. in 1986, which demonstrated the synthesis of insulin by cultured rat brain neuronal and astrocyte glial cells and their release of insulin in primary culture. The insulin release after membrane depolarization of the neurons was biphasic, in a manner similar to that of pancreatic beta cells (58). In 1990s, Schechter et al. provided both *in vivo* and *in vitro* evidence from mammalian brains supporting the *de novo* synthesis of insulin. *In vitro* evidence included the demonstration of preproinsulin I and II mRNA in neuron cell cultures of fetal rat brains (59). From *in vivo* studies, presence of preproinsulin I and II mRNAs and insulin immunoreaction was detected within the rough endoplasmic reticulum, the Golgi apparatus, cytoplasm, axon, synapsis, and dendrites of the rat fetal brain (40).

Summarily, as can be seen in **Figure 1**, whether insulin is derived from the periphery, local sources or both, insulin is present in the CNS, where it subserves many functions and contributes to neurobiological processes.

ACTIVATION OF INSULIN RECEPTORS IN THE BRAIN

As in peripheral tissues, insulin signaling in the brain occurs mainly via the IR pathway (**Figure 2**), which contains several critical nodes of interaction with other signaling pathways (60). Activation of the insulin signaling cascade starts with binding of the insulin ligand to the IR, which belongs to the family of tyrosine kinase receptors, auto phosphorylation of which is essential for their activation. Upon activation, the IR phosphorylates insulin receptor substrate (IRS) proteins. IRS proteins are also activated upon binding of the IGF-1 ligand to its cognate receptor. Thus, IRS proteins represent a critical node of conversion of the insulin and IGF-1 signaling cascades, and their crosstalk with other pathways, such as cytokine signaling. In addition to its activation of the Ras–mitogen-activated protein kinase (MAPK) pathway, activated IRS proteins serve as docking sites for the assembly and activation of, among others, phospho-inositol-3 kinase (PI3K), which generates the lipid second messenger phosphatidylinositol 3,4,5-triphosphate (PIP3). PI3K represents another critical node of crosstalk with other signaling pathways, including the c-Jun-N-terminal kinase (JNK) stress signaling pathway. Elevated levels of PIP3 activate phosphoinositide-dependent protein kinase-1

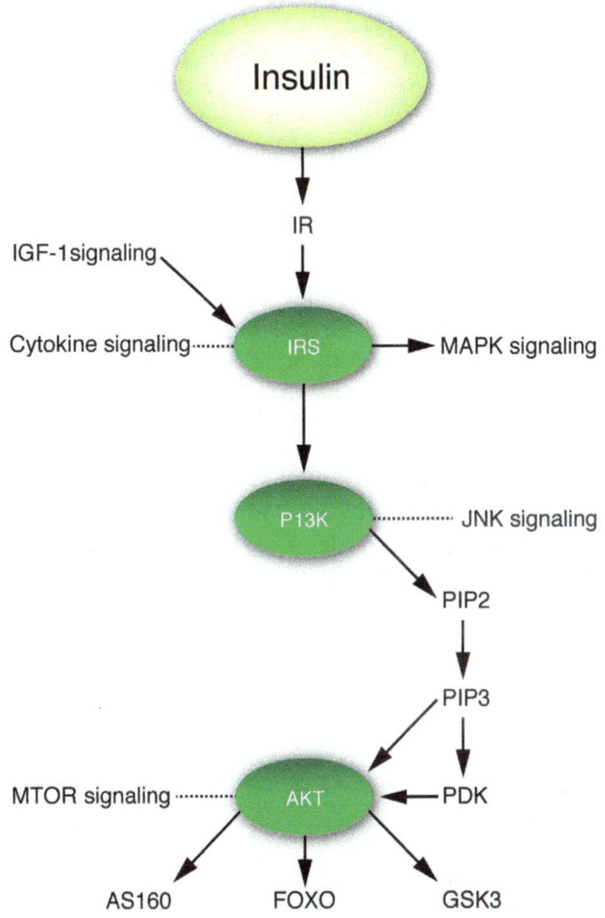

FIGURE 2 | Insulin–IRS–P13K–AKT signaling cascade and its crosstalk with other signaling pathways. Figure denotes three critical nodes in insulin signaling that are important for the interaction of insulin signaling with other pathways relevant to this review.

(PDK1) and AKT. AKT represents yet another critical node of interaction with the mammalian target of rapamycin (mTOR) nutrient signaling pathway. AKT targets include glycogen synthase kinase 3 (GSK3), Akt substrate of 160 kDa (AS160, phosphorylation of which is required for translocation of the glucose transporter GLUT4 to the plasma membrane) and forkhead transcription factors (FOXOs) (**Figure 2**). Phosphorylation of FOXOs induces their translocation from the nucleus, which causes profound changes in the transcription of key factors implicated in metabolism, cell cycle regulation, apoptosis, and resistance to oxidative stress (61).

DISTRIBUTION OF INSULIN RECEPTORS IN THE BRAIN

In higher mammals and humans, IRs are widely distributed throughout peripheral tissues, with their main function being to transport glucose into cells, inhibit glucose production and increase glucose uptake by triggering signaling pathways in the liver, muscle, and fat (62). The IR consists of a tetramer, with two alpha subunits and two beta subunits. Brain IR subunits differ structurally from peripheral IR subunits in that they have a lower molecular weight (63) and can withstand exposure to high concentrations of insulin without undergoing down-regulation (64, 65). The mammalian brain has specific IRs (29, 66), which are of two types. One is the neuronal/neuron-specific type, which is abundant in the neuron (67), while the second type is the non-neuronal/peripheral-like type, with lower density in glial cells (38, 66, 68). Insulin receptors are highly abundant in the neurons, with high protein concentrations in cell bodies and synapses, and less abundant in the glia. Brain IRs are abundant in the brain, but are highly enriched in the olfactory bulb, hypothalamus, hippocampus, cerebellum, amygdala, and cerebral cortex (12).

Growing but controversial evidence suggests that the specific regional concentrations of IR reflect different IR functions associated with particular brain regions. IR enrichment in the hypothalamus and limbic system including the hippocampus, pyriform cortex, and amygdala, areas that reciprocally connect and communicate with each other, has been proposed to be suggestive of a role in emotion and higher cognitive functions, particularly learning and memory (69, 70). Higher IR concentrations are found in the hippocampus, which is critically involved in spatial memory processing, suggesting insulin's role in learning and declarative memory (69). Evidence that synthesis of IR may be increased in these hippocampal areas as a result of learning is supported by the up-regulation and the changes in distribution patterns of IR mRNA in the hippocampus and dentate gyrus following water maze training in rats (70). Insulin is involved in the regulation of food intake, which is consistent with the high concentrations of IR in the olfactory bulb and the hypothalamus. Furthermore, the high concentration of IR in the choroid plexus suggests that it may be required for transport of peripheral insulin across the blood–CSF barrier (70).

FUNCTIONAL SIGNIFICANCE OF INSULIN IN THE BRAIN

As the most potent anabolic hormone yet identified, insulin has both metabolic and non-metabolic functions. Insulin regulates food intake, as well as glucose, lipid, and energy homeostasis and stimulates synthesis (as well as inhibition of breakdown) of glycogen, triglycerides, and most proteins. It is also involved in regulation of hedonic behavior and non-homeostatic control of intake of food and other substances via reward processing.

NON-METABOLIC FUNCTIONS

The presence of insulin and IRs in the brain indicates that the brain is a target organ for insulin. Insulin plays a key role in synaptic plasticity, apoptosis, mood, learning, reproduction, and growth (37, 71–74). Insulin and IR expression in the brain has been suggested to exert neurotrophic effects on CNS neurons (75). Insulin has been considered to support neuronal protein synthesis and cytoskeletal protein expression (75), neurite outgrowth (76, 77), migration, and differentiation in the absence of other growth factors (78, 79), and nascent synapse formation (75, 80). It promotes growth and regeneration of axonal sprouts, especially small sized sensory neurons (81), neuronal survival, circuit development, synaptic plasticity (82), and postsynaptic neurotransmitter receptor trafficking (80). Evidence in favor of insulin's role as a neurotransmitter in the CNS includes the observations that (i) insulin is present in neurons (67), (ii) neurons contain specific IRs (64), and (iii) insulin affects neuronal firing and catecholamine metabolism (83–85). Insulin also has effects on BBB function, including ability to affect the transport of other substances. Binding sites for insulin have been described at both the choroid plexus and on brain endothelial cells (86, 87). Insulin also has neuro-protective properties (88–90). Central insulin plays a role in cognitive processes such as attention, executive functioning, learning, and memory (91), and direct application of insulin to the CNS in humans has been shown to improve memory and cognition (92, 93). Thus, insulin is involved in attributes that are essential for healthy aging.

METABOLIC FUNCTIONS

The brain plays a key role in maintenance of homeostasis, or the ability to maintain vital parameters of the internal environment within narrow limits, despite fluctuations in the external environment. Metabolic homeostasis requires the integration of numerous cues reflecting energy availability by the hypothalamus and nearby brain structures, to mount a coordinated response to adapt fuel flux so as to maintain energy homeostasis. Insulin is one of the many cues informing the brain about energy status. Research on insulin signaling has primarily focused on insulin-mediated processes in the classical insulin target organs. These include glucose uptake into skeletal muscle, inhibition of glucose production by the liver, and inhibition of lipolysis in adipose tissue. However, in 1979, a role for insulin in the central regulation of energy homeostasis was suggested based on the observations that insulin levels circulate in proportion to fat mass in most mammals and that intra-cerebroventricular insulin administration results in a dose dependent reduction in food intake and body weight in monkeys (94). In line, IRs are expressed throughout the mammalian brain (29). Metabolic syndrome and diabetes have traditionally been considered as peripheral metabolic diseases. Recently, various non-invasive brain-imaging techniques have revealed structural and functional abnormalities that are associated with diabetes. Critical autonomic regulatory neurons in the hypothalamus and brainstem are responsible for maintenance of energy homeostasis and functional changes in these areas are associated with the development of diabetes (95). It was also shown that after hepatic branch vagotomy the suppression of hepatic gluconeogenesis induced by increasing circulating insulin levels was reduced by half (96). Mechanistically, binding of insulin to the IR and activation of the PI3K pathway in hypothalamic glucose-responsive neurons, which was shown to induce their hyperpolarization by opening of ATP-dependent potassium channels (97), has been implicated in the central effects of insulin on hepatic glucose production (96). Recently, it was shown that ingestion of a glucose solution resulted in a prolonged and significant blood oxygen dependent decrease in activity in the hypothalamus of healthy subjects, but not in type 2 diabetic patients (98). Insulin is also involved in regulation of energy homeostasis via IR in the ventromedial hypothalamus and acts on the brain to suppress feeding (99). Thus, insulin acts as a satiety factor, a finding supported by the observation that the response of glucose-excited neurons in the ventrolateral and ventromedial hypothalamic nucleus to decreased glucose is blunted by insulin (100).

Taken together, these data indicate that, beside peripheral insulin resistance, reduced brain insulin action may also contribute to loss of maintenance of metabolic control. Indeed, brain specific deletion of the IR was shown to result in enhanced food intake in female mice; and in mild obesity, hyperleptinemia, insulin resistance, and hypertriglyceridemia in both male and female mice (101). In line with these findings, in rats, decreasing hypothalamic IRs caused overeating and insulin resistance and hypothalamic insulin signaling was shown to be required for inhibition of glucose production (102). High-fat diet-induced obesity is associated with reduced brain insulin transport and an impairment of insulin action when given directly into the CNS, suggesting a loss of the effectiveness of insulin in the CNS to provide feedback signaling in circumstances of chronic hyperinsulinemia (103). Upon aging, peripheral insulin resistance progressively increases, inducing compensatory chronic elevations in circulating insulin levels. Therefore, central insulin action will be discussed in the context of models of delayed and accelerated aging.

INSULIN AND THE BRAIN: MODELS OF DELAYED AGING

NEMATODE MODELS OF DELAYED AGING

There is an impressive body of literature implicating insulin/IGF-1 like ligands and insulin/IGF-1 signaling in the regulation of metabolism, development, and longevity in the roundworm *C. elegans* (104). In response to unfavorable stressful environmental conditions, *C. elegans* larvae can transiently exit the cycle of growth and development to sexual maturity by transformation into developmentally arrested, non-feeding, stress resistant, and long-lived dauer larvae (105, 106). It was found that several dauer formation defective (daf) mutants are also long-lived, possibly because these mutants display specific key features of the dauer stage while developing in sexually mature adults, such as enhanced resistance to multiple stresses due to induction of cytoprotective pathways (107). Of the many long-lived daf mutants in nematodes, the ones that are best characterized comprise the *daf-2*, *age-1 (daf 23)*, *daf-16*, and *daf-18* mutants. Cloning and sequencing of the loci affected in long-lived daf mutants has revealed that these show strong sequence homology with evolutionarily conserved components of the mammalian insulin/insulin-like growth factor-1 signal transduction cascade (108–110). For example, the *daf-2* gene that has been shown to regulate lifespan in *C. elegans*, and the related tyrosine kinase receptors InR in *Drosophila melanogaster* (*D. melanogaster*) encode components that are homologous to the mammalian insulin and insulin-like growth factor-1 receptors. In response to food or the perception of food, multiple insulin-like ligands are secreted from neurosecretory cells in the brain of *C. elegans* (111) and *D. melanogaster* (112), indicating that in these invertebrates, the CNS plays a key role in insulin signaling mediated regulation of physiology and lifespan in response to environmental cues. Moreover, more than 10 years ago, Wolkow et al. (17) demonstrated that restoration of the daf-2 pathway of insulin-like signaling in neurons alone was sufficient to restore wildtype lifespan in *C. elegans*, and thus provided further evidence as to the role of insulin in the nervous system as a central regulator of animal longevity.

MOUSE MODELS OF DELAYED AGING

In mammals, the insulin/insulin-like growth factor-1 signaling cascade exhibits some striking differences compared to the insulin/insulin-like growth factor-1 signaling cascade in invertebrates (113). These differences include the acquisition of GH as a main regulator of IGF-1 production by the liver, and the acquisition of separate receptors for insulin and IGF-1. Again, several of the existing long-lived mammalian mutants with defects in insulin/IGF-1 signaling point to a role of the CNS in the regulation of mammalian longevity. The mutations that have thus far been most consistently and most strongly associated with increases in lifespan in mice comprise the *Prop-1* mutation displayed by Ames dwarf mice (114) and the *Pit-1* mutation displayed by Snell dwarf mice (115). These two mutations confer a defect in the development of the anterior pituitary gland, which causes a lifelong combined hormonal deficiency in growth hormone, thyroid stimulating hormone, and prolactin. In these as well as other long-lived mice, longevity has been strongly correlated with enhanced insulin sensitivity (116). In addition to the Ames and Snell dwarf mice, many other mouse mutants with defects in insulin/IGF-1 signaling have been described to display a longevity phenotype, which strongly implicates the insulin/IGF-1 signaling pathway in the regulation of rodent longevity. Involvement of both insulin signaling and IGF-1 signaling in mouse longevity was suggested by the long-lived phenotypes displayed by mice with selective disruption of the IR in adipose tissue (4) and mice heterozygous for mutation of IGF-1R (1). Summarily, improved insulin control (of carbohydrate homeostasis) has been identified as one of the pathways implicated in the remarkable extension of longevity in long-lived mouse mutants (117).

HUMAN MODELS OF DELAYED AGING

Also in humans, preserved insulin sensitivity has been associated with longevity. Insulin resistance has been shown to predict the development of age-related diseases, including hypertension, coronary heart disease, stroke, cancer, and type 2 diabetes (118). In the general population, the association between aging and decline in insulin sensitivity (119–123) has been demonstrated in several studies (**Figure 3**). Mechanisms suggested to contribute to decreased insulin sensitivity in the elderly include (i) age-related receptor and post-receptor defects in insulin action (124, 125), (ii) an age-related decrease in insulin stimulated whole body glucose oxidation (126), (iii) an age-related reduction in beta cell response to glucose (126), and (iv) impaired insulin-mediated glucose uptake, and inability to suppress hepatic glucose output (127, 128). In contrast, centenarians, which exhibit exceptional longevity, seem protected against the age-related decline in insulin sensitivity when compared to a group of advanced middle-aged individuals. (11) Of note, a methodological difficulty that is associated with the comparison of groups that differ in calendar age is potential confounding by the changes that occur in body composition and endocrine function with advancing age. Moreover, differences may exist between different birth cohorts in environmental impacts, including differences in the availability vaccinations or medications (e.g., antibiotics).

The relationship between longevity and preserved insulin action has also been observed in studies of familial longevity. In the Leiden longevity study, offspring of long-lived nonagenarian siblings, having inherited on average 50% of the genetic propensity of their long-lived parent were included together with the partners of the offspring (129), with whom they have shared the same socioeconomic and geographical environment for decades and who are of a similar age. We showed that already at middle age the offspring from these long-lived siblings displayed a decreased mortality risk suggesting that there is indeed evidence for genetic enrichment for longevity (129). Moreover, human offspring of exceptionally long-lived siblings, when compared to their partners showed a remarkably lower prevalence of metabolic syndrome (130) and diabetes (131). After exclusion of diabetic patients, the offspring of exceptionally long-lived siblings displayed lower circulating levels of glucose and slightly lower circulating insulin levels (7). Using hyperinsulinemic euglycemic clamps studies, we could show that the offspring of long-lived siblings specifically displayed enhanced peripheral insulin sensitivity compared to age matched controls (8). A study using high field (7-T) MR spectroscopy of the tibialis anterior muscle indicated that the enhanced peripheral insulin sensitivity of offspring is associated with lower intramyocellular lipid content, which may be indicative of better mitochondrial capacity (132).

The mechanisms underlying the preserved insulin action in centenarians as well as in offspring of nonagenarian siblings remain unclear. However, suggested mechanisms include genetic enrichment for favorable features related to body fat and lipoprotein distribution, reduced plasma free radical concentrations, and enhanced cellular response to oxidative stress and immune function (11, 133, 134). Taken together, these results suggest that maintenance of insulin sensitivity is a key feature of healthy longevity.

INSULIN AND THE BRAIN: MODELS OF ACCELERATED AGING

OBESITY AS A MODEL FOR ACCELERATED AGING

The most common acquired factors causing insulin resistance are obesity and a sedentary lifestyle. Obesity and the associated increase in body fat are the consequences of chronic, long-term nutrient excess. In Western societies, the prevalence of obesity continues to increase and numerous studies have demonstrated an association between obesity and enhanced mortality risk (135). The relationship between obesity and excess mortality is consistent with evidence that obese individuals are at increased risk of essential hypertension, type 2 diabetes mellitus (DM2), and cardiovascular disease (CVD). It has been suggested that insulin

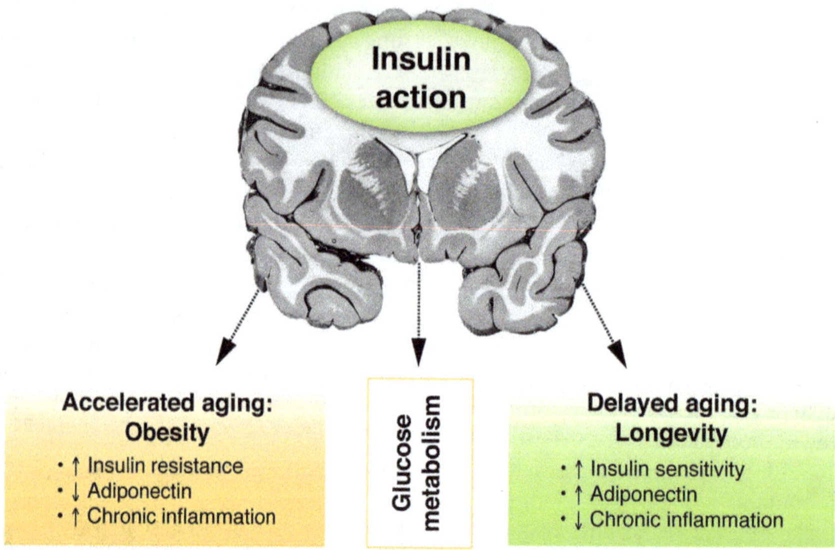

FIGURE 3 | Insulin and the brain: models of accelerated and delayed aging. Figure showing the putative relationship between central insulin action and glucose metabolism in models of accelerated or delayed aging. Obesity as a model for accelerated aging is associated with peripheral insulin resistance, decreased adiponectin levels, and enhanced chronic inflammation. Opposite features are observed in healthy longevity as a model of delayed aging.

resistance is the major contributor to clinical outcomes associated with obesity (136).

It is not known why some obese individuals develop insulin resistance while others remain insulin sensitive (137). A potential mechanism that might explain the association between excess adiposity and peripheral insulin resistance is impaired adipogenesis and reduced lipogenesis in subcutaneous fat, which would lead to enhanced deposition of fat in the visceral depots and larger sizes of visceral adipocytes (137, 138). Increased visceral adiposity is associated with enhanced secretion of inflammatory cytokines and induction of insulin resistance (139). Nutrient excess results in enhanced exposure of cells and tissues to high levels of circulatory glucose and fatty acids. These exposures can activate various intracellular inflammatory pathways and lead to mitochondrial dysfunction, reactive oxygen species (ROS), ER stress, and the associated unfolded protein response that induce resistance to both leptin and insulin (140). ROS can have both stimulatory and inhibitory effects on insulin signaling. It was shown that under normal physiological conditions, optimal activation of the IR requires redox priming by IR mediated activation of NAD(P)H oxidase (NOX) in many cell types (141). In addition, mild bursts in intracellular ROS can activate the IR receptor independent of insulin, allowing for ROS mediated ligand activation bypass of IR signaling (142). In contrast, increased levels of ROS or prolonged exposure to oxidative stress have been shown to inhibit insulin signaling and to induce insulin resistance (143). Enhanced exposure of skeletal muscle to high levels of fatty acids in circulation can result in enhanced levels of intramyocellular triglyceride storage. Because intramyocellular lipid droplets are stored in close vicinity to mitochondria, which constitute the main intracellular source of ROS, intramyocellular triglycerides are very vulnerable to oxidation. Upon peroxidation of intramyocellular triglycerides toxic lipid species are generated, including diacylglycerol (DAG), ceramide, and long-chain fatty acyl-CoA, which impair insulin signaling (143). Both enhanced influx, as a consequence of nutrient excess, and reduced efflux, as a result reduced oxidative capacity and mitochondrial dysfunction have been implicated in the accumulation of toxic intramyocellular lipids (144, 145). In support of a role of reduced efflux due to mitochondrial dysfunction, non-obese, insulin sensitive first degree relatives of patients with type 2 diabetes were shown to display impaired ability to switch to fat oxidation after high-fat intake (146), as well as higher levels of intramyocellular lipids and reduced oxidative capacity (147). These data implicate ROS and mitochondrial dysfunction in the development of insulin resistance.

It is unknown via which mechanisms insulin resistance is associated with a shortening of lifespan. If peripheral organs, such as skeletal muscle and adipose tissue become less responsive to insulin, euglycemia will be maintained by the capacity of the pancreas to hypersecrete insulin so as to overcome insulin resistance at peripheral organs. Exposure to continuous surges of hyperinsulinemia may overstimulate other tissues that have remained normally responsive to insulin, such as the liver, resulting in a pro-atherogenic lipid profile (148). Other data implicate adiponectin in the association between insulin resistance and lifespan. Adiponectin, an anti-inflammatory adipokine secreted by adipose tissue (149) was found to be negatively correlated with adipocyte size and obesity (150). Interestingly, elevated adiponectin levels have been observed in long-lived mice, such as the Ames dwarf mice (151) as well as in long-lived humans, such as centenarians (152–154). Recently, effects of adiponectin on peripheral insulin sensitivity also implicate central effects on reduction of high-fat diet-induced hypothalamic inflammation and insulin resistance (155).

INFLAMMATION AND THE BRAIN

INFLAMMATION AND AGING: INFLAMMAGING

Inflammaging is characterized by the increase in chronic, low-grade inflammation in the absence of overt infection that occurs with aging (156). Inflammaging as well as the circulatory markers that characterize this state, including C-reactive protein (CRP), interleukin-6 (IL-6), tumor necrosis factor α (TNF-α), and interleukin 1 beta (IL1beta) are strong risk factors for many age-related diseases and mortality. It is thought that part of these circulatory factors are produced locally, after which these leak into the circulation. Different sources that contribute to the state of inflammaging include the accumulation of cellular debris and organelle components, accumulation of senescent cells, immunosenescence, changes in the gut microbiome and deregulation of the coagulation system.

Macromolecules, cells, and tissues are continuously damaged and repaired. Chronic inflammation is part of regular tissue remodeling as it facilitates tissue repair and turnover. However, a persistent inflammatory response can lead to tissue degeneration by activated leukocytes, cytokines, or collagen deposition. In literature, one key structure where links between inflammation and aging are emerging is the hypothalamus.

HYPOTHALAMIC INFLAMMATION

The hypothalamus is the seat of control of various metabolic and non-metabolic processes in the body, and is responsible for maintenance of homeostasis from early life through to aging. Besides its role in the synthesis and secretion of neurohormones, the hypothalamus regulates energy balance, stress responsiveness, as well as lipid and glucose metabolism. Diet-induced obesity has been shown to be associated with central leptin and insulin resistance (157). High-fat feeding has been shown to induce hypothalamic inflammation, which has been linked to the development of insulin resistance and obesity (157–159). In 2005, De Souza et al. demonstrated that 6 weeks of high-fat feeding induced impaired functional and molecular activation of the insulin-signaling pathway, with accompanying expression of several pro-inflammatory cytokines (IL-1β, TNFα, and IL-6) and inflammatory responsive proteins in the hypothalamus (158). Moreover, hypothalamic inflammation was shown to decrease the efficacy of central insulin administration to inhibit lipolysis, even before the onset of peripheral insulin resistance in white adipose tissue (160). Recently, a series of experiments in mice has demonstrated that hypothalamic inflammation occurs rapidly after high-fat feeding and is mediated by hyper activation of hypothalamic microglia, which was associated with gliosis in the ARC nucleus and eventual reduction in the number of POMC neurons, which are key in the regulation of energy homeostasis and adiposity (161).

Microglia are resident macrophages that play an important role in the clearance of cell debris via phagocytosis and the release of pro-inflammatory cytokines to recruit other immune responsive cells to the sites of injury in the CNS, including blood-borne macrophages. It is pivotal for tissue homeostasis and repair that the initial inflammatory immune response is followed by an active phase of resolution of inflammation and scar tissue. Recently, it has been shown that after insult, monocyte-derived M2-like macrophages are recruited to the site of injury and that these have an essential role as inflammation-resolving cells in recovery from acute CNS injury. The anti-inflammatory activity displayed by M2-like macrophages, notably their IL10 expression, is required for regulation of the activated microglia (162, 163). In addition, their expression of matrix degrading enzymes favors axonal regrowth by degradation of the glial scar (164). CNS specific T cells facilitate recruitment of blood-borne M2-like macrophages to the CNS through the choroid plexus within the blood–CSF barrier (165). Age-related Th2 inflammation is associated with chronically elevated IL4 levels, which can disrupt choroid plexus barrier functions and thus prevent the resolution of pro-inflammatory processes and induce a state of CNS inflammaging.

THERAPEUTIC MEASURES AND FUTURE PROSPECTS

Since brain insulin has been linked with aging, two possible mechanisms can be proffered for enhancing brain insulin action (**Figure 4**). Enhanced insulin efficacy might occur through measures aimed at minimizing inflammation; and enhanced delivery might be promoted to the brain areas that are crucial for healthy longevity.

Inflammation, including that occurring in the hypothalamus, has been linked to age-related decline in insulin sensitivity. It has been shown that hypothalamic microglia hyperactivation is regulated by metabolic hormones [leptin, glucagon-like peptide 1 (GLP-1)] and diet but not by body weight *per se* (166). Inflammaging may be treatable and preventable through changes in lifestyle. Interventions that are currently applied to reduce the state of low-grade chronic inflammaging include low dosing of aspirin or statins, weight loss, and exercise. Notably, a lower intake of calories and food that is rich in saturated fat and carbohydrates has been shown to reduce inflammaging (167). In mice, it was shown that hypothalamic inflammation can be resolved by central administration of omega3 and omega9 fatty acids after which body weight regulation and food intake were normalized (168). Physical exercise is known to be protective against numerous diseases and reduction of inflammation has been implicated in the health benefits conferred by exercise (169). Recently, in mice, exercise has also been shown to protect against hypothalamic inflammation induced by high-fat diet (170). Future research may focus on hypothalamic microglia as relevant targets for prevention and treatment of metabolic disorders.

The strong blood glucose lowering effects of intravenously administered insulin have hampered research on the role of insulin in the brain. These hypoglycemic effects can be circumvented by intranasal administration of insulin, which is an innovative way to enhance insulin concentration in the brain without affecting insulin concentration in the circulation (171). Intranasal administration of insulin was shown to be safe and effective in numerous studies in healthy humans and in patients with metabolic disease or cognitive impairment (172). Sub-chronic intranasal insulin application in humans was shown to decrease food intake and weight gain (92) in healthy young men, and to improve declarative memory and mood (173). Moreover, sub-chronic intranasal insulin application in humans was also shown to decrease HPA activation in response to a social stress test. It was shown that insulin may also influence meal-induced thermogenesis and postprandial insulin levels (174). Future research may focus on unraveling the effects of intranasal insulin on other aspects of energy and glucose metabolism in different age groups.

CONCLUSION

Insulin is the most powerful anabolic hormone discovered to date. Besides the well-established action of insulin in peripheral organs, such as liver, muscle, and adipose tissue, it is becoming

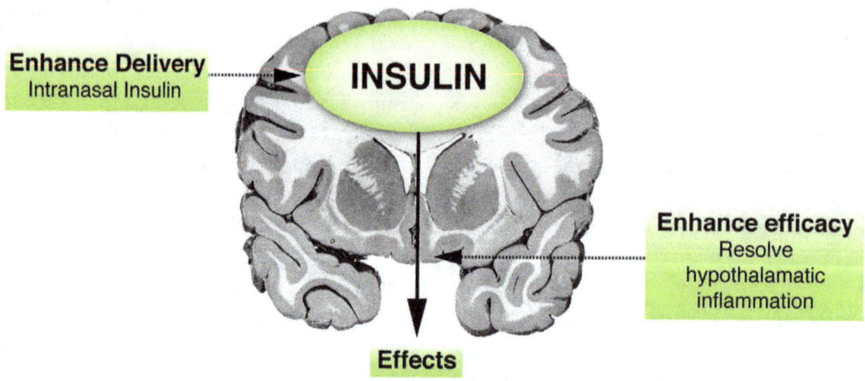

FIGURE 4 | Insulin and the brain: therapeutic implications. Hypothetical figure presenting two possibilities of enhancing brain insulin action. First, a way of increasing insulin concentrations in the brain is via enhanced delivery, such as delivery via the intranasal route, which has been shown to have some beneficial effects. Second, insulin action could probably also be augmented by enhancing its efficacy, for example, via resolution of brain (hypothalamic) inflammation.

increasingly clear that insulin affects important features of glucose metabolism via central mechanisms. Insulin signaling has been linked to longevity in organisms ranging from nematodes to mammals. While insulin is clearly a neuropeptide in nematodes, it is not yet clear how central insulin contributes to the differences in glucose metabolism that are observed in the context of conditions that are associated with accelerated aging, such as obesity, and delayed aging, such as healthy human longevity. However, novel data indicate that obesity is associated with reduced brain insulin action. Potential mechanisms that contribute to deficits in brain insulin action are impaired transport of insulin from the periphery to the brain and reduced brain insulin sensitivity due to hypothalamic inflammation. In contrast, we speculate that healthy longevity is associated with preserved brain insulin action, and discuss potential ways of enhancing brain insulin action in old age. Given the increasing prevalence of population aging, improving brain insulin action may represent an important therapeutic option to facilitate health in old age.

ACKNOWLEDGMENTS

The authors would like to thank Gerrit Kracht for his valuable contributions to the production of the figures contained in this review. This work was supported by the European Commission funded projects Switchbox (FP7, Health-F2-2010-2597772) and HUMAN (Health-2013-INNOVATION-1-602757).

REFERENCES

Holzenberger M, Dupont J, Ducos B, Leneuve P, Geloen A, Even PC, et al. IGF- 1 receptor regulates lifespan and resistance to oxidative stress in mice. *Nature* (2003) 421(6919):182–7. doi:10.1038/nature01298

Iser WB, Gami MS, Wolkow CA. Insulin signaling in *Caenorhabditis elegans* regulates both endocrine-like and cell-autonomous outputs. *Dev Biol* (2007) 303(2):434–47. doi:10.1016/j.ydbio.2006.04.467

Bartke A, Chandrashekar V, Dominici F, Turyn D, Kinney B, Steger R, et al. Insulin-like growth factor 1 (IGF-1) and aging: controversies and new insights. *Biogerontology* (2003) 4(1):1–8. doi:10.1023/A:1022448532248

Bluher M, Kahn BB, Kahn CR. Extended longevity in mice lacking the insulin receptor in adipose tissue. *Science* (2003) 299(5606):572–4. doi:10. 1126/science.1078223

Fulop T, Larbi A, Douziech N. Insulin receptor and ageing. *Pathol Biol* (2003) 51(10):574–80. doi:10.1016/j.patbio.2003.09.007

Fulop T Jr, Nagy JT, Worum I, Foris G, Mudri K, Varga P, et al. Glucose intolerance and insulin resistance with aging – studies on insulin recep- tors and post-receptor events. *Arch Gerontol Geriatr* (1987) 6(2):107–15. doi:10.1016/0167-4943(87)90003-3

Rozing MP, Westendorp RG, Frolich M, de Craen AJ, Beekman M, Heijmans BT, et al. Human insulin/IGF-1 and familial longevity at middle age. *Aging* (2009) 1(8):714–22.

Wijsman CA, Rozing MP, Streefland TC, le Cessie S, Mooijaart SP, Slagboom PE, et al. Familial longevity is marked by enhanced insulin sensitivity. *Aging Cell* (2011) 10(1):114–21. doi:10.1111/j.1474-9726.2010.00650.x

Barbieri M, Gambardella A, Paolisso G, Varricchio M. Metabolic aspects of the extreme longevity. *Exp Gerontol* (2008) 43(2):74–8. doi:10.1016/j.exger.2007. 06.003

Barbieri M, Rizzo MR, Manzella D, Grella R, Ragno E, Carbonella M, et al. Glucose regulation and oxidative stress in healthy centenarians. *Exp Gerontol* (2003) 38(1–2):137–43. doi:10.1016/S0531-5565(02)00153-5

Paolisso G, Gambardella A, Ammendola S, D'Amore A, Balbi V, Varricchio M, et al. Glucose tolerance and insulin action in healthy centenarians. *Am J Physiol* (1996) 270(5 Pt 1):E890–4.

Duarte AI, Moreira PI, Oliveira CR. Insulin in central nervous system: more than just a peripheral hormone. *J Aging Res* (2012) 2012:384017. doi:10.1155/2012/384017

Schwartz MW, Seeley RJ, Tschop MH, Woods SC, Morton GJ, Myers MG, et al. Cooperation between brain and islet in glucose homeostasis and diabetes. *Nature* (2013) 503(7474):59–66. doi:10.1038/nature12709

Gerozissis K. Brain insulin: regulation, mechanisms of action and functions. *Cell Mol Neurobiol* (2003) 23(1):1–25. doi:10.1023/A:1025021529347

Derakhshan F, Toth C. Insulin and the brain. *Curr Diabetes Rev* (2013) 9(2):102–16. doi:10.2174/1573399811309020002

Anisimov VN. Insulin/IGF-1 signaling pathway driving aging and cancer as a target for pharmacological intervention. *Exp Gerontol* (2003) 38(10):1041–9. doi:10.1016/S0531-5565(03)00169-4

Wolkow CA, Kimura KD, Lee MS, Ruvkun G. Regulation of *C. elegans* life-span by insulinlike signaling in the nervous system. *Science* (2000) 290(5489):147–50. doi:10.1126/science.290.5489.147

Taguchi A, Wartschow LM, White MF. Brain IRS2 signaling coordinates life span and nutrient homeostasis. *Science* (2007) 317(5836):369–72. doi:10.1126/science.1142179

Houston DK, Nicklas BJ, Zizza CA. Weighty concerns: the growing preva- lence of obesity among older adults. *J Am Diet Assoc* (2009) 109(11):1886–95. doi:10.1016/j.jada.2009.08.014

Mozumdar A, Liguori G. Persistent increase of prevalence of metabolic syn- drome among U.S. adults: NHANES III to NHANES 1999-2006. *Diabetes Care* (2011) 34(1):216–9. doi:10.2337/dc10-0879

Centers for Disease Control and Prevention. *National diabetes fact sheet: national estimates and general information on diabetes and prediabetes in the United States, 2011*. Atlanta, GA: U.S. Department of Health and Human Services, Centers for Disease Control and Prevention (2011).

Alzheimer's Association. 2011 Alzheimer's disease facts and figures. *Alzheimer Dement* (2011) 7(2):208–44. doi:10.1016/j.jalz.2011.02.004

Schwartz MW, Porte D Jr. Diabetes, obesity, and the brain. *Science* (2005) 307(5708):375–9. doi:10.1126/science.1104344

Sherlock M, Toogood AA. Aging and the growth hormone/insulin like growth factor-I axis. *Pituitary* (2007) 10(2):189–203. doi:10.1007/s11102-007-0039-5

Frolich L, Blum-Degen D, Bernstein HG, Engelsberger S, Humrich J, Laufer S, et al. Brain insulin and insulin receptors in aging and sporadic Alzheimer's disease. *J Neural Transm* (1998) 105(4–5):423–38. doi:10.1007/s007020050068

Zeyda M, Stulnig TM. Obesity, inflammation, and insulin resistance – a mini- review. *Gerontology* (2009) 55(4):379–86. doi:10.1159/000212758

Haugaard N, Vaughan M, Haugaard ES, Stadie WC. Studies of radioactive injected labeled insulin. *J Biol Chem* (1954) 208(2):549–63.

Margolis RU, Altszuler N. Insulin in the cerebrospinal fluid. *Nature* (1967) 215(5108):1375–6. doi:10.1038/2151375a0

Havrankova J, Roth J, Brownstein M. Insulin receptors are widely distrib- uted in the central nervous system of the rat. *Nature* (1978) 272(5656):827–9. doi:10.1038/272827a0

Havrankova J, Schmechel D, Roth J, Brownstein M. Identification of insulin in rat brain. *Proc Natl Acad Sci U S A* (1978) 75(11):5737–41. doi:10.1073/pnas. 75.11.5737

Dorn A, Rinne A, Bernstein HG, Hahn HJ, Ziegler M. Insulin and C-peptide in human brain neurons (insulin/C-peptide/brain peptides/ immunohistochemistry/radioimmunoassay). *J Hirnforsch* (1983) 24(5): 495–9.

Dorn A, Bernstein HG, Rinne A, Ziegler M, Hahn HJ, Ansorge S. Insulin- and glucagon-like peptides in the brain. *Anat Rec* (1983) 207(1):69–77. doi:10.1002/ar.1092070108

Baskin DG, Woods SC, West DB, van Houten M, Posner BI, Dorsa DM, et al. Immunocytochemical detection of insulin in rat hypothalamus and its pos- sible uptake from cerebrospinal fluid. *Endocrinology* (1983) 113(5):1818–25. doi:10.1210/endo-113-5-1818

Wallum BJ, Taborsky GJ Jr, Porte D Jr, Figlewicz DP, Jacobson L, Beard JC, et al. Cerebrospinal fluid insulin levels increase during intravenous insulin infu- sions in man. *J Clin Endocrinol Metab* (1987) 64(1):190–4. doi:10.1210/jcem-64-1-190

Schechter R, Whitmire J, Holtzclaw L, George M, Harlow R, Devaskar SU. Developmental regulation of insulin in the mammalian central nervous sys- tem. *Brain Res* (1992) 582(1):27–37. doi:10.1016/0006-8993(92)90313-X

Hallschmid M, Schultes B. Central nervous insulin resistance: a promising tar- get in the treatment of metabolic and cognitive disorders? *Diabetologia* (2009) 52(11):2264–9. doi:10.1007/s00125-009-1501-x

Abraham MA, Filippi BM, Kang GM, Kim MS, Lam TK. Insulin action in the hypothalamus and dorsal vagal complex. *Exp Physiol* (2014) 99(9):1104–9. doi:10.1113/expphysiol.2014.079962

Frank HJ, Pardridge WM. A direct in vitro demonstration of insulin binding to isolated brain microvessels. *Diabetes* (1981) 30(9):757–61. doi:10.2337/diab.30.9.757

Havrankova J, Roth J, Brownstein MJ. Concentrations of insulin and insulin receptors in the brain are independent of peripheral insulin levels. Studies of obese and streptozotocin-treated rodents. *J Clin Invest* (1979) 64(2):636–42. doi:10.1172/JCI109504

Schechter R, Beju D, Gaffney T, Schaefer F, Whetsell L. Preproinsulin I and II mRNAs and insulin electron microscopic immunoreaction are present within the rat fetal nervous system. *Brain Res* (1996) 736(1–2):16–27. doi:10.1016/0006-8993(96)00664-6

Banks WA, Kastin AJ. Differential permeability of the blood-brain barrier to two pancreatic peptides: insulin and amylin. *Peptides* (1998) 19(5):883–9. doi:10.1016/S0196-9781(98)00018-7

Devaskar SU, Holekamp N, Karycki L, Devaskar UP. Ontogenesis of the insulin receptor in the rabbit brain. *Horm Res* (1986) 24(4):319–27. doi:10.1159/000180573

Banks WA. The source of cerebral insulin. *Eur J Pharmacol* (2004) 490(1– 3):5–12. doi:10.1016/j.ejphar.2004.02.040

Baura GD, Foster DM, Porte D Jr, Kahn SE, Bergman RN, Cobelli C, et al. Saturable transport of insulin from plasma into the central nervous system of dogs in vivo. A mechanism for regulated insulin delivery to the brain. *J Clin Invest* (1993) 92(4):1824–30. doi:10.1172/JCI116773

Duffy KR, Pardridge WM. Blood-brain barrier transcytosis of insulin in developing rabbits. *Brain Res* (1987) 420(1):32–8. doi:10.1016/0006-8993(87)90236-8

Frank HJ, Jankovic-Vokes T, Pardridge WM, Morris WL. Enhanced insulin binding to blood-brain barrier in vivo and to brain microvessels in vitro in newborn rabbits. *Diabetes* (1985) 34(8):728–33. doi:10.2337/diab.34.8.728

Frank HJ, Pardridge WM. Insulin binding to brain microvessels. *Adv Metab Disord* (1983) 10:291–302. doi:10.1016/B978-0-12-027310-2.50016-5

Freude S, Plum L, Schnitker J, Leeser U, Udelhoven M, Krone W, et al. Periph- eral hyperinsulinemia promotes tau phosphorylation in vivo. *Diabetes* (2005) 54(12):3343–8. doi:10.2337/diabetes.54.12.3343

Pardridge WM. Receptor-mediated peptide transport through the blood-brain barrier. *Endocr Rev* (1986) 7(3):314–30. doi:10.1210/edrv-7-3-314

Pardridge WM, Eisenberg J, Yang J. Human blood-brain barrier insulin receptor. *J Neurochem* (1985) 44(6):1771–8. doi:10.1111/j.1471-4159.1985.tb07167.x

Banks WA, Jaspan JB, Kastin AJ. Selective, physiological transport of insulin across the blood-brain barrier: novel demonstration by species- specific radioimmunoassays. *Peptides* (1997) 18(8):1257–62. doi:10.1016/S0196-9781(97)00198-8

Porte D Jr, Seeley RJ, Woods SC, Baskin DG, Figlewicz DP, Schwartz MW. Obe- sity, diabetes and the central nervous system. *Diabetologia* (1998) 41(8):863–81. doi:10.1007/s001250051002

Sankar R, Thamotharan S, Shin D, Moley KH, Devaskar SU. Insulin-responsive glucose transporters-GLUT8 and GLUT4 are expressed in the developing mam- malian brain. *Brain Res Mol Brain Res* (2002) 107(2):157–65. doi:10.1016/ S0169-328X(02)00487-4

Weindl A, Sofroniew MV. Relation of neuropeptides to mammalian circum- ventricular organs. *Adv Biochem Psychopharmacol* (1981) 28:303–20.

Pardridge WM. Transport of insulin-related peptides and glucose across the blood-brain barrier. *Ann N Y Acad Sci* (1993) 692:126–37. doi:10.1111/j.1749-6632.1993.tb26211.x

Blasberg RG, Patlak C, Fenstermacher JD. Intrathecal chemotherapy: brain tis- sue profiles after ventriculocisternal perfusion. *J Pharmacol Exp Ther* (1975) 195(1):73–83.

Burbach JP. Neuropeptides from concept to online database www.neuropeptides.nl. *Eur J Pharmacol* (2010) 626(1):27–48. doi:10.1016/j.ejphar. 2009.10.015

Clarke DW, Mudd L, Boyd FT Jr, Fields M, Raizada MK. Insulin is released from rat brain neuronal cells in culture. *J Neurochem* (1986) 47(3):831–6. doi:10.1111/j.1471-4159.1986.tb00686.x

Schechter R, Yanovitch T, Abboud M, Johnson G III, Gaskins J. Effects of brain endogenous insulin on neurofilament and MAPK in fetal rat neuron cell cultures. *Brain Res* (1998) 808(2):270–8. doi:10.1016/S0006-8993(98) 00842-7

Taniguchi CM, Emanuelli B, Kahn CR. Critical nodes in signalling path- ways: insights into insulin action. *Nat Rev Mol Cell Biol* (2006) 7(2):85–96. doi:10.1038/nrm1837

Eijkelenboom A, Burgering BM. FOXOs: signalling integrators for homeostasis maintenance. *Nat Rev Mol Cell Biol* (2013) 14(2):83–97. doi:10. 1038/nrm3507

Saltiel AR, Kahn CR. Insulin signalling and the regulation of glucose and lipid metabolism. *Nature* (2001) 414(6865):799–806. doi:10.1038/414799a

Heidenreich KA, Zahniser NR, Berhanu P, Brandenburg D, Olefsky JM. Struc- tural differences between insulin receptors in the brain and peripheral target tissues. *J Biol Chem* (1983) 258(14):8527–30.

Boyd FT Jr, Raizada MK. Effects of insulin and tunicamycin on neuronal insulin receptors in culture. *Am J Physiol* (1983) 245(3):C283–7.

Zahniser NR, Goens MB, Hanaway PJ, Vinych JV. Characterization and reg- ulation of insulin receptors in rat brain. *J Neurochem* (1984) 42(5):1354–62. doi:10.1111/j.1471-4159.1984.tb02795.x

van Houten M, Posner BI. Insulin binds to brain blood vessels in vivo. *Nature* (1979) 282(5739):623–5. doi:10.1038/282623a0

Raizada MK, Yang JW, Fellows RE. Binding of [125I]insulin to specific receptors and stimulation of nucleotide incorporation in cells cultured from rat brain. *Brain Res* (1980) 200(2):389–400. doi:10.1016/0006-8993(80)90929-4

van Houten M, Posner BI, Kopriwa BM, Brawer JR. Insulin binding sites local- ized to nerve terminals in rat median eminence and arcuate nucleus. *Science* (1980) 207(4435):1081–3. doi:10.1126/science.6986652

Wickelgren I. Tracking insulin to the mind. *Science* (1998) 280(5363):517–9. doi:10.1126/science.280.5363.517

Zhao W, Chen H, Xu H, Moore E, Meiri N, Quon MJ, et al. Brain insulin receptors and spatial memory. Correlated changes in gene expression, tyrosine phosphorylation, and signaling molecules in the hippocampus of water maze trained rats. *J Biol Chem* (1999) 274(49):34893–902. doi:10.1074/jbc.274.49. 34893

Zhao WQ, Chen H, Quon MJ, Alkon DL. Insulin and the insulin receptor in experimental models of learning and memory. *Eur J Pharmacol* (2004) 490(1– 3):71–81. doi:10.1016/j.ejphar.2004.02.045

de la Monte SM, Wands JR. Review of insulin and insulin-like growth factor expression, signaling, and malfunction in the central nervous system: relevance to Alzheimer's disease. *J Alzheimer Dis* (2005) 7(1):45–61.

Avogaro A, de Kreutzenberg SV, Fadini GP. Insulin signaling and life span. *Pflugers Arch* (2010) 459(2):301–14. doi:10.1007/s00424-009-0721-8

Plum L, Schubert M, Bruning JC. The role of insulin receptor signaling in the brain. *Trends Endocrinol Metab* (2005) 16(2):59–65. doi:10.1016/j.tem.2005. 01.008

Schulingkamp RJ, Pagano TC, Hung D, Raffa RB. Insulin receptors and insulin action in the brain: review and clinical implications. *Neurosci Biobehav Rev* (2000) 24(8):855–72. doi:10.1016/S0149-7634(00)00040-3

Dickson BJ. Development. Wiring the brain with insulin. *Science* (2003) 300(5618):440–1. doi:10.1126/science.1084513

Song J, Wu L, Chen Z, Kohanski RA, Pick L. Axons guided by insulin recep- tor in *Drosophila* visual system. *Science* (2003) 300(5618):502–5. doi:10.1126/science.1081203

Torres-Aleman I. Insulin-like growth factors as mediators of functional plas- ticity in the adult brain. *Horm Metab Res* (1999) 31(2–3):114–9. doi:10.1055/ s-2007-978707

Recio-Pinto E, Rechler MM, Ishii DN. Effects of insulin, insulin-like growth factor-II, and nerve growth factor on neurite formation and survival in cultured sympathetic and sensory neurons. *J Neurosci* (1986) 6(5):1211–9.

Puro DG, Agardh E. Insulin-mediated regulation of neuronal maturation. *Sci- ence* (1984) 225(4667):1170–2. doi:10.1126/science.6089343

Sugimoto K, Baba M, Suda T, Yasujima M, Yagihashi S. Peripheral neuropa- thy and microangiopathy in rats with insulinoma: association with chronic hyperinsulinemia. *Diabetes Metab Res Rev* (2003) 19(5):392–400. doi:10.1002/ dmrr.395

Kremerskothen J, Wendholt D, Teber I, Barnekow A. Insulin-induced expression of the activity-regulated cytoskeleton-associated gene (ARC) in human neuroblastoma cells requires p21(ras), mitogen-activated protein kinase/ extracellular regulated kinase and src tyrosine kinases but is protein kinase C-independent. *Neurosci Lett* (2002) 321(3):153–6.

Palovcik RA, Phillips MI, Kappy MS, Raizada MK. Insulin inhibits pyramidal neurons in hippocampal slices. *Brain Res* (1984) 309(1):187–91. doi:10.1016/0006-8993(84)91028-X

Barbaccia ML, Chuang DM, Costa E. Is insulin a neuromodulator? *Adv Biochem Psychopharmacol* (1982) 33:511–8.

Boyd FT Jr, Clarke DW, Muther TF, Raizada MK. Insulin receptors and insulin modulation of norepinephrine uptake in neuronal cultures from rat brain. *J Biol Chem* (1985) 260(29):15880–4.

Baskin DG, Brewitt B, Davidson DA, Corp E, Paquette T, Figlewicz DP, et al. Quantitative autoradiographic evidence for insulin receptors in the choroid plexus of the rat brain. *Diabetes* (1986) 35(2):246–9. doi:10.2337/diab.35.2.246

Miller DW, Keller BT, Borchardt RT. Identification and distribution of insulin receptors on cultured bovine brain microvessel endothelial cells: possible func- tion in insulin processing in the blood-brain barrier. *J Cell Physiol* (1994) 161(2):333–41. doi:10.1002/jcp.1041610218

Dudek H, Datta SR, Franke TF, Birnbaum MJ, Yao R, Cooper GM, et al. Regu- lation of neuronal survival by the serine-threonine protein kinase Akt. *Science* (1997) 275(5300):661–5. doi:10.1126/science.275.5300.661

Takadera T, Sakura N, Mohri T, Hashimoto T. Toxic effect of a beta-amyloid peptide (beta 22-35) on the hippocampal neuron and its prevention. *Neurosci Lett* (1993) 161(1):41–4. doi:10.1016/0304-3940(93)90135-8

Tanaka M, Sawada M, Yoshida S, Hanaoka F, Marunouchi T. Insulin prevents apoptosis of external granular layer neurons in rat cerebellar slice cultures. *Neurosci Lett* (1995) 199(1):37–40. doi:10.1016/0304-3940(95)12009-S

Kern W, Peters A, Fruehwald-Schultes B, Deininger E, Born J, Fehm HL. Improving influence of insulin on cognitive functions in humans. *Neuroen- docrinology* (2001) 74(4):270–80. doi:10.1159/000054694

Hallschmid M, Benedict C, Schultes B, Fehm HL, Born J, Kern W. Intranasal insulin reduces body fat in men but not in women. *Diabetes* (2004) 53(11):3024–9. doi:10.2337/diabetes.53.11.3024

Benedict C, Hallschmid M, Schultes B, Born J, Kern W. Intranasal insulin to improve memory function in humans. *Neuroendocrinology* (2007) 86(2):136–42. doi:10.1159/000106378

Woods SC, Lotter EC, McKay LD, Porte D Jr. Chronic intracerebroventricular infusion of insulin reduces food intake and body weight of baboons. *Nature* (1979) 282(5738):503–5. doi:10.1038/282503a0

Eikelis N, Esler M. The neurobiology of human obesity. *Exp Physiol* (2005) 90(5):673–82. doi:10.1113/expphysiol.2005.031385

Pocai A, Lam TK, Gutierrez-Juarez R, Obici S, Schwartz GJ, Bryan J, et al. Hypo- thalamic K(ATP) channels control hepatic glucose production. *Nature* (2005) 434(7036):1026–31. doi:10.1038/nature03439

Spanswick D, Smith MA, Mirshamsi S, Routh VH, Ashford ML. Insulin acti- vates ATP-sensitive K+ channels in hypothalamic neurons of lean, but not obese rats. *Nat Neurosci* (2000) 3(8):757–8. doi:10.1038/77660

Vidarsdottir S, Smeets PA, Eichelsheim DL, van Osch MJ, Viergever MA, Romijn JA, et al. Glucose ingestion fails to inhibit hypothalamic neuronal activity in patients with type 2 diabetes. *Diabetes* (2007) 56(10):2547–50. doi:10.2337/db07-0193

Schwartz MW, Sipols AJ, Marks JL, Sanacora G, White JD, Scheurink A, et al. Inhibition of hypothalamic neuropeptide Y gene expression by insulin. *Endocrinology* (1992) 130(6):3608–16. doi:10.1210/en.130.6.3608

Cotero VE, Routh VH. Insulin blunts the response of glucose-excited neurons in the ventrolateral-ventromedial hypothalamic nucleus to decreased glucose. *Am J Physiol Endocrinol Metab* (2009) 296(5):E1101–9. doi:10.1152/ajpendo. 90932.2008

Bruning JC, Gautam D, Burks DJ, Gillette J, Schubert M, Orban PC, et al. Role of brain insulin receptor in control of body weight and reproduction. *Science* (2000) 289(5487):2122–5. doi:10.1126/science.289.5487.2122

Obici S, Zhang BB, Karkanias G, Rossetti L. Hypothalamic insulin signaling is required for inhibition of glucose production. *Nat Med* (2002) 8(12):1376–82. doi:10.1038/nm1202-798

Kaiyala KJ, Prigeon RL, Kahn SE, Woods SC, Schwartz MW. Obesity induced by a high-fat diet is associated with reduced brain insulin transport in dogs. *Diabetes* (2000) 49(9):1525–33. doi:10.2337/diabetes.49.9.1525

Kenyon CJ. The genetics of ageing. *Nature* (2010) 464(7288):504–12. doi:10. 1038/nature08980

Braendle C, Milloz J, Felix MA. Mechanisms and evolution of environmen- tal responses in *Caenorhabditis elegans*. *Curr Top Dev Biol* (2008) 80:171–207. doi:10.1016/S0070-2153(07)80005-6

Klass M, Hirsh D. Non-ageing developmental variant of *Caenorhabditis elegans*. *Nature* (1976) 260(5551):523–5. doi:10.1038/260523a0

Shore DE, Carr CE, Ruvkun G. Induction of cytoprotective pathways is central to the extension of lifespan conferred by multiple longevity pathways. *PLoS Genet* (2012) 8(7):e1002792. doi:10.1371/journal.pgen.1002792

Kimura KD, Tissenbaum HA, Liu Y, Ruvkun G. daf-2, an insulin receptor-like gene that regulates longevity and diapause in *Caenorhabditis elegans*. *Science* (1997) 277(5328):942–6. doi:10.1126/science.277.5328.942

Lin K, Dorman JB, Rodan A, Kenyon C. daf-16: an HNF-3/forkhead family member that can function to double the life-span of *Caenorhabditis elegans*. *Science* (1997) 278(5341):1319–22. doi:10.1126/science.278.5341.1319

Ogg S, Paradis S, Gottlieb S, Patterson GI, Lee L, Tissenbaum HA, et al. The Fork head transcription factor DAF-16 transduces insulin-like meta- bolic and longevity signals in *C. elegans*. *Nature* (1997) 389(6654):994–9. doi:10.1038/40194

Apfeld J, Kenyon C. Regulation of lifespan by sensory perception in *Caenorhab- ditis elegans*. *Nature* (1999) 402(6763):804–9. doi:10.1038/45544

Broughton SJ, Slack C, Alic N, Metaxakis A, Bass TM, Driege Y, et al. DILP-producing median neurosecretory cells in the *Drosophila* brain medi- ate the response of lifespan to nutrition. *Aging Cell* (2010) 9(3):336–46. doi:10.1111/j.1474-9726.2010.00558.x

van Heemst D. Insulin, IGF-1 and longevity. *Aging Dis* (2010) 1(2):147–57.

Brown-Borg HM, Borg KE, Meliska CJ, Bartke A. Dwarf mice and the ageing process. *Nature* (1996) 384(6604):33. doi:10.1038/384033a0

Flurkey K, Papaconstantinou J, Miller RA, Harrison DE. Lifespan extension and delayed immune and collagen aging in mutant mice with defects in growth hormone production. *Proc Natl Acad Sci U S A* (2001) 98(12):6736–41. doi:10.1073/pnas.111158898

Masternak MM, Panici JA, Bonkowski MS, Hughes LF, Bartke A. Insulin sensi- tivity as a key mediator of growth hormone actions on longevity. *J Gerontol A Biol Sci Med Sci* (2009) 64(5):516–21. doi:10.1093/gerona/glp024

Bartke A, Westbrook R. Metabolic characteristics of long-lived mice. *Front Genet* (2012) 3:288. doi:10.3389/fgene.2012.00288

Facchini FS, Hua N, Abbasi F, Reaven GM. Insulin resistance as a predic- tor of age-related diseases. *J Clin Endocrinol Metab* (2001) 86(8):3574–8. doi:10.1210/jcem.86.8.7763

Paolisso G, Scheen A, Lefebvre P. Glucose handling, diabetes and ageing. *Horm Res* (1995) 43(1–3):52–7. doi:10.1159/000184237

Bourey RE, Kohrt WM, Kirwan JP, Staten MA, King DS, Holloszy JO. Rela- tionship between glucose tolerance and glucose-stimulated insulin response in 65-year-olds. *J Gerontol* (1993) 48(4):M122–7. doi:10.1093/geronj/48.4.M122

Elahi D, Muller DC, McAloon-Dyke M, Tobin JD, Andres R. The effect of age on insulin response and glucose utilization during four hyperglycemic plateaus. *Exp Gerontol* (1993) 28(4–5):393–409. doi:10.1016/0531-5565(93)90066-M

Pratley RE, Coon PJ, Muller DC, Rogus EM, Goldberg AP. The effects of single and sequential insulin infusions on glucose disposal in older men. *Exp Gerontol* (1993) 28(4–5):381–91. doi:10.1016/0531-5565(93)90065-L

Couet C, Delarue J, Constans T, Lamisse F. Age-related insulin resistance: a review. *Horm Res* (1992) 38(1–2):46–50. doi:10.1159/000182483

Fink RI, Kolterman OG, Griffin J, Olefsky JM. Mechanisms of insulin resistance in aging. *J Clin Invest* (1983) 71(6):1523–35. doi:10.1172/JCI110908

Rowe JW, Minaker KL, Pallotta JA, Flier JS. Characterization of the insulin resistance of aging. *J Clin Invest* (1983) 71(6):1581–7. doi:10.1172/JCI110914

Gumbiner B, Thorburn AW, Ditzler TM, Bulacan F, Henry RR. Role of impaired intracellular glucose metabolism in the insulin resistance of aging. *Metabolism* (1992) 41(10):1115–21. doi:10.1016/0026-0495(92)90296-M

Meneilly GS, Elahi D, Minaker KL, Sclater AL, Rowe JW. Impairment of noninsulin-mediated glucose disposal in the elderly. *J Clin Endocrinol Metab* (1989) 68(3):566–71. doi:10.1210/jcem-68-3-566

Paolisso G, Marrazzo G, de Riu S, Sgambato S, Varricchio M, d'Onofrio F, et al. Effects of mild-to-moderate hyperglycaemia per se on glucose production and uptake in the elderly. *Eur J Med* (1992) 1(1):6–12.

Schoenmaker M, de Craen AJ, de Meijer PH, Beekman M, Blauw GJ, Slagboom PE, et al. Evidence of genetic enrichment for exceptional survival using a family approach: the Leiden longevity study. *Eur J Hum Genet* (2006) 14(1):79–84. doi:10.1038/sj.ejhg.5201508

Rozing MP, Westendorp RG, de Craen AJ, Frolich M, de Goeij MC, Heijmans BT, et al. Favorable glucose tolerance and lower prevalence of metabolic syn- drome in offspring without diabetes mellitus of nonagenarian siblings: the Leiden longevity study. *J Am Geriatr Soc* (2010) 58(3):564–9. doi:10.1111/j.1532-5415.2010.02725.x

Westendorp RG, van Heemst D, Rozing MP, Frolich M, Mooijaart SP, Blauw GJ, et al. Nonagenarian siblings and their offspring display lower risk of mortality and morbidity than sporadic nonagenarians: the Leiden Longevity Study. *J Am Geriatr Soc* (2009) 57(9):1634–7. doi:10.1111/j.1532-5415.2009.02381.x

Wijsman CA, van Opstal AM, Kan HE, Maier AB, Westendorp RG, Slag- boom PE, et al. Proton magnetic resonance spectroscopy shows lower intramyocellular lipid accumulation in middle-aged subjects predisposed to familial longevity. *Am J Physiol Endocrinol Metab* (2012) 302(3):E344–8. doi:10.1152/ajpendo.00455.2011

Dekker P, Maier AB, van Heemst D, de Koning-Treurniet C, Blom J, Dirks RW, et al. Stress-induced responses of human skin fibroblasts in vitro reflect human longevity. *Aging Cell* (2009) 8(5):595–603. doi:10.1111/j.1474-9726.2009.00506.x

Heijmans BT, Beekman M, Houwing-Duistermaat JJ, Cobain MR, Powell J, Blauw GJ, et al. Lipoprotein particle profiles mark familial and sporadic human longevity. *PLoS Med* (2006) 3(12):e495. doi:10.1371/journal.pmed.0030495

Hu FB, Willett WC, Li T, Stampfer MJ, Colditz GA, Manson JE. Adiposity as compared with physical activity in predicting mortality among women. *N Engl J Med* (2004) 351(26):2694–703. doi:10.1056/NEJMoa042135

McLaughlin T, Abbasi F, Lamendola C, Reaven G. Heterogeneity in the preva- lence of risk factors for cardiovascular disease and type 2 diabetes mellitus in obese individuals: effect of differences in insulin sensitivity. *Arch Intern Med* (2007) 167(7):642–8. doi:10.1001/archinte.167.7.642

McLaughlin T, Sherman A, Tsao P, Gonzalez O, Yee G, Lamendola C, et al. Enhanced proportion of small adipose cells in insulin-resistant vs insulin- sensitive obese individuals implicates impaired adipogenesis. *Diabetologia* (2007) 50(8):1707–15. doi:10.1007/s00125-007-0708-y

Salans LB, Knittle JL, Hirsch J. The role of adipose cell size and adipose tissue insulin sensitivity in the carbohydrate intolerance of human obesity. *J Clin Invest* (1968) 47(1):153–65. doi:10.1172/JCI105705

Fontana L, Eagon JC, Trujillo ME, Scherer PE, Klein S. Visceral fat adipokine secretion is associated with systemic inflammation in obese humans. *Diabetes* (2007) 56(4):1010–3. doi:10.2337/db06-1656

Hotamisligil GS. Inflammation and metabolic disorders. *Nature* (2006) 444(7121):860–7. doi:10.1038/nature05485

Goldstein BJ, Mahadev K, Wu X. Redox paradox: insulin action is facilitated by insulin-stimulated reactive oxygen species with multiple potential signaling targets. *Diabetes* (2005) 54(2):311–21. doi:10.2337/diabetes.54.2.311

Papaconstantinou J. Insulin/IGF-1 and ROS signaling pathway cross-talk in aging and longevity determination. *Mol Cell Endocrinol* (2009) 299(1):89–100. doi:10.1016/j.mce.2008.11.025

Houstis N, Rosen ED, Lander ES. Reactive oxygen species have a causal role in multiple forms of insulin resistance. *Nature* (2006) 440(7086):944–8. doi:10.1038/nature04634

Samocha-Bonet D, Heilbronn LK, Lichtenberg D, Campbell LV. Does skele- tal muscle oxidative stress initiate insulin resistance in genetically predisposed individuals? *Trends Endocrinol Metab* (2010) 21(2):83–8. doi:10.1016/j.tem. 2009.09.008

Moro C, Galgani JE, Luu L, Pasarica M, Mairal A, Bajpeyi S, et al. Influence of gender, obesity, and muscle lipase activity on intramyocellular lipids in sedentary individuals. *J Clin Endocrinol Metab* (2009) 94(9): 3440–7. doi:10.1210/jc. 2009-0053

Heilbronn LK, Gregersen S, Shirkhedkar D, Hu D, Campbell LV. Impaired fat oxidation after a single high-fat meal in insulin-sensitive nondiabetic individ- uals with a family history of type 2 diabetes. *Diabetes* (2007) 56(8):2046–53. doi:10.2337/db06-1687

Petersen KF, Dufour S, Befroy D, Garcia R, Shulman GI. Impaired mitochon- drial activity in the insulin-resistant offspring of patients with type 2 diabetes. *N Engl J Med* (2004) 350(7):664–71. doi:10.1056/NEJMoa031314

Reaven GM. Compensatory hyperinsulinemia and the development of an atherogenic lipoprotein profile: the price paid to maintain glucose homeosta- sis in insulin-resistant individuals. *Endocrinol Metab Clin North Am* (2005) 34(1):49–62. doi:10.1016/j.ecl.2004.12.001

Combs TP, Berg AH, Obici S, Scherer PE, Rossetti L. Endogenous glucose pro- duction is inhibited by the adipose-derived protein Acrp30. *J Clin Invest* (2001) 108(12):1875–81. doi:10.1172/JCI14120

Bahceci M, Gokalp D, Bahceci S, Tuzcu A, Atmaca S, Arikan S. The cor- relation between adiposity and adiponectin, tumor necrosis factor alpha, interleukin-6 and high sensitivity C-reactive protein levels. Is adipocyte size associated with inflammation in adults? *J Endocrinol Invest* (2007) 30(3):210–4. doi:10.1007/BF03347427

Wang Z, Al-Regaiey KA, Masternak MM, Bartke A. Adipocytokines and lipid levels in Ames dwarf and calorie-restricted mice. *J Gerontol A Biol Sci Med Sci* (2006) 61(4):323–31. doi:10.1093/gerona/61.4.323

Atzmon G, Pollin TI, Crandall J, Tanner K, Schechter CB, Scherer PE, et al. Adiponectin levels and genotype: a potential regulator of life span in humans. *J Gerontol A Biol Sci Med Sci* (2008) 63(5):447–53. doi:10.1093/ gerona/63.5.447

Bik W, Baranowska-Bik A, Wolinska-Witort E, Martynska L, Chmielowska M, Szybinska A, et al. The relationship between adiponectin levels and metabolic status in centenarian, early elderly, young and obese women. *Neuro Endocrinol Lett* (2006) 27(4):493–500.

Arai Y, Nakazawa S, Kojima T, Takayama M, Ebihara Y, Shimizu K-I, et al. High adiponectin concentration and its role for longevity in female centenarians. *Geriatr Gerontol Int* (2006) 6:32–9. doi:10.1111/j.1447-0594.2006.00304.x

Koch CE, Lowe C, Legler K, Benzler J, Boucsein A, Bottiger G, et al. Central adiponectin acutely improves glucose tolerance in male mice. *Endocrinology* (2014) 155(5):1806–16. doi:10.1210/en.2013-1734

Franceschi C, Campisi J. Chronic inflammation (inflammaging) and its poten- tial contribution to age-associated diseases. *J Gerontol A Biol Sci Med Sci* (2014) 69(Suppl 1):S4–9. doi:10.1093/gerona/glu057

Zhang X, Zhang G, Zhang H, Karin M, Bai H, Cai D. Hypothalamic IKKbeta/NF-kappaB and ER stress link overnutrition to energy imbalance and obesity. *Cell* (2008) 135(1):61–73. doi:10.1016/j.cell.2008.07.043

Cani PD, Amar J, Iglesias MA, Poggi M, Knauf C, Bastelica D, et al. Meta- bolic endotoxemia initiates obesity and insulin resistance. *Diabetes* (2007) 56(7):1761–72. doi:10.2337/db06-1491

Kleinridders A, Schenten D, Konner AC, Belgardt BF, Mauer J, Okamura T, et al. MyD88 signaling in the CNS is required for development of fatty acid-induced leptin resistance and diet-induced obesity. *Cell Metab* (2009) 10(4):249–59. doi:10.1016/j.cmet.2009.08.013

Scherer T, Lindtner C, Zielinski E, O'Hare J, Filatova N, Buettner C. Short term voluntary overfeeding disrupts brain insulin control of adipose tissue lipolysis. *J Biol Chem* (2012) 287(39):33061–9. doi:10.1074/jbc.M111.307348

Thaler JP, Yi CX, Schur EA, Guyenet SJ, Hwang BH, Dietrich MO, et al. Obesity is associated with hypothalamic injury in rodents and humans. *J Clin Invest* (2012) 122(1):153–62. doi:10.1172/JCI59660

Rapalino O, Lazarov-Spiegler O, Agranov E, Velan GJ, Yoles E, Fraidakis M, et al. Implantation of stimulated homologous macrophages results in par- tial recovery of paraplegic rats. *Nat Med* (1998) 4(7):814–21. doi:10.1038/nm0798-814

Shechter R, London A, Varol C, Raposo C, Cusimano M, Yovel G, et al. Infiltrating blood-derived macrophages are vital cells playing an anti- inflammatory role in recovery from spinal cord injury in mice. *PLoS Med* (2009) 6(7):e1000113. doi:10.1371/journal.pmed.1000113

Shechter R, Raposo C, London A, Sagi I, Schwartz M. The glial scar-monocyte interplay: a pivotal resolution phase in spinal cord repair. *PLoS One* (2011) 6(12):e27969. doi:10.1371/journal.pone.0027969

Kunis G, Baruch K, Rosenzweig N,

Kertser A, Miller O, Berkutzki T, et al. IFN- gamma-dependent activation of the brain's choroid plexus for CNS immune surveillance and repair. *Brain* (2013) 136(Pt 11):3427–40. doi:10.1093/brain/ awt259

Gao Y, Ottaway N, Schriever SC, Legutko B, Garcia-Caceres C, de la Fuente E, et al. Hormones and diet, but not body weight, control hypothalamic microglial activity. *Glia* (2014) 62(1):17–25. doi:10.1002/glia.22580

Fontana L. Neuroendocrine factors in the regulation of inflammation: exces- sive adiposity and calorie restriction. *Exp Gerontol* (2009) 44(1–2):41–5. doi:10.1016/j.exger.2008.04.005

Cintra DE, Ropelle ER, Moraes JC, Pauli JR, Morari J, Souza CT, et al. Unsat- urated fatty acids revert diet-induced hypothalamic inflammation in obesity. *PLoS One* (2012) 7(1):e30571. doi:10.1371/journal.pone.0030571

Ford ES. Does exercise reduce inflammation? Physical activity and C-reactive protein among U.S. adults. *Epidemiology* (2002) 13(5):561–8. doi:10.1097/00001648-200209000-00012

Yi CX, Al-Massadi O, Donelan E, Lehti M, Weber J, Ress C, et al. Exercise pro- tects against high-fat diet-induced hypothalamic inflammation. *Physiol Behav* (2012) 106(4):485–90. doi:10.1016/j.physbeh.2012.03.021

Born J, Lange T, Kern W, McGregor GP, Bickel U, Fehm HL. Sniffing neu- ropeptides: a transnasal approach to the human brain. *Nat Neurosci* (2002) 5(6):514–6. doi:10.1038/nn0602-849

Benedict C, Dodt C, Hallschmid M, Lepiorz M, Fehm HL, Born J, et al. Immedi- ate but not long-term intranasal administration of insulin raises blood pressure in human beings. *Metabolism* (2005) 54(10):1356–61. doi:10.1016/j.metabol. 2005.04.026

Benedict C, Hallschmid M, Hatke A, Schultes B, Fehm HL, Born J, et al. Intranasal insulin improves memory in humans. *Psychoneuroendocrinology* (2004) 29(10):1326–34. doi:10.1016/j.psyneuen.2004.04.003

Benedict C, Brede S, Schioth HB, Lehnert H, Schultes B, Born J, et al. Intranasal insulin enhances postprandial thermogenesis and lowers post- prandial serum insulin levels in healthy men. *Diabetes* (2011) 60(1):114–8. doi:10.2337/db10-0329

17

Neuroendocrine role for VGF

Jo E. Lewis[1], John M. Brameld[2] and Preeti H. Jethwa[2]*

[1] Queen's Medical Centre, School of Life Sciences, University of Nottingham Medical School, Nottingham, UK
[2] Division of Nutritional Sciences, School of Biosciences, University of Nottingham, Loughborough, UK

Edited by:
Hubert Vaudry, University of Rouen, France

Reviewed by:
Alena Sumova, Academy of Sciences of the Czech Republic, Czech Republic
Ruud Buijs, Universidad Autónoma de México, Mexico

***Correspondence:**
Preeti H. Jethwa, Division of Nutritional Sciences, School of Biosciences, University of Nottingham, Sutton Bonington Campus, Loughborough, LE12 5RD, UK
e-mail: preeti.jethwa@nottingham.ac.uk

The *vgf* gene (non-acronymic) is highly conserved and was identified on the basis of its rapid induction *in vitro* by nerve growth factor, although can also be induced by brain-derived neurotrophic factor, and glial-derived growth factor. The VGF gene gives rise to a 68 kDa precursor polypeptide, which is induced robustly, relatively selectively and is synthesized exclusively in neuronal and neuroendocrine cells. Post-translational processing by neuroendocrine specific prohormone convertases in these cells results in the production of a number of smaller peptides. The VGF gene and peptides are widely expressed throughout the brain, particularly in the hypothalamus and hippocampus, in peripheral tissues including the pituitary gland, the adrenal glands, and the pancreas, and in the gastrointestinal tract in both the myenteric plexus and in endocrine cells. VGF peptides have been associated with a number of neuroendocrine roles, and in this review, we aim to describe these roles to highlight the importance of VGF as therapeutic target for a number of disorders, particularly those associated with energy metabolism, pain, reproduction, and cognition.

Keywords: VGF, energy homeostasis, pain, cognition, reproduction

INTRODUCTION

VGF (non-acronymic) is a neurotrophin-induced gene, which was first identified as VGF8a, NGF33.1, and a2 on the basis of its rapid induction in PC12 cells treated with nerve growth factor (NGF) (1–3). Subsequent studies demonstrated that VGF is similarly upregulated by numerous neurotrophins, including brain-derived neurotrophic factor (BDNF) and neurotrophin-3 (NT-3), in neuronal targets such as cortical or hippocampal neurons (4). However, VGF mRNA levels are only marginally increased by other growth factors including epidermal growth factor (EGF), fibroblast growth factor (FGF), interleukin-6 (IL-6), and insulin, despite the capacity of these proteins to robustly induce transcription of other immediate early genes in the PC12 cell line (3, 5, 6).

The VGF polypeptide, which is robustly and exclusively synthesized in neuronal and neuroendocrine cells (1, 3, 7, 8), is processed by the prohormone convertases (PC), PC1/3 and PC2 (9). VGF derived peptides with specific neuronal bioactivities include TLQP-62, TLQP-21, HHPD-41, AQEE-30, AQEE-11, LQEQ-19, and neuroendocrine regulatory peptides-1 and -2 (NERP-1 and -2; 9–11). Studies have shown that TLQP-62 and AQEE-30 increase the firing rate of hippocampal neurons, induce neurogenesis, and have anti-depressive properties (4, 12, 13), whereas HHPD-41, AQEE-30, AQEE-11, and LQEQ-19 stimulate sympathetic outflow and facilitate penile erection in rats (14–16); and TLQP-21 and NERP-2 regulate energy balance (17–20). Furthermore, TLQP-21 regulates contractile activity in the gastrointestinal tract, has analgesic properties, reduces neuronal apoptosis *in vitro* and decreases rodent blood pressure (21–23) and NERP-1 and -2 regulate water homeostasis and suppress vasopressin release (11, 20, 24). Here, we review the regulation of VGF and the neuroendocrine role of its derived peptides.

THE TRANSCRIPTIONAL REGULATION OF VGF

IN VITRO

The gene itself is highly conserved among mammalian species in respect to the coding region and the promoter sequence (25). The VGF promoter region contains a CCAAT box, various specificity protein 1 (SP-1), and activating protein 2 (AP-2) sites and a silencer element similar to the one involved in tissue-specific expression of neuronal genes (3, 25). Furthermore, it contains a cyclic AMP response element (CRE), which is embedded within a 14bp palindromic sequence, mutations of which abolish NGF and cAMP responses (6). VGF expression in response to neurotrophins that requires the combined actions of several regulator complexes; in addition to the CRE, the CCAAT box was shown to be important for NGF induction (26), possibly in association with the activity of a large complex containing a CRE binding protein (CREB), mammalian achaete-scute homolog-1 (MASH-1), and p300 (27).

IN VIVO

A genomic fragment extending from 800-bp 5' to the transcriptional start site and including the first 700-bp of 5'-untranslated sequence results in reporter gene expression in a tissue-restricted pattern similar to that of the endogenous VGF gene (28). Interestingly, this region of the promoter contains a putative silencer element that is located 400-bp 5' to the transcriptional start site, which prevents expression in non-neuronal cell lines (25). VGF mRNA in the hypothalamus alters in response to feeding/fasting (14, 15, 20), salt loading (29), adrenalectomy (30), and seasonal rhythms (31). Furthermore, VGF mRNA varies in the pituitary during the estrous cycle (32) and in the suprachiasmatic nucleus (SCN) according to circadian rhythmicity (33); while gastric damage increases VGF mRNA in the nucleus tractus solitarius (NTS) and dorsomedial nucleus of the vagus (34). VGF mRNA is also modulated in other diverse conditions, which have been well described elsewhere (35).

THE STRUCTURE AND PROCESSING OF THE VGF POLYPEPTIDE

VGF is a 68 kDa polypeptide comprising 615 (human) or 617 (mouse/rat) amino acids with a typical secretory leader sequence of 22 amino acids at the N-terminal of VGF, which promotes translocation to the endoplasmic reticulum (ER) (36). Subsequent sequencing of the polypeptide in the mouse, horse, and bovine has confirmed extensive sequence conservation with approximately >85% identity (35). The most prominent VGF-derived peptides have apparent molecular masses of 20 (NAPP-129) and 10 kDa (TLQP-62), respectively (9) (**Figure 1**). However, the mouse and human sequences contain a minimum of 10 conserved regions of basic amino acid residues, which represent potential PC cleavage sites (37) (**Figure 2**). Indeed cleavage at the Arg-Pro-Arg555 sequence in the rat has been shown to give rise to the TLQP peptides (9). It is possible, however, that the number and function of VGF derived peptides are greater than currently known (38). The extensive review by Ferri et al. (35) describes this in more detail.

DISTRIBUTION OF VGF AND ITS DERIVED PEPTIDES

VGF mRNA

VGF mRNA is widely expressed throughout the nervous system. During embryogenesis VGF mRNA is expressed in distinct neurotrophin-responsive targets in the central and peripheral nervous system (CNS and PNS, respectively) in the rat (39, 40). At birth, VGF mRNA is expressed in neurons throughout the brain and in peripheral endocrine and neuroendocrine tissues. While in the adult brain VGF mRNA has the highest expression in the hypothalamus and the granular layer of the cerebellum, it is also expressed in a number of other brain areas including the main and accessory olfactory bulbs, hippocampus, cortex, basal ganglia, thalamus, amygdala, midbrain, and the brainstem. Within the hypothalamus, the highest concentrations of VGF mRNA have been found in the ventromedial hypothalamus, in particular the arcuate nucleus (ARC), as well as in the SCN (7, 39, 41). VGF mRNA expression in the mouse is similar to the rat (14).

VGF PEPTIDES

VGF and its derived peptides are found in dense core vesicles and are released in response to depolarizing signals from neuronal and neuroendocrine cells through the regulated secretory pathway (10, 42, 43). Antibodies raised to synthetic peptides corresponding to the C- or N-termini of potential or actual cleavage products have been utilized to study VGF derived peptide distribution. In animal tissues, VGF immunoreactivity was restricted to central and peripheral neurons (41, 44), as well as to endocrine cells of the pituitary, adrenal medulla, gut, and pancreas (44). The highest concentrations of VGF immunoreactivity have correspondingly been found in the medial hypothalamus, particularly in the ARC, in the SCN, and in the parvocellular and magnocellular cells of the paraventricular nucleus (PVN) and the supraoptic nucleus (SON) (41). Weak immunoreactivity was also detected in the hippocampus, amygdala, thalamus, and cerebral cortex (41). VGF immunoreactivity was also displayed in the female rat in the pars distalis, mainly with C-terminal antibodies (32). This, however, disappeared in accordance with the estrous peak of luteinizing hormone (LH) secretion, along with an induction of VGF mRNA in the pituitary. Additionally, VGF-derived peptides are prominent in the adult spinal cord, in α- and γ-motor neurons of the ventral horn and in the dorsal horn neurons, as well as cells of the inner nuclear and ganglion cell layers of the retina (45). In the PNS, both sympathetic ganglia and dorsal root ganglia of primary sensory neurons are important sites of localization of VGF-derived

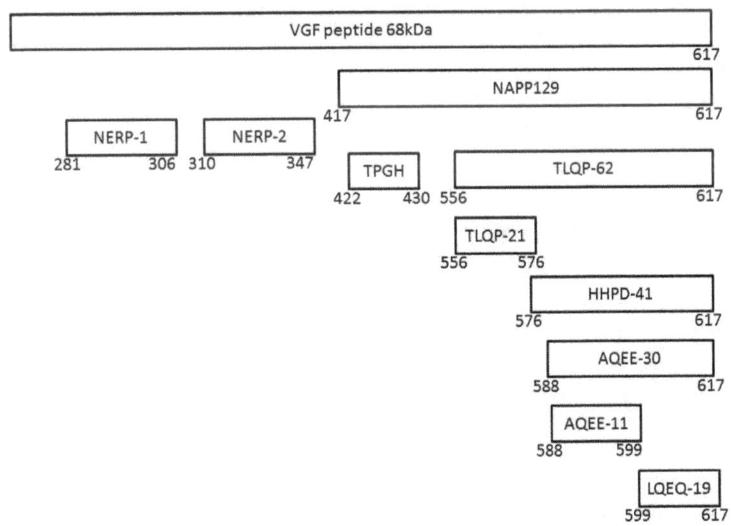

FIGURE 1 | The *vgf* gene and its derived peptides. The VGF polypeptide is the precursor of several biologically active peptides, which are released and play a role in intercellular communication. The gene contains a number of specific sequences, which are highly conserved between the species and these represent potential cleavage sites for the convertases of the kexin/subtilisin-like series proteinases family, namely prohormone convertases-1/3 and -2.

```
Human MKALRLSASALFC-LLLINGLGAAPPGRPEAQPPPLSSEHKEPVAGDAVPGPKDGSAPEV 59
Mouse MKTFTLPASVLFCFLLLIQGLGAAPPGRPDVFPPPLSSEHNGQVAEDAVSRPKDDGVPEV 60
      **:: *.**.*** ****:**********:. ********:  ** ***. ***...***

Human RGARNSEPQDEGELFQGVDPRALAAVLLQALDRPASPP-APSGSQQGPEEEAAEALLTET 118
Mouse RAARNPEPQDQGELFQGVDPRALASVLLQALDRPASPPSVPGGSQQGTPEEAAEALLTES 120
      *.***.****:*************:*************  .*.*****. **********:

Human VRSQTHSLPAPESPEP-AAPPRPQTPENGPEASDPSEELEALASLLQELRDFSPSSAKRQ 177
Mouse VRSQTHSLPAPEIQAPAVAPPRPQTQDRDPEEDDRSEELEALASLLQELRDFSPSNAKRQ 180
      ************    * .******* :..** .* ********************.****

Human QETAAAETETRTHTLTRVNLESPGPERVWRASWGEFQARVPERAPLPPPAPSQFQARMPD 237
Mouse QETAAAETETRTHTLTRVNLESPGPERVWRASWGEFQARVPERAPLPPPVPSQFQARMSE 240
      *************************************************.********.:

Human SGPLPETHKFGEGVSSPKTHLGEALAPLSKAYQGVAAPFPKARRPESALLGGSEAGERLL 297
Mouse SAPLPETHQFGEGVSSPKTHLGETLTPLSKAYQSLGGPFPKVRRLEGSFLGGSEAGERLL 300
      *.******:**************:*:*******.:..****.** *.::***********

Human QQGLAQVEAGRRQAEATRQAAAQEERLADLASDLLLQYLLQGGARQRGLGGRGLQEAAEE 357
Mouse QQGLAQVEAGRRQAEATRQAAAQEERLADLASDLLLQYLLQGGARQRDLGGRELQETQQE 360
      ***********************************************.**** ***: :*

Human RESAREEEEAEQERRGG-EERVGEEDEEAAEAEAEAEEAERARQNALLFAEEEDGEAGAE 416
Mouse RENEREEE-AEQERRGGGEDDVGEEDEEAAEAEAEAEEAERARQNALLFAEEEDGEAGAE 419
      **. **** ******** *: ***************************************

Human DKRSQEETPGHRRKEAEGTEEGGEEEDD-EEMDPQTIDSLIELSTKLHLPADDVVSIIEE 475
Mouse DKRSQEEAPGHRRKDAEGAEEGGEEDDDDEEMDPQTIDSLIELSTKLHLPADDVVSIIEE 479
      *******:******:***:******:** *******************************

Human VEEKRKRKKNAPPEPVPPPRAAPAPTHVRSPQPPPPAPAPARDELPDWNEVLPPWDREED 535
Mouse VEEKRKRKKNAPPEPVPPPRAAPAPTHVRSPQPPP--PAPARDELPDWNEVLPPWDREED 537
      ***********************************  ***********************

Human EVYPPGPYHPFPNYIRPRTLQPPSALRRRHYHHALPPSRHYPGREAQARRAQEEAEAEER 595
Mouse EVFPPGPYHPFPNYIRPRTLQPPASSRRRHFHHALPPARHHPDLEAQARRAQEEADAEER 597
      **:*********************:: ****:******:**:*. ***************:***

Human RLQEQEELENYIEHVLLRRP 615
Mouse RLQEQEELENYIEHVLLHRP 617
      *****************:**
```

FIGURE 2 | Comparison of the human and mouse VGF polypeptide sequences. * indicates the position which have a single, fully conserved residue. ":" indicates conservation between groups of strongly similar properties scoring >0.5 in the Gonnect PAM 250 matrix. "." indicates conservation between groups of weakly similar properties scoring <0.5 in the Gonnect PAM 250 matrix. Clusters of basic amino acids, which represent potential cleavage sites, are boxed. Sequence identity was >85%.

peptides (40). This is comparable to the expression of neuropeptide Y (NPY), ghrelin, and cholecystokinin (CCK), all of which regulate feeding and in some cases, gastrointestinal motility (46, 47). VGF-derived peptides are also present in mouse brown adipose tissue (BAT), where they are reduced in response to a high fat diet (HFD) (48).

VGF RECEPTORS

Of all the VGF derived peptides, TLQP-21 has had the most interest (17, 19, 23, 49–52). Previously, TLQP-21 was shown to bind to adipocyte membranes in a saturable manner, (53) and atomic force microscopy of living cells revealed the existence of a single class of binding sites for TLQP-21 (54). Taken together these results suggested a cell surface receptor for TLQP-21. Two possible receptors have recently been identified for TLQP-21. Chen et al. (55) identified gC1qR, showing that TLQP-21 activated rat macrophages through gC1qR, which then caused mechanical hypersensitivity in rats. gC1qR protein was expressed by both brain and spinal cord derived microglia (55) and is indispensable for adipogenesis and insulin signaling (56). Furthermore, obese mice fed a HFD demonstrated increased density of TLQP-21 binding in adipose tissues (54). However, neither TLQP-62 nor LQEQ-19 elicited a response in their experimental model, both of which had been previously implicated in pain processing (22, 57). This supports the hypothesis of different receptors for the VGF derived peptides. Hannedouche et al. (58) reported the complement receptor, C3A receptor-1 (C3AR1), as a receptor for TLQP-21, which mediated activity for TLQP-21 in two different rodent cell lines. C3AR1 was originally thought to be restricted to the innate immune response, its role limited to the complement cascade. However, it has subsequently been shown to have a role in cancer (59), neurogenesis (60), and hormone release from the pituitary gland (61). However, C3AR1$^{-/-}$ mice are transiently resistant to diet-induced obesity (DIO) and are protected against HFD-induced insulin resistance (62). The discovery of these receptors will help identify the mechanisms by which TLQP-21 and possible other derived peptide may modulate its actions.

PHYSIOLOGICAL ROLES OF VGF GENE AND DERIVED PEPTIDES

ENERGY BALANCE

The high expression of VGF in the hypothalamus and the change in expression of the *vgf* gene in the ARC following acute altered energy balance first suggested the importance of VGF in the regulation of energy balance (14, 20). Indeed fasting has been shown to increase VGF mRNA expression, while administration of leptin prevents the fasting induced increase in VGF mRNA (15). These changes in VGF can be observed in models of chronic energy imbalance; VGF mRNA levels resemble that of fasted wild-type mice in the ARC of the leptin deficient *ob/ob* mouse and in the leptin resistance *db/db* mouse (15). It is well known that the ARC has two neuronal populations that respond to the fed and fasted state as well as to leptin signaling, the pro-opiomelanocortin (POMC) and neuropeptide Y (NPY) neurons (63). VGF immunoreactivity has been shown to be co-localized with both these neuronal populations in the ARC, however, expression is modulated with energy state. In the *ad libitum* fed state and re-fed animals, VGF mRNA is co-localized with POMC (15, 64). On the other hand, fasting increases co-localization of VGF in the NPY neurons (64).

Energy balance and lack of functional VGF

The function of VGF and its extension derived peptides was first assessed through the development of mice lacking a functional copy of the *vgf* gene (VGF$^{-/-}$) via homologous recombination (14). At birth, the homozygous VGF$^{-/-}$ mice are indistinguishable from either their heterozygous or wild-type littermates. No defects in development were detected in either the CNS or the PNS. However, in the weeks following birth, the VGF$^{-/-}$ mice were visibly smaller than their wild-type littermates and adults were found to weigh 50-70% less due to a 50% reduction in adiposity compared to wild-type littermates (14). Consistent with the reduction in adiposity, leptin levels, serum glucose and insulin levels, and liver glycogen were reduced (48). The mice consumed considerably more calories per gram body weight, but this increase in food intake was not sufficient to maintain the same body weight as wild-type mice. The VGF$^{-/-}$ mice utilized twice as much oxygen at rest and displayed increased locomotor activity compared to wild-type littermates (14). Overall, the major change in VGF$^{-/-}$ mice is an increase in energy consumption; indeed *vgf* gene deletion did not block obesity via monosodium glutamate administration (15) suggesting that the thermogenic pathways resulting in the VGF$^{-/-}$ phenotype are blocked. These initial observations led Hahm et al. (14) to suggest that VGF may play a non-redundant role in the regulation of energy homeostasis and antagonism of the gene may constitute a basis for the treatment of obesity. Furthermore, *vgf* gene deletion blocked the development of obesity as a result of a HFD, gold thioglucose treatment, as well as in the *agouti* mouse, and suggesting that VGF functions in outflow pathways regulating energy expenditure downstream of the hypothalamic melanocortin receptors (15).

Energy balance and VGF-derived peptides

Thus from the phenotype of the VGF$^{-/-}$ mice one might predict that VGF promotes an anabolic drive. Surprisingly, this view has not been supported by subsequent studies in mice and Siberian hamsters. Chronic intracerebroventricular (ICV) infusion of TLQP-21 in mice fed a normal lab chow resulted in a small increase in resting energy expenditure and rectal temperature (17). The changes in metabolic parameters were mirrored by increased epinephrine content in BAT, upregulation of BAT β2-adrenergic receptor (AR), uncoupling protein 1 (UCP-1) mRNA, higher expression of peroxisome proliferator-activated receptor-δ (PPAR-δ), and β3-AR in white adipose tissue (WAT). However, hypothalamic expressions of agouti-related protein (AgRP), NPY, α-melanocyte-stimulating hormone (α-MSH), POMC, and corticotrophin-releasing hormone (CRH) were unchanged (17). In mice, switched to a HFD treatment with TLQP-21 halted the expected increase in body weight and WAT, attenuated rises in leptin, and normalized ghrelin levels (17). In rats, ICV infusion of TLQP-21 significantly decreased gastric emptying, an effect that was blocked by ICV infusion of indomethacin, which blocks prostaglandin release (65).

A similar catabolic effect was noted in Siberian hamsters, a seasonal model of energy balance. Not only is VGF mRNA significantly increased in the winter weight-loss state in the dorsal medial posterior arcuate nucleus (dmpArc) (31) but ICV infusion of TLQP-21 at the onset of the dark phase was found to significantly and dose dependently decrease food intake and body weight (19). However, there was no effect on energy expenditure as Siberian hamsters pair-fed to the treated group lost a similar amount of body weight (19). Weight loss was, therefore, attributable to reduced caloric intake rather than energy expenditure.

One of the possible explanations for this contradiction between the functional *in vivo* studies and the VGF$^{-/-}$ mice, where all the VGF peptides have been ablated, is that some of these peptides may have opposing roles in energy balance. Interestingly, Bartolomucci et al. (66) have suggested that HHPD-41 increased food intake following ICV infusion, and more recently ICV infusion of NERP-2 in rats has been shown to increase food intake, body temperature, oxygen consumption, and locomotor activity (20). Furthermore, intravenous administration of NERP-2 significantly augmented glucose stimulated insulin secretion in anesthetized rats or following intraperitoneal injection to conscious mice (67). Thus VGF may have a biphasic role in the regulation of energy balance and further characterization of the other VGF-derived peptides is required.

Energy balance and circadian rhythm

It is well known that food intake and energy metabolism in mammals are regulated by their circadian clock, and food intake is one such signal that can entrain the circadian clock (68). As previously described, VGF is expressed in the SCN, the circadian pacemaker in animals, while the E-box contained in the *vgf* gene promoter region is similar to the many clock genes such as the *per* gene (33). Therefore, it is not unexpected that the *vgf* gene exhibits circadian rhythm in the SCN even under constant dark conditions, while VGF mRNA levels are increased in response to light simulation in the SCN when light would be expected to cause a phase shift in locomotor rhythms (33). Indeed VGF$^{-/-}$ mice can maintain circadian rhythm of wheel running in constant darkness, however, the period length was found to be slightly but significantly shorter than wild-type littermates (14). Thus, this raises the question could the metabolic phenotype of the VGF$^{-/-}$ mice be attributed, in part, to the disruption of the circadian system.

VGF AND WATER BALANCE

Water deprivation and salt loading in rats increases VGF mRNA levels in both the SON and PVN, along with vasopressin mRNA (29). ICV injection of NERP-1 and NERP-2 suppresses hypertonic saline or angiotensin II induced increases in plasma vasopressin in rats (69). Additionally, ICV infusion of NERP-1 and -2 attenuated the increase in vasopressin as a result of water deprivation in rats, an effect which was reversed following immunoneutralisation by ICV infusion of anti-NERP-1 and -2 antibodies (69). Taken together, these data suggest that NERP-1 and -2 may be involved in the central control of body fluid balance.

VGF AND REPRODUCTION

The role of VGF signaling in reproduction was inferred from the observation that VGF gene deletion resulted in infertility in both male and female mice (14). In male VGF$^{-/-}$ mice, the onset of puberty and sexual maturation was delayed, and the weights of the testes, albeit having mobile spermatozoa in the lumen, were significantly lower than those of wild-type littermates (14). While in the female VGF$^{-/-}$ mice histological examination revealed no mature follicles or corpus lutea, and the ovaries, oviduct, and uteri weighed 30% less than those of the wild-type littermates (14). However, transplanting ovaries from VGF$^{-/-}$ mice into ovariectomized wild-type females restored fertility, suggesting that the reproductive deficits of VGF$^{-/-}$ mice were not the result of pathology but arose from deficits in the hypothalamic-pituitary-gonadal axis (14). However, Ferri et al. (32) showed that VGF gene expression varied during estrous; there was an increase in VGF mRNA and VGF peptide/s degranulation, suggesting perturbation of anterior pituitary function.

It is common knowledge that alterations in energy metabolism and fat stores can affect reproductive function. VGF$^{-/-}$ mice have reduced leptin and altered energy status, therefore, it could be suggested that the deficit may be due to gonadotropin releasing hormone (GnRH) synthesis or secretion. However, while GnRH levels are not affected, LH and follicle-stimulating hormone (FSH) mRNA levels were reduced in VGF$^{-/-}$ mice (14) suggesting decreased GnRH secretion. Indeed it has been shown that central administration of TLQP-21 in female rats during the pubertal transition advanced the timing of vaginal opening and increased the number of animals with signs of ovulation (70). These effects of TLQP-21 may be via stimulation of the GnRH release, as TLQP-21 has been shown to induce LH secretion *in vitro* (71). Furthermore, Pinilla et al. (71) have shown that chronic administration of TLQP-21 was able to prevent the hypogonadotropic state induced by food deprivation.

There is further evidence of VGF peptides and a possible role in the regulation of reproduction. While HHPD-41, AQEE-30, and LQEQ-19 have been shown to induce penile erection in rats following infusion into the PVN in a dose dependent manner, NERP-1 has a pro-erectile effect when injected into the lateral ventricles or the ARC of rats (72). The effect on penile erection is thought to be via nitric oxide mediated activation of oxytocinergic pathways (16).

VGF AND PAIN

VGF is a gene commonly upregulated in sensory neurons in clinically relevant models of neuropathic pain, namely, varicella zoster infection, HIV-associated neuropathy, and peripheral nerve trauma (55). Furthermore, VGF has been shown to be upregulated in the dorsal root ganglia and spinal cord in a number of neuropathic and inflammatory pain models (22, 57, 73–76). In these areas, VGF is co-localized with substance P, calcitonin gene related peptide, TrkA, and P2 × 3 (22, 51). A functional role for VGF-derived peptides has been identified in pain pathways. Indeed intrathecal infusion of TLQP-62 results in cold behavioral hypersensitivity in rats; while injection of TLQP-21 into the hind paw of mice resulted in hypersensitivity in both control animals and the formalin model of inflammatory pain (51) as well as inducing thermal hyperalgesia in the warm-water immersion tail-withdrawal test (77). Additionally, both LQEQ-19 and AQEE-30 have been shown to induce p38 MAP kinase phosphorylation in spinal microglia (22), suggesting that VGF-derived peptides have pro-nociceptive and hyperalgesic functions.

VGF AND MEMORY AND LEARNING

As previously stated VGF mRNA is expressed in the hippocampus, and it has been shown that VGF transcription is accompanied by translation within 3 hours of BDNF exposure in hippocampal slices *in vitro* (4). Additionally, VGF mRNA has been shown to be upregulated by activities, such as memory and learning (8), while VGF$^{-/-}$ mice have demonstrated impaired hippocampal-dependent spatial learning and contextual fear conditioning tasks (78). Indeed more recently, TLQP-62 has been shown to induce transient potentiation in hippocampal slices (78), enhance synaptic activity (4), and increase neurogenesis in early phase neural progenitor cells in the adult hippocampus (12, 79), as well as shown to have effect on cognitive mechanism (80), thus suggesting that VGF may be important in memory processes.

To further support this notion, proteomic studies have demonstrated a reduction in VGF-derived peptides in the cerebrospinal fluid of patients affected by Alzheimer's disease (AD) (81–83). Similarly, there was a reduction in VGF-derived peptides in the parietal cortex of AD patients (84) and a reduction in TPGH and NERP-1 in the parietal cortex of Parkinson's disease patients (84).

VGF AND DEPRESSION

VGF protein expression is reduced in both the learned helplessness and forced swim test depression paradigms (85), while VGF is increased by antidepressant drugs and voluntary exercise (12). Exercise regulates VGF mRNA and protein expression in the rodent hippocampus and induces an antidepressant response; an opposing phenotype is observed in the heterozygous VGF$^{-/+}$ mouse (86). Recently, inhibition of phosphodiesterase-4 or -5 was shown to result in increases in cAMP, activating CREB, BDNF, and VGF, which produces antidepressant-like effects on behavior in mice (87). Similarly, microinjection of TLQP-62 into the hippocampal CA1 regions demonstrated antidepressant-like behavioral effects in mice (88), possibly via a BDNF-dependent mechanism (78).

CONCLUSION

The evidence presented in this review indicates that the gene and gene product have a key neuroendocrine role and that VGF or its derived peptides may act as biomarkers or therapeutic targets in a number of disorders such as obesity, dementia, depression, and pain. The mechanisms by which VGF and its derived peptides are involved remains to be identified, however, the discovery of the new receptors will help advancements in this area both *in vitro* and *in vivo*.

ACKNOWLEDGMENTS

We thank Professor Francis Ebling and Dr. Perry Barrett for their continued support.

REFERENCES

Levi A, Eldridge JD, Paterson BM. Molecular cloning of a gene sequence reg- ulated by nerve growth factor. *Science* (1985) 229:393–5. doi:10.1126/science.3839317

Cho KO, Skarnes WC, Minsk B, Palmieri S, Jackson-Grusby L, Wagner JA. Nerve growth factor regulates gene expression by several distinct mechanisms. *Mol Cell Biol* (1989) 9:135–43.

Salton SR, Fischberg DJ, Dong KW. Structure of the gene encoding VGF, a ner- vous system-specific mRNA that is rapidly and selectively induced by nerve growth factor in PC12 cells. *Mol Cell Biol* (1991) 11:2335–49.

Alder J, Thakker-Varia S, Bangasser DA, Kuroiwa M, Plummer MR, Shors TJ. Brain-derived neurotrophic factor-induced gene expression reveals novel actions of VGF in hippocampal synaptic plasticity. *J Neurosci* (2003) 23:10800–8.

Possenti R, Di Rocco G, Nasi S, Levi A. Regulatory elements in the promoter region of vgf, a nerve growth factor-inducible gene. *Proc Natl Acad Sci U S A* (1992) 89:3815–9. doi:10.1073/pnas.89.9.3815

Hawley RJ, Scheibe RJ, Wagner JA. NGF induces the expression of the VGF gene through a cAMP response element. *J Neurosci* (1992) 12:2573–81.

van den Pol AN, Bina K, Decavel C, Ghosh P. VGF expression in the brain. *J Comp Neurol* (1994) 347:455–69. doi:10.1002/cne.903470311

Snyder SE, Cheng HW, Murray KD, Isackson PJ, McNeill TH, Salton SR. The messenger RNA encoding VGF, a neuronal peptide precursor, is rapidly regu- lated in the rat central nervous system by neuronal activity, seizure and lesion. *Neuroscience* (1998) 82:7–19. doi:10.1016/S0306-4522(97)00280-7

Trani E, Giorgi A, Canu N, Amadoro G, Rinaldi AM, Halban PA. Isola- tion and characterization of VGF peptides in rat brain. Role of PC1/3 and PC2 in the maturation of VGF precursor. *J Neurochem* (2002) 81:565–74. doi:10.1046/j.1471-4159.2002.00842.x

Possenti R, Eldridge JD, Paterson BM, Grasso A, Levi A. A protein induced by NGF in PC12 cells is stored in secretory vesicles and released through the regulated pathway. *EMBO J* (1989) 8:2217–23.

Yamaguchi H, Sasaki K, Satomi Y, Shimbara T, Kageyama H, Mondal MS. Peptidomic identification and biological validation of neuroendocrine reg- ulatory peptide-1 and -2. *J Biol Chem* (2007) 282(26354–60):M701665200. doi:10.1074/jbc.M701665200

Thakker-Varia S, Alder J. Neuropeptides in depression: role of VGF. *Behav Brain Res* (2009) 197:262–78. doi:10.1016/j.bbr.2008.10.006

Cattaneo A, Sesta A, Calabrese F, Nielsen G, Riva MA, Gennarelli M. The expression of VGF is reduced in leukocytes of depressed patients and it is restored by effective antidepressant treatment. *Neuropsychopharmacology* (2010) 35:1423–8. doi:10.1038/npp.2010.11

Hahm S, Mizuno TM, Wu TJ, Wisor JP, Priest CA, Kozak CA. Targeted dele- tion of the Vgf gene indicates that the encoded secretory peptide precursor plays a novel role in the regulation of energy balance. *Neuron* (1999) 23:537–48. doi:10.1016/S0896-6273(00)80806-5

Hahm S, Fekete C, Mizuno TM, Windsor J, Yan H, Boozer CN. VGF is required for obesity induced by diet, gold thioglucose treatment, and agouti and is differentially regulated in pro-opiomelanocortin- and neuropeptide Y-containing arcuate neurons in response to fasting. *J Neurosci* (2002) 22:6929–38.

Succu S, Cocco C, Mascia MS, Melis T, Melis MR, Possenti R. Pro-VGF-derived peptides induce penile erection in male rats: possible involvement of oxytocin. *Eur J Neurosci* (2004) 20:3035–40. doi:10.1111/j.1460-9568.2004.03781.x

Bartolomucci A, La Corte G, Possenti R, Locatelli V, Rigamonti AE, Torsello A. TLQP-21, a VGF-derived peptide, increases energy expenditure and prevents the early phase of diet-induced obesity. *Proc Natl Acad Sci U S A* (2006) 103:14584–9. doi:10.1073/pnas.0606102103

Jethwa PH, Warner A, Brameld JM, Keyte JW, Nilaweera NK, Morgan PJ. The role of a VGF derived peptide in the regulation of food intake in a seasonal rodent. *Front Neuroendocrinol* (2006) 27:5–6. doi:10.1016/j.yfrne.2006. 03.012

Jethwa PH, Warner A, Nilaweera KN, Brameld JM, Keyte JW, Carter WG. VGF- derived peptide, TLQP-21, regulates food intake and body weight in Siberian hamsters. *Endocrinology* (2007) 148:4044–55. doi:10.1210/en.2007-0038

Toshinai K, Yamaguchi H, Kageyama H, Matsuo T, Koshinaka K, Sasaki K. Neu- roendocrine regulatory peptide-2 regulates feeding behavior via the orexin system in the hypothalamus. *Am J Physiol Endocrinol Metab* (2010) 299:E394–401. doi:10.1152/ajpendo.00768.2009

Severini C, Ciotti MT, Biondini L, Quaresima S, Rinaldi AM, Levi A. TLQP-21, a neuroendocrine VGF-derived peptide, prevents cerebellar granule cells death induced by serum and potassium deprivation. *J Neurochem* (2008) 104:534–44. doi:10.1111/j.1471-4159.2007.05068.x

Riedl MS, Braun PD, Kitto KF, Roiko SA, Anderson LB, Honda CN. Proteomic analysis uncovers novel actions of the neurosecretory protein VGF in nociceptive processing. *J Neurosci* (2009) 29:13377–88. doi:10.1523/JNEUROSCI.1127-09. 2009

Fargali S, Garcia AL, Sadahiro M, Jiang C, Janssen WG, Lin WJ. The granin VGF promotes genesis of secretory vesicles, and regulates circulating catecholamine levels and blood pressure. *FASEB J* (2014) 28:2120–33. doi:10.1096/fj.13-239509

D'Amato F, Cocco C, Noli B, Cabras T, Messana I, Ferri GL. VGF peptides upon osmotic stimuli: changes in neuroendocrine regulatory peptides 1 and 2 in the hypothalamic-pituitary-axis and plasma. *J Chem Neuroanat* (2012) 44:57–65. doi:10.1016/j.jchemneu.2012.05.001

Canu N, Possenti R, Rinaldi AM, Trani E, Levi A. Molecular cloning and charac- terization of the human VGF promoter region. *J Neurochem* (1997) 68:1390–9. doi:10.1046/j.1471-4159.1997.68041390.x

D'Arcangelo G, Habas R, Wang S, Halegoua S, Salton SR. Activation of code- pendent transcription factors is required for transcriptional induction of the vgf gene by nerve growth factor and Ras. *Mol Cell Biol* (1996) 16:4621–31.

Mandolesi G, Gargano S, Pennuto M, Illi B, Molfetta R, Soucek L. NGF-dependent and tissue-specific transcription of vgf is regulated by a CREB-p300 and bHLH factor interaction. *FEBS Lett* (2002) 510:50–6. doi:10.1016/S0014-5793(01)03227-6

Piccioli P, Di Luzio A, Amann R, Schuligoi R, Surani MA, Donnerer J. Neu- roantibodies: ectopic expression of a recombinant anti-substance P antibody in the central nervous system of transgenic mice. *Neuron* (1995)

15:373–84. doi:10.1016/0896-6273(95)90041-1

Mahata SK, Mahata M, Fischer-Colbrie R, Winkler H. In situ hybridization: mRNA levels of secretogranin II, VGF and peptidylglycine alpha-amidating monooxygenase in brain of salt-loaded rats. *Histochemistry* (1993) 99:287–93. doi:10.1007/BF00269101

Mahata SK, Mahata M, Hortnag H, Fischer-Colbrie R, Steiner HJ, Dietze O. Concomitant changes of messenger ribonucleic acid levels of secretogranin II, VGF, vasopressin and oxytocin in the paraventricular nucleus of rats after adrenalectomy and during lactation. *J Neuroendocrinol* (1993) 5:323–30. doi:10.1111/j.1365-2826.1993.tb00489.x

Barrett P, Ross AW, Balik A, Littlewood PA, Mercer JG, Moar KM. Photoperiodic regulation of histamine H3 receptor and VGF messenger ribonucleic acid in the arcuate nucleus of the Siberian hamster. *Endocrinology* (2005) 146:1930–9. doi:10.1210/en.2004-1452

Ferri GL, Gaudio RM, Cossu M, Rinaldi AM, Polak JM, Berger P. The "VGF" protein in rat adenohypophysis: sex differences and changes during the estrous cycle and after gonadectomy. *Endocrinology* (1995) 136:2244–51. doi:10.1210/endo.136.5.7720674

Wisor JP, Takahashi JS. Regulation of the vgf gene in the golden hamster suprachiasmatic nucleus by light and by the circadian clock. *J Comp Neurol* (1997) 378:229–38. doi:10.1002/(SICI)1096-9861(19970210)378:2<229::AID-CNE6>3.3.CO;2-6

Kanemasa K, Okamura H, Kodama T, Ibata Y. Induction of VGF mRNA in neu- rons of the rat nucleus tractus solitarius and the dorsal motor nucleus of vagus in duodenal ulceration by cysteamine. *Brain Res Mol Brain Res* (1995) 32:55–62. doi:10.1016/0169-328X(95)00059-2

Ferri GL, Noli B, Brancia C, D'Amato F, Cocco C. VGF: an inducible gene product, precursor of a diverse array of neuro-endocrine peptides and tissue- specific disease biomarkers. *J Chem Neuroanat* (2011) 42:249–61. doi:10.1016/j.jchemneu.2011.05.007

Jethwa PH, Ebling FJP. Role of VGF-derived peptides in the control of food intake, body weight and reproduction. *Neuroendocrinology* (2008) 88:80–7. doi:10.1159/000127319

Salton SR, Ferri GL, Hahm S, Snyder SE, Wilson AJ, Possenti R, et al. VGF: a novel role for this neuronal and neuroendocrine polypeptide in the regulation of energy balance. *Front Neuroendocrinology* (2000) 21:199–219. doi:10.1006/ frne.2000.0199

Levi A, Ferri GL, Watson E, Possenti R, Salton SR. Processing, distribution, and function of VGF, a neuronal and endocrine peptide precursor. *Cell Mol Neurobiol* (2004) 24:517–33. doi:10.1023/B:CEMN.0000023627.79947.22

Snyder SE, Salton SR. Expression of VGF mRNA in the adult rat central nervous system. *J Comp Neurol* (1998) 394:91–105. doi:10.1002/(SICI)1096-9861(19980427)394:1<91::AID-CNE7>3.3.CO;2-B

Snyder SE, Pintar JE, Salton SR. Developmental expression of VGF mRNA in the prenatal and postnatal rat. *J Comp Neurol* (1998) 394:64–90. doi:10.1002/ (SICI)1096-9861(19980427)394:1<64::AID-CNE6>3.0.CO;2-F

van den Pol AN, Decavel C, Levi A, Paterson B. Hypothalamic expression of a novel gene product, VGF: immunocytochemical analysis. *J Neurosci* (1989) 9:4122–37.

Laslop A, Mahata SK, Wolkersdorfer M, Mahata M, Srivastava M, Seidah NG. Large dense-core vesicles in rat adrenal after reserpine: levels of mRNAs of sol- uble and membrane-bound constituents in chromaffin and ganglion cells indi- cate a biosynthesis of vesicles with higher secretory quanta. *J Neurochem* (1994) 62:2448–56. doi:10.1046/j.1471-4159.1994.62062448.x

Benson DL, Salton SR. Expression and polarization of VGF in developing hip- pocampal neurons. *Brain Res Dev Brain Res* (1996) 96:219–28. doi:10.1016/ 0165-3806(96)00108-3

Ferri GL, Levi A, Possenti R. A novel neuroendocrine gene product: selec- tive VGF8a gene expression and immuno-localisation of the VGF protein in endocrine and neuronal populations. *Brain Res Mol Brain Res* (1992) 13:139–43. doi:10.1016/0169-328X(92)90053-E

Zhao Z, Lange DJ, Ho L, Bonini S, Shao B, Salton SR. Vgf is a novel bio- marker associated with muscle weakness in amyotrophic lateral sclerosis (ALS), with a potential role in disease pathogenesis. *Int J Med Sci* (2008) 5:92–9. doi:10.7150/ijms.5.92

Wren AM, Small CJ, Ward HL, Murphy KG, Dakin CL, Taheri S. The novel hypothalamic peptide ghrelin stimulates food intake and growth hormone secretion. *Endocrinology* (2000) 141:4325–8. doi:10.1210/endo.141. 11.7873

Wren AM, Small CJ, Abbott CR, Jethwa PH, Kennedy AR, Murphy KG. Hypothalamic actions of neuromedin U. *Endocrinology* (2002) 143:4227–34. doi:10.1210/en.2002-220308

Watson E, Fargali S, Okamoto H, Sadahiro M, Gordon RE, Chakraborty T. Analysis of knockout mice suggests a role for VGF in the control of fat storage and energy expenditure. *BMC Physiol* (2009) 9:19. doi:10.1186/1472-6793-9-19

Bartolomucci A, Rigamonti AE, Bulgarelli I, Torsello A, Locatelli V, Pavone F. Chronic intracerebroventricular TLQP-21 delivery does not modulate the GH/IGF-1-axis and muscle strength in mice. *Growth Horm IGF Res* (2007) 17:342–5. doi:10.1016/j.ghir.2007.02.002

Bartolomucci A, Moles A, Levi A, Possenti R. Pathophysiological role of TLQP-21: gastrointestinal and metabolic functions. *Eat Weight Disord* (2008) 13:e49–54.

Rizzi R, Bartolomucci A, Moles A, D'Amato F, Sacerdote P, Levi A. The VGF- derived peptide TLQP-21: a new modulatory peptide for inflammatory pain. *Neurosci Lett* (2008) 441:129–33. doi:10.1016/j.neulet.2008.06.018

Brancia C, Cocco C, D'Amato F, Noli B, Sanna F, Possenti R. Selective expression of TLQP-21 and other VGF peptides in gastric neuroendocrine cells and mod- ulation by feeding. *J Endocrinol* (2010) 207:329–41. doi:10.1677/JOE-10-0189

Possenti R, Muccioli G, Petrocchi P, Cero C, Cabassi A, Vulchanova L. Char- acterization of a novel peripheral pro-lipolytic mechanism in mice: role of VGF-derived peptide TLQP-21. *Biochem J* (2012) 441:511–22. doi:10.1042/BJ20111165

Cassina V, Torsello A, Tempestini A, Salerno D, Brogioli D, Tamiazzo L. Biophys- ical characterization of a binding site for TLQP-21, a naturally occurring peptide which induces resistance to obesity. *Biochim Biophys Acta* (2013) 1828:455–60. doi:10.1016/j.bbamem.2012.10.023

Chen YC, Pristera A, Ayub M, Swanwick RS, Karu K, Hamada Y. Identification of a receptor for neuropeptide VGF and its role in neuropathic pain. *J Biol Chem* (2013) 288:34638–46. doi:10.1074/jbc.M113.510917

Kim KB, Kim BW, Choo HJ, Kwon YC, Ahn BY, Choi JS. Proteome analysis of adipocyte lipid rafts reveals that gC1qR plays essential roles in adipogene- sis and insulin signal transduction. *Proteomics* (2009) 9:2373–82. doi:10.1002/pmic.200800811

Moss A, Ingram R, Koch S, Theodorou A, Low L, Baccei M. Origins, actions and dynamic expression patterns of the neuropeptide VGF in rat peripheral and central sensory neurones following peripheral nerve injury. *Mol Pain* (2008) 4:62. doi:10.1186/1744-8069-4-62

Hannedouche S, Beck V, Leighton-Davies J, Beibel M, Roma G, Oakeley EJ. Identification of the C3a receptor (C3AR1) as the target of the VGF- derived peptide TLQP-21 in rodent cells. *J Biol Chem* (2013) 288:27434–43. doi:10.1074/jbc.M113.497214

Opstal-van Winden AW, Vermeulen RC, Peeters PH, Beijnen JH, van Gils CH. Early diagnostic protein biomarkers for breast cancer: how far have we come? *Breast Cancer Res Treat* (2012) 134:1–12. doi:10.1007/s10549-011-1907-2

Klos A, Tenner AJ, Johswich KO, Ager RR, Reis ES, Kohl J. The role of the anaphylatoxins in health and disease. *Mol Immunol* (2009) 46:2753–66. doi:10.1016/j.molimm.2009.04.027

Francis K, Lewis BM, Akatsu H, Monk PN, Cain SA, Scanlon MF. Complement C3a receptors in the pituitary gland: a novel pathway by which an innate immune molecule releases hormones involved in the control of inflammation. *FASEB J* (2003) 17:2266–8. doi:10.1096/fj.02-1103fje

Mamane Y, Chung Chan C, Lavallee G, Morin N, Xu LJ, Huang J. The C3a anaphylatoxin receptor is a key mediator of insulin resistance and functions by modulating adipose tissue macrophage infiltration and activation. *Diabetes* (2009) 58:2006–17. doi:10.2337/db09-0323

Schwartz MW, Woods SC, Porte D Jr, Seeley RJ, Baskin DG. Central nervous system control of food intake. *Nature* (2000) 404:661–71. doi:10.1038/35007534

Saderi N, Buijs FN, Salgado-Delgado R, Merkenstein M, Basualdo MC, Ferri GL. A role for VGF in the hypothalamic arcuate and paraventricular nuclei in the control of energy homeostasis. *Neuroscience* (2014) 265:184–95. doi:10.1016/j.neuroscience.2014.01.060

Severini C, La Corte G, Improta G, Broccardo M, Agostini S, Petrella C. In vitro and in vivo pharmacological role of TLQP-21, a VGF-derived peptide, in the regulation of rat gastric motor functions. *Br J Pharmacol* (2009) 157:984–93. doi:10.1111/j.1476-5381.2009.00192.x

Bartolomucci A, Possenti R, Levi A, Pavone F, Moles A. The role of the vgf gene and VGF-derived peptides in nutrition and metabolism. *Genes Nutr* (2007) 2:169–80. doi:10.1007/s12263-007-0047-0

Moin AS, Yamaguchi H, Rhee M, Kim JW, Toshinai K, Waise TM. Neu- roendocrine regulatory peptide-2 stimulates glucose-induced insulin secre- tion in vivo and in vitro. *Biochem Biophys Res Commun* (2012) 428:512–7. doi:10.1016/j.bbrc.2012.10.073

Turek FW, Joshu C, Kohsaka A, Lin E, Ivanova G, McDearmon E. Obesity and metabolic syndrome in circadian clock mutant mice. *Science* (2005) 308:1043–5. doi:10.1126/science.1108750

Toshinai K, Nakazato M. Neuroendocrine regulatory peptide-1 and -2: novel bioactive peptides processed from VGF. *Cell Mol Life Sci* (2009) 66:1939–45. doi:10.1007/s00018-009-8796-0

Aguilar E, Pineda R, Gaytan F, Sanchez-Garrido MA, Romero M, Romero- Ruiz A. Characterization of the reproductive effects of the Vgf-derived peptide TLQP-21 in female rats: in vivo and in vitro studies. *Neuroendocrinology* (2013) 98:38–50. doi:10.1159/000350323

Pinilla L, Pineda R, Gaytan F, Romero M, Garcia-Galiano D, Sanchez-Garrido MA. Characterization of the reproductive effects of the anorexi- genic VGF-derived peptide TLQP-21: in vivo and in vitro studies in male rats. *Am J Physiol Endocrinol Metab* (2011) 300:E837–47. doi:10.1152/ajpendo. 00598.2010

Melis MR, Sanna F, Succu S, Ferri GL, Argiolas A. Neuroendocrine regula- tory peptide-1 and neuroendocrine regulatory peptide-2 influence differentially feeding and penile erection in male rats: sites of action in the brain. *Regul Pept* (2012) 177:46–52. doi:10.1016/j.regpep.2012.04.007

Costigan M, Befort K, Karchewski L, Griffin RS, D'Urso D, Allchorne A. Repli- cate high-density rat genome oligonucleotide microarrays reveal hundreds of regulated genes in the dorsal root ganglion after peripheral nerve injury. *BMC Neurosci* (2002) 3:16. doi:10.1186/1471-2202-3-16

Wang H, Sun H, Della Penna K, Benz RJ, Xu J, Gerhold DL. Chronic neuro- pathic pain is accompanied by global changes in gene expression and shares pathobiology with neurodegenerative diseases. *Neuroscience* (2002) 114:529–46. doi:10.1016/S0306-4522(02)00341-X

Valder CR, Liu JJ, Song YH, Luo ZD. Coupling gene chip analyses and rat genetic variances in identifying potential target genes that may contribute to neuro- pathic allodynia development. *J Neurochem* (2003) 87:560–73. doi:10.1046/j.1471-4159.2003.02016.x

Maratou K, Wallace VC, Hasnie FS, Okuse K, Hosseini R, Jina N. Comparison of dorsal root ganglion gene expression in rat models of traumatic and HIV- associated neuropathic pain. *Eur J Pain* (2009) 13:387–98. doi:10.1016/j.ejpain. 2008.05.011

Fairbanks CA, Peterson CD, Speltz RH, Riedl MS, Kitto KF, Dykstra JA. The VGF- derived peptide TLQP-21 contributes to inflammatory and nerve injury-induced hypersensitivity. *Pain* (2014) 155:1229–37. doi:10.1016/j.pain.2014.03.012

Bozdagi O, Rich E, Tronel S, Sadahiro M, Patterson K, Shapiro ML. The neurotrophin-inducible gene Vgf regulates hippocampal function and behavior through a brain-derived neurotrophic factor-dependent mechanism. *J Neurosci* (2008) 28:9857–69. doi:10.1523/JNEUROSCI.3145-08.2008

Thakker-Varia S, Behnke J, Doobin D, Dalal V, Thakkar K, Khadim F. VGF (TLQP-62)-induced neurogenesis targets early phase neural progenitor cells in the adult hippocampus and requires glutamate and BDNF signaling. *Stem Cell Res* (2014) 12:762–77. doi:10.1016/j.scr.2014.03.005

Brouillette J, Young D, During MJ, Quirion R. Hippocampal gene expres- sion profiling reveals the possible involvement of Homer1 and GABA(B) receptors in scopolamine-induced amnesia. *J Neurochem* (2007) 102:1978–89. doi:10.1111/j.1471-4159.2007.04666.x

Carrette O, Demalte I, Scherl A, Yalkinoglu O, Corthals G, Burkhard P. A panel of cerebrospinal fluid potential biomarkers for the diagnosis of Alzheimer's disease. *Proteomics* (2003) 3:1486–94. doi:10.1002/pmic.200300470

Ruetschi U, Zetterberg H, Podust VN, Gottfries J, Li S, Hviid Simonsen A. Iden- tification of CSF biomarkers for frontotemporal dementia using SELDI-TOF. *Exp Neurol* (2005) 196:273–81. doi:10.1016/j.expneurol.2005.08.002

Selle H, Lamerz J, Buerger K, Dessauer A, Hager K, Hampel H. Identification of novel biomarker candidates by differential peptidomics analysis of cere- brospinal fluid in Alzheimer's disease. *Comb Chem High Throughput Screen* (2005) 8:801–6. doi:10.2174/138620705774962391

Cocco C, D'Amato F, Noli B, Ledda A, Brancia C, Bongioanni P. Distribution of VGF peptides in the human cortex and their selective changes in Parkinson's and Alzheimer's diseases. *J Anat* (2010) 217:683–93. doi:10.1111/j.1469-7580.2010.01309.x

Thakker-Varia S, Krol JJ, Nettleton J, Bilimoria PM, Bangasser DA, Shors TJ. The neuropeptide VGF produces antidepressant-like behavioral effects and enhances proliferation in the hippocampus. *J Neurosci* (2007) 27:12156–67. doi:10.1523/JNEUROSCI.1898-07.2007

Hunsberger JG, Newton SS, Bennett AH, Duman CH, Russell DS, Salton SR. Antidepressant actions of the exercise-regulated gene VGF. *Nat Med* (2007) 13:1476–82. doi:10.1038/nm1669

Wang C, Zhang J, Lu Y, Lin P, Pan T, Zhao X. Antidepressant-like effects of the phosphodiesterase-4 inhibitor etazolate and phosphodiesterase-5 inhibitor sildenafil via cyclic AMP or cyclic GMP signaling in mice. *Metab Brain Dis* (2014) 29:673–82. doi:10.1007/s11011-014-9533-4

Lin P, Wang C, Xu B, Gao S, Guo J, Zhao X. The VGF-derived peptide TLQP62 produces antidepressant-like effects in mice via the BDNF/TrkB/CREB signaling pathway. *Pharmacol Biochem Behav* (2014) 120:140–8. doi:10.1016/j.pbb.2014. 03.003

18

Neuropeptides in the gonads: from evolution to pharmacology

Nicolette L. McGuire[1] and George E. Bentley[1,2]*

[1] Laboratory of Reproductive Neuroendocrinology, Department of Integrative Biology, University of California at Berkeley, Berkeley, CA, USA
[2] Helen Wills Neuroscience Institute, University of California at Berkeley, Berkeley, CA, USA

Edited by:
George J. Christ, Wake Forest University School of Medicine, USA

Reviewed by:
Randy J. Nelson, The Ohio State University, USA
Kazuyoshi Tsutsui, Waseda University, Japan

***Correspondence:**
George E. Bentley, 3060 VLSB #3140, Department of Integrative Biology, University of California at Berkeley, Berkeley, CA 94720, USA.
e-mail: gb7@berkeley.edu

Vertebrate gonads are the sites of synthesis and binding of many peptides that were initially classified as neuropeptides. These gonadal neuropeptide systems are neither well understood in isolation, nor in their interactions with other neuropeptide systems. Further, our knowledge of the control of these gonadal neuropeptides by peripheral hormones that bind to the gonads, and which themselves are under regulation by true neuropeptide systems from the hypothalamus, is relatively meager. This review discusses the existence of a variety of neuropeptides and their receptors which have been discovered in vertebrate gonads, and the possible way in which such systems could have evolved. We then focus on two key neuropeptides for regulation of the hypothalamo-pituitary-gonadal axis: gonadotropin-releasing hormone (GnRH) and gonadotropin-inhibitory hormone (GnIH). Comparative studies have provided us with a degree of understanding as to how a gonadal GnRH system might have evolved, and they have been responsible for the discovery of GnIH and its gonadal counterpart. We attempt to highlight what is known about these two key gonadal neuropeptides, how their actions differ from their hypothalamic counterparts, and how we might learn from comparative studies of them and other gonadal neuropeptides in terms of pharmacology, reproductive physiology and evolutionary biology.

Keywords: GnRH, GnIH, RFRP, testes, ovary, vertebrate, primate

INTRODUCTION

"What's in a name? That which we call a rose
By any other name would smell as sweet."
Romeo and Juliet (Act 2, scene 2)

Neuropeptides appear to be appropriately named: they are peptides synthesized by neurons in the central nervous system. However, what matters is what they do, not what they are called, and we shall see in this review that neither the synthesis nor actions of neuropeptides are limited to the brain. This article focuses on "neuropeptides" in the gonads of vertebrates, with special emphasis on what we can learn from pharmacological experiments on gonadal tissue and then apply to our understanding of an animal's ecology in the wild.

Investigating the presence of neuropeptides in the gonads of a diverse array of species will provide us with information as to the possible evolutionary origins, adaptations, interactions and functions of what we are choosing to term "gonadal neuropeptide" systems. The conservation of localized gonadal regulation by gonadal neuropeptides across vertebrates has important implications for understanding the evolution, reproductive physiology and ecology of animals, along with the study and practice of reproductive health and medicine, both clinical and veterinary.

NEUROPEPTIDES IN THE GONADS

Many neuronally produced hormones with important endocrine, behavioral, sensory and autonomic roles in the vertebrate brain are also expressed by and may act directly within the gonads (**Table 1**; neuropeptide Y (NPY), Achi et al., 1995; bradykinin, Singh et al., 2007; corticotropin releasing factor (CRF), Huang et al., 1995; gonadotropin-releasing hormone (GnRH), Jones and Hsueh, 1981; Bahk et al., 1995; Pati and Habibi, 1998; gonadotropin-inhibitory hormone (GnIH), Hinuma et al., 2000; Bentley et al., 2008; kisspeptin, Castellano et al., 2006). The presence of neuropeptide receptors in the gonads: GnRH-R in mammals (Jones et al., 1980; Whitelaw et al., 1995; Schirman-Hildesheim et al., 2005)and fish, (von Schalburg et al., 1999; Bogerd et al., 2002); galanin receptor in mammals (Romanelli et al., 1998); vasoactive intestinal peptide receptor (VIP-R) in birds and mammals (Johnson and Tilly, 1988; Kawashima, 1995; El-Gehani et al., 1998; Bajo et al., 2000; Vaccari et al., 2006); NPY-R in mammals (Kopp et al., 1997); CRF-R in mammals (Heinrich et al., 1998; Waser et al., 2006), urocortin receptor in mammals (Florio et al., 2004) and kisspeptin receptor (GPR54) in mammals (Shahed and Young, 2009), supports this function. See **Table 1** for further clarification.

In the same way that synthesis and actions of steroids in the brain or other, non-gonadal tissues are often overlooked (Schmidt et al., 2008), so are the synthesis and actions of gonadal neuropeptides. It is likely that the synthesis and actions of these hormones are often not taken into consideration in endocrine studies because they fall outside the classic endocrine axes (for example, the hypothalamo-pituitary-gonadal [HPG] axis). It is also sometimes harder to manipulate these systems in isolation within the gonads or brain than as intact components of the classic axes. Generally, neural or gonadal tissue needs to be cultured *ex vivo* in order to gain some understanding of the hormone of interest that they produce, which of course limits interpretation. Furthermore, although it is somewhat logical to assume that the brain is able to interpret environmental and physiological cues and regulate its own steroid production, it is harder to understand

Table 1 | Presence of neuropeptides in the gonads of vertebrates. GnRH isoforms appear to be highly conserved across vertebrates, but there are large gaps in our knowledge of the evolution of other gonadal neuropeptides.

Neuropeptide	Protochordates	Agnathans	Fish	Amphibians	Reptiles	Birds	Mammals
lGnRH-I/ lGnRH-III		Gazourian et al. (1997)					
sGnRH			Madigou et al. (2002)				
cGnRH-II	Di Fiore et al. (2000)		Andreyu-Vieyra (2000)			Sun et al. (2001)	Kang et al. (2001)
mGnRH/ GnRH-I	Di Fiore et al. (2000)			Hsueh et al. (1981)	Minucci et al. (1986)	Hertelendy et al. (1982)	Clayton et al. (1979)
GnIH						Bentley et al. (2008)	Zhao et al. (2010)
CRH			Garcia-Reyero (2009)				Huang et al. (1995)
TRH						Geris et al. (2000)	Pekary et al. (1980)
GHRH			McRory et al. (1995)				Campbell and Scanes (1992)
VIP							El-Gehani et al. (1998)
Oxytocin	Kawada et al. (2008)						Nicholson et al. (1984)
PACAP			McRory et al. (1995)				Arimura et al. (1991)
POMC			Masini et al. (1997)	Shen et al. (2003)	Endo and Park (2004)	Takeuchi et al. (1999)	Pintar et al. (1984)
ANP							Akiho et al. (1995)
NPY			MacDonald and Volkoff (2009)	Achi et al. (1995)			Terado (2006)
Secretin							Ohta et al. (1992)
Substance P							Schulze et al. (1987)

GnRH, Gonadotropin-releasing hormone; lGnRH, isoforms from lamprey; sGnRH, salmon; cGnRH-II, chicken; mGnRH/GnRH-I, mammals; GnIH, Gonadotropin inhibiting hormone; CRH, Corticotropin releasing hormone, TRH, Thyrotropin releasing hormone; GHRH, Growth hormone releasing hormone; VIP, Vasoactive intestinal peptide; PACAP, Pituitary adenylate cyclase activating peptide; POMC, Pro-opiomelanocortin; ANP, Atrial natriuretic peptide; NPY, Neuropeptide Y.

how the gonads might respond to similar cues outside of the framework of the classic HPG axis. How, for example, does a gonad regulate its own GnRH production? Can a gonad respond to changes in day length, or social stimuli, or stress? How are these stimuli perceived?

Another consideration is that it might seem hard to understand why a gonadal neuropeptide system exists and how it evolved? The primary functions of gonads are to synthesize gonadal steroids and produce gametes, both of which appear to be exquisitely regulated and accomplished by the H-P components of the HPG axis. An additional, internal regulatory system in the gonad appears at first glance to be superfluous. It is possible that in early vertebrates, neural tissue containing neuropeptides and gonadal tissue were not as disparate as they are in modern vertebrates. It is thought that before the evolution of the vertebrate pituitary gland, GnRH neurons might have released GnRH directly into the bloodstream very close to the gonads and acted directly on the gonads (Powell et al., 1996). More evidence for this scenario comes from bivalve mollusks (Pazos and Mathieu, 1999). The vertebrate gonads may thus have retained the capability of at least responding to neuropeptides directly, but this does not enlighten us as to how the gonads have retained (or acquired) the capability of synthesizing neuropeptides such as GnRH. Additionally, all isoforms of GnRH are bioactive (affect DNA synthesis) in the molluskan gonad. The protochordate *Ciona intestinalis*, synthesizes two isoforms of GnRH, mammalian GnRH (mGnRH) and chicken GnRH-II (cGnRH-II), in its gonads (Di Fiore et al., 2000). *Ciona* gonads cultured in vitro with both isoforms show an increase in sex steroid synthesis and release. The gonads of vertebrates may thus have retained the capability of producing and responding to neuropeptides directly. As well, in higher vertebrates, local control of the gonads may have been retained for rapid, transient responsiveness to environmental and physiological stimuli. It is less clear what the regulatory mechanisms governing the synthesis of these gonadal neuropeptides might be.

NEUROPEPTIDES OF THE HPG AXIS IN THE GONADS

Vertebrate gonadal tissues typically synthesize and contain receptors for several hormones that are classified as neuropeptides. For example, GnRH, a key hormone for vertebrate reproduction, and its receptor are present in the gonads of fish, amphibians, birds, reptile and mammals (Hsueh and Jones, 1981; Oikawa et al., 1990; Bahk et al., 1995; Grober et al., 1995; Di Matteo et al., 1996; Dong et al., 1996; Lin and Peter, 1996; Pati and Habibi, 1998; von Schalburg et al., 1999; Sun et al., 2001; Bogerd et al., 2002; Ikemoto and Park, 2007). Gonadal GnRH most likely plays an autocrine/paracrine function in the regulation of gonadal development and activity. For example, its action includes testicular steroidogenesis in rats and frogs (Hsueh et al., 1983; D'Antonio et al., 1992), spermatogenesis in fish (Andreu-Vieyra and Habibi, 2001; Andreu-Vieyra et al., 2005) and oocyte meiosis and follicular steroidogenesis in fish (Pati and Habibi, 2000). There is also variation in the expression of GnRH and GnRH-R across the estrus cycle and in a circadian manner in rats (Schirman-Hildesheim et al., 2005, 2006), although specific function has yet to be assigned to this variation.

Along with GnRH, this article will place emphasis on another neuropeptide involved in the HPG axis: GnIH. This neuropeptide was discovered 10 years ago in Japanese quail (Tsutsui et al., 2000), when it was isolated and found to inhibit pituitary luteinizing hormone (LH) release. It is now known that GnIH is a regulator of pituitary gonadotropin synthesis and release in birds and mammals (Tsutsui et al., 2000, 2007; Ciccone et al., 2004; Osugi et al., 2004; Bentley et al., 2006a; Kriegsfeld et al., 2006; Tsutsui and Ukena, 2006; Ubuka et al., 2006; Johnson et al., 2007; Clarke et al., 2009; Sari et al., 2009).

GnRH IN THE GONADS

Gonadotropin-releasing hormone was initially characterized as a hypothalamic neuroendocrine regulator of LH and follicle stimulating hormone (FSH) synthesis and release from the anterior pituitary gland (Ling et al., 1973; Schally et al., 1971). Evidence now exists that GnRH is also produced in, binds to and exerts a local action on the gonads. Several isoforms of GnRH (identified by both species letters and isoform numbers) and GnRH receptor are present in the gonads of vertebrates and will be discussed below. Many species possess multiple isoforms, including isoforms named as a result of their initial discovery in other species.

GnRH-I and GnRH type 1 receptor (GnRH-I R) are expressed in the mammalian gonads. This isoform is also known as mammalian GnRH (mGnRH). GnRH-I mRNA and GnRH-I R mRNA have been identified in granulosa and luteal cells of adult female rats (Oikawa et al., 1990; Whitelaw et al., 1995) and humans (Peng et al., 1994). In males, GnRH-I mRNA is present in Sertoli cells and germ cells of adult rats and humans, while the interstitial layer of the testis expresses GnRH-I R mRNA (Bahk et al., 1995). Gonadal GnRH is also expressed in fetal rats (Botté et al., 1998). In addition to GnRH-I, primate testes and ovaries express a second GnRH isoform, first characterized in chicken (cGnRH-II) and its receptor, GnRH type 2 receptor.

In addition to mammals, protochordates, fish, amphibians, reptiles and birds also express isoforms of GnRH and GnRH-R in their testes and ovaries (von Schalburg et al., 1999; Di Fiore et al., 2000; Sun et al., 2001; Canosa et al., 2002; Ikemoto and Park, 2007). See **Table 1**.

EFFECTS OF GONADAL GnRH ARE ISOFORM-, SPECIES- AND SEX-DEPENDENT IN NON-MAMMALIAN VERTEBRATES

The gonadal GnRH system has a diversity of functions in non-mammalian vertebrates. As mentioned earlier, the gonads of the protochordate *Ciona intestinalis*, synthesize both mGnRH and cGnRH-II (Di Fiore et al., 2000). *Ciona* gonads cultured in vitro with these isoforms show an increase in testosterone, progesterone and estradiol synthesis and release. A lamprey isoform of GnRH (lGnRH-III) significantly stimulates basal estradiol production and ovulation in the ovary and significantly increases estradiol and progesterone production in the testes of lampreys *in vitro* (Gazourian et al., 1997). In a later study, two isoforms of lGnRH, lGnRH-I and –III, independently stimulated estradiol production by lamprey testis *in vitro*, with lGnRH-III being the more potent of the two GnRH isoforms used. In contrast to their earlier study, the authors conclude there is no direct effect of either form of lGnRH on the ovary in this study, although the authors do state that "lamprey GnRH-III at 1000 ng/ml directly stimulated the ovaries incubated at 14°C ($P < 0.05$) (data not shown)" (Gazourian et al., 2000). Taken together, it seems that the lGnRHs are capable of acting directly on male and female lamprey gonads to elicit steroid production.

The differential expression of GnRH isoforms and their cognate receptors in rainbow trout gonads indicates a role for these peptides in paracrine/autocrine regulation of gonadal function in this species. In the rainbow trout (*Oncorhynchus mykiss*), salmon GnRH (sGnRH) mRNA from whole testes increases as the spermatogenic cycle proceeds while chicken GnRH (cGnRH-II) mRNA decreases (Madigou et al., 2002). GnRH-R mRNA 1, which putatively codes for the receptor that binds sGnRH, also increases in whole testes as spermatogenesis progresses (Madigou et al., 2002). Stage-specific expression indicates sGnRH may be associated with spermatogenic development while cGnRH-II may hinder it. In whole ovaries, GnRH-R type 1 mRNA was undetectable in the same study, but sGnRH, cGnRH-II and GnRH-R type 2 mRNA were expressed from the beginning of vitellogenesis to post-ovulation (Madigou et al., 2002). Although the manner of this regulation remains unclear, when combined with functional evidence from goldfish- sGnRH and cGnRH-II inhibit gonadotropin-stimulated oocyte meiosis and follicular testosterone production (Pati and Habibi, 2000)- sGnRH and cGnRH-II are most probably involved in regulation of follicular hierarchy and/or maturation via inhibitory actions.

In toads (*Bufo arenarum*), mammalian GnRH (mGnRH or GnRH-I) inhibits basal and human chorionic gonadotropin (hCG)-stimulated testosterone release in the testes by decreasing the activity of cytochrome P450c17 (steroid 17 alpha-hydroxylase/17,20 lyase) (Hsueh et al., 1981). In leopard frogs, *Rana pipiens*, and bullfrogs, *R. catesbeiana*, no action of 1000 ng/ml GnRH was observed on testosterone or progesterone secretion from mature follicles coincidently incubated with pituitary homogenate or with bullfrog LH (Hubbard and Licht, 1985). Which isoform of GnRH used here is not clear from this study, but we assume that it was mGnRH- this is important as different isoforms appear to have different effects. This may be one reason why some studies show inhibition while others show stimulation. In another, contrasting study on ovaries of frog (*Rana esculenta*), lizard (*Podarcis sicula sicula*) and fish (*Torpedo ocellata* and *Gobius paganellus*) indicated that the action of GnRH in the gonads may be species-dependent. In frogs, a GnRH agonist (GnRHa, HOE766) inhibited LH-induced progesterone release (Minucci et al., 1986) whereas in lizards, GnRHa stimulated progesterone production in preovulatory follicles. In both fish species studied no effects of GnRHa or ovine LH were seen. However, in a later study on goldfish (*Carassius auratus*), sGnRH and cGnRH-II increased testicular apoptosis, indicating a paracrine role for GnRH in the control of apoptosis. This effect of sGnRH and cGnRH-II on apoptosis was also observed in goldfish ovaries (Andreu-Vieyra and Habibi, 2000).

In cockerels (*Gallus domesticus*), both cGnRH-II and cGnRH-R are expressed in the testes in addition to the brain and although its regulatory role has not been tested, estrogen treatment appears to reduce the concentration of cGnRH-II in the testes (Sun et al., 2001). GnRH can directly alter steroid biosynthesis in chicken ovaries: LH- stimulated progesterone production is increased by GnRH in isolated granulosa cells of domestic chickens (Hertelendy et al., 1982). Differences in the stimulatory/inhibitory properties of GnRH in non-mammalian vertebrate gonads appear to be isoform-, species- and sex-dependent.

EFFECTS OF GONADAL GnRH ON STEROID BIOSYNTHESIS IN THE MAMMALIAN TESTES

GnRH immunoreactivity was first identified in the rat testis in 1981 (Paull et al., 1981) and rats have since been consistently used as a mammalian model for studies on the activity of gonadal GnRH-I. The GnRH-I R (GnRH type 1 receptor) in rat gonad is structurally identical to that in the pituitary (Moumni et al., 1994). Functionally, in immature rat testicular cells, GnRH decreases hCG/FSH- stimulated androstanediol and androsterone production, but not steroidogenic acute regulatory (StAR) protein and progesterone production (Hsueh et al., 1981). The short-term (4 h) effect of the GnRH agonist LHRH ethylamide on Leydig cells is to stimulate steroidogenesis, but in contrast, 24-h stimulation with the agonist inhibits responsiveness to LH and hCG (Sharpe et al., 1982). In another study using adult rat primary testis culture, GnRH agonist decreased testosterone (T), androstenedione and 17a-OH progesterone (Hsueh et al., 1983). In yet another study, GnRH agonists inhibited LH-dependent steroid production in a dose-dependent fashion and abolished the acute testosterone rise in response to hCG. The expression of functional GnRH receptor during culture and its suppression by LH suggest that there is an interaction between pituitary gonadotropins and the gonadal GnRH system. It is likely that pituitary gonadotropins exert a tonic inhibitory effect upon testicular GnRH receptors. The presence of a functional GnRH receptor and inhibitory actions of GnRH agonists in cultured fetal and neonatal Leydig cells indicates that GnRH-related peptides can influence the actions of gonadotropins on the fetal Leydig cell population (Dufau and Knox, 1985).

EFFECTS OF GONADAL GnRH ON STEROID BIOSYNTHESIS IN THE MAMMALIAN OVARY

In female rats, GnRH-I is highly expressed and functional in the corpus luteum and in granulosa cells. Pharmacological levels of GnRH-I (0.5 uM) decrease basal luteal progesterone synthesis, but hCG (at concentrations greater than 10^{-13} M) is able to rescue this effect (Clayton et al., 1979). Cultured rat granulosa cells experience a significant reduction in estradiol (E2) and progesterone production stimulated by FSH in the presence of GnRH-I. No change in total mass occurs, apparently precluding an effect of GnRH in cell death (Hsueh and Erickson, 1979), although GnRH agonists have since been implicated in the promotion of ovarian apoptosis (Takekida et al., 2003). A later experiment by Hsueh et al. (1980) showed that GnRH reduces E2 production by preventing the FSH-induced 12-fold increase in LH/hCG receptor expression in granulosa cells. If GnRH indirectly reduces E2 production via reduced LH/hCG receptors in the ovary, ovarian androgen production should be directly reduced as well. Prepubertal female rat ovaries cultured with hCG, LH and leuprolide acetate, a GnRH agonist, show a concomitant decrease in both androsterone and P450(C17) enzyme activity relative to ovaries treated with hCG/LH alone (Irusta et al., 2007). As we have already mentioned, GnRH-I inhibits P450(C17) in toad (*Bufo arenarum*) testes, resulting in decreased testosterone secretion (Canosa, 2002). Thus this property may be evolutionarily conserved. GnRH-I also appears to inhibit FSH-stimulated aromatase activity in addition to P450(C17) inhibition in rat granulosa, but not Sertoli cells (Gore-Langton et al., 1981). The sex difference is likely due to the lack of GnRH-I R on male rat Sertoli cells. Again, there appears to be a sex and/or tissue difference, where GnRH is acting upstream of progesterone synthesis in the female corpus luteum but downstream of progesterone synthesis in male Leydig cells. Interestingly, the inhibitory effect of GnRH agonist on 17β-estradiol and progesterone secretion occurred in granulosa cells from large but not from small and medium follicles. The stimulatory effect of GnRH agonist on apoptosis was, however, uniform regardless of the stages of follicular growth (Takekida et al., 2003). Thus GnRH-I potentially exerts diverse actions on granulosa cells over the course of follicular growth. One is to downregulate granulosa cell proliferation in immature follicles as well as steroidogenesis in mature follicles, and the other is to upregulate apoptosis of granulosa cells, regardless of the stage of follicular growth.

Functionally, local GnRH action on estrogen synthesis may not be needed to regulate estrogen production in males, as estrogen has a much larger contribution to gametogenesis in females and would require tighter control in that sex. GnRH-I inhibits both androgen and consequently estrogen production in rat ovaries. In rat testes, GnRH-I primarily inhibits testosterone production. In both sexes, local GnRH modulates and primarily limits the major steroid supporting gamete maturation.

GONADAL GnRH IN PRIMATES

Humans and other primates express both mammalian GnRH (mGnRH/GnRH-I) and cGnRH-II and their cognate receptors (GnRH type 1 receptor/GnRH-I R and GnRH type 2 receptor/

GnRH-II R), in the testes and ovary (Bahk et al., 1995; Millar et al., 2001; Neill, 2002). Both receptors are members of the seven transmembrane family of G protein-coupled receptors and associated with Gαq protein. GnRH-II R contains a c-terminal tail consistent with receptors able to internalize in response to high ligand concentration, while GnRH-I R lacks this tail and does not undergo receptor desensitization (Neill, 2002). Although rats have been used a pharmacological and medical model, the presence of cGnRH-II and its receptor have not been identified in rat gonads. In fact, the transcripts of cGnRH-II and GnRH-II R appear to be truncated in rat cDNA libraries generated from other tissues (Stewart et al., 2009). Thus it is hypothesized rats do not code for a functional GnRH-II R, and thus receptor densitization is a moot point for them. In human granulosa-luteal cells, GnRH-I inhibits progesterone production (as it does in rats), and this effect is completely reversed by the MEK1 inhibitor PD98059, indicating GnRH-I acts through the MAP kinase signaling pathway (Kang et al., 2000). cGnRH-II also inhibits basal and hCG-stimulated progesterone production and LH/FSH receptor expression (Kang et al., 2001). GnRH-I agonists have also been implicated in causing apoptosis in granulosa-luteal cells (Zhao et al., 2000). If gonadal GnRH decreases LH/FSH receptors, inhibits basal and hCG-stimulated progesterone production and increases apoptosis in the corpus luteum, it may serve a functional role in luteolysis. GnRH-I and cGnRH-II expression have been mapped across the luteal phase in primates and their comparative mRNA levels are consistent with this projection. GnRH-I mRNA expression is maximal at luteal regression, although GnRH-I R mRNA remains low throughout the luteal phase (Chakrabarti et al., 2008). An enhanced explanation of GnRH actions on the ovary during follicular development can be seen in **Figure 1**.

Less is known about the functional significance of GnRH-I and cGnRH-II and their receptors in the human and non-human primate testes. This is probably due to the greater availability of and higher occurrence of treatment on female reproductive tissues in fertility treatments. Although the bioactivity of systemically delivered GnRH antagonists has been studied for 25 years in primates in anticipation of their use as a male contraceptive (Weinbauer et al., 1984) and chemotherapy protectant (cetrorelix, Boekelheide et al., 2005), the testicular effects of GnRH-I and cGnRH-II are highly dependent upon reduced LH and FSH secretion from the pituitary and there have been no attempts to quantify direct effects of GnRH *ex vivo*. lGnRH and sGnRH transcripts have not been identified in primate gonads.

COMPARING THE ACTIONS OF HYPOTHALAMIC AND GONADAL GnRH: WHAT CAN WE INFER?

Gonadal GnRH appears to act non-genomically, modifying enzyme activity through inositol phosphate breakdown via stimulation of its Gαq receptor (Davis et al., 1986). This is also the mechanism used by hypothalamic GnRH on the pituitary for LH/FSH secretion. However differences between gonadotropes and granulosa/luteal/interstitial cells cause the action of GnRH to be classified as "stimulatory" to reproduction in the pituitary and "inhibitory" to reproduction in the gonads.

GnIH IN GONADS

Gonadotropin-inhibitory hormone was so named for its discovery as an inhibitor of LH release from the pituitary of Japanese quail (Tsutsui et al., 2000). Later work has shown that GnIH inhibits both LH and FSH synthesis and secretion from the pituitary of birds and mammals (Kriegsfeld et al., 2006; Tsutsui et al., 2007). GnIH not only acts at the level of the pituitary gland to influence gonadotropin synthesis and release, but also within the brain of birds and mammals to inhibit GnRH neurons (see Bentley et al., 2006a, 2009; Tsutsui et al., 2009 for reviews). Therefore, there are several lines of evidence that GnIH can act directly on multiple components of the HPG axis.

Motivated by the direct action of GnIH on the other tissues of the HPG axis, we investigated the possibility that GnIH and/or its receptor are present in and act directly on the gonads of vertebrates. It is now clear that GnIH and GnIH-R are expressed in the gonads of birds and mammals, suggesting that GnIH acts directly elsewhere in the reproductive system. Further, our experimental evidence from pharmacological manipulations indicates that gonadal GnIH is responsive to cues from peripheral hormones and influences gonadal steroid release. These findings are important for us to understand the endocrine-behavior interactions when considering an animal's behavioral ecology. Further, a localized regulatory system in reproductive tissues is an important consideration/target for reproductive/contraceptive therapies.

CONSERVATION OF GONADAL GnIH EXPRESSION AND ACTIONS

A role for a local action of GnIH in vertebrate gonads was first hypothesized when systemic receptor fluorography revealed binding sites for GnIH on the thecal and granulosa layers of the ovary and within the interstitium and seminiferous tubules of the testes of white crowned sparrows (*Zonotrichia leucophrys*; Wingfield et al., 2004). Building upon this initial finding, gonadal GnIH was first characterized in European starlings and Japanese quail, species of two different orders of birds (Bentley et al., 2008). Transcripts for GnIH and GnIH-R were found in the quail and starling testes, quail epididymis, starling vas deferens and starling ovary and oviduct, indicating its potential as a paracrine/autocrine regulator within reproductive tissues. Immunohistochemistry and *in situ* hybridization further localized production sites of GnIH and GnIH-R to specific cell types involved in steroid biosynthesis and gamete maturation in the gonads. GnIH-immunoreactivity (GnIH-ir), indicating the presence of mature peptide, was detected in thecal and granulosa cells of starling ovaries and in the interstitium of the testes and psuedostratified columnar epithelium of the epididymus of quail testes (Bentley et al., 2008). In house sparrow testes, GnIH mRNA is present in the interstitium (McGuire and Bentley, 2010). GnIH-R mRNA was localized to the germ cells and interstitium of starling and house sparrow (*Passer domesticus*) testes (Bentley et al., 2008; McGuire and Bentley, 2010). In house sparrows, germ cell expression of GnIH-R was further characterized as secondary spermatocyte expression (McGuire and Bentley, 2010). In the ovary of chickens (*Gallus domesticus*), GnIH-R mRNA was detected in the thecal and granulosa layers by RT-PCR (Maddineni et al., 2008). GnIH mRNA has not been detected in chicken ovary (Maddineni et al., 2008), although sequencing of PCR products confirms the presence of transcripts for GnIH in the ovaries of the other bird species studied (McGuire and Bentley, 2010; McGuire et al., 2010). It is possible these birds carry an ovarian transcript not detectable by our current methods.

The sites of GnIH-R synthesis across birds are consistent with fluorescent GnIH binding observed in the first white crowned sparrow study. Thus GnIH-R transcript detection is most likely associated with functional receptors and appears conserved across passeriform and galliform birds.

Expression of GnIH mRNA and presence of GnIH peptide in steroid biosynthetic cells of the ovary and the testes, coupled with the presence of its Gαi protein-coupled receptor there, provide the potential for this system to act in a paracrine/autocrine fashion to regulate steroid biosynthesis. As well, these findings indicate gonadal GnIH may be an important target for steroid production therapies. Furthermore, the expression of these components on germ cells indicates the gonadal GnIH system may be an important consideration in the development of gamete maturation therapies.

The mammalian ortholog of GnIH, RFRP, and its receptor are also present in the gonads of mammals. Syrian hamster spermatocytes and round to early elongated spermatids are immunoreactive for RFRP and its putative rodent receptors, GPR-147 and GPR-74 (Zhao et al., 2010). The two receptors are differentially present across the spermatogenic cycle; GPR 147 is present at all stages, while GPR-74 immunoreactivity is observable in late elongated spermatids only, indicating their expression may be stage-regulated. The sequential expression of RFRP and GPR-74 across different spermatogenic stages would allow a role for RFRP in the differentiation of germ cells in the testes.

GONADAL GnIH IN PRIMATES

The sperm development patterns of rodents and primates are quite similar (Clermont, 1972). Thus data garnered from the expression patterns of RFRP and GPR-74 across the spermatogenesic cycle of hamsters provide an excellent model for studies of sperm development issues in humans. Although the gonadal expression of RFRP and OT7T022, its human cognate receptor, have not been studied in humans, RFRP and OT7T022 are expressed in the human hypothalamus (Ubuka et al., 2009).

RFRP is not observed in the interstitium of Syrian hamsters. However, RFRP-ir and mRNA are present in the steroid biosynthetic cells as well as the germ cells of the rhesus macaque (*Macaca*

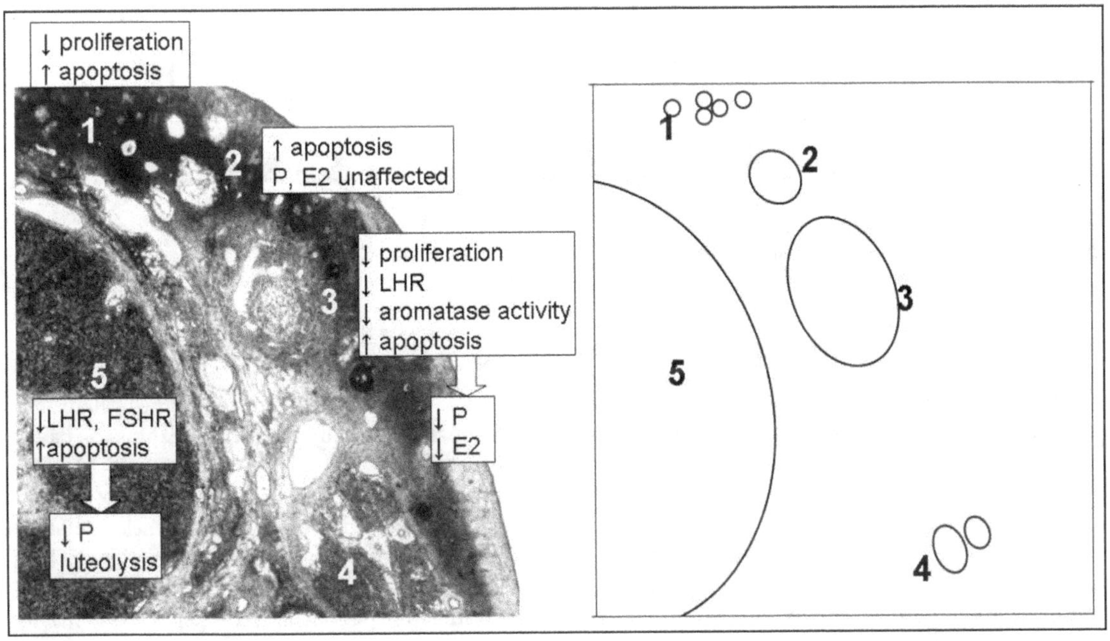

FIGURE 1 | Theoretical construct of local gonadotropin-releasing hormone (GnRH) action on follicular development in the mammalian ovary, based on experimental evidence. GnRH and GnRH receptor (GnRH-R) are expressed on granulosa cells at all stages of follicular development and on granulosa-luteal cells of corpora lutea. *Prehierarchical follicles* (1) are not stimulated by Follicle stimulating hormone (FSH) and gonadal GnRH reduces granulosa cell numbers by reducing proliferation and increasing apoptosis in these follicles (Takekida et al., 2003). As follicles gain the ability to respond to FSH, they overcome this inhibition and grow into *small/medium hierarchical follicles* (2). GnRH increases apoptosis of granulosa cells in these follicles, but this does not cause a significant reduction in the secretion of already low levels of estradiol (E2) and progesterone (P) (Takekida et al., 2003). FSH, P and E2 enhance the growth of these follicles into *large hierarchical follicles* (3). GnRH reduces granulosa cell proliferation, aromatase activity (Gore-Langton et al., 1981) and luteinizing hormone receptor (LH-R) expression (Hsueh et al., 1980) while continuing to increase granulosa cell apoptosis (Takekida et al., 2003). All of these factors contribute to a significant decrease in the secretion of E2 and P from these follicles (Hsueh et al., 1980; Takekida et al., 2003). The reduction in LH-R also makes the follicle less able to respond to the LH surge with ovulation. If large hierarchical follicles are not able to overcome this inhibition, their growth will cease and they would become *atretic* (4). If a large hierarchical follicle does overcome inhibition by GnRH it can become the *corpus luteum* (5) post-ovulation. GnRH decreases LH-R and FSH-R expression in, reduces secretion of progesterone from and increases apoptosis of granulosa-luteal cells (Kang et al., 2000, 2001; Zhao et al., 2000). The highest expression of GnRH and GnRH-R occurs at the end of the luteal phase (Chakrabarti et al., 2008), indicating GnRH may be a contributing factor to luteolysis. The diagram on the right is a representation of the photomicrograph on left, showing the relative location of each follicular stage for clarity.

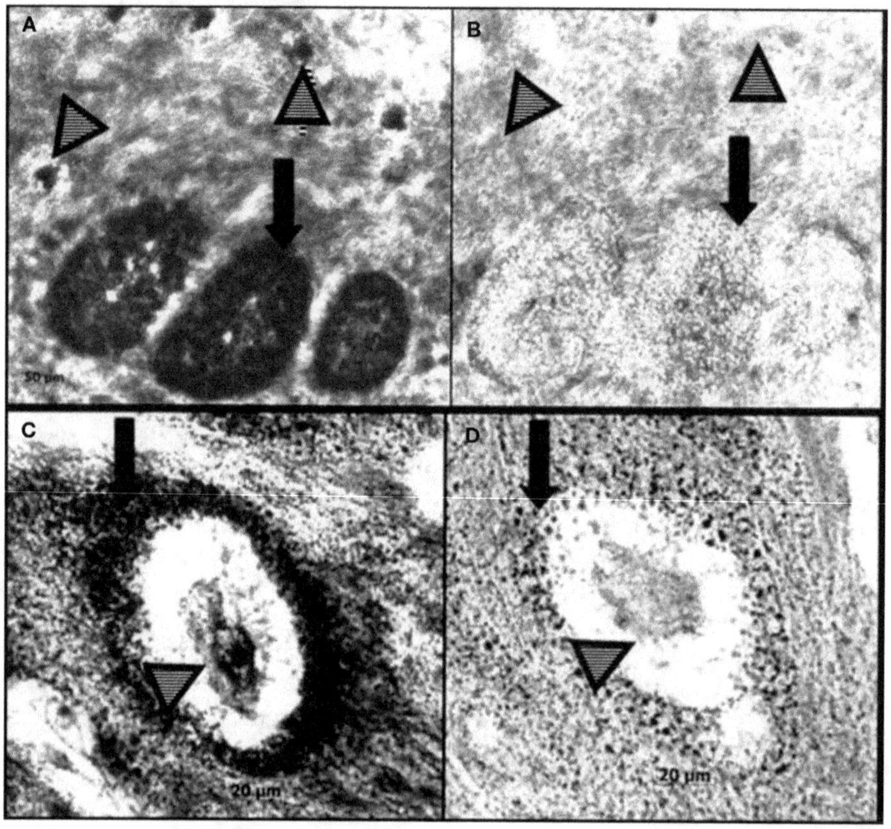

FIGURE 2 | *In situ* hybridization for RF-amide related peptide (RFRP) and its receptor (OT7T022) in rhesus macaque (*Macaca mulatta*) ovary. RFRP antisense probe labels mRNA in granulosa cells and oocytes **(A)**. An adjacent section incubated with RFRP sense probe (control) is shown in **(B)**. OT7T022 antisense probe labels mRNA in granulosa cells and oocytes **(C)**. An adjacent section incubated with OT7T022 sense probe (control) is shown in **(D)**. Black arrows, granulosa cells. Striped arrowheads, oocytes.

mulatta) testes. mRNA for OT7T022, the putative macaque RFRP receptor, is also expressed there (**Figure 2**). *In situ* hybridization reveals the presence of transcripts for RFRP in Leydig cells, spermatogonia, and spermatocytes. The location of OT7T022 mRNA on spermatogonia, spermatocytes and Sertoli cells and Leydig cells (**Figure 3**). RFRP and OT7T022 are also expressed on rhesus macaque ovarian tissue. RFRP-ir and mRNA and OT7T022 mRNA are present on granulosa cells and oocytes of preantral follicles (**Figure 2**). Non-hierarchical follicles and corpora lutea were not tested. Cell types were identified based on rhesus macaque gonadal morphology (Gougeon, 1996; Boekelheide et al., 2005), and with concurrent sections labeled with hematoxylin and eosin stain (data not shown). RFRP thus has the potential to act as a regulator of steroid biosynthetic cells and gametes in rhesus macaque testes and ovaries.

The expression pattern of RFRP and OT7T022 in primate gonads appears to be more closely related to that observed in seasonally-breeding songbirds than to hamsters (**Table 2**). Like house sparrows and hamsters, rhesus macaques undergo seasonal cycles of gonadal growth and regression characterized by significant changes in sex steroids and gametogenesis (Riesen et al., 1971; Gupta et al., 2000; Bansode et al., 2003), in which the gonadal GnIH system may play a regulatory role. It is not at present clear why hamsters differ from songbirds and rhesus macaques in the expression patterns of GnIH and its receptor.

Although human reproductive cycles are not thought to be regulated by photoperiod or rain, they nonetheless retain the ability to modulate their reproductive output during times of food restriction and stress (Vigersky et al., 1977; Vermeulen, 1993; Ferin, 1999). The conserved nature of gonadal neuropeptide systems makes it likely that this mechanism allowing for enhanced reproductive responsiveness is most likely conserved in humans as well.

COMPARING THE ACTIONS OF HYPOTHALAMIC AND GONADAL GnIH: WHAT CAN WE INFER?

Although the expression sites/pattern of GnIH and its receptor are suggestive of a role in steroid synthesis and gamete maturation, a general inhibitory action for the peptide cannot be inferred simply based on direct inhibition of GnRH (Ducret et al., 2009) and LH/FSH (Tsutsui et al., 2000) by its more characterized counterpart in the hypothalamus. However, GnIH-R has the same sequence, is recognized by the same antibodies and mRNA probes and binds fluorescently-labeled GnIH identically to pituitary GnIH-R (Wingfield et al., 2004; Bentley et al., 2008; Maddineni et al., 2008; McGuire

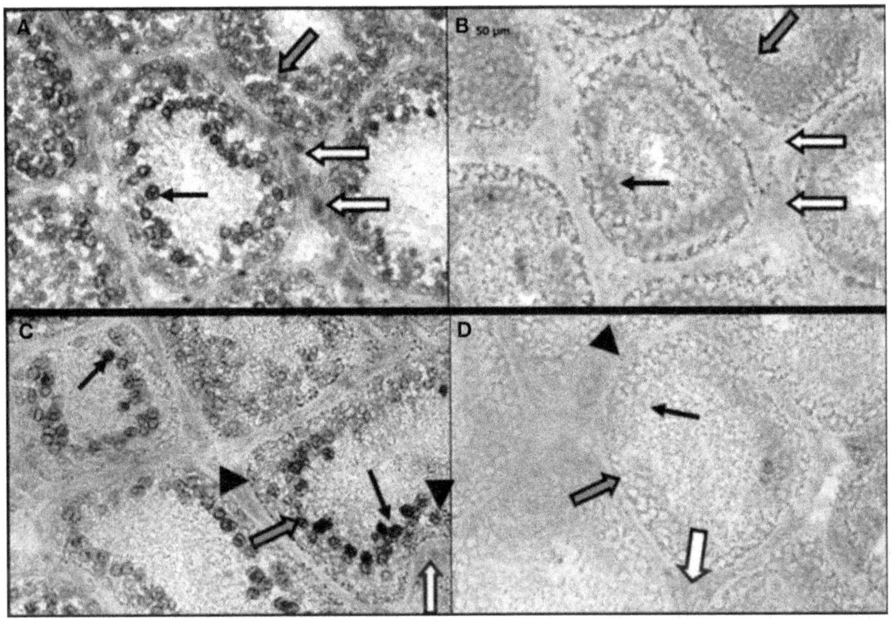

FIGURE 3 | *In situ* hybridization for RF-amide related peptide (RFRP) and its receptor (OT7T022) in rhesus macaque (*Macaca mulatta*) testis. RFRP antisense probe labels mRNA in Leydig cells, spermatogonia and spermatocytes **(A)**. An adjacent section incubated with RFRP sense probe (control) is shown in **(B)**. OT7T022 antisense probe labels mRNA in Leydig cells, Sertoli cells, spermatogonia and spermatocytes **(C)**. An adjacent section incubated with OT7T022 sense probe (control) is shown in **(D)**. White arrows, Leydig cells. Gray arrows, spermatogonia. Black arrows, spermatocytes. Black arrowheads, Sertoli cells. All figures to scale, scale bar = 50 μm.

Table 2 | Summary of RFRP and OT7T022 mRNA and peptide localization in rhesus macaques.

Cell type	Macaque RFRP	Macaque OT7T022	Avian GnIH	Avian GnIH-R	Rodent RFRP	Rodent GPR74
Spermatogonia	✓	✓	✓	✓	✓	
Spermatocytes	✓	✓	✓	✓	✓	
Spermatids	-	-	-	-	✓	✓
Spermatozoa	-	-	-	-	✓	✓
Sertoli cells	-	✓	-	-	-	-
Leydig cells	✓	✓				
Seminiferous tubules	✓	✓	✓	✓	✓	✓
Interstitium	✓	✓	✓	✓	-	-
Oocytes	✓	✓	-	-		
Granulosa cells	✓	✓	✓	✓		
Thecal cells	-	-	✓	✓		

Avian GnIH mRNA and peptide and GnIH-R mRNA and binding sites characterized in European starlings (Sturnus vulgaris, Bentley et al., 2008), house sparrows (Passer domesticus, McGuire and Bentley, 2010), Japanese quail (Coturnix japonica, Bentley et al., 2008) and domestic chicken (Gallus gallus, Maddineni et al., 2008). Rodent RFRP and GPR74 peptides characterized in hamster (Mesocricetus auratus, Zhao et al., 2010). Checkmarks indicate presence in the cell type, dashes denote lack of mRNA, peptide or binding sites and blank spaces indicate lack of evidence.

et al., 2010). Yin et al. (2005) identified GnIH-R in quail pituitary as a member of the GPCR family coupled to Gαi/o. Thus agonist binding of this receptor causes inhibition of adenylate cyclase. Hinuma et al. (2000) showed that agonist binding of rat RFRP receptor reduced the forskolin-induced cAMP response in transfected Chinese hamster ovary (CHO) cells. Inhibition of forskolin- stimulated adenylate cyclase and consequent decreased cAMP accumulation was later confirmed in chicken pituitary (Shimizu and Bédécarrats, 2010). Thus it is likely that binding of GnIH/RFRP to it receptor in the gonads also reduces cAMP accumulation and inhibits transcription of proteins with cAMP responsive elements.

GONADAL GnIH AND TESTOSTERONE SYNTHESIS

GnIH has the potential to, but does it actually directly affect testosterone synthesis in the testes? Systemic (intraperitoneal) administration of GnIH to male quail reduced plasma testosterone and caused apoptosis in testicular germ cells (Ubuka et al., 2006). These researchers concluded that the effects were caused by a reduction in LH secretion from the pituitary. However, the administration route for GnIH (i.p. via osmotic pumps) did not prevent its action elsewhere in the HPG axis. GnIH could be acting both to decrease LH secretion from the pituitary (indirectly effecting testosterone secretion) and by binding its receptor in the gonads and directly decreasing testosterone. The presence of GnIH receptor was later identified in quail testes (Bentley et al., 2008), specifically on germ cells and in the interstitium. A parsimonious explanation of these data is that significant apoptosis in germ cells of GnIH-treated birds versus saline control birds resulted from lack of testosterone support (testosterone reduced by lower LH stimulation *and* higher direct GnIH inhibition) and/or direct action of GnIH on germ cells. Additionally, the observed reduction in testosterone was the result of both reduced gonadotropin support and direct action of GnIH in the interstitium. New evidence from house sparrows suggests that GnIH can directly reduce testosterone secretion from the testes. 1 and 10 uM doses of GnIH significantly reduced the amount of testosterone secreted from LH/FSH- stimulated house sparrow testes cultured *in vitro* (McGuire and Bentley, 2010). GnIH does not have a significant effect on basal testosterone synthesis, suggesting the gonadal GnIH system acts to regulate high levels of testosterone secretion and would have the greatest regulatory capability in post-pubertal males. Thus GnIH can reduce testosterone via two mechanisms: GnIH reduces LH/FSH secretion from the pituitary, decreasing stimulation to produce testosterone and GnIH inhibits testosterone secretion in the testes directly, in the presence of LH/FSH stimulation.

Why would such a system be necessary? Why not constantly support tonically high levels of testosterone, the highest sperm production levels and the highest frequency of reproductive displays possible? High testosterone levels are associated with a number of pathologies in vertebrates, including prostate cancer and immunocompromise (Gann et al., 1996; Roberts et al., 2007). The brain already controls a mechanism whereby high levels of gonadal steroids limit further secretion of the hormones that stimulate their synthesis, but this process requires a lengthy and time-consuming feedback loop. Fine-tuning of testosterone secretion on-site is highly adaptive in species with temporally or socially constrained breeding - especially if that system (in this case the gonad) is able to respond directly to environmental cues.

GONADAL GnIH AND ESTRADIOL SYNTHESIS

Based on its distribution, GnIH has the potential to, but does it actually directly affect estradiol synthesis in the ovary? The viability of granulosa cells from chicken ovaries was significantly reduced when cultured with GnIH alone but not when FSH was present in the culture medium (Maddineni et al., 2008). Dispersion culture of whole European starling ovary reveals that GnIH reduces basal, but not LH/FSH-stimulated estradiol production (McGuire et al., 2010). Taken together, these data suggest that GnIH affects basal estradiol synthesis in the ovary by reducing viability of granulosa cells and this effect is rescued by FSH.

The expression pattern of GnIH-R in ovaries is consistent with the observed reduction of basal, but not gonadotropin-stimulated estradiol production. Sexually immature chickens express significantly more ovarian GnIH-R mRNA compared to sexually mature chicken ovaries (Maddineni et al., 2008). Among mature hens, GnIH-R mRNA is significantly decreased by estradiol and progesterone alone and in combination (Maddineni et al., 2008). Like the differential expression of RFRP and GPR-74 in Syrian hamster testes, ovarian GnIH-R/OT7T022 has hierarchical expression in the ovary. GnIH-R mRNA is expressed on both prehierarchical and preovulatory follicles in hens (Maddineni et al., 2008) and on preantral follicles in macaque (**Figure 2**). There is no difference in the relative levels of GnIH-R mRNA on granulosa cells between the two stages of hen follicles, although prehierarchical follicles express significantly more GnIH-R mRNA on their thecal cells than do preovulatory follicles. We therefore propose this scenario: in the absence of FSH stimulation, GnIH reduces granulosa cell viability in follicles (which would all be prehierarchical in the absence of FSH), reducing estradiol secretion and inhibiting their maturation. As follicles mature, expression of GnIH-R mRNA on the theca is reduced, allowing them to respond to an LH surge with ovulation and progesterone production. Post-ovulation, granulosa cell numbers of hierarchical follicles that did not ovulate are reduced in the absence of FSH and presence of unchanged levels of GnIH-R, causing follicular atresia. Overall, evidence suggests ovarian GnIH has the greatest regulatory capability in prepubertal hens and in the prehierarchical or atretic follicles of sexually mature hens, in contrast to the effects seen in males.

The mechanism and timing of regulation by gonadal GnIH may be very different in male and female gonads. In males, GnIH acts as a regulator of stimulated testosterone production and possibly gamete maturation. In females, GnIH has a role in the prevention of follicle maturation and ovulation. As with gonadal GnRH, there appear to be sex differences in the actions of gonadal GnIH.

GONADAL GnIH AND THE ORGANISM'S ENVIRONMENT

Is the gonadal GnIH system able to directly respond to environmental cues? New evidence from starling testes and ovaries indicates that LH/FSH-stimulated testosterone and estradiol levels are directly reduced by cortisol and melatonin (McGuire et al., 2010, unpublished observation). Cultures treated with cortisol and melatonin also show higher levels of GnIH mRNA relative to LH/FSH-stimulated cells (McGuire et al., 2010, unpublished observation). Thus it is likely that the gonads directly respond to stress and an endocrine proxy of day length. Although changes in seasonal day length are not cause for concern in most humans, these results point toward significant effects in shift workers, pilots/flight attendants and those who self-medicate with over-the-counter melatonin. The stress-related hormone cortisol may act on GnIH and other factors to reduce follicle maturation. This might have evolved as an adaptive process, allowing an organism to wait to breed until conditions are more favorable – but it may be one mechanism in stress-induced infertility. Additionally, corticosteroid pharmaceuticals may have biologically significant effects on estradiol production and ovarian function. Recently, we found that female rats express glucocorticoid receptor (GR) transcripts in their ovaries, even when not stressed (McGuire et al., unpublished observation). However, they still significantly increase GR mRNA in the ovary in response to chronic, but not acute stress. This indicates that the ovaries are highly responsive to levels of the stress hormone cortisol in the plasma and that they may become increasingly responsive to stressful events with repeated exposure.

CURRENT PHARMACOLOGY OF GONADAL GnRH AND GnIH

Why do transient increases in GnIH or GnRH and decreases in testosterone and estradiol matter? Repeated events which stimulate or inhibit this system over time may lead to decreased fertility or increased cancer risk. Can pharmacological treatments manipulate this ratio favorably? Will pharmacological treatments inadvertently manipulate this ratio unfavorably? Should gonadal GnIH and GnRH be considered in the development of new contraceptives/ fertility treatments/cancer therapies?

GnRH AND OVARIAN CANCER LINES

The stimulatory potential of GnRH-I has already made it a target of oncology. For example, GnRH antagonists and cytotoxic GnRH analogues have been used to inhibit the pituitary and retard growth of ovarian and prostate cancers (Schally, 1999). However, the assumed function of these systemic treatments precludes the ability of GnRH to act directly on the ovary. In the case of GnRH antagonists, the therapy may in fact further proliferation within the gonad and reduce programmed cell death. The direct inhibitory capability of GnRH analogs on granulosa cells of the ovaries of a variety of species indicates that there is the potential for some therapies to be more localized: direct application of GnRH agonists or cytotoxic GnRH at the gonadal tumor site to reduce proliferation and cause apoptosis locally, while sparing the rest of the ovary. Further research is needed to determine GnRH receptor expression in cancerous cells. GnRH-II has been less well studied than GnRH-I.. However, GnRH-II and its receptor are expressed in human ovarian cancer cell lines and native GnRH-II dose- and time-dependently reduces proliferation in those cancer cells (Gründker et al., 2002). The observed effect is significantly more potent than the anti-proliferative ability of GnRH-I. As well, these researchers showed GnRH-II was able to reduce proliferation in another ovarian cancer cell line, SK-OV-3, which is not responsive to GnRH-I. Development of GnRH-II analogues will further this line of research.

GnIH ANTAGONIST

RF9 is a recently reported agent that blocks opiod-induced hyperalgesia by antagonizing the NPFF receptor. RF9 also antagonizes the closely related RFRP receptor, preventing regulation of the HPG axis by RFRP. A pharmacological dose of RF9, delivered in a single bolus ICV injection, causes robust secretion of LH and FSH in diestrus-1 and estrus female rats (Pineda et al., 2010). These profiles are stronger and longer lasting than those induced by kisspeptin administered ICV. In male rats, RF9 causes a robust, but transient increase in LH secretion. Thus, pharmacological doses of this chronic pain treatment antagonize RFRP receptor and remove its inhibitory action from LH/FSH secretion. The researchers point out that the downstream activation of the HPG axis, as a side effect of using RF9 in chronic pain management, should be carefully considered. Given the local action of GnIH on the gonads themselves, direct action of RF9 in the testes and ovaries may be highly consequential as well. RF9 action on the gonads could cause overproduction of sperm, benign prostatic hyperplasia, ovarian cysts or high synthesis of testosterone and estradiol, which may predispose the patient to increased risk of breast, prostate or uterine cancer over time. Conversely, it may be a positive therapy in infertile patients.

CONCLUDING REMARKS

It is clear from the differences in action of GnRH, and sites of synthesis and receptor binding of GnIH in different study organisms even within the same vertebrate class that it would be unwise to create any sweeping generalizations about the gonadal actions of these peptides. The take-home message is that despite our knowledge of the existence of many gonadal neuroeptide systems (see **Table 1**) we still only have a vague understanding of how they operate and are regulated. It is also clear that we cannot assume that a gonadal neuropeptide will operate in a similar manner to its hypothalamic counterpart. Given that GnRH is the most well-studied gonadal neuropeptide our knowledge of it is rather poor. However, study of gonadal GnRH has provided us with some ideas as to how the HPG axis might have evolved from a common ancestor, and some important insights as to its gonadal actions. **Table 1** indicates the large gaps in our knowledge of the existence of gonadal neuropeptides in different vertebrate classes; further comparative studies can only be beneficial in terms of creating a framework of knowledge upon which we can build and create novel therapeutic drugs, deepen our understanding of the evolution of the vertebrate reproductive system, and provide us with clues as to how the gonadal neuropeptides have adapted to the ecology of different vertebrates. In part, the naming of these peptides as neuropeptides creates immediate bias in terms of our consideration that they might exist in the gonads. Further, the functional names given to the gonadal counterparts of the neuropeptides in question might also bias us as to our consideration of their actions -with possible detriment to science and medicine. We feel that the time is ripe for further exploration of the gonads in terms of discovering new gonadal neuropeptides in different vertebrate classes as well as elucidating the actions of those already known to exist.

ACKNOWLEDGMENTS

Funded by NSF IOS 0641188 and 0920753 to George E. Bentley and National Science Foundation Graduate Research Fellowship to Nicolette L. McGuire.

REFERENCES

Achi, M. V., Figueroa, J. M., González Nicolini, V., Villar, M. J., and Tramezzani, J. H. (1995). NPY- and CGRP-like immunoreactive nerve fibers in the testis and mesorchium of the toad (Bufo arenarum). *Cell Tissue Res.* 281, 375–378.

Akiho, H., Chijiiwa, Y., Okabe, H., Harada, N., and Nawata, H. (1995). Interaction between atrial natriuretic peptide and vasoactive intestinal peptide in guinea pig cecal smooth muscle. *Gastroenterology* 109, 1105–1112.

Andreu-Vieyra, C. V., Buret, A. G., and Habibi, H. R. (2005). Gonadotropin-releasing hormone induction of apoptosis in the testes of goldfish (*Carassius auratus*). *Endocrinology* 146, 1588–1596.

Andreu-Vieyra, C. V, Habibi, H. R. (2000). Factors controlling ovarian apoptosis. *Can. J. Physiol. Pharmacol.* 78, 1003–1012.

Andreu-Vieyra,, C. V., and Habibi, H. R. (2001). Effects of salmon GnRH and chicken GnRH-II on testicular apoptosis in goldfish (*Carassius auratus*). *Comp. Biochem. Physiol. B, Biochem. Mol. Biol.* 129, 483–487.

Arimura, A., Somogyvári-Vigh, A., Miyata, A., Mizuno, K., Coy, D. H., and Kitada, C. (1991). Tissue distribution of PACAP as determined by RIA: highly abundant in the rat brain and testes. *Endocrinology* 129, 2787–2789.

Bahk, J. Y., Hyun, J. S., Chung, S. H., Lee, H., Kim, M. O., Lee, B. H., and Choi, W. S. (1995). Stage specific identification of the expression of GnRH mRNA and localization of the GnRH receptor in mature rat and adult human testis. *J. Urol.* 154, 1958–1961.

Bajo, A. M, Juarranz, M. G., Valenzuela, P., Martínez, P., Prieto, J. C., and Guijarro, L. G. (2000). Expression of vasoactive intestinal peptide (VIP) receptors in human uterus. *Peptides* 21, 1383–1388.

Bansode, F. W., Chowdhury, S. R., and Dhar, J. D. (2003). Seasonal changes in the seminiferous epithelium of rhesus and bonnet monkeys. *J. Med. Primatol.* 32, 170–177.

Bentley, G. E., Kriegsfeld, L. J., Osugi, T., Ukena, K., O'Brien, S., Perfito, N., Moore, I. T., Tsutsui, K., and Wingfield, J. C. (2006a). Interactions of gonadotropin-releasing hormone (GnRH) and gonadotropin-inhibitory hormone (GnIH) in birds and mammals. *J. Exp. Zoolog. Part A Comp. Exp. Biol.* 305, 807–814.

Bentley, G. E., Jensen, J. P., Kaur, G. J., Wacker, D. W., Tsutsui, K., and Wingfield, J. C. (2006b). Rapid inhibition of female sexual behavior by gonadotropin-inhibitory hormone (GnIH). *Horm. Behav.* 49, 550–555.

Bentley, G. E., Ubuka, T., McGuire, N. L., Calisi, R. M., Perfito, N., Kriegsfeld, L. J., WIngfield, J. C., and Tsutsui, K. (2009). GnIH: a multifunctional neuropeptide. *J. Neuroendocrinol.* 21, 276–281.

Bentley, G. E., Ubuka, T., McGuire, N. L., Chowdhury, V. S., Morita,, Y., Yano T., Hasunuma, I., Binns, M., Wingfield, J. C., and Tsutsui, K. (2008). Gonadotropin-inhibitory hormone and its receptor in the avian reproductive system. *Gen. Comp. Endocrinol.* 156, 34–43.

Boekelheide, K., Schoenfeld, H. A., Hall, S. J., Weng, C. C., Shetty, G., Leith, J., Harper, J., Sigman, M., Hess, D. L., and Meistrich, M. L. (2005). Gonadotropin-releasing hormone antagonist (Cetrorelix) therapy fails to protect nonhuman primates (*Macaca arctoides*) from radiation-induced spermatogenic failure. *J. Androl.* 26, 222–234.

Bogerd, J., Diepenbroek, W. B., Hund, E., van Oosterhout, F., Teves, A. C., Leurs, R., and Blomenröhr, M. (2002). Two gonadotropin-releasing hormone receptors in the African catfish: no differences in ligand selectivity, but differences in tissue distribution. *Endocrinology* 143, 4673–4682.

Botté, M. C., Chamagne, A. M., Carré, M. C., Counis, R., and Kottler, M. L. (1998). Fetal expression of GnRH and GnRH receptor genes in rat testis and ovary. *J. Endocrinol.* 159, 179–189.

Campbell, R. M., and Scanes, C. G. (1992). Evolution of the growth hormone-releasing factor (GRF) family of peptides. *Growth Regul.* 2, 175–191.

Castellano, J. M., Gaytan, M., Roa, J., Vigo, E., Navarro, V. M., Bellido, C., Dieguez, C., Aguilar, E, Sánchez-Criado, J. E., Pellicer, A., Pinilla, L., Gaytan, F., and Tena-Sempere, M. (2006). Expression of KiSS-1 in rat ovary: putative local regulator of ovulation? *Endocrinology* 147, 4852–4862.

Chakrabarti, N., Subbarao, T., Sengupta, A., Xu, F., Stouffer, R. L., and Sridaran, R. (2008). Expression of mRNA and proteins for GnRH I and II and their receptors in primate corpus luteum during menstrual cycle. *Mol. Reprod. Dev.* 75, 1567–1577.

Ciccone, N. A., Dunn, I. C., Boswell, T., Tsutsui, K., Ubuka, T., Ukena, K., and Sharp, P. J. (2004). Gonadotrophin inhibitory hormone depresses gonadotrophin alpha and follicle-stimulating hormone beta subunit expression in the pituitary of the domestic chicken. *J. Neuroendocrinol.* 16, 999–1006.

Clarke, I. J., Qi, Y., Puspita Sari, I., and Smith, J. T. (2009). Evidence that RF-amide related peptides are inhibitors of reproduction in mammals. *Front. Neuroendocrinol.* 30, 371–378.

Clayton, R. N., Harwood, J. P., and Catt, K. J. (1979). Gonadotropin-releasing hormone analogue binds to luteal cells and inhibits progesterone production. *Nature* 282, 90–92.

Clermont, Y. (1972). Kinetics of spermatogenesis in mammals: seminiferous epithelium cycle and spermatogonial renewal. *Physiol. Rev.* 52, 198–236.

D'Antonio, M., Fasano, S., de Leeuw, R., and Pierantoni, R. (1992). Effects of gonadotropin-releasing hormone variants on plasma and testicular androgen levels in intact and hypophysectomized male frogs, Rana esculenta. *J. Exp. Zool.* 261, 34–39.

Davis, J. S., West, L. A., and Farese, R. V. (1986). Gonadotropin-releasing hormone (GnRH) rapidly stimulates the formation of inositol phosphates and diacyglycerol in rat granulosa cells: further evidence for the involvement of Ca2+ and protein kinase C in the action of GnRH. *Endocrinology* 118, 2561–2571.

Di Fiore, M. M., Rastogi, R. K., Ceciliani, F., Messi, E., Botte, V., Botte, L., Pinelli, C., D'Aniello, B., and D'Aniello, A. (2000). Mammalian and chicken I forms of gonadotropin-releasing hormone in the gonads of a protochordate, Ciona intestinalis. *Proc. Natl. Acad. Sci. U.S.A.* 97, 2343–2348.

Di Matteo, L., Vallarino, M., and Pierantoni, R. (1996). Localization of GnRH molecular forms in the brain, pituitary, and testis of the frog, Rana esculenta. *J. Exp. Zool.* 274, 33–40.

Dong, K. W., Duval, P., Zeng, Z., Gordon, K., Williams, R. F., Hodgen, G. D., Jones, G., Kerdelhue, B., and Roberts, J. L. (1996). Multiple transcription start sites for the GnRH gene in rhesus and cynomolgus monkeys: a non-human primate model for studying GnRH gene regulation. *Mol. Cell. Endocrinol.* 117, 121–130.

Ducret, E., Anderson, G. M., and Herbison, A. E. (2009). RFamide-related peptide-3, amammalian gonadotropin-inhibitory hormone ortholog, regulates gonadotropin-releasing hormone neuron firing in the mouse. *Endocrinology* 150, 2799–2804.

Dufau, M. L., and Knox, G. F. (1985). Fetal Leydig cell culture–an in vitro system for the study of trophic hormone and GnRH receptors and actions. *J. Steroid Biochem.* 23, 743–755.

El-Gehani, F., Tena-Sempere, M., and Huhtaniemi, I. (1998). Vasoactive intestinal peptide stimulates testosterone production by cultured fetal rat testicular cells. *Mol. Cell. Endocrinol.* 140, 175–178.

Endo, D., and Park, M. K. (2004). Molecular characterization of the leopard gecko POMC gene and expressional change in the testis by acclimation to low temperature and with a short photoperiod. *Gen. Comp. Endocrinol.* 138, 70–77.

Ferin, M. (1999). Clinical review 105: stress and the reproductive cycle. *J. Clin. Endocrinol. Metab.* 84, 1768–1774.

Florio, P., Vale, W., and Petraglia, F. (2004). Urocortins in human reproduction. *Peptides* 25, 1751–1757.

Gann, P. H., Hennekens, C. H., Ma, J., Longcope, C., and Stampfer, M. J. (1996). Prospective study of sex hormone levels and risk of prostate cancer. *J. Natl. Cancer Inst.* 88, 1118–1126.

Garcia-Reyero, N., Villeneuve, D. L., Kroll, K. J., Liu, L., Orlando, E. F., Watanabe, K. H., Sepúlveda, M. S., Ankley, G. T., and Denslow, N. D. (2009). Expression signatures for a model androgen and antiandrogen in the fathead minnow (*Pimephales promelas*) ovary. *Environ. Sci. Technol.* 43, 2614–2619.

Gazourian, L., Deragon, K. L., Chase, C. F., Pati, D., Habibi, H. R., and Sower, S. A. (1997). Characteristics of GnRH binding in the gonads and effects of lamprey GnRH-I and -III on reproduction in the adult sea lamprey. *Gen. Comp. Endocrinol.* 108, 327–339.

Gazourian, L., Evans, E. L., Hanson, L., Chase, C. F., and Sower, S. A. (2000). The effects of lamprey GnRH-I, -III and analogs on steroidogenesis in the sea lamprey (Petromyzon marinus). *Aquaculture* 188, 147–165.

Geris, K. L., Meeussen, G., Kühn, E. R., and Darras, V. M. (2000). Distribution of somatostatin in the brain and of somatostatin and thyrotropin-releasing hormone in peripheral tissues of the chicken. *Brain Res.* 873, 306–309.

Gore-Langton, R. E., Lacroix, M., and Dorrington, J. H. (1981). Differential effects of luteinizing hormone-releasing hormone on follicle-stimulating hormone-dependent responses in rat granulosa cells and Sertoli cells in vitro. *Endocrinology* 108, 812–819.

Gougeon, A. (1996). Regulation of ovarian follicular development in primates: Facts and hypotheses. *Endocr. Rev.* 17, 121–155.

Grober, M. S., Myers, T. R., Marchaterre, M. A., Bass, A. H., and Myers, D. A. (1995). Structure, localization, and molecular phylogeny of a GnRH cDNA from a paracanthopterygian fish, the plainfin midshipman (*Porichthys notatus*). *Gen. Comp. Endocrinol.* 99, 85–99.

Gründker, C., Günthert, A. R., Millar, R. P., and Emons, G. (2002). Expression of gonadotropin-releasing hormone II (GnRH-II) receptor in human endometrial and ovarian cancer cells and effects of GnRH-II on tumor cell proliferation. *J. Clin. Endocrinol. Metab.* 87, 1427–1430.

Gupta, G., Maikhuri, J. P., Setty, B. S., and Dhar, J. D. (2000). Seasonal variations in daily sperm production rate of rhesus and bonnet monkeys. *J. Med. Primatol.* 29, 411–414.

Heinrich, N., Meyer, M. R., Furkert, J., Sasse, A., Beyermann, M., Bönigk, W., and Berger, H. (1998). Corticotropin-releasing factor (CRF) agonists stimulate testosterone production in mouse leydig cells through CRF receptor-1. *Endocrinoly* 139, 651–658.

Hertelendy, F., Lintner, F., Asem, E. K., and Raab, B. (1982). Synergistic effect of gonadotropin releasing hormone on LH-stimulated progesterone production in granulosa cells of the domestic fowl (*Gallus domesticus*). *Gen. Comp. Endocrinol.* 48, 117–122.

Hinuma, S., Shintani, Y., Fukusumi, S., Iijima, N., Matsumoto, Y., Hosoya, M., Fujii, R., Watanabe, T., Kikuchi, K., Terao, Y., Yano, T., Yamamoto, T., Kawamata, Y., Habata, Y., Asada, M., Kitada, C., Kurokawa, T., Onda, H., Nishimura, O., Tanaka, M., Ibata, Y., and Fujino, M. (2000). New neuropeptides containing carboxy-terminal RFamide and their receptor in mammals. *Nat. Cell Biol.* 2, 703–708.

Hsueh, A. J., Bambino, T. H., Zhuang, L. Z., Welsh, T. H. Jr., and Ling, N. C. (1983). Mechanism of the direct action of gonadotropin-releasing hormone and its antagonist on androgen biosynthesis by cultured rat testicular cells. *Endocrinology* 112, 1653–1661.

Hsueh, A. J., and Erickson, G. F. (1979). Extra-pituitary inhibition of testicular function by luteinising hormone releasing hormone. *Nature* 81, 66–67.

Hsueh, A. J., and Jones, P. B. (1981). Extrapituitary actions of gonadotropin-releasing hormone. *Endocr. Rev.* 2, 437–461.

Hsueh, A. J., Schreiber, J. R., and Erickson, G. F. (1981). Inhibitory effect of gonadotropin releasing hormone upon cultured testicular cells. *Mol. Cell. Endocrinol.* 21, 43–49.

Hsueh, A. J., Wang, C., and Erickson, G. F. (1980). Direct inhibitory effect of gonadotropin-releasing hormone upon follicle-stimulating hormone induction of luteinizing hormone receptor, and aromatase activity in rat granulosa cells. *Endocrinolgy* 106, 1697–1705.

Huang, B. M., Stocco, D. M., Hutson, J. C., and Norman, R. L. (1995). Corticotropin-releasing hormone stimulates steroidogenesis in mouse Leydig cells. *Biol. Reprod.* 53, 620–626.

Hubbard, G. M., and Licht, P. (1985). In vitro study of the direct ovarian effects of gonadotropin-releasing hormone (GnRH) in the frogs, Rana pipiens and Rana catesbeiana. *Gen. Comp. Endocrinol.* 60, 154–161.

Ikemoto, T., and Park, M. K. (2007). Comparative analysis of the pituitary and ovarian GnRH systems in the leopard gecko: signaling crosstalk between multiple receptor subtypes in ovarian follicles. *J. Mol. Endocrinol.* 38, 289–304.

Irusta, G., Parborell, F., and Tesone, M. (2007). Inhibition of cytochrome P-450 C17 enzyme by a GnRH agonist in ovarian follicles from gonadotropin-stimulated rats. *Am. J. Physiol. Endocrinol. Metab.* 292, E1456–E1464.

Johnson, A. L., and Tilly, J. L. (1988). Effects of vasoactive intestinal peptide on steroid secretion and plasminogen activator activity in granulosa cells of the hen. *Biol. Reprod.* 38, 296–303.

Johnson, M. A., Tsutsui, K., and Fraley, G. S. (2007). Rat RFamide-related peptide-3 stimulates GH secretion, inhibits LH secretion, and has variable effects on sex behavior in the adult male rat. *Horm. Behav.* 51, 171–180.

Jones, P. B., Conn, P. M., Marian, J., and Hsueh, A. J. (1980). Binding of gonadotropin releasing hormone agonist to rat ovarian granulose cells. *Life Sci.* 27, 2125–2132.

Jones, P. B., and Hsueh, A. J. (1981). Direct effects of gonadotropin releasing hormone and its antagonist upon ovarian functions stimulated by FSH, prolactin, ans LH. *Biol. Reprod.* 24, 747.

Kang, S. K., Tai, C. J., Cheng, K. W., and Leung, P. C. (2000). Gonadotropin-releasing hormone activates mitogen-activated protein kinase in human ovarian and placental cells. *Mol. Cell. Endocrinol.* 170, 143–151.

Kang, S. K., Tai, C. J., Nathwani, P. S., and Leung, P. C. (2001). Differential regulation of two forms of gonadotropin-releasing hormone messenger ribonucleic acid in human granulosa-luteal cells. *Endocrinolgy* 142, 182–192.

Kawada, T., Sekiguchi, T., Itoh, Y., Ogasawara, M., and Satake, H. (2008). Characterization of a novel vasopressin/oxytocin superfamily peptide and its receptor from an ascidian, Ciona intestinalis. *Peptides* 29, 1672–1678.

Kawashima, M., Takahashi, T., Yasuoka, T., Kamiyoshi, M., and Tanaka, K. (1995). A vasoactive intestinal peptide binding component in hen granulose cells. *Proc. Soc. Exp. Biol. Med.* 209, 387–391.

Kopp, J., Zhang, X., and Hökfelt, T. (1997). Neuropeptide Y1 receptors in the rat genital tract. *Regul. Pept.* 70, 149–160.

Kriegsfeld, L. J., Mei, D. F., Bentley, G. E., Ubuka, T., Mason, A. O., Inoue, K., Ukena, K., Tsutsui, K., and Silver, R. (2006). Identification and characterization of a gonadotropin-inhibitory system in the brains of mammals. *Proc. Natl. Acad. Sci. U.S.A.* 103, 2410–2415.

Lin, X. W., and Peter, R. E. (1996). Expression of salmon gonadotropin-releasing hormone (GnRH) and chicken GnRH-II precursor messenger ribonucleic acids in the brain and ovary of goldfish. *Gen. Comp. Endocrinol.* 101, 282–296.

MacDonald, E., and Volkoff, H. (2009). Neuropeptide Y (NPY), cocaine- and amphetamine-regulated transcript (CART) and cholecystokinin (CCK) in winter skate (*Raja ocellata*): cDNA cloning, tissue distribution and mRNA expression responses to fasting. *Gen. Comp. Endocrinol.* 161, 252–261.

Maddineni, S. R., Ocón-Grove, O. M., Krzysik-Walker, S. M., and Hendricks, G. L. 3rd, Ramachandran, R. (2008). Gonadotropin-inhibitory hormone (GnIH) receptor gene is expressed in the chicken ovary: potential role of GnIH in follicular maturation. *Reproduction* 135, 267–274.

Madigou, T., Uzbekova, S., Lareyre, J. J., and Kah, O. (2002). Two messenger RNA isoforms of the gonadotrophin-releasing hormone receptor, generated by alternative splicing and/or promoter usage, are differentially expressed in rainbow trout gonads during gametogenesis. *Mol. Reprod. Dev.* 63, 151–160.

Masini, M. A., Sturla, M., Pestarino, M., Gallinelli, A., Facchinetti, F., and Uva, B. M. (1997). Pro-opiomelanocortin (POMC) expression and immunolocalization of POMC-related peptides in the ovary of *Protopterus annectens*, an African lungfish. *Peptides* 18, 1411–1414.

McGuire, N. L., and Bentley, G. E. (2010). A functional neuropeptide system in vertebrate gonads: Gonadotropin-inhibitory hormone and its receptor in testes of field-caught house sparrow (Passer domesticus). *Gen. Comp. Endocrinol.* 166, 565–572.

McGuire, N. L., Kangas, K. K, and Bentley, G. E. (2010). Direct regulation of the gonadal GnIH system and steroid biosynthesis in the European starling (*Sturnus vulgaris*) testes and ovary by melatonin. *Endocrinology* (Submitted).

McRory, J. E., Parker, D. B., Ngamvongchon, S., and Sherwood, N. M. (1995). Sequence and expression of cDNA for pituitary adenylate cyclase activating polypeptide (PACAP) and growth hormone-releasing hormone (GHRH)-like peptide in catfish. *Mol. Cell. Endocrinol.* 108, 169–177.

Millar, R., Lowe, S., Conklin, D., Pawson, A., Maudsley, S., Troskie, B., Ott, T., Millar, M., Lincoln, G., Sellar, R., Faurholm, B., Scobie, G., Kuestner, R., Terasawa, E., and Katz, A. (2001). A novel mammalian receptor for the evolutionarily conserved type II GnRH. *Proc. Natl. Acad. Sci. U.S.A.* 98, 9636–9641.

Minucci, S., Di Matteo, L., Pierantoni, R., Varriale, B., Rastogi, R. K., and Chieffi, G. (1986). In vivo and in vitro stimulatory effect of a gonadotropin-releasing hormone analog (HOE 766) on spermatogonial multiplication in the frog, *Rana esculenta*. *Endocrinology* 119, 731–736.

Moumni, M., Kottler, M. L., and Counis, R. (1994). Nucleotide sequence analysis of mRNA predicts that rat pituitary and gonadal gonadotropin-releasing hormone receptor proteins have identical primary structure. *Biochem. Biophys. Res. Commun.*. 200, 1359–1366.

Neill, J. D. (2002). GnRH and GnRH receptor genes in the human genome. *Endocrinology* 143, 737–743.

Nicholson, H. D., Swann, R. W., Burford, G. D., Wathes, D. C., Porter, D. G., and Pickering, B. T. (1984). Identification of oxytocin and vasopressin in the testis and in adrenal tissue. *Regul. Pept.* 8, 141–146.

Ohta, M., Funakoshi, S., Kawasaki, T., and Itoh, N. (1992). Tissue-specific expression of the rat secretin precursor gene. *Biochem. Biophys. Res. Commun.* 183, 390–395.

Oikawa, M., Dargan, C., Ny, T., and Hsueh, A. J. (1990). Expression of gonadotropin-releasing hormone and prothymosin-alpha messenger ribonucleic acid in the ovary. *Endocrinology* 127, 2350–2356.

Osugi, T., Ukena, K., Bentley, G. E., O'Brien, S., Moore, I. T., Wingfield, J. C., and Tsutsui, K. (2004). Gonadotropin-inhibitory hormone in Gambel's white-crowned sparrow (Zonotrichia leucophrys gambelii): cDNA identification, transcript localization and functional effects in laboratory and field experiments. *J. Endocrinol.* 182, 33–42.

Pati, D., and Habibi, H. R. (1998). Presence of salmon gonadotropin-releasing hormone (GnRH) and compounds with GnRH-like activity in the ovary of goldfish. *Endocrinology* 139, 2015–2024.

Pati, D., and Habibi, H. R. (2000). Direct action of GnRH variants on goldfish oocyte meiosis and follicular steroidogenesis. *Mol. Cell. Endocrinol.* 160, 75–88.

Paull, W. K., Turkelson, C. M., Thomas, C. R., and Arimura, A. (1981). Immunohistochemical demonstration of a testicular substance related to luteinizing hormone-releasing hormone. *Science* 213, 1263–1264.

Pazos, A. J., and Mathieu, M. (1999). Effects of five natural gonadotropin-releasing hormones on cell suspensions of marine bivalve gonad: stimulation of gonial DNA synthesis. *Gen. Comp. Endocrinol.* 113, 112–120.

Pekary, A. E., Meyer, N. V., Vaillant, C., and Hershman, J. M. (1980). Thyrotropin-releasing hormone and a homologous peptide in the male rat reproductive system. *Biochem. Biophys. Res. Commun.* 95, 993–1000.

Peng, C., Fan, N. C., Ligier, M., Väänänen, J., and Leung, P. C. (1994). Expression and regulation of gonadotropin-releasing hormone (GnRH) and GnRH receptor messenger ribonucleic acids in human granulosa-luteal cells. *Endocrinology* 135, 1740–1746.

Pineda, R., Garcia-Galiano, D., Sanchez-Garrido, M. A., Romero, M., Ruiz-Pino, F., Aguilar, E., Dijcks, F. A., Blomenröhr, M., Pinilla, L., van Noort, P. I., and Tena-Sempere, M. (2010). Characterization of the potent gonadotropin-releasing activity of RF9, a selective antagonist of RF-amide-related peptides and neuropeptide FF receptors: physiological and pharmacological implications. *Endocrinology* 151, 1902–1913.

Pintar, J. E., Schachter, B. S., Herman, A. B., Durgerian, S., and Krieger, D. T. (1984). Characterization and localization of proopiomelanocortin messenger RNA in the adult rat testis. *Science* 225, 632–634.

Powell, J. F., Reska-Skinner, S. M., Prakash, M. O., Fischer, W. H., Park, M., Rivier, J. E., Craig, A. G., Mackie, G. O., and Sherwood, N. M. (1996). Two new forms of gonadotropin-releasing hormone in a protochordate and the evolutionary implications. *Proc. Natl. Acad. Sci. U.S.A.* 93, 10461–10464.

Riesen, J. W., Meyer, R. K., and Wolf, R. C. (1971). The effect of season on occurrence of ovulation in the rhesus monkey. *Biol. Reprod.* 5, 111–114.

Roberts, M. L., Buchanan, K. L., Hasselquist, D., and Evans, M. R. (2007). Effects of testosterone and corticosterone on immunocompetence in the zebra finch. *Horm. Behav.* 51, 126–134.

Romanelli, F., Fillo, S., Isidori, A., Gaudino, S., and Conte, D. (1998). Galanin stimulates steroidogenesis in rat Leydig cells. *Life Sci.* 63, 255–263.

Sari, I. P., Rao, A., Smith, J. T., Tilbrook, A. J., and Clarke, I. J. (2009). Effect of RF-amide-related peptide-3 on luteinizing hormone and follicle-stimulating hormone synthesis and secretion in ovine pituitary gonadotropes. *Endocrinology* 150, 5549–5556.

Schally, A. V. (1999). Luteinizing hormone-releasing hormone analogs: their impact on the control of tumorigenesis. *Peptides* 20, 1247–1262.

Schally, A. V., Arimura, A., Kastin, A. J., Matsuo, H., Baba, Y., Redding, T. W., Nair, R. M., Debeljuk, L., and White, W. F. (1971). Gonadotropin-releasing hormone: one polypeptide regulates secretion of luteinizing and follicle-stimulating hormones. *Science* 173, 1036–1038.

Schirman-Hildesheim, T. D., Bar, T., Ben-Aroya, N., and Koch, Y. (2005). Differential gonadotropin-releasing hormone (GnRH) and GnRH receptor messenger ribonucleic acid expression patterns in different tissues of the female rat across the estrous cycle. *Endocrinology* 146, 3401–3408.

Schirman-Hildesheim, T. D., Ben-Aroya, N., and Koch, Y. (2006). Daily GnRH and GnRH-receptor mRNA expression in the ovariectomized and intact rat. *Mol. Cell. Endocrinol.* 252, 120–125.

Schmidt, K. L., Pradhan, D. S., Shah, A. H., Charlier, T. D., Chin, E. H., and Soma, K. K. (2008). Neurosteroids, immunosteroids, and the Balkanization of endocrinology. *Gen. Comp. Endocrinol.* 157, 266–274.

Schulze, W., Davidoff, M. S., and Holstein, A. F. (1987). Are Leydig cells of neural origin? Substance P-like immunoreactivity in human testicular tissue. *Acta Endocrinol.* 115, 373–377.

Shahed A., and Young, K. A. (2009). Differential ovarian expression of KiSS-1 and GPR-54 during the estrous cycle and photoperiod induced recrudescence in siberian hamsters (*Phodopus sungorus*). *Mol. Reprod. Dev.* 76, 444–452.

Sharpe, R. M., Doogan, D. G., and Cooper, I. (1982). Stimulation of Leydig cell testosterone secretion in vitro and in vivo in hypophysectomized rats by an agonist of luteinizing hormone releasing hormone. *Biochem. Biophys. Res. Commun.* 106, 1210–1217.

Shen, S. T., Lu, L. M., Chen, J. R., Chien, J. T., and Yu, J. Y. (2003). Molecular cloning of proopiomelanocortin (POMC) cDNA from mud turtle, *Pelodiscus sinensis*. *Gen. Comp. Endocrinol.* 131, 192–201.

Shimizu, M., and Bédécarrats, G. Y. (2010). Activation of the chicken gonadotropin-inhibitory hormone receptor reduces gonadotropin releasing hormone receptor signaling. *Gen. Comp. Endocrinol.* 67, 331–337.

Singh, P., Krishna, A., and Sridaran, R. (2007). Localization of gonadotrophin-releasing hormone I, bradykinin and their receptors in the ovaries of non-mammalian vertebrates. *Reproduction* 133, 969–981.

Stewart, A. J., Katz, A. A., Millar, R. P., and Morgan, K. (2009). Retention and silencing of prepro-GnRH-II and type II GnRH receptor genes in mammals. *Neuroendocrinology* 90, 416–432.

Sun, Y. M., Dunn, I. C., Baines, E., Talbot, R. T., Illing, N., Millar, R. P., and Sharp, P. J. (2001). Distribution and regulation by oestrogen of fully processed and variant transcripts of gonadotropin releasing hormone I and gonadotropin releasing hormone receptor mRNAs in the male chicken. *J. Neuroendocrinol.* 13, 37–49.

Takekida, S., Matsuo, H., and Maruo, T. (2003). GnRH agonist action on granulosa cells at varying follicular stages. *Mol. Cell. Endocrinol.* 202, 155–164.

Takeuchi, S., Teshigawara, K., and Takahashi, S. (1999). Molecular cloning and characterization of the chicken pro-opiomelanocortin (POMC) gene. *Biochim. Biophys. Acta* 1450, 452–459.

Terado, M., Nomura, M., Mineta, K., Fujimoto, N., and Matsumoto, T. (2006). Expression of neuropeptide Y gene in mouse testes during testicular development. *Asian J. Androl.* 8, 443–449.

Tsutsui, K., Bentley, G. E., Ubuka, T., Saigoh, E., Yin, H., Osugi, T., Inoue, K., Chowdhury, V. S., Ukena, K., Ciccone, N., Sharp, P. J., and Wingfield, J. C. (2007). The general and comparative biology of gonadotropin-inhibitory hormone (GnIH). *Gen. Comp. Endocrinol.* 153, 365–370.

Tsutsui, K., Saigoh, E., Ukena, K., Teranishi, H., Fujisawa, Y., Kikuchi, M., Ishii, S., and Sharp, P. J. (2000). A novel avian hypothalamic peptide inhibiting gonadotropin release. *Biochem. Biophys. Res. Commun.* 275, 661–667.

Tsutsui, K., Saigoh, E., Yin, H., Ubuka, T., Chowdhury, V. S., Osugi, T., Ukena, K., Sharp, P. J., Wingfield, J. C., and Bentley, G. E. (2009). A new key neurohormone controlling reproduction, gonadotropin-inhibitory hormone (GnIH) in birds: discovery, progress and prospect. *J. Neuroendocrinol.* 21, 271–275.

Tsutsui, K., and Ukena, K. (2006). Hypothalamic LPXRF-amide peptides in vertebrates: identification, localization and hypophysiotropic activity. *Peptides* 1121–1129.

Ubuka, T, Morgan, K., Pawson, A. J., Osugi, T., Chowdhury, V. S., Minakata, H., Tsutsui, K., Millar, R. P., and Bentley, G. E. (2009). Identification of human GnIH homologs, RFRP-1 and RFRP-3, and the cognate receptor, GPR147 in the human hypothalamic pituitary axis. *PLoS ONE* 4, e8400. doi:10.1371/journal.pone.0008400.

Ubuka, T., Ukena, K., Sharp, P. J., Bentley, G. E., and Tsutsui, K. (2006). Gonadotropin-inhibitory hormone inhibits gonadal development and maintenance by decreasing gonadotropin synthesis and release in male quail. *Endocrinolgy* 147, 1187–1194.

Vaccari, S., Latini, S., Barberi, M., Teti, A., Stefanini, M., and Canipari, R. (2006). Characterization and expression of different pituitary adenylate cyclase-activating polypeptide/vasoactive intestinal polypeptide receptors in rat ovarian follicles. *J. Endocrinol.* 191, 287–299.

Vermeulen, A. (1993). Environment, human reproduction, menopause, and andropause. *Environ. Health Perspect.* 101(Suppl. 2), 91–100.

Vigersky, R. A., Andersen, A. E., Thompson, R. H., and Loriaux, D. L. (1977). Hypothalamic dysfunction in secondary amenorrhea associated with simple weight loss. *N. Engl. J. Med.* 297, 1141–1145.

von Schalburg, K. R., Harrower, W. L., and Sherwood, N. M. (1999). Regulation and expression of gonadotropin-releasing hormone in salmon embryo and gonad. *Mol. Cell. Endocrinol.* 157, 41–54.

Waser, B., Rehmann, R., Rivier, J., Vale, W., and Reubi, J. C. (2006). CRF receptors in the rodent and human cardiovascular systems: species differences. *Peptides* 27, 3029–3038.

Weinbauer, G. F., Surmann, F. J., Akhtar, F. B., Shah, G. V., Vickery, B. H., and Nieschlag, E. (1984). Reversible inhibition of testicular function by a gonadotropin hormone-releasing hormone antagonist in monkeys (*Macaca fascicularis*). *Fertil. Steril.* 42, 906–914.

Whitelaw, P. F., Eidne, K. A., Sellar, R., Smyth, C. D., and Hillier, S. G. (1995). Gonadotropin-releasing hormone receptor messenger ribonucleic acid expression in rat ovary. *Endocrinology* 136, 172–179.

Wingfield, J. C., Ukena, K., Tsutsui, K., and Bentley, G. E. (2004). Photoperiod effects on plasma gonadotropin-inhibitory hormone (GnIH), and evidence for peripheral GnIH binding sites in white-crowned sparrows. *Abstract 885.9 presented at the 34th Annual Meeting for the Society for Neuroscience*, San Diego, CA.

Yin, H., Ukena, K., Ubuka, T., and Tsutsui, K. (2005). A novel G protein-coupled receptor for gonadotropin-inhibitory hormone in the Japanese quail (*Coturnix japonica*): identification, expression and binding activity. *J. Endocrinol.* 184, 257–266.

Zhao, S., Saito, H., Wang, X., Saito, T., Kaneko, T., and Hiroi, M. (2000). Effects of gonadotropin-releasing hormone agonist on the incidence of apoptosis in porcine and human granulosa cells. *Gynecol. Obstet. Invest.* 49, 52–56.

Zhao, S., Zhu, E., Yang, C., Bentley, G. E., Tsutsui, K., and Kriegsfeld, L. J. (2010). RFamide-related peptide and messenger ribonucleic acid expression in mammalian testis: association with the spermatogenic cycle. *Endocrinology* 151, 617–627.

Glutamatergic signaling and low prodynorphin expression are associated with intact memory and reduced anxiety in rat models of healthy aging

Caroline Ménard[1,2,3,4], *Rémi Quirion*[1,2], *Sylvain Bouchard*[5], *Guylaine Ferland*[6,7] *and Pierrette Gaudreau*[3,4]*

[1] Neuroscience Division, Douglas Mental Health University Institute Research Center, Montreal, QC, Canada
[2] Department of Psychiatry, McGill University, Montreal, QC, Canada
[3] Laboratory of Neuroendocrinology of Aging, Centre Hospitalier de l'Université de Montréal Research Center, Montreal, QC, Canada
[4] Department of Medicine, University of Montreal, Montreal, QC, Canada
[5] Faculty of Medicine, University of Montreal, Montreal, QC, Canada
[6] Hôpital du Sacré-Coeur de Montréal Research Center, Montreal, QC, Canada
[7] Department of Nutrition, University of Montreal, Montreal, QC, Canada

Edited by:
Merce Pallas, University of Barcelona, Spain

Reviewed by:
Emmanuel Planel, Centre Hospitalier de l'Université Laval, Canada
Jacques Epelbaum, Université Paris Descartes, France
Isao Shimokawa, Nagasaki University School of Medicine, Japan

***Correspondence:**
Pierrette Gaudreau, Laboratory of Neuroendocrinology of Aging, Centre Hospitalier de l'Université de Montréal Research Center, 900 St-Denis Street, Viger Tower, Montreal, QC H2X 0A9, Canada
e-mail: pierrette.gaudreau@umontreal.ca

The LOU/C/Jall (LOU) rat strain is considered a model of healthy aging due to its increased longevity, maintenance of stable body weight (BW) throughout life and low incidence of age-related diseases. However, aging LOU rat cognitive and anxiety status has yet to be investigated. In the present study, male and female LOU rat cognitive performances (6–42 months) were assessed using novel object recognition and Morris Water Maze tasks. Recognition memory remained intact in all LOU rats up to 42 months of age. As for spatial memory, old LOU rat performed similarly as young animals for learning acquisition, reversal learning, and retention. While LOU rat BW remained stable despite aging, 20-month-old *ad-libitum*-fed (OAL) male Sprague Dawley rats become obese. We determined if long-term caloric restriction (LTCR) prevents age-related BW increase and cognitive deficits in this rat strain, as observed in the obesity-resistant LOU rats. Compared to young animals, recognition memory was impaired in OAL but intact in 20-month-old calorie-restricted (OCR) rats. Similarly, OAL spatial learning acquisition was impaired but LTCR prevented the deficits. Exacerbated stress responses may favor age-related cognitive decline. In the elevated plus maze and open field tasks, LOU and OCR rats exhibited high levels of exploratory activity whereas OAL rats displayed anxious behaviors. Expression of prodynorphin (Pdyn), an endogenous peptide involved in stress-related memory impairments, was increased in the hippocampus of OAL rats. Group 1 metabotropic glutamate receptor 5 and immediate early genes *Homer 1a* and *Arc* expression, both associated with successful cognitive aging, were unaltered in aging LOU rats but lower in OAL than OCR rats. Altogether, our results, supported by principal component analysis and correlation matrix, suggest that intact memory and low anxiety are associated with glutamatergic signaling and low Pdyn expression in the hippocampus of non-obese aging rats.

Keywords: aging, cognition, anxiety, caloric restriction, obesity, glutamate receptors

INTRODUCTION

Chronic conditions such as diabetes and obesity have become a growing concern in public health around the world and its prevalence is rising in different age groups, including older adults (Mathus-Vliegen, 2012). High fat and calorie intakes not only lead to metabolic disorders but could also accelerate age-related cognitive decline (Williamson et al., 2012; Fadel et al., 2013). Epidemiological studies suggest that type 2 diabetes and obesity increase the risk of dementias (Williamson et al., 2012). Stress exposure over the lifespan may also accelerate cellular aging and promote cognitive dysfunction (Lupien et al., 2009; O'Donovan et al., 2013).

Animal models of healthy aging could help increase our understanding of the impact of obesity on cellular and molecular processes underlying cognitive dysfunctions and anxious status. The LOU/C/Jall (LOU) rat strain is characterized by increased longevity (median lifespan of 29 and 34 months for males and females, respectively), a low and stable adipose tissue mass and a reduced incidence of common age-related diseases (Alliot et al., 2002). To date, no study has examined the changes in recognition and spatial memory and anxiety behavioral components in young adult (6 months) to very old (38–42 months) male and female LOU rats. The single neurobehavioral study performed to date on LOU rats, investigating exclusively recognition memory in young and 24-month-old male LOU rat, showed no change with age (Kollen et al., 2010).

Hippocampus-dependent memory involves glutamatergic transmission (Baudry et al., 2011; Menard and Quirion, 2012a). Notably, cognitive decline is characterized by a decrease in glutamate receptor levels altering synaptic plasticity in the aged mouse brain (Zhao et al., 2009). Spatial memory can be rescued when the expression of N-methyl-D-aspartate (NMDA) receptor NR2B subunit is enhanced (Brim et al., 2012). Group 1 metabotropic glutamate receptors (mGluR) were recently correlated with successful cognitive aging in Long–Evans male rats (Menard and Quirion, 2012b; Yang et al., 2013). Their activation plays crucial roles in the formation of both spatial (Lu et al., 1997; Balschun et al., 1999; Menard and Quirion, 2012b) and recognition memory (Barker et al., 2006; Christoffersen et al., 2008) in rodents.

In the present study, the effects of aging and body mass on recognition and spatial memory, anxious behaviors and related synaptic plasticity was investigated using two models of successful aging: the obesity-resistant LOU rat (Alliot et al., 2002) and the Sprague Dawley (SD) rat subjected to long-term caloric restriction (LTCR) (Bedard et al., 2010, 2013; Moyse et al., 2012). LTCR, the most powerful nutritional intervention known to increase longevity in good health, has been associated with enhanced hippocampal plasticity in rodents (Stranahan and Mattson, 2011). Altogether our results indicate that intact memory, glutamate receptor levels, and immediate early gene (IEG) expression were observed in LOU rats up to 42 month-old while age-related memory deficits were partially prevented by LTCR. Synaptic plasticity was altered and anxious behaviors significantly increased in obese old *ad-libitum*-fed (OAL) rats compared to the other groups. It might be linked to higher prodynorphin (Pdyn) expression, a neuropeptide associated with age-related memory impairment and stress-induced disorders (Menard et al., 2013).

MATERIALS AND METHODS

ANIMALS

Young adult (Y: 6 months, $n = 12$: 6 males, 6 females), mature (M: 12 months, $n = 15$: 7 males, 8 females), old (O: 24 months, $n = 12$: 7 males, 5 females) and old-old (O/O: 38–42-months, $n = 13$: 3 males, 10 females) LOU rats, and young adult *ad-libitum*-fed (AL) (YAL: 3 months, $n = 8$), old AL (OAL: 20 months, $n = 5$), and old calorie-restricted (CR) (OCR: 20 months, $n = 11$) male SD rats were obtained from the Quebec Network for Research on Aging rat colonies. Sampling size was determined according to a published study comparing novel object recognition performances in 24-month-old LOU and SD rats (Kollen et al., 2010). Rats had free access to chow, except for CR rats, and water. At 7.5 months, SD rats were subjected or not to 20% caloric restriction for 2 weeks and 40% thereafter until death (Bedard et al., 2010, 2013; Moyse et al., 2012). AL and CR SD rats were fed chow Teklad control diet TD04088 and fortified TD 04089, respectively, to ensure that the two groups receive equivalent amounts of minerals and vitamins (Harlan Teklad, Madison, WI), as previously described (Moyse et al., 2012). LOU rats were fed chow A03 SAFE growing diet for 3 weeks after weaning and the maintenance A04 SAFE diet thereafter (Perotech, Toronto, CA) (Veyrat-Durebex et al., 2005). All rats were fed between 07:00 and 08:00 h. SD (1/cage) and LOU (2–3/cage) rats were housed in plastic cages in temperature-, humidity-, and lighting-controlled rooms (12:12-h light-dark cycles; lights on at 07:00 h). Food intake and body weight (BW) were recorded regularly. BW and serum corticosterone (CORT) levels of each group are shown in Supplemental Table 1. To control for possible effects of circadian rhythms, all trials were performed during an established time frame (10:00–15:00). For behavioral experiments, animals were trained in two successive groups. The first included all SD rats and very old male and female LOU rats whereas the second one included young, mature and old male and female LOU rats. Upon completion of behavioral testing, non-fasted unaesthetized rats were quickly sacrificed by rapid decapitation for *ex vivo* analyses (Whittington et al., 2013). Animal care, surgery and handling procedures were approved by the CHUM Research Center Animal Care Committees in compliance with the Canadian Council for Animal Care.

NOVEL OBJECT RECOGNITION (NOR)

This task was used to evaluate episodic and reference memory. The rats were first exposed to the empty arena (41 × 41 × 21 cm DietScan clear plexiglass cage; AccuScan Instruments Inc., Columbus, OH) for 5 min (day 0) under bright light, to minimize stress related to a novel environment. On day 1, the rats were allowed to interact with two objects for 5 min. Sixty minutes later, the animals were re-introduced into the arena for 3 min, this time with one familiar and one novel object. The position of the objects was always the same in the arena to remove any spatial memory component from the task. Twenty-four h later (day 2), the rats were again exposed to the familiar object and another novel object for 3 min. Finally, 5 min later, the animal was exposed once more to the familiar object and another novel object for 3 min. The animals were filmed with a camera (Sony Handycam DCR-SX45) and the interaction time (nose at 2 cm or less in the object's direction) with the novel and familiar objects, and distance traveled (cm) were analyzed with the Top Scan 2.0 tracking software (Clever Systems Inc., Heston, VI, USA).

ELEVATED PLUS MAZE (EPM)

On day 3, animals were placed in the center of the EPM apparatus (maze: 100 × 100 cm, arms: 10 × 45 cm) and tested for 5 min to evaluate anxiety and explorative behaviors. This task opposes rodents' innate fear of open bright spaces to their desire to explore new environments. Security was provided by the closed arms whereas the open arms offer exploratory values. Distances traveled (cm), as derived from the tracking system (Panlab), were compared.

OPEN FIELD (OF)

Like EPM, this task opposes the conflict between rodents' innate fear of the open bright center area of the arena (90 × 90 × 40 cm, black plastic) vs. their desire to explore a new environment (day 4). Distances traveled (cm) in the areas of the maze derived from the tracking system (Panlab) were compared. Security was provided by the walls of the arena.

MORRIS WATER MAZE (MWM)

Following the first week of behavioral testing (NOR, EPM, OF), the animals were allowed to rest for 2 days. Then, the long-term reference memory version of the MWM, a hippocampus-dependent behavioral task, was used to investigate spatial memory. A cued test, including three trials of 60 s in which the platform was visible and positioned in the middle of the pool, was conducted on day 0 to assess age-related visual deficits and motivation to escape from water. A flag was positioned on the platform as a visual cue. On day 1, the rats were required to find in a pool (diameter: 150 cm; height: 60 cm) a submerged platform (15 cm in diameter) located 2 cm below the surface of water (24°C), rendered opaque by the addition of non-allergenic white gouache paint. Animals were pseudo-randomly started from a different position on each trial and used distal visual-spatial cues to find the hidden escape platform that remained in the middle of the same quadrant throughout training. The rats were given three trials of 90 s per day for four consecutive days (day 1–4). Animals were guided to the platform if it was not localized within 90 s. All the rats remained on the platform for 15 s before removal. Sixty minutes after the acquisition phase on day 4, the rats were given one probe trial of 90 s for which the platform was removed from the pool to assess short-term memory (learning probe). The distance traveled in each quadrant was measured using a video tracking system. At the end of the probe test, the visible platform was re-introduced into the pool to confirm motivation to escape water, visual acuity and ruled out thigmotaxis.

After 1 day of rest (day 5), all animals were submitted to a reverse memory paradigm to evaluate reversal learning. Briefly, the platform was moved to the opposite quadrant while the position of visual cues stayed the same. The rats were then trained to find the new hidden platform location for four consecutive days, as described above. A second probe test for which the platform was removed was conducted at the end of day 9 (reverse probe). Following the reversal probe trial, the visible platform was re-introduced. Finally, a third probe test was done 7 days later to reactivate long-term memory processes. Animals were sacrificed by quick decapitation 2–3 h after the last MWM probe test to allow IEG expression (day 16). After each trial, the rats were immediately placed under a heat lamp to dry and prevent hypothermia. Data derived from the MWM task were recorded on computer using a video tracking system and analyzed with the SMART 2.0 software (Panlab/Harvard Apparatus, Barcelona, Spain).

MWM exclusion criteria

If the performances of old rats in the cued test third trial exceeded by two times the standard deviation of the representative mean of young rats, individuals were excluded for a lack of motivation to escape water. Only one 38-month-old female LOU rat of the O/O group showed motivation to escape water (**Figure 2B**) therefore the entire age group was excluded. Three rats of the OCR group (3/11) also lacked motivation to escape water during the cued test and were excluded from the analysis.

Swimming speed was also used as a control for motor function, a parameter that could potentially be altered by aging. One out of three 38-month-old male LOU rats had intact motor function for swimming (average swim speed >15 cm/s) so this group was excluded. Moreover, the CHUM Research Center Animal Care Committee did not allow MWM testing on the 42-month-old female LOU rats ($n = 3$). O/O LOU rats with intact visual and motor function (7 females, 38 months old) swam every day along with other age groups. Two 20-month-old SD rats (one OAL, one OCR) did not swim properly (average swim speed <15 cm/s) and were excluded from the analysis.

TISSUE PREPARATION AND BIOCHEMICAL ANALYSIS

The hippocampus and adjacent cortex (entorhinal, perirhinal, and portions of adjacent neocortices) from one half-brain were isolated for immunoblotting, snap frozen and stored at −80°C. The other half-brain was fixed in 4% paraformaldehyde for 24 h, cryoprotected in 30% sucrose for 48 h, and stored at −80°C for immunochemistry. Blood was collected at sacrifice (13:00–16:00) to measure immunoreactive serum CORT concentrations.

CORTICOSTERONE MEASUREMENTS

Blood was quickly centrifuged at 5000 × g for 5 min to separate and collect the serums. The CORT level was quantified for each animal in duplicate with an enzyme immunoassay (EIA, Immunodiagnostic Systems, Boldon, UK) (Veyrat-Durebex et al., 2009). Briefly, the EIA is a competitive assay utilizing a polyclonal CORT antibody, horseradish peroxidase and chromogenic substrate. The concentration of CORT was calculated from a calibration curve and samples had to be diluted by 10 with the Sample Diluent provided.

IMMUNOBLOTTING

Tissues were randomly chosen for both rat strains with equal number of male and female LOU rats (except for the very old group). Brain tissues were homogenized with a polytron in 2 ml of Tris-acetate buffer (50 mM, pH 7.4) containing 100 μM EGTA and protease inhibitors (leupeptin 5 μM, phenylmethylsulfonyl fluoride 200 μM, N-tosyl-L-phenylalanine chloromethyl ketone 1 μg/ml; Sigma-Aldrich Canada, Oakville, ON, Canada). Protein concentrations were determined using the bicinchoninic acid protein assay kit (Pierce, Rockford, IL, USA). Western blot analysis was carried out on aliquots of homogenates obtained from both aging SD and LOU rats. Ten-μg protein samples were loaded on 4–20% Tris-Glycine gels and subjected to sodium dodecyl sulfate polyacrylamide gel electrophoresis on denaturing NuPAGE® Novex 4–20% Bis-Tris gel (Invitrogen, Carlsbad, CA, USA). Proteins were transferred onto Hybond-C nitrocellulose membranes (Amersham Biosciences, Little Chalfont, UK). To block non-specific sites, membranes were first incubated for 1 h at room temperature (RT) in phosphate-buffered saline (PBS) containing 2% bovine serum albumin (BSA). Membranes were next incubated with primary antibodies directed against AMPA (GluR1 and GluR2, Abcam, Cambridge, MA, USA), NMDA (NR1, Santa Cruz Biotechnology, Santa Cruz, CA, USA; NR2A and NR2B, Abcam), group 1 mGluR (mGluR1α and mGluR5, Millipore, Billerica, MA, USA), Homer 1a (Santa Cruz Biotechnology), Arc (Cell Signaling, Danvers, MA, USA), or Zif268 proteins (Abcam) in PBS containing 2% BSA. Bands corresponding to proteins were detected with a peroxidase-conjugated secondary antibody (Santa

Cruz Biotechnology) and Western Lightning Chemiluminescence Reagent Plus (Perkin Elmer, Boston, MA, USA) on Kodak BioMax MS film (Amersham Biosciences). Non-specific labeling was assessed by replacing the primary antibody with an equivalent volume of PBS-BSA. Immunoreactive levels of actin were used as a loading control. Immunoblots were placed on a Northern light illuminator and computer-generated images were analyzed semi-quantitatively by densitometry with a microcomputer imaging system (Imaging Research, MCID, St. Catharines, ON, Canada).

Pdyn AND mGluR5 IMMUNOHISTOCHEMISTRY (IHC)

Half-brains from both rat strains were randomly chosen for sectioning. Twenty-μm coronal sections of fixed brains at the level of the dorsal hippocampus were mounted on Superfrost Plus slides (Thermo Scientific, Portsmouth, NH, USA) and processed for IHC. Briefly, the slices were washed in PBS (pH 7.4) for 5 min then immersed in methanol containing 0.3% H_2O_2 for 30 min at RT to quench endogenous peroxidases. After PBS washes (3 × 5 min), sections were preincubated with 10% normal goat serum (NGS) in PBS at RT for 1 h, followed by incubation with the polyclonal mGluR5 (dilution 1/5000, Millipore) or Pdyn (dilution 1/1000, Millipore) primary antibodies (in PBS with 1% NGS) overnight at 4°C. Subsequently, sections were washed 3 times in PBS and incubated with biotinylated anti-guinea pig (Pdyn) or anti-rabbit (mGluR5) IgGs (1:1000; Vector Laboratories, Burlingame, CA, USA) in 1% NGS for 30 min at RT. After washing in PBS (4 × 10 min), sections were incubated with the avidin biotinylated enzyme complex (ABC reagent, Vector Laboratories) in PBS for 30 min. The peroxidase reaction was carried out with 0.02% $H_2O_2$and 3,3′-diaminobenzidine tetrahydrochloride (0.1% in 100 mM Tris-HCl buffer, pH 7.4). Sections were then washed in tap water, cleaned, and coverslipped. IHC staining was visualized using bright-field microscopy (Nikon Eclipse, Melville, NY, USA) at 4 × and 20 × magnification and quantified with MCID (Imaging Research). Controls were performed using the same labeling procedure, without the primary or secondary antibodies and preadsorbtion of primary antibodies with specific peptides (data not shown).

IEG IMMUNOFLUORESCENCE

Half-brains for both rat strains were randomly chosen for sectioning. Twenty-μm coronal sections of fixed brains at the level of the dorsal hippocampus were mounted, then washed in PBS (pH 7.4) for 5 min. Sections were permeabilized with 0.2% Tween 20 in PBS (PBST) for 10 min at RT then processed for immunofluorescence labeling. In brief, sections were incubated in 10% NGS (or normal horse serum for Homer 1a) diluted in 0.1 M PBS with 0.05% Tween 20 (PBST) and 1% BSA for 60 min at RT, followed by overnight incubation with each primary antibody (1/100 for Homer 1a and Arc, and 1/500 for the neuronal marker MAP2, Abcam) at 4°C in 0.1 M PBST containing 1% serum and BSA. After 3 washes in PBS, sections were incubated with corresponding secondary antibodies (1:500, Invitrogen, Carlsbad, CA, USA) conjugated with Alexa Fluor 488 or Alexa Fluor 568 in PBST containing 1% BSA for 2 h at RT in the dark. Sections were washed in PBS (3 × 5 min each, in the dark). Nuclei were stained with Hoechst solution (2 μg/ml, Invitrogen) for 5 min, and the sections were washed and coverslipped using fluoromount-G (Southern Biotech, Birmingham, AL, USA). Pictures were taken at 40 × magnification with an Axio Observer microscope with Apotome (Carl Zeiss MicroImaging GmbH, Jena, Germany).

STATISTICS

All data are expressed as the mean ± s.e.m. ANOVA followed by Bonferroni's *post-hoc* test was used to assess the level of significance between groups for NOR, MWM, EPM, and OF parameters and protein levels. Correlation between serum CORT levels and age was analyzed using the two-tailed Pearson's test (Prism 4, GraphPad Software Inc., La Jolla, CA). Significance was established at $p < 0.05$.

Principal component analysis (PCA) was used to examine patterns of intercorrelations between the variables (Moura et al., 2010). Principal components produced by PCA are linear combinations of the original measures reflecting independent characteristics (or dimensions) underlying the correlation matrix. The first component explains most of the variance (expressed in terms of the first eigenvalue), the second component explains most of the remaining variation, and so forth. The loading of each measure on a principal component represents the correlation between the latent characteristic and the original measure and thus indicates the importance of a measure for a principal component. Measures with high loadings on the same principal component of the same sign are positively correlated, and loadings of the opposite sign are negatively correlated. Original data sets of each individual rat ($n = 50$) containing 16 variables (age, BW, NOR average, EPM open arms, OF center, serum CORT, GluR1, GluR2, NR1, NR2A, NR2B, mGluR1α, mGluR5, Homer 1a, Arc, and Zif268) were standardized using z-scores and analyzed to obtain the correlation matrix and PCA. Multivariate analyses were performed using the MATLAB software. MWM data were omitted as no reliable data could be obtained in O/O LOU rats.

RESULTS

AGING MARGINALLY AFFECTS LOU RATS' BW AND RECOGNITION MEMORY IS INTACT IN MALE AND FEMALE LOU RATS UP TO 38 AND 42 MONTHS OF AGE, RESPECTIVELY

Increased longevity has been reported for the LOU rat strain (Alliot et al., 2002). In our study, median survival age was evaluated at 38.2 months for females vs. 34.3 months for males LOU rats (**Figure 1A**, curves comparison: $p = 0.0181$). To evaluate survivability, only natural deaths were considered ($n =$ 28–39/group); sacrifices for experimentation and deaths related to surgeries were excluded. Survival proportions were similar between males and females groups up to 24 months of age. Then, the male population slowly decline while that of females remained stable up to 32 months of age. Aging is generally associated with a large BW gain in rodents. In male LOU rats, a 19% increase was observed between 6- and 12 months but BW was stable thereafter, even at a very advanced age (**Figure 1B**, $n = 3$–7). In females, BW changes were even slighter (**Figure 1B**, $n = 5$–10).

Intact recognition memory has previously been observed in 24-month-old male LOU rats (Kollen et al., 2010). Here, we

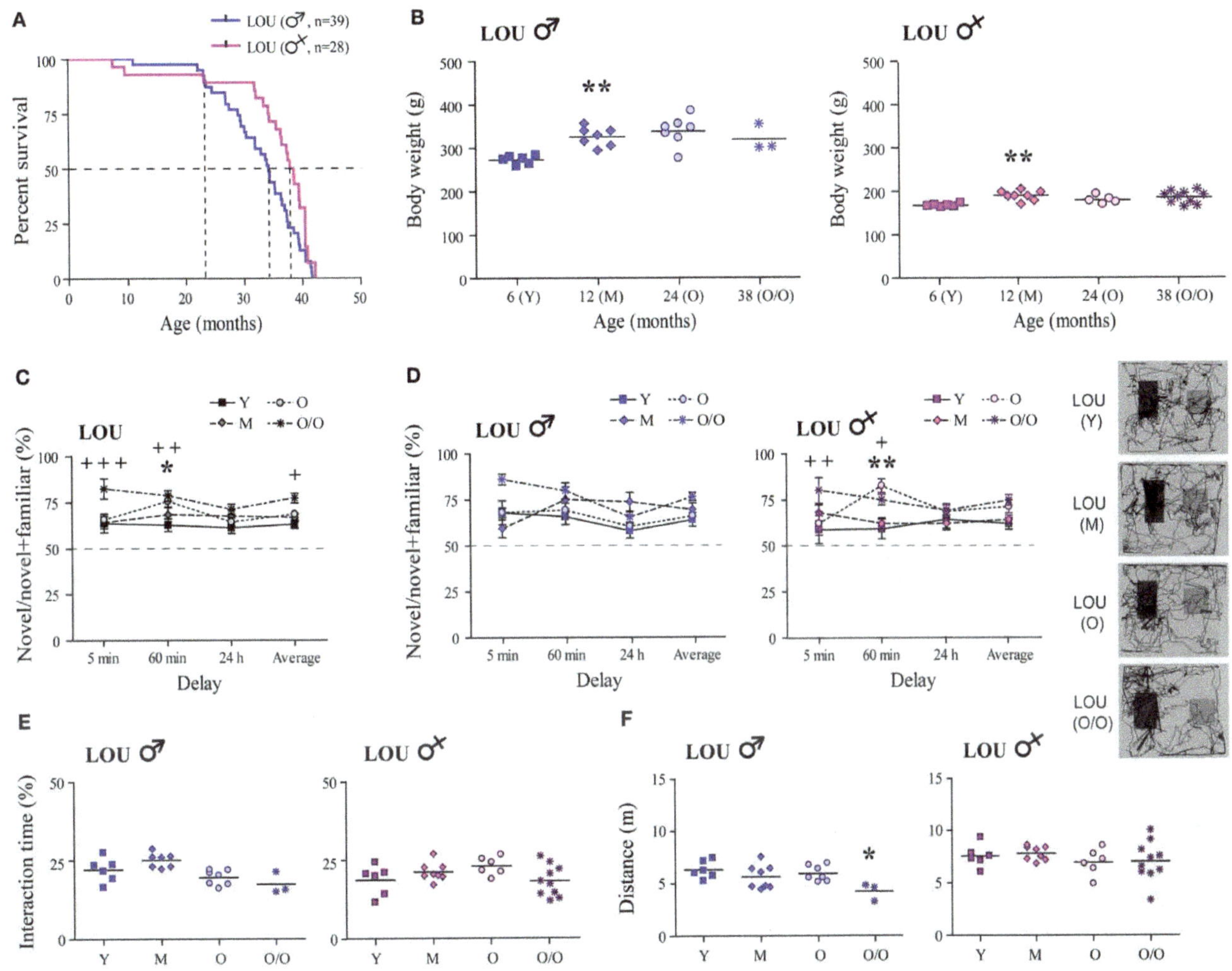

FIGURE 1 | Male and female LOU rats are characterized by high longevity, stable body weight, and intact recognition memory. (A) Median survival age was 38.2 months for females vs. 34.3 months for males LOU rats. **(B)** BW of male and female LOU rats increased only slightly in the course of aging (Y, young adult; M, mature; O, old; O/O, old/old). **(C)** Amount of time spent interacting with novel objects did not decrease with age in LOU rats, and O/O rats spent significantly more time with novel objects on average and after the 5- and 60-min delay than young rats. **(D)** Recognition memory is intact in males and females LOU rats up to 38 and 42 months of age, respectively, with significant differences only for females. Representative paths (60 min delay) are shown with novel object on the right side. **(E)** Average interacting time with the objects was similar at different ages. **(F)** Distance traveled in the arena was not different between LOU age groups for females but lower for O/O males. Values are means ± s.e.m.; $n = 12$–15/age group. Significance of changes was determined by One-Way ANOVA (Two-Way for NOR), followed by Bonferroni post-test, Y vs. O: $^{*}p < 0.05$, $^{**}p < 0.01$; Y vs. O/O: $^{+}p < 0.05$, $^{++}p < 0.01$, $^{+++}p < 0.001$.

report for the first time that up to 38–42 months, male and female LOU rats spent significantly more time with novel objects at every delay tested (**Figure 1C**, $n = 12$–15), suggesting the maintenance of an intact recognition memory in this strain at advanced age. O/O rats interact even more with the novel objects than young rats [age effect Y vs. O/O: Two-Way ANOVA, $F_{(1, 69)} = 17.77$, $p = 0.0003$, $n = 12$–13]. Time delays of novel object exposure affected old and very old male LOU rats with higher percentage of time interacting with the novel object after the 5-min delay [**Figure 1D**, delay effect Y vs. O: Two-Way ANOVA, $F_{(3, 33)} = 4.12$, $p = 0.0138$, $n = 6$–7; Y vs. O/O: $F_{(3, 21)} = 6.09$, $p = 0.0039$, $n = 3$–6]. No significant difference was observed for aging female LOU rats. Total interaction times with the objects remained similar at all ages in male and female LOU rats (**Figure 1E**). Aging had no effect on motor function in female LOU rats however total distance traveled in the NOR arena was reduced by 33% in very old males compared to young animals [**Figure 1F**; One-Way ANOVA, $F_{(3, 20)} = 3.601$, $p = 0.0315$, $n = 3$–6].

SPATIAL MEMORY IS INTACT IN 24-MONTH-OLD MALE AND FEMALE LOU RATS

We next examined whether or not hippocampus-dependent spatial memory was preserved in aging male and female LOU rats, using the MWM reference task. First, a cued test for which the platform was visible was conducted to assess swimming ability, motivation, visual, and motor functions. O/O LOU rats lack motivation to escape water and did not improve their performance during the cued test (**Figure 2A**, trial 1: 47.5 s ± 8.3 s, trial 3: 46.3 s ± 7.6 s, $n = 8$–15), therefore this group was excluded from the analysis (see Materials and Methods, MWM Exclusion

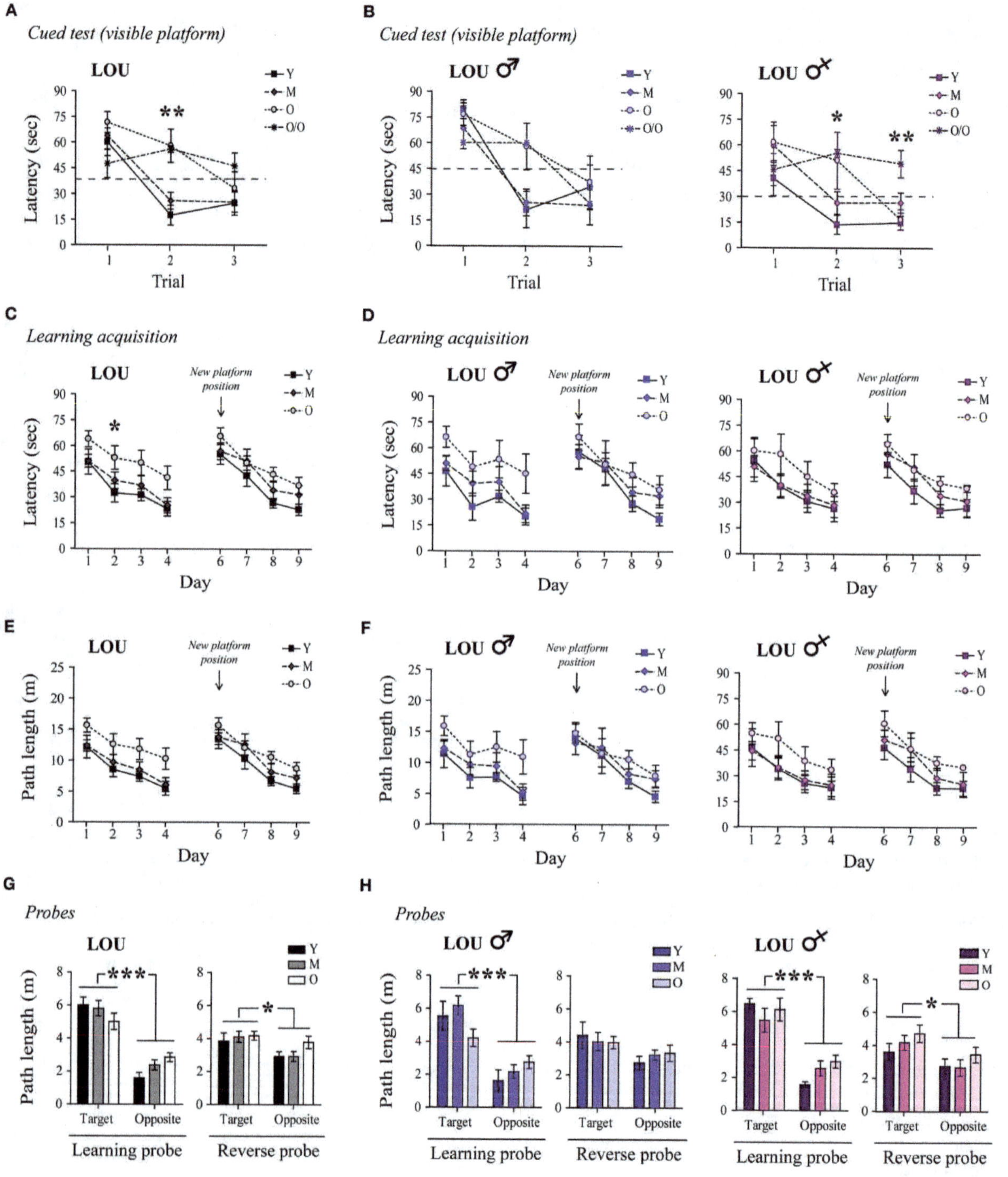

FIGURE 2 | Spatial memory acquisition is intact in old LOU rats. (A) All animals except the O/O LOU rats learned to swim to the visible platform to escape the water after three trials of 60 s (delay of 30 min between each trial, see Materials and Methods, for exclusion criteria). A flag was positioned on the platform as a visual cue. **(B)** Very old female LOU rats lacked motivation to escape water. **(C)** Morris Water Maze (MWM) learning acquisition curves of aging LOU rats (day 1–4, three trials per day). Old LOU rats took more time to find the platform only on day 2. After 1 day of rest, the platform was moved to the opposite quadrant to assess inhibitory learning acquisition (day 6–9, three trials per day). Performances were similar for all LOU rats despite aging. **(D)** No significant difference was observed when individual performances were analyzed by gender. **(E,F)** To rule out an effect of motor function, path lengths to reach the platform were compared. Again, performances were similar for all LOU rats. **(G)** Aging did not affect LOU rat performances in the retention probe tests conducted 60 min after the last trial on day 4 (learning) and 9 (reverse), as distance swum in target quadrants was similar for all groups but significantly higher when compared to the opposite quadrant. **(H)** Female LOU rats performed better in the reverse probe test. Values are means ± s.e.m.; $n = 12$–15/age group. Significance of changes for latencies and path length was determined by Two-Way ANOVA followed by Bonferroni post-test, $^{*}p < 0.05$, $^{**}p < 0.01$, $^{***}p < 0.001$.

Criteria section). Conversely, LOU rats in other age groups learned to escape the pool after three trials [time effect: Two-Way ANOVA, $F_{(2, 72)} = 26.01, p < 0.0001, n = 12–15$].

Likewise, old LOU rats appeared to take more time to acquire the task and find the hidden platform (day 1–4) compared to young LOU rats [**Figure 2C**, age effect: Two-Way ANOVA, $F_{(2, 108)} = 8.05, p = 0.0013, n = 12–15$]. Nevertheless, old LOU rat latencies consistently decreased as in young animals, suggesting slower learning speed but efficient spatial memory (linear regression young: slope = −8.31, $R^2 = 0.8642$; old: slope = −7.05, $R^2 = 0.9590$, $n = 12–15$). Our group and others have shown that reversal learning and memory is affected by aging. Old mice, rats, and monkeys cannot discriminate between two related tasks as well as adult animals (Burke et al., 2011; Menard and Quirion, 2012b; Menard et al., 2013). To evaluate reverse spatial memory function, the platform was moved to the opposite quadrant of the pool on day 6 and learning was studied for four consecutive days (day 6–9). For this task, no significant difference was observed between the LOU rat age groups, suggesting intact reversal learning acquisition despite aging (**Figure 2C**). We also examined if gender differentially affects spatial learning acquisition in old LOU rats. As shown on **Figure 2D**, learning acquisition was slower for 24-month-old male LOU rats [age effect: Two-Way ANOVA, $F_{(2, 51)} = 5.50, p = 0.0144, n = 6–7$] but no significant difference was observed for reversal learning [age effect: Two-Way ANOVA, $F_{(2, 51)} = 0.94, p = 0.4108, n = 6–7$]. In contrast, old female LOU rats successfully learned both tasks. Swim speed may decline with age thus we compared path lengths to reach the platform on training trials (**Figure 2E**). We obtained similar results with an effect of aging only for the learning acquisition task (day 1–4) of old male LOU rats [**Figure 2F**, Two-Way ANOVA, $F_{(2, 51)} = 4.82, p = 0.0219, n = 6–7$]. Finally, memory retention was measured by conducting probe trials with the platform removed 60 min after the last hidden platform training on day 4 of learning and day 9 of reverse acquisition tasks. LOU rats favored the target quadrant in both probe tests [**Figure 2G**, Two-Way ANOVA learning quadrant: $F_{(1, 36)} = 72.23$, $p < 0.0001$; reverse quadrant: $F_{(1, 36)} = 5.74$, $p = 0.0219$, $n = 12–15$], confirming efficient spatial memory. While both male and female LOU rats favored the target quadrant in the learning probe test [**Figure 2H**, Two-Way ANOVA quadrant effect males: $F_{(1, 17)} = 30.42, p < 0.0001$; females: $F_{(1, 16)} = 44.02, p < 0.0001$], the difference was significant only for females during the reverse probe trial [males: $F_{(1, 17)} = 4.03$, $p = 0.0608$; females: $F_{(1, 16)} = 5.60$, $p = 0.031$].

LTCR PREVENTS AGE-RELATED BW GAIN AND RECOGNITION MEMORY DEFICITS IN SD RATS

Cognitive functions generally decline with aging in humans and metabolic disturbances related to diabetes and obesity can exacerbate these deficits. In fact, diabetes has been associated with declining cognitive performance in aging (Umegaki et al., 2013), and elevated levels of circulating glucose and insulin, as found in OAL SD rats, are prevented by LTCR (Bedard et al., 2010). In AL male SD rats, aging was associated with a large BW gain as previously reported (Bedard et al., 2010, 2013; Moyse et al., 2012). In 20-month-old AL rats, BW was 216% higher than in YAL rats, and LTCR prevented this increase [**Figure 3A**, One-Way ANOVA, $F_{(2, 21)} = 73.49, p < 0.0001, n = 5–11$].

In the NOR task, 20-month-old AL SD rats spent 32, 12, and 26% less time with the novel objects than YAL rats after 5-min, 60-min, and 24-h delays, respectively (**Figure 3B**). Interestingly, LTCR prevented this decline [diet effect: Two-Way ANOVA, $F_{(1, 42)} = 16.55, p = 0.0012, n = 5–11$]. OAL SD rats' total interaction time with the objects decreased by 5–10% compared to YAL and OCR rats [**Figure 3C**, One-Way ANOVA, $F_{(2, 21)} = 7.343$, $p = 0.0038$, $n = 5–11$]. The decreases observed in OAL SD rats were not related to lower exploratory behavior, since no difference was observed in the total distance traveled in the NOR arena between age groups [**Figure 3D**; One-Way ANOVA, $F_{(2, 21)} = 0.2844, p = 0.7553, n = 5–11$].

We next evaluated if aging and diet affects spatial memory in this rat strain using the MWM task. In the cued test, all SD rats learned to escape the pool after three trials [**Figure 3F**, time effect: Two-Way ANOVA, $F_{(2, 32)} = 10.39$, $p = 0.0003$, $n = 4–8$]. As shown in **Figure 3E**, YAL SD rats quickly learned to find the hidden platform (day 1–4). However, aging affected OAL rat performances, as this group exhibit longer escape latencies than younger rats on day 4 [One-Way ANOVA, $F_{(2, 16)} = 8.226$, $p = 0.0035$, $n = 4–8$]. The learning acquisition curve was significantly different for the OAL group compared to young animals [age effect: Two-Way ANOVA, $F_{(1, 30)} = 12.23$, $p = 0.0058$, $n = 4–8$], and LTCR appeared ineffective to improve spatial memory in old SD rats [diet effect: Two-Way ANOVA, $F_{(1, 27)} = 0.03$, $p = 0.8641$, $n = 4–7$]. However, a comparison of curve slopes revealed similar learning patterns for young and OCR rats (linear regression YAL: slope = −10.53, $R^2 = 0.8787$; OCR: slope = −11.69, $R^2 = 0.9402$, $n = 7–8$) while OAL latencies increased on day 4, affecting learning progress (linear regression OAL: slope = −10.15, $R^2 = 0.3241$, $n = 4$). In the reverse learning task, YAL SD rats quickly swam to the new hidden platform position (**Figure 3E**). Conversely, both OAL and OCR rats performed poorly [YAL vs. OAL: Two-Way ANOVA, $F_{(1, 30)} = 6.04$, $p = 0.0338$; YAL vs. OCR: Two-Way ANOVA, $F_{(1, 39)} = 5.82, p = 0.0314$, $n = 4–8$]. Comparison of curve slopes and coefficient of determination confirmed reverse memory deficits in old SD rats (linear regression YAL: slope = −8.42, $R^2 = 0.9397$; OAL: slope = −2.05, $R^2 = 0.1199$; OCR: slope = 0.09, $R^2 = 0.0004$, $n = 4–10$). Nonetheless, only OAL rats took significantly more time to escape the pool on day 9 in comparison to young animals [**Figure 3E**, One-Way ANOVA, $F_{(2, 16)} = 4.923, p = 0.0216$, $n = 4–8$]. Path lengths to reach the platform on training trials confirmed memory impairments for OAL rats with significant differences on day 4 [**Figure 3G**, One-Way ANOVA, $F_{(2, 16)} = 9.151, p = 0.0022, n = 4–8$] and 9 [One-Way ANOVA, $F_{(2, 16)} = 4.762$, $p = 0.0238$, $n = 4–8$]. In comparison to young animals, path length in the target quadrant was significantly lower for OCR rats in the learning probe test but distance traveled in the target quadrant was significantly higher for all SD rat groups when compared to the opposite quadrant [**Figure 3H**, Two-Way ANOVA learning quadrant: $F_{(1, 16)} = 68.87$, $p < 0.0001$], indicating intact memory retention. No significant difference was seen in the reverse probe test. Overall these results suggest that obese 20-month-old SD rat recognition memory is impaired and

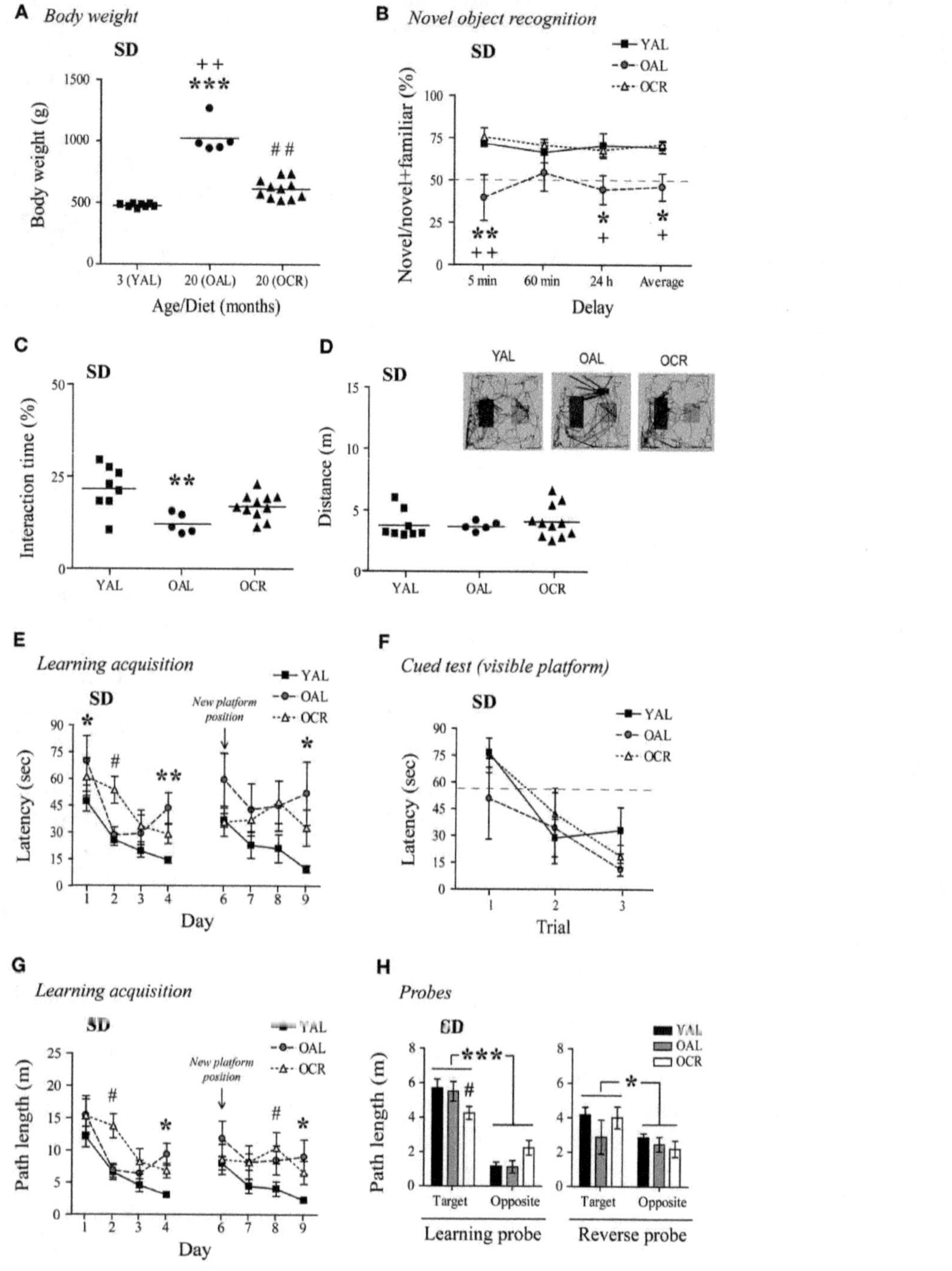

FIGURE 3 | Long-term caloric restriction prevents age-related body weight increase and minimizes the cognitive deficits observed in old AL male SD rats. (A) The age-related increase in BW is prevented by LTCR in SD rats (YAL, young *ad-libitum*-fed; OAL, old *ad-libitum*-fed; OCR, old calorie-restricted). **(B)** OAL SD rats spent less time interacting with novel objects on average and after a 5-min or 24-h delay compared to YAL and OCR rats. **(C)** OAL SD rats spent less time interacting with the objects during the test compared to YAL rats. **(D)** Distance traveled in the arena was not different between SD age groups. Representative paths (60 min delay) are shown with novel object on the right side. **(E)** MWM learning acquisition curves of the YAL, OAL, and OCR SD rats (three trials per day). Performances were significantly different when compared to YAL for OAL on day 1, 4, and 9, and OCR on day 2. These differences were not related to visual deficits, motor function, or lack of motivation to escape water as assessed by the cued test **(F)**. **(G)** Longer path lengths on the last day of both learning (day 4) and reversal learning (day 9) acquisition confirmed memory deficits in the OAL group. **(H)** Path length in the target quadrant was lower in OCR for the learning probe test (conducted 60 min after the last trial on day 4), while no difference was seen for the reverse probe test (60 min after the last trial on day 9). Path lengths were also significantly higher when compared to the opposite quadrant. Values are means ± s.e.m.; $n = 5$–11/age group ($n = 4$–8/age group for MWM, see Materials and Methods, for exclusion criteria). Significance of changes in BW, total interaction times, and distances traveled were determined by One-Way ANOVA followed by Bonferroni post-test. Significance of changes in percentages of time spent with novel objects, latencies, and path lengths were determined by Two-Way ANOVA followed by Bonferroni post-test, YAL vs. OAL: $^{*}p < 0.05$, $^{**}p < 0.01$, $^{***}p < 0.001$; YAL vs. OCR: $^{\#}p < 0.05$, $^{\#\#}p < 0.01$; OAL vs. OCR: $^{+}p < 0.05$, $^{++}p < 0.01$.

spatial memory acquisition less efficient in comparison to young animals. Interestingly, LTCR partially prevented these deficits.

ANXIETY IS LOW IN AGING LOU RATS AND REDUCED IN OLD CR SD RATS

Normal aging is associated with increased anxiety and cognitive decline in mice (Menard et al., 2013) and humans (Bunce et al., 2012). In adult mice, caloric restriction reduces anxiety-related behaviors (Yamamoto et al., 2009). Therefore, we studied stress responses and explorative behavior in both aging rat models, using the EPM and OF tasks. In EPM, anxiety-like behaviors and exploration were measured by the distance traveled in the open arms of the maze. In the LOU rat strain, mature animals exhibited the highest exploratory behavior in the EPM open arms [**Figure 4A**, One-Way ANOVA, $F_{(3,\ 48)} = 4.061$, $p = 0.0119$] and aging did not increase their levels of anxiety (Y: 132.33 ± 38.27 cm, O/O: 184.64 ± 42.16 cm, $n = 12$–15). Male and female aging LOU rat exploratory activity was similar in this task (**Figure 4B**). Locomotor activity gradually increased with age to become significantly different for O/O LOU rats compared to other age groups [**Figure 4C**, One-Way ANOVA, $F_{(3,\ 48)} = 10.66$, $p < 0.0001$, $n = 12$–15]. This difference was associated with the female group (**Figure 4D**). In contrast, none of the AL 20-month-old SD rats explored the EPM open arms (**Figure 4E**, YAL: 16.50 ± 11.22 cm, OAL: 0 ± 0 cm, $n = 5$–8) despite intact locomotor activity (**Figure 4F**, YAL: 1388.2 ± 89.72 cm, OAL: 1499.05 ± 117.48 cm, $n = 5$–8). Interestingly, caloric restriction significantly enhanced both exploratory behavior [**Figure 4E**, One-Way ANOVA, $F_{(2,\ 21)} = 3.867$, $p = 0.0390$, 112.91 ± 46.68 cm, $n = 5$–11] and locomotor activity [**Figure 4F**, One-Way ANOVA, $F_{(2,\ 21)} = 7.163$, $p = 0.0042$, 1860.75 ± 92.58 cm, $n = 5$–11].

In contrast to EPM results, the distance traveled in the center area of the OF arena decreased with aging in LOU rats [**Figure 5A**, One-Way ANOVA, $F_{(3,\ 48)} = 12.03$, $p < 0.0001$, Y: 531.00 ± 57.21 cm, M: 438.92 ± 50.71 cm, O: 387.79 ± 36.31 cm,

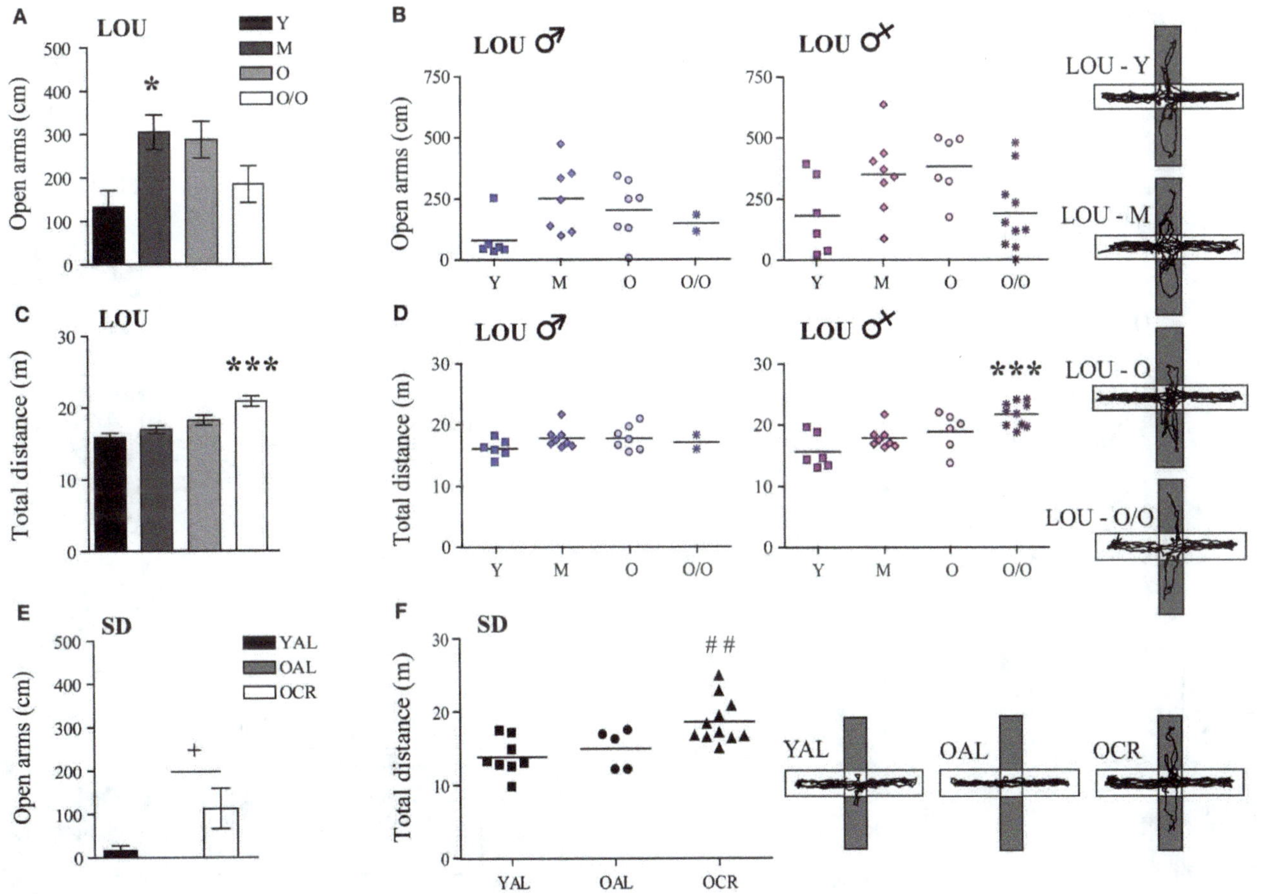

FIGURE 4 | LOU rats exhibit a low anxiety phenotype in the elevated plus maze task and LTCR reduces anxious behavior in old SD rats. (A) LOU rats traveled over 100 cm on the EPM open arms, revealing high explorative behaviors and low anxiety. **(B)** No significant difference was observed between aging male and female LOU rats. **(C)** Locomotor activity increased with age for the LOU rats to become significantly different in O/O rats. **(D)** This effect is specific to females. **(E)** OAL SD rats did not explore the EPM open arms, indicating stress-related anxious behaviors. LTCR enhanced explorative behaviors in old SD rats. **(F)** OCR SD rats traveled a higher total distance in the EPM arena compared to YAL rats, suggesting lower anxiety and higher explorative behavior in a bright environment. Representative paths are shown (open arms in gray). Values are means ± s.e.m.; *n SD* = 5–11/age group; *n LOU* = 12–15/age group. Significance of changes for distances traveled in the open arms and total distances were determined by One-Way ANOVA followed by Bonferroni post-test, $^{*}p < 0.05$, $^{***}p < 0.001$; YAL vs. OCR: $^{\#\#}p < 0.01$; OAL vs. OCR: $^{+}p < 0.05$.

O/O: 138.91 ± 37.29 cm, $n = 12–15$]. Both male and female O/O LOU rats displayed anxious behaviors (**Figure 5B**) although their locomotor activity remained stable [**Figure 5C**, One-Way ANOVA, $F_{(3, 48)} = 1.075$, $p = 0.3685$, $n = 12–15$] with no gender difference (**Figure 5D**). Nevertheless, in comparison to OAL SD rats, mean distances traveled in the center area were significantly higher for LOU rats up to 42 months of age [One-Way ANOVA, $F_{(4, 52)} = 16.01$, $p < 0.0001$, $n = 5–15$]. In fact, none of the OAL SD rats reached the center of the arena, suggesting a high anxiety state [**Figure 5E**, One-Way ANOVA, $F_{(2, 21)} = 5.922$, $p = 0.0091$, YAL: 222.78 ± 51.87 cm, OAL: 0 ± 0 cm, OCR: 91.68 ± 35.91 cm, $n = 5–11$]. Locomotor activity did not change significantly between SD groups [**Figure 5F**, One-Way ANOVA, $F_{(2, 21)} = 2.949$, $p = 0.0743$, $n = 5–11$]. Our results suggest that LTCR reduces anxiety-related behaviors associated with aging and that the obesity-resistant LOU rat strain could be considered as a low-anxiety phenotype.

CIRCULATING CORTICOSTERONE LEVELS ARE STABLE IN MATURE TO VERY OLD LOU RATS AND INCREASED IN AGING SD RATS WHILE PRODYNORPHIN IS OVEREXPRESSED IN THE HIPPOCAMPUS AND ENTORHINAL CORTEX OF OLD AL SD RATS

Stressful events inducing the release of glucocorticoids (GC) have been associated with memory impairments in older adults (Lupien et al., 2005). Exaggerated anxiety responses, as observed in OAL SD rats, may affect memory formation and consolidation by promoting GC production. Notably, plasma CORT levels have been correlated with cognitive ability in young mice (Harrison et al., 2009). As shown in **Figure 6A**, CORT level was increased in 12-months-old LOU rats compared to young animals; however, it remained stable thereafter up to 38 months [**Figure 6A**, age effect: One-Way ANOVA, $F_{(3, 44)} = 2.354$, $p = 0.0850$, $n = 10–15$]. Serum CORT was elevated in old SD rats with a significant difference for OCR SD rats [One-Way ANOVA, $F_{(2, 18)} = 2.823$, $p = 0.0858$, $n = 4–10$; YAL vs. OCR: $p < 0.05$, $n = 7–10$]

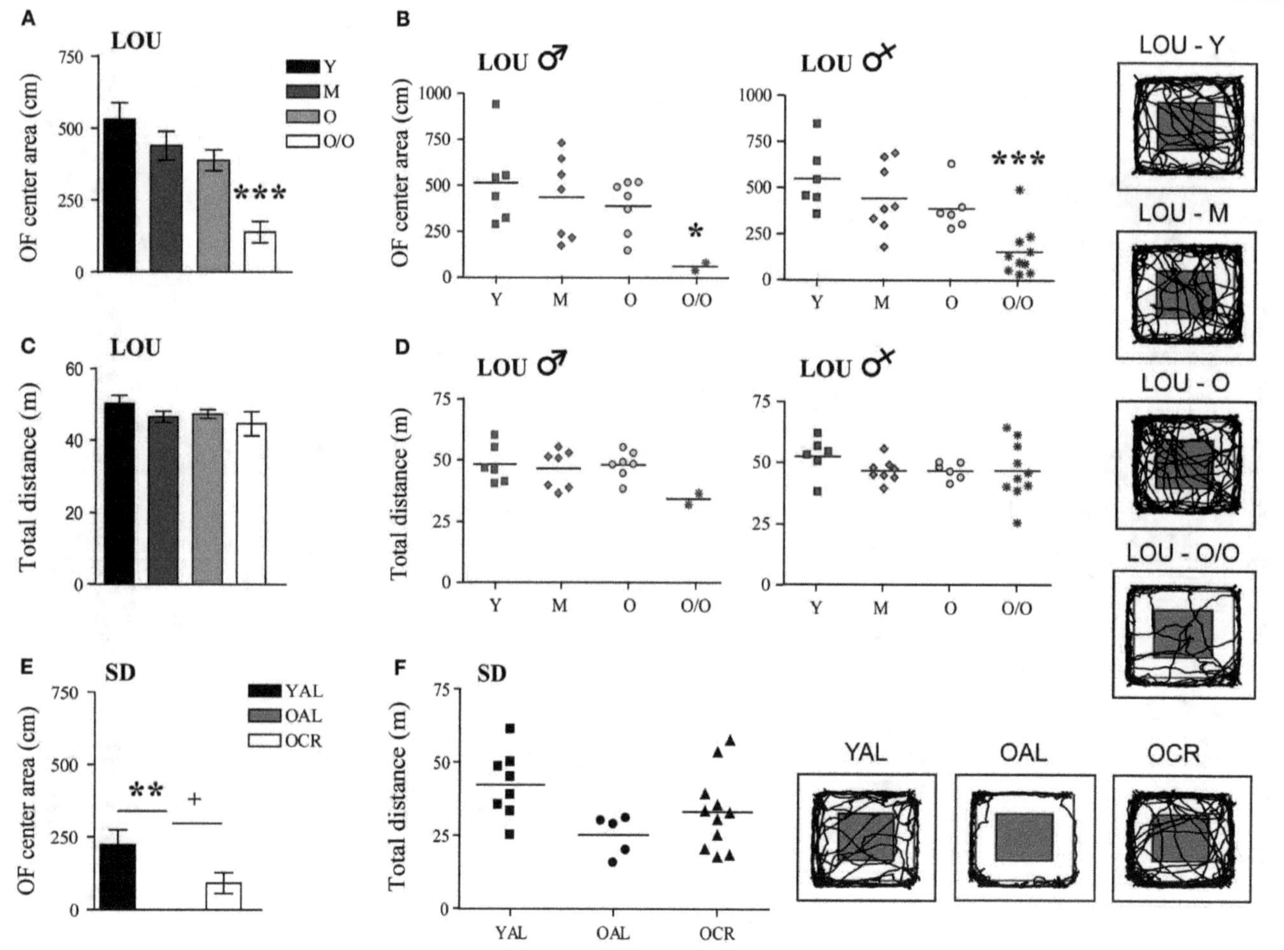

FIGURE 5 | Decreased anxiety-related behavior is observed in old LOU and CR SD rats in the open field task. (A) In contrast to EPM results, O/O LOU rat exploratory behavior in the OF center area of the arena was significantly reduced. **(B)** This difference was observed in both O/O males and females. Representative paths are shown (center area in gray). Neither aging **(C)** nor gender **(D)** affected total distances traveled. **(E)** OAL SD rats did not explore the center area, suggesting high anxiety as in the EPM test. LTCR prevented the development of anxious behavior as observed in OCR SD rats. **(F)** The total distance traveled was not significantly different between the three groups. Representative paths are shown. Values are means ± s.e.m.; n SD = 5–11/group; n LOU = 12–15/group. Significance of changes in distances traveled in the OF center area and total distances were determined by One-Way ANOVA followed by Bonferroni post-test, *$p < 0.05$, **$p < 0.01$, ***$p < 0.001$; OAL vs. OCR: $^{+}p < 0.05$.

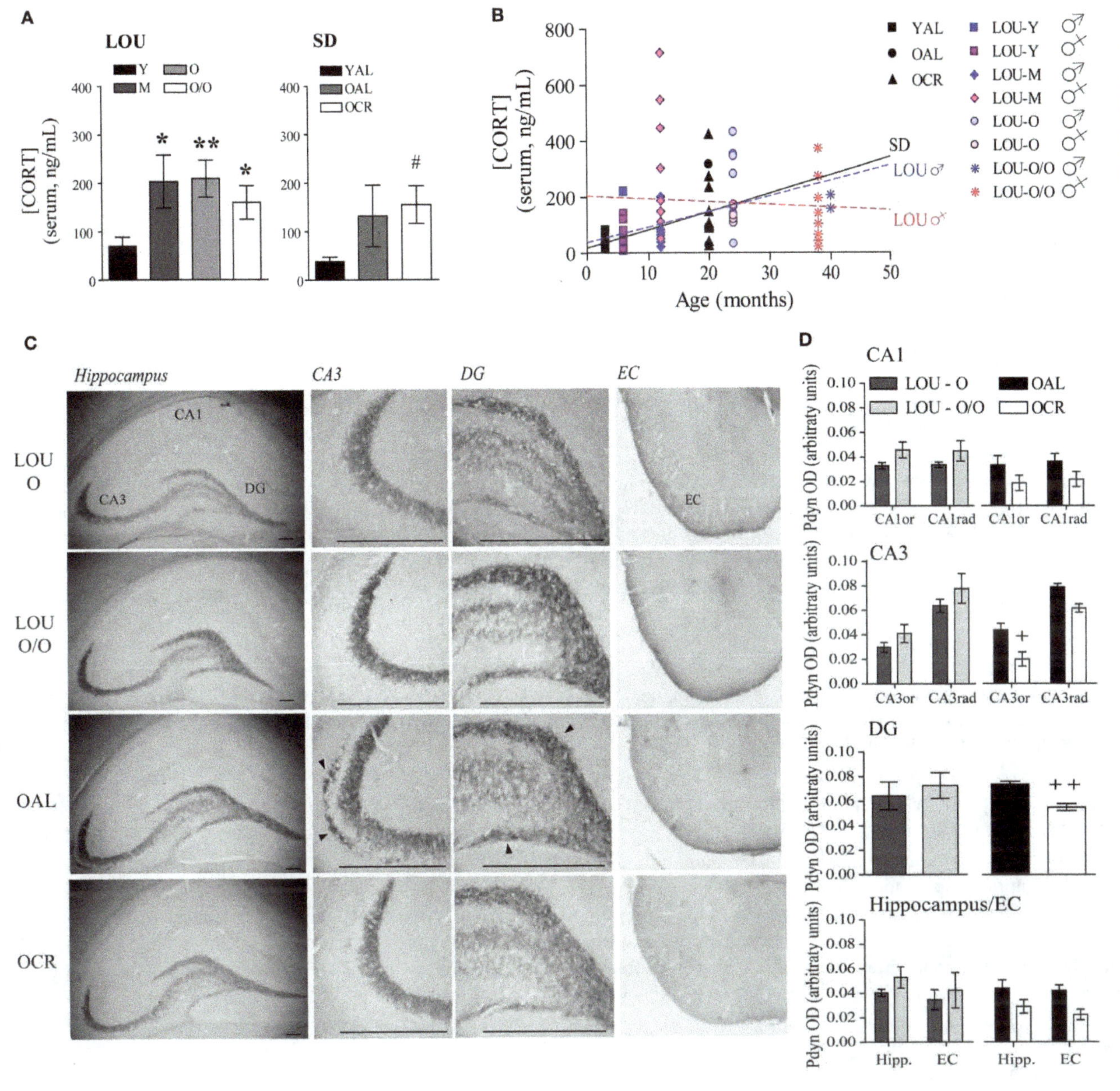

FIGURE 6 | The endogenous opioid prodynorphin is overexpressed in OAL SD rat hippocampus and entorhinal cortex. (A) Enhancement of circulating CORT was observed in 12-month-old LOU rats but remained stable thereafter. CORT levels increased in old SD rats and were significantly correlated with age in male SD and male LOU rats **(B)**. **(C)** Pdyn immunostaining is localized in the CA3 and DG hippocampal areas and entorhinal cortex. Scale bar at 500 μm. Arrowheads indicate Pdyn-positive cells. **(D)** While Pdyn is highly expressed in the hippocampus CA3 and DG of OAL SD rats in comparison to OCR animals, no difference was observed between O and O/O LOU rats. Values are means ± s.e.m.; $n = 15$ slices from three animals/group. Significance of changes in CORT levels was determined by One-Way ANOVA in each strain. Association of CORT levels with age was performed was assessed using Pearson's correlation. Changes in the intensity of immunostaining were determined using *t*-test for DG and Two-Way ANOVA followed by Bonferroni post-test for other brain regions, $^{*}p < 0.05$, $^{**}p < 0.01$; OAL vs. OCR: $^{+}p < 0.05$, $^{++}p < 0.01$.

consistent with previous findings in naive OCR rats (Bedard et al., 2010). We then examined the correlation between age and circulating CORT in each strain. While serum CORT significantly increased in 20-month-old SD rats in comparison to 3-month-old animals (**Figure 6B**, $p = 0.0268$, $R^2 = 0.2327$), no correlation was observed for young and aging LOU rats ($p = 0.3329$, $R^2 = 0.0203$). Interestingly, the correlation between CORT levels and age was significant for males ($p = 0.0154$, $R^2 = 0.2489$) but not females ($p = 0.7224$, $R^2 = 0.0056$) LOU rats.

The endogenous opioid peptides dynorphins are released during stress response and enhance anxiety-related behaviors (Wittmann et al., 2009; Bilkei-Gorzo et al., 2012). Since *Pdyn* gene expression generally increases in normal aging (Kotz et al., 2004) and has been associated with age-related cognitive deficits

(Nguyen et al., 2005; Menard et al., 2013), we examined the effect of LTCR on Pdyn levels in old SD brain. Strong Pdyn immunostaining was observed in the hippocampal CA3 region and dentate gyrus (DG) regions, as previously reported (Schwarzer, 2009) (**Figure 6C**). No significant difference was observed for LOU rats despite aging (**Figure 6D**, Two-Way ANOVA, O vs. O/O: CA1: $p = 0.1978$; CA3: $p = 0.3085$; DG: $p = 0.6176$; hippocampus/EC: $p = 0.4641$). However, quantification of immunostaining revealed a significant effect of LTCR on Pdyn expression in CA3 neurons [**Figure 6D**, OAL vs. OCR: Two-Way ANOVA, $F_{(1, 4)} = 13.72$, $p = 0.0208$, $n = 15$ slices from 3 rats/group] and DG (two-tailed *t*-test, $p = 0.0067$, $n = 15$ slices from 3 rats/group), in line with reduced anxiety-related behaviors. In comparison to OCR animals, Pdyn immunostaining was significantly higher in OAL hippocampus and EC [**Figure 6D**, Two-Way ANOVA, $F_{(1, 4)} = 24.50$, $p = 0.0078$, $n = 15$ slices from 3 rats/group]. Comparison of Pdyn expression between LOU and OCR rats revealed no significant difference between O, O/O LOU, and OCR rats [Two-Way ANOVA, CA1: $p = 0.0554$; CA3: $p = 0.1483$; DG: $p = 0.2755$; hippocampus/EC: $p = 0.1929$]. The hippocampal CA3 region is essential for encoding novelty and pattern separation (Kesner, 2007) and glutamate receptor function in this area was recently tied to individual differences in cognitive aging (Yang et al., 2013). In contrast, EC has been closely associated with working memory (Traissard et al., 2007; Newmark et al., 2013). Higher Pdyn expression in these brain areas could reduce glutamatergic transmission (Wagner et al., 1993) and impaired synaptic plasticity underlying memory processes in the OAL SD rat brain.

GLUTAMATE RECEPTOR LEVELS REMAIN UNCHANGED IN AGING LOU RATS AND ARE INCREASED IN OLD CR SD RATS

Therefore, we assessed AMPA and NMDA receptor subunit levels in the hippocampus and adjacent cortices of aging LOU and SD rats. Tissue preparation included the whole hippocampus and adjacent cortices, since recognition memory has been related to the perirhinal cortex (Burke et al., 2011). Moreover, behavioral training was performed on a 4-week schedule, which implies consolidation of memories in the cortices (Frankland and Bontempi, 2005). Glutamate receptor protein levels were unaffected in the aging obesity-resistant LOU rat strain (**Figure 7A**). Moreover, no significant variation was observed between males and females (data not shown). In contrast, NMDA receptor subunit levels increased significantly in the brains of OCR SD rats compared to age-matched OAL rats [**Figure 7B**, Two-Way ANOVA, $F_{(1, 30)} = 4.66$, $p = 0.0390$, $n = 4–8$]. Metabotropic group 1 mGluRs play a crucial role in memory processes in the aging brain (Xu et al., 2009; Menard and Quirion, 2012a; Menard et al., 2013) and like ionotropic glutamate receptors mGluR1α and mGluR5 protein levels were maintained in the brain of aging LOU rats (**Figure 7A**). In contrast, protein levels of mGluR5 were significantly lower in the brain of OAL compared to OCR SD rats [**Figure 7B**, Two-Way ANOVA, $F_{(1, 20)} = 5.75$, $p = 0.0263$, $n = 4–8$] and young rats [Two-Way ANOVA, $F_{(1, 20)} = 6.69$, $p = 0.0177$, $n = 4–8$]. Moreover, higher protein levels were observed overall in old LOU rats compared to OAL SD rats [Two-Way ANOVA, $F_{(1, 60)} = 5.28$, $p = 0.0444$, $n = 4–8$] while the difference was not significant between old LOU and OCR SD rats [Two-Way ANOVA, $F_{(1, 84)} = 0.09$, $p = 0.7629$, $n = 8$], indicating that LTCR may insure memory protection by preventing age-related decrease of glutamate receptor expression. We investigated further expression pattern of glutamatergic synaptic markers independently between young LOU vs. SD rats. We obtained a significant difference for GluR1 ($p < 0.05$) when we analyzed AMPA receptor expression. Protein levels of NMDA NR2 subunits were also significantly increased in young LOU rats when compared to young SD rats ($p = 0.0392$).

mGluR5 receptors are enriched in the CA1 region of the hippocampus, which is crucial for working and spatial memory processing. Using immunohistochemistry, we compared mGluR5 staining in old LOU and SD rats. As shown in **Figure 7C**, mGluR5 immunoreactivity revealed intensely stained pyramidal neurons in the hippocampal CA1 region. mGluR5 staining was slightly increased in the CA1 *stratum radiatum* of O/O LOU rats compared to O LOU rats [CA1, O vs. O/O, Two-Way ANOVA, $F_{(1, 4)} = 4.64$, $p = 0.0976$, $n = 15$ slices/group from 3 animals]. Immunoreactivity was significantly higher in the CA1 pyramidal neurons of OCR in comparison to those of OAL SD rats [OAL vs. OCR, Two-Way ANOVA, $F_{(1, 4)} = 26.00$, $p = 0.0070$, $n = 15$ slices/group from 3 animals]. Finally, mGluR5 immunostaining was significantly enriched in the whole hippocampus and entorhinal cortex of OCR SD rats [**Figure 7C**, OAL vs. OCR, Two-Way ANOVA, $F_{(1, 4)} = 20.99$, $p = 0.0102$, $n = 15$ slices/group from 3 animals], while no difference was observed for LOU rats (**Figure 7C**).

Homer 1a AND Arc IMMEDIATE EARLY GENES ARE INVOLVED IN THE MAINTENANCE OF MEMORY FUNCTIONS IN AGING LOU RATS AND OLD CR SD RATS

Activation of glutamate receptors following behavioral training should lead to expression of IEG necessary to consolidate memories (Inoue et al., 2009; Czerniawski et al., 2011). In fact, down-regulation of IEG expression has been associated with memory impairments in aged rats (Rowe et al., 2007; Benoit et al., 2011; Penner et al., 2011; Menard and Quirion, 2012b). Scaffolding protein Homer 1a regulates group 1 mGluR activation and reduced levels have been associated with memory impairments (Menard and Quirion, 2012b; Kaja et al., 2013). On the other hand, IEG *Arc* is considered a master regulator of synaptic plasticity (Shepherd and Bear, 2011). Along with youthful levels of glutamate receptor and intact cognitive abilities, Homer 1a and Arc protein levels were unaltered in the hippocampal formation and adjacent cortices of aging LOU rats (**Figure 8A**). No significant variation was observed between males and females (data not shown). In line with cognitive deficits, both Homer 1a and Arc levels were significantly lower in the brains of OAL SD rats when compared to young animals [**Figure 8B**, YAL vs. OAL, Two-Way ANOVA, $F_{(1, 20)} = 9.63$, $p = 0.0056$, $n = 4–8$] and LTCR prevented this change [**Figure 8B**, OAL vs. OCR, Two-Way ANOVA, $F_{(1, 20)} = 13.01$, $p = 0.0018$, $n = 4–8$]. Zif 268, another IEG involved in the early steps of memory consolidation (Alberini, 2009), was unaltered in aging LOU and SD rats (**Figures 8A,B**). Homer 1a (**Figure 8C**)

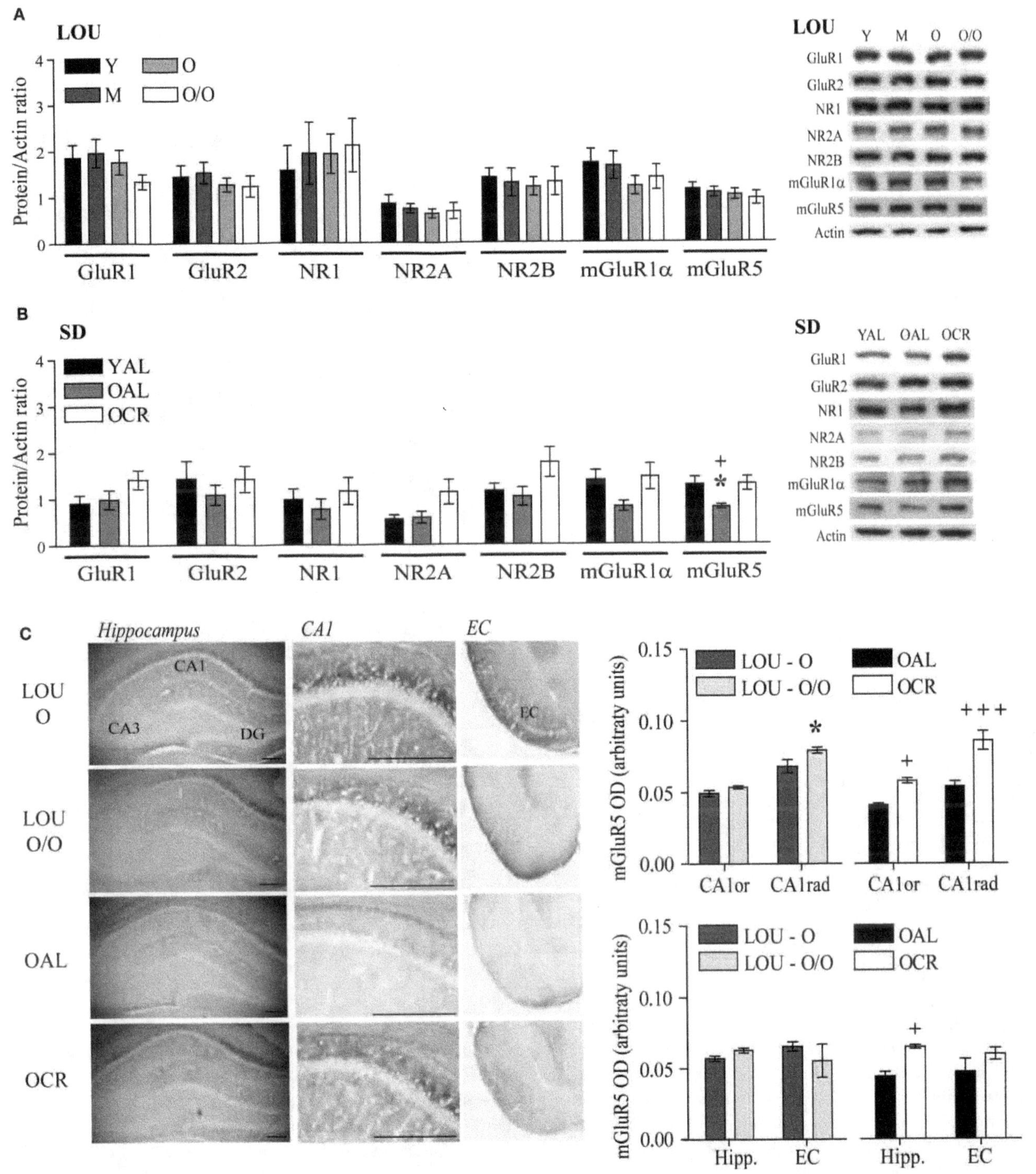

FIGURE 7 | Glutamate receptor levels are unaltered in aging LOU rats and mGluR5 expression is increased by LTCR in the hippocampus of old SD rats. (A) No change for ionotropic AMPA GluR1, GluR2, NMDA NR1, NR2A, NR2B, and metabotropic mGluR1α and mGluR5 protein level was observed in LOU rat hippocampal formation up to 38–42 months of age. **(B)** mGluR5 receptor level was significantly reduced in OAL compared to young and OCR SD rats. **(C)** Quantification of immunostaining revealed higher mGluR5 expression in CA1 and overall hippocampus of OCR rats compared to OAL and a slight increase in the CA1 *stratum radiatum* (CA1rad) of O/O LOU rats. Western blot values are means ± s.e.m. of eight individual experiments and data are expressed as protein/actin ratio. Representative blots of glutamate receptor subunits and actin loading control are shown for each rat group. *n LOU* = 8/age group, *n SD* = 4–8/age group. For immunohistochemistry, values are means ± s.e.m.; *n* = 15 slices from three animals/group. Scale bar at 500 μm. Significance of changes was determined by Two-Way ANOVA followed by Bonferroni post-test, $^{*}p < 0.05$; OAL vs. OCR: $^{+}p < 0.05$, $^{+++}p < 0.001$.

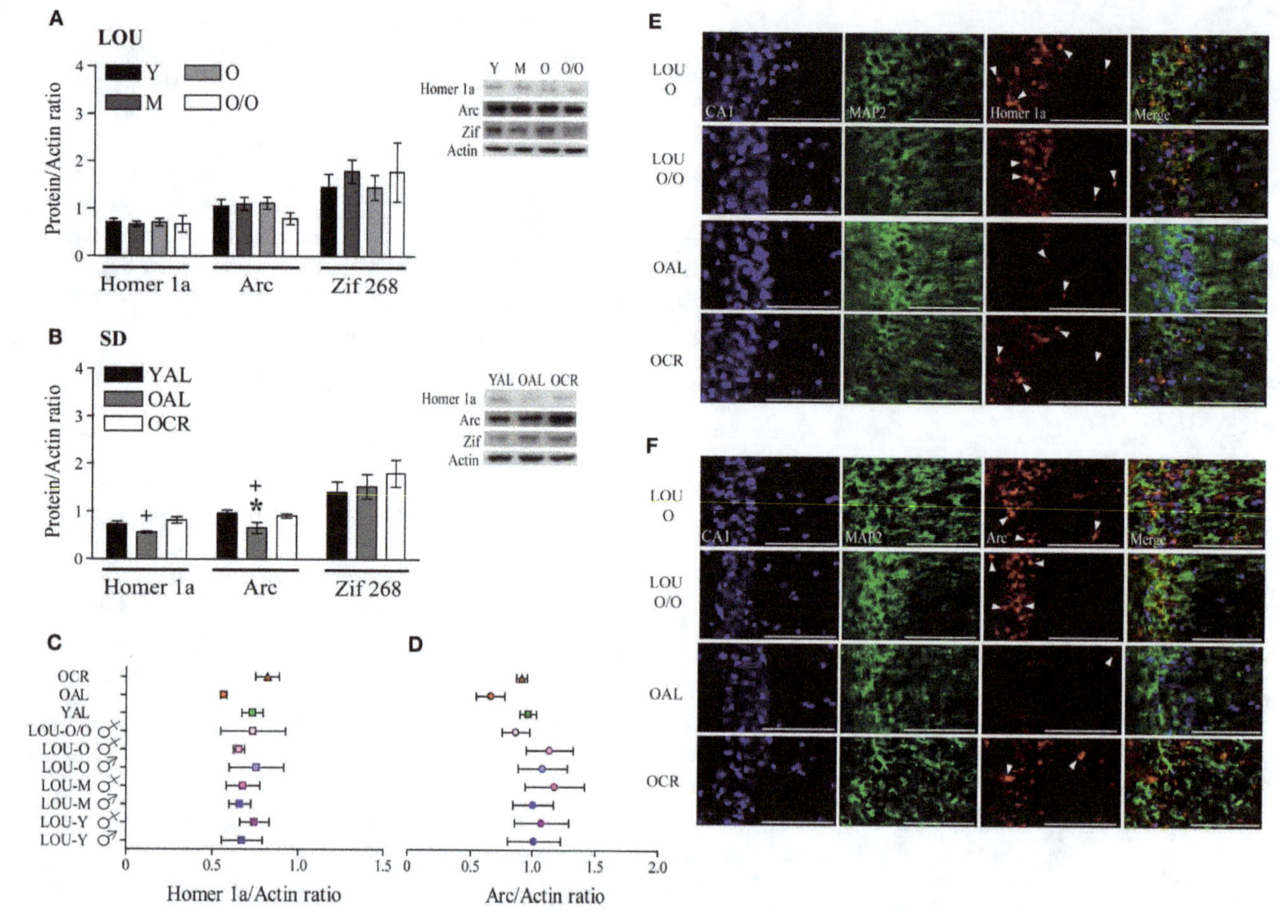

FIGURE 8 | Immediate early genes *Homer 1a* and *Arc* protein levels are maintained in the hippocampal formation of O and O/O LOU and OCR SD rats. (A) In line with intact cognition and youthful levels of glutamate receptors, Homer 1a, Arc, and Zif 268 expression remained unchanged in aging LOU rats after MWM reactivation. **(B)** Conversely, both Homer 1a and Arc expression was decreased in old AL memory-impaired SD rats, in comparison to OCR rats which are characterized by intact recognition memory and spatial learning acquisition. Representative blots of IEG protein levels and actin loading control are shown for each rat group. Comparison of IEG protein levels between all rat groups is shown for Homer 1a **(C)** and Arc **(D)**. **(E)** Homer 1a co-immunolabeling with the neuronal marker microtubule-associated protein 2 (MAP2) confirmed higher expression of this IEG in aging LOU and OCR SD rats pyramidal cells compared to OAL SD rats. **(F)** Arc staining was also enhanced in the CA1 area of these rats compared to that of OAL SD rats. Western blot values are means ± s.e.m. of eight separate experiments and data are expressed as ratio of protein/actin levels. *n LOU* = 8/age group; *n SD* = 4–8/age group. Scale bar at 100 μm. Arrowheads indicate IEG-positive cells. Significance of changes for IEG protein levels were determined by Two-Way ANOVA followed by Bonferroni post-test, YAL vs. OAL: $^{*}p < 0.05$; OAL vs. OCR: $^{+}p < 0.05$.

and Arc (**Figure 8D**) protein levels are similar in all rat groups except for the OAL SD rats. An age-related decrease of *Arc* gene transcription has been reported in the pyramidal cells of the hippocampus CA1 region of memory-impaired Fischer-344 rats (Penner et al., 2011). Since glutamate receptors mGluR5 are enriched in this area (**Figure 7C**) alterations of *Homer 1a* expression following behavioral training could be expected as well. Co-localization of Homer 1a with the neuronal marker microtubule-associated protein 2 (MAP2) revealed more positive cells in the CA1 region of old and very old LOU and OCR SD rats than in OAL animals (**Figure 8E**), which is in line with better cognitive performances. Similarly, Arc expression was lower in the CA1 region of OAL SD rats compared to other groups (**Figure 8F**).

COGNITIVE PERFORMANCES AND ANXIOUS BEHAVIORS ARE ASSOCIATED WITH GLUTAMATERGIC SIGNALING AND STRESS-RELATED MARKERS

We studied the association between physiological parameters (age, BW), cognition (NOR average), anxious behaviors (EPM open arms, OF center), serum CORT, glutamatergic receptors levels (GluR1, GluR2, NR1, NR2A, NR2B, mGluR1α, mGluR5), and IEG expression (Homer 1a, Arc, Zif268) using PCA. When data from all LOU and SD rats were pooled, 51.7% of the overall variance was explained by the first three components (**Figure 9A**). The main component, corresponding to 27.6% of the variance, was characterized by 13 out of 16 variables on the positive side (**Figure 9B**), with the exception of age, BW, and Zif268. Next, the impact of rat strain on the correlation matrix was assessed

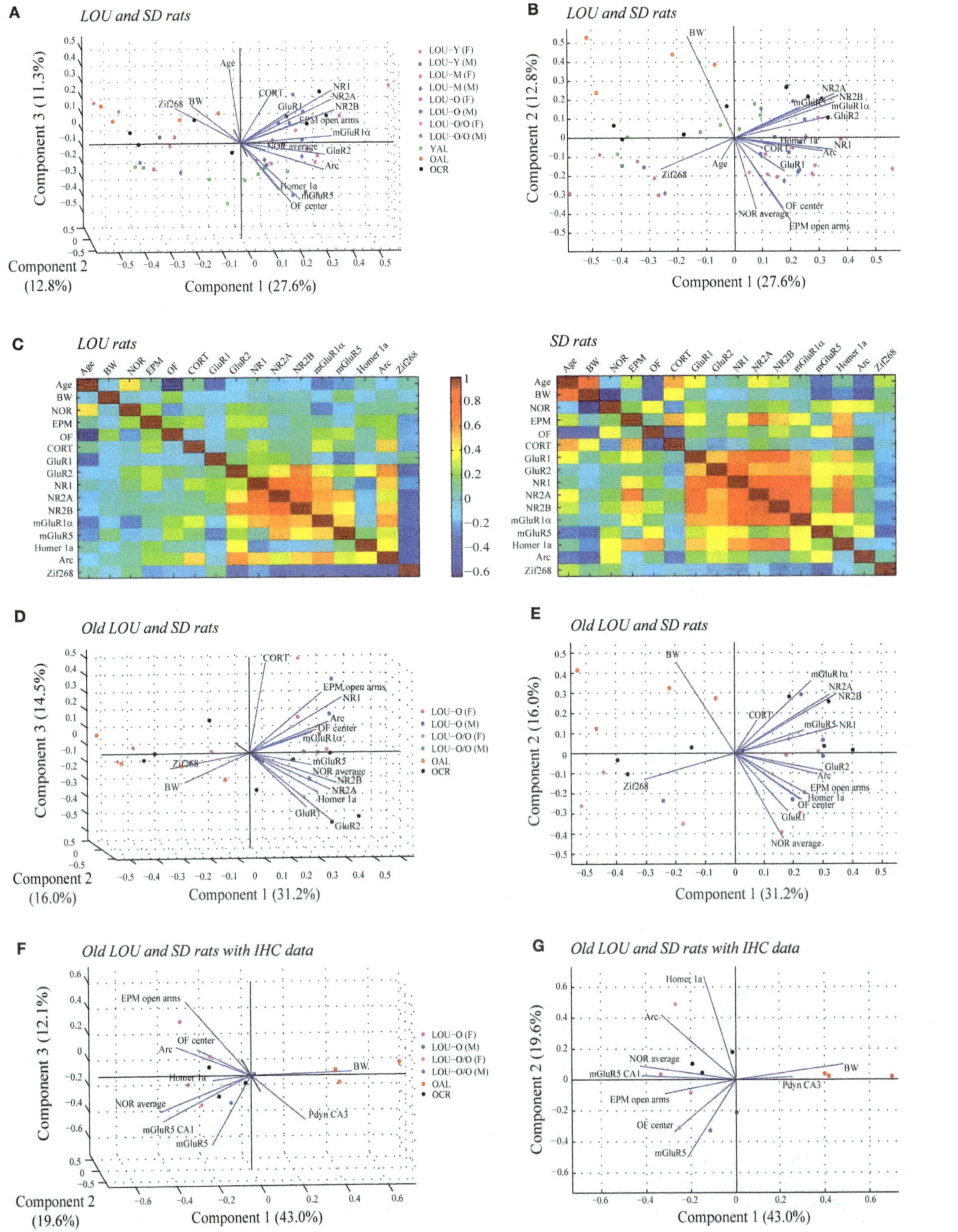

FIGURE 9 | Associations between physiological parameters, cognition, anxious behaviors, glutamatergic signaling, and stress-related markers in aging LOU and SD rats. (A) Biplot of the principal component coefficients and scores (first three components) of all LOU and SD rats data sets for 16 variables including physiological parameters (age, BW), cognition (NOR average), anxious behaviors (EPM open arms, OF center), stress marker (serum CORT), glutamatergic receptor levels (GluR1, GluR2, NR1, NR2A,

(Continued)

FIGURE 9 | Continued
NR2B, mGluR1α, mGluR5), and IEG expression (Homer 1a, Arc, Zif268) ($n = 50$, 16 variables). **(B)** Two-dimensional view of the first and second components of **(A)**. **(C)** Correlation matrix for pairs of variables for each rat strain. **(D)** Biplot showing the result of the PCA of old LOU (O, O/O) and SD (OAL, OCR) rats for the 16 variables except age ($n = 26$, 15 variables). **(E)** Two-dimensional view of the first and second component of **(D)**. **(F)** PCA analysis of the 12 rats with IHC data for Pdyn and mGluR5 expression in the hippocampus. Variables include BW as physiological parameter, NOR average for cognition, EPM and OF performances as anxious behaviors, stress-related precursor protein Pdyn and glutamatergic signaling (mGluR5, Homer 1a, Arc) ($n = 12$, 9 variables). **(G)** Two-dimensional view of the first and second component of **(F)**.

for the 16 variables. As shown on **Figure 9C**, variation is greater in SD rats then LOU rats. Interestingly, there is a strong association among glutamatergic receptor levels and to some extent between glutamatergic receptor and IEG expression in both rat strains (LOU: positive with Arc, negative with Zif268; SD: positive with Homer 1a, negative with Zif268). In LOU rats, NOR and OF performances were affected by aging while BW had no significant impact. Conversely, BW had a strong negative correlative impact on NOR, OF, mGluR5, and Arc in SD rats. Age also affected serum CORT and ionotropic glutamate receptor levels in this strain. When PCA was repeated using only the aged rodents (O and O/O LOU rats, OAL and OCR SD rats), 61.7% of the overall variance was explained by the first three components (**Figure 9D**). The main component, corresponding to 31.2% of the variance, was again characterized by all variables being on the positive side, except for BW and Zif268 (**Figure 9E**). Finally, we tested our conceptual framework using only the 12 rats for which we had IHC data. We studied the association between BW, cognition, anxious behaviors, stress-related precursor protein Pdyn expression in CA3, and glutamatergic signaling (mGluR5, mGluR5 in CA1, Homer 1a and Arc). The first three components of the PCA explained 74.7% of the overall variance with the main component corresponding to 43.0% of the variance (**Figure 9F**). Increased BW and hippocampal Pdyn expression appears to have a negative effect on behaviors and mGluR5 receptor level and related IEG (**Figure 9G**). Finally, as shown in **Table 1**, the main contributors of the first component are BW, cognition, anxious behaviors, Pdyn level, mGluR5 expression in CA1, and IEG Arc, leading us to suggest an association between these variables in healthy aging.

Table 1 | Major contributions to the overall variance on the first, second, and third principal components resulting from the principal component analysis (PCA, Figures 9F,G) applied to old and very old male and female LOU rats ($n = 6$) and old SD rats ($n = 6$) with IHC data.

	Components		
	1st (43.0%)	2nd (19.6%)	3rd (12.1%)
PHYSIOLOGICAL PARAMETER			
BW	**0.481**	0.101	0.010
COGNITION			
NOR average	**−0.425**	0.091	−0.294
EMOTIONAL BEHAVIORS			
EPM open arms	**−0.315**	−0.089	**0.592**
OF center	**−0.273**	**−0.334**	**0.262**
STRESS-RELATED MARKER			
Pdyn CA3	**0.256**	0.019	**−0.348**
GLUTAMATERGIC SIGNALING			
mGluR5	−0.214	**−0.497**	**−0.447**
mGluR5 CA1	**−0.418**	0.026	**−0.357**
Homer 1a	−0.139	**0.663**	−0.155
Arc	**−0.329**	**0.417**	0.150

Higher loading factors (> ±0.25) for each component of the PCA are indicated in bold.

DISCUSSION

In the present study, obesity-resistant LOU rats were characterized by intact recognition and spatial memory, high levels of hippocampal and EC glutamate receptor and related IEG as well as low anxiety and *Pdyn* expression despite aging. LTCR prevented high BW and favor an increase of glutamate receptor and IEG expression, facilitating memory consolidation. Anxious behaviors were associated with elevated *Pdyn* expression in OAL SD rat hippocampus/EC.

Age-related recognition memory decline is common in animal models and humans (Burke et al., 2012) but somehow remains controversial in rats (Markowska et al., 1998; Shukitt-Hale et al., 2001; Carter et al., 2009). Intact recognition memory was reported in 24-month-old male LOU rats and related to unaltered NMDA-mediated synaptic plasticity in the CA1 hippocampal region (Kollen et al., 2010). Here, the impact of aging on memory was investigated in detail, both in male and female rats from adulthood up to very old age. Since median lifespan of LOU rats is higher than common rat strains (Alliot et al., 2002), memory impairments could be expected to occur at a more advanced age. However, intact recognition memory was observed up to 42 months of age in line with stable expression of glutamate receptor subunits. In addition, we report the performances of aging LOU rats for learning acquisition, reversal learning, and memory retention in the MWM reference task, which is extensively used to discriminate memory-impaired from memory-unimpaired aged rats (Burke et al., 2012; Menard and Quirion, 2012b; Yang et al., 2013). All LOU rats performed well in the MWM task except the 24-month-old male in the learning acquisition task. Nevertheless, improvement was similar to young animals and an extra day of training might be required in future studies to confirm whether or not this function in impaired in old male LOU rats. In contrast, 24-month-old AL male SD rats were shown to develop memory impairments and to exhibit lower NMDA receptor levels and function compared to young rats (Kollen et al., 2010). We observed significant recognition memory impairments in 20-month-old AL SD rats and this deficit was prevented by LTCR. Caloric restriction was shown to facilitate learning consolidation through mechanisms dependent of NMDA receptors in adult mice (Fontan-Lozano et al., 2007). In $F_{344} \times$ BN rats, LTCR stabilizes age-related decreases of ionotropic glutamate receptors (Adams et al., 2008). Here we report a strong association between AMPA GluR1 and GluR2, NMDA NR1, NR2A, NR2B, and mGluR1α protein levels in SD rats. In contrast, LOU rat correlation matrix revealed an association between NMDA and group 1 mGluR levels and to some extent, GluR2, but not with GluR1. Moreover, GluR1 level was positively associated with cognition and low anxious behaviors in SD but not in LOU rats. NMDA-mediated synaptic plasticity involves efficient AMPA receptor trafficking (Huganir and Nicoll, 2013). However, insertion of GluR1 homomeric receptors in synaptic membranes can lead to AMPA-mediated excitotoxicity (Menard et al., 2007) as GluR2 subunits are recognized to confer calcium impermeability to AMPA receptors (Sommer et al., 1991; Geiger et al., 1995). Strain-related differences in hippocampal learning tasks and regulation of AMPA receptors have been previously reported in mice (Upchurch and Wehner, 1988, 1989; Rossi-Arnaud and Ammassari-Teule, 1998; Menard et al., 2004) but, to our knowledge, not in rats yet. In addition, we found that the memory status of OAL SD rats varies between individuals as well as the impact of LTCR. Variability of age-associated memory decline within the SD rat strain has previously been described and seems to appear only with increasing age (Kollen et al., 2010). Furthermore, individual differences are known to exist in aging rat populations (Zyzak et al., 1995; Menard and Quirion, 2012b). Accordingly, in our study variations are very low for both recognition and spatial memory tasks in young SD but increase with aging. Here, we show that LTCR improved spatial memory performances of old SD rats but did not completely prevent age-related cognitive deficits despite maintenance of youthful NMDA receptor expression. The impact of caloric restriction on cognitive aging seems to be highly dependent of the rat strain and genetic variance (Markowska and Savonenko, 2002).

Group 1 mGluR function and signaling in the hippocampus CA1 and CA3 regions correlates with successful cognitive aging in rats (Lee et al., 2005; Menard and Quirion, 2012b; Yang et al., 2013), and mGluR5$^{-/-}$ mice show impairments in inhibitory learning and spatial memory (Xu et al., 2009). In line with intact memory, mGluR5 expression was maintained throughout life in LOU rats. Interestingly, LTCR prevented the decrease of mGluR5 observed in the hippocampus of old SD rats. A reduction of hypothalamic mGluR5 activation was shown to mediate appetite and BW increase in mGluR5$^{-/-}$ mice (Bradbury et al., 2005). Thus, a lack of mGluR5 might reduce susceptibility to diet-induced insulin resistance, since mGluR5$^{-/-}$ mice show decreased plasma levels of leptin and insulin, despite a 10-week high-fat diet (Bradbury et al., 2005). Improved leptin sensitivity has been reported in the young LOU rat (Veyrat-Durebex et al., 2013) and could be related to unaltered BW despite aging. Our group recently showed that age-related recognition and spatial memory deficits can be reversed following injections of an mGluR5 agonist (Menard et al., 2013). While young adult animals seem to rely on NMDA receptor function to establish and consolidate memories, mGluR function becomes crucial in the old hippocampus (Menard et al., 2013; Yang et al., 2013). Thus, a lower mGluR5 expression in OAL SD rat brain might be a consequence of obesity, affecting memory processes at advanced age.

To our knowledge, this study is also the first one to examine the impact of age-related obesity on the expression of IEG linked to memory formation and consolidation. *Homer 1a* is a dominant negative modulator of group 1 mGluR activity (Kammermeier and Worley, 2007), and its expression is experience-dependent (Nikbakht et al., 2012). Both reduction (Menard and Quirion, 2012b; Kaja et al., 2013) and overexpression (Klugmann et al., 2005) of Homer 1a levels have been associated with memory deficits, highlighting a tightly regulated expression. Here we report a strong association in SD rats between protein levels of Homer 1a, AMPA GluR1, and NMDA receptor subunits. *Homer 1a* modulates the efficacy of synaptic transmission (Inoue et al., 2007) and may facilitate NMDA-mediated synaptic plasticity in aging SD rats. LTCR could help maintaining youthful levels of ionotropic glutamate receptors and Homer 1a, favoring activity-induced synaptic plasticity and then prevent, to some extent, age-related memory-impairments in OCR rats. Interestingly, Homer 1a expression was also positively correlated with exploratory behaviors in the EPM and OF tasks in this strain. Our group recently reported low anxious behaviors and elevated Homer 1a expression in the hippocampus of aged Pdyn KO mice (Menard et al., 2013). The IEG *Arc* is necessary for memory consolidation and successful cognitive aging in rodents (Penner et al., 2011; Menard and Quirion, 2012b; Menard et al., 2013), and post-training disruption of Arc expression impairs long-term memory (Holloway and McIntyre, 2011). LTCR prevented age-related reduction of Homer 1a and Arc expression following behavioral training in SD rats, in line with better cognitive performances. LOU rats were characterized by a strong association between NMDA receptor subunits, mGluR5 and Arc levels which were all negatively correlated to Zif268 expression. Intact NMDA-mediated synaptic plasticity was reported in the CA1 hippocampal region of 24-month-old LOU rats (Kollen et al., 2010). On the other hand, group 1 mGluR-mediated synaptic plasticity has been associated with successful cognitive aging (Menard et al., 2013; Yang et al., 2013), formation of spatial (Lu et al., 1997; Balschun et al., 1999; Menard and Quirion, 2012b; Menard et al., 2013) and recognition memory (Barker et al., 2006; Christoffersen et al., 2008; Menard et al., 2013). Maintenance of both forms of synaptic plasticity in aging LOU rats could protect memory function up to a very advanced age. Following neuronal activity, Arc encoding mRNA is quickly transported to the dendrites and then translated (Bramham et al., 2008; Shepherd and Bear, 2011). This IEG has been associated to synapse-specific homeostatic plasticity (Beique et al., 2011) which is crucial for learning and memory processes and seems to be intact in the aging LOU rats. Strong association of Arc with glutamatergic receptor levels may explain better performances in the MWM reversal learning task for the LOU rat groups. Indeed, expression of this IEG is positively correlated with hippocampus-dependent spatial reversal learning (Guzowski et al., 2001). While the role of Arc in synaptic plasticity may cover several phases of memory formation, Zif268 is more important in the early steps of memory consolidation (Alberini, 2009). Prolonged training might decrease its expression in memory-unimpaired animals, such as the LOU rats. Interestingly, Zif268 expression is negatively correlated with mGluR5 in both rat strains, suggesting a strong interaction between those in successful cognitive processes in the aged brain.

Obesity-resistant LOU rats were also characterized by low hippocampal and EC Pdyn expression and stable circulating CORT. Low CORT has been reported in 20-week-old LOU rats

(Veyrat-Durebex et al., 2009). We found that serum CORT levels were higher in 12-month-old and older male rats than young ones but remained stable in females. This sexual dimorphism may explain, at least in part, the differences observed in spatial learning acquisition and reverse probe test. Older LOU rats may also be less sensitive to CORT than other rat strains (Marissal-Arvy et al., 2007) which would dampen stress-induced learning and memory deficits. Caloric restriction increases CORT release in adult (Levay et al., 2010) and old animals (Bedard et al., 2010). Beneficial effects provided by dietary restriction can be enhanced by reducing GC production (Qiu et al., 2012), suggesting that lowering circulating CORT in old SD rats may help preventing spatial memory impairments. Anxiety-related behaviors in the EPM task can be reduced after 8 days of caloric restriction in adult mice (Yamamoto et al., 2009). Here, we provide the first evidence that age-related exacerbated anxiety can be prevented by LTCR. Short-term food deprivation reduces Pdyn level in the arcuate nucleus (Kim et al., 1996), and we found that LTCR significantly decreases this stress-related peptide expression in the aged hippocampus. Therefore, LOU rats might be more resilient to stressful events (Russo et al., 2012). Resilience has been associated with increased lifespan (Vahia et al., 2011), which is a characteristic of this rat strain, as shown by Alliot et al. (2002) and extended here.

Stress and elevated circulating CORT can induce cognitive impairments (Landfield et al., 1981; Bodnoff et al., 1995; Lupien et al., 2005; Sandi, 2011). Enhanced serum CORT were found in naïve 20-month-old CR SD rats but not in age-matched AL rats (Bedard et al., 2010), raising the hypothesis that behavioral training might promote sustained threat perception in OAL SD rats, exacerbating basal levels of stress response effectors (O'Donovan et al., 2013). Accordingly, *Pdyn* expression was significantly increased in OAL hippocampus and EC. Activation of κ-opioid receptors (KOR), the main target of dynorphins, suppresses glutamate release (Simmons et al., 1994), and KOR activation mediates stress-induced memory deficits (Carey et al., 2009). Reduction of *Pdyn* gene expression protects old mice from cognitive impairments and anxious behaviors through upregulation of group 1 mGluR expression and function (Menard et al., 2013) and may favor AMPA GluR1 and NMDA NR2B expression in the aged brain (Menard et al., 2014). Both group 1 mGluR function and *Homer 1* expression have been associated with stress-induced cognitive deficits (Tronson et al., 2010; Menard et al., 2013; Wagner et al., 2013), and anxious behaviors are exacerbated by aging in the mGluR5$^{-/-}$ mice (Inta et al., 2013). Age-related obesity, as observed in OAL SD rats, could affect multiple neurotransmitters and modulators leading to exacerbated anxiety and memory deficits. In contrast, LOU rats may be protected from these alterations through a better regulation of brain plasticity-related genes during aging (Paban et al., 2012).

In summary, intact recognition and spatial memory in the obese-resistant LOU rat strain is associated with low anxiety responses, low levels of the stress-related *Pdyn* in the hippocampus and EC and enhanced expression of synaptic plasticity effectors at the cellular and molecular level. On the other hand, age-related weight gain affects lifespan, glutamate receptors and IEG expression, exacerbates anxiety and induced memory deficits. Nutritional intervention such as adult-onset LTCR can prevent age-induced reduction of glutamate receptor expression and signaling in SD rats, in line with the results obtained for the LOU rats but does not allow to completely preserve youthful spatial memory. Future studies will therefore be necessary to confirm if LTCR has the same effect on other rat strains including Wistar rats since LOU rats are thought to be of Wistar origin (Alliot et al., 2002). Whole genome or exome sequencing of the LOU rat will also have to be performed to allow determining if this strain is indeed originating from the Wistar stain. Another set of interesting experiments would be to evaluate if high-fat diet can induce obesity in aging LOU rats and affect cognition and/or lifespan. Finally, whether or not preservation of healthy memory functions in the aging LOU rat is related to a general or tissue-specific mechanism will deserve further attention. However, our results support a novel conceptual framework and highlight potential pharmacological targets to treat cognitive decline and anxious behaviors associated with aging-related obesity.

AUTHOR CONTRIBUTIONS

Caroline Ménard, Rémi Quirion, Guylaine Ferland, and Pierrette Gaudreau designed research; Caroline Ménard performed research; Caroline Ménard and Sylvain Bouchard analyzed data; Caroline Ménard, Sylvain Bouchard, and Pierrette Gaudreau interpreted the data; Caroline Ménard, Rémi Quirion, Guylaine Ferland, and Pierrette Gaudreau wrote the paper.

ACKNOWLEDGMENTS

This research was supported by grants from the Canadian Institutes of Health Research (CIHR) to Rémi Quirion and the Quebec Network for Research on Aging (a network funded by the *Fonds de recherche du Québec – Santé*) to Pierrette Gaudreau and Guylaine Ferland. Caroline Menard was the recipient of a postdoctoral fellowship from the CIHR. The authors are deeply grateful to Professor Josette Alliot (Université Blaise Pascal, Clermont-Ferrant, FR) for providing the Quebec Network for Research on Aging with male and female LOU/C/jall rats to start the network LOU rat colony. They also thank Julie Bédard and Cordélia Cadieux for technical assistance.

REFERENCES

Adams, M. M., Shi, L., Linville, M. C., Forbes, M. E., Long, A. B., Bennett, C., et al. (2008). Caloric restriction and age affect synaptic proteins in hip- pocampal CA3 and spatial learning ability. *Exp. Neurol.* 211, 141–149. doi: 10.1016/j.expneurol.2008.01.016

Alberini, C. M. (2009). Transcription factors in long-term memory and synaptic plasticity. *Physiol. Rev.* 89, 121–145. doi: 10.1152/physrev.00017.2008

Alliot, J., Boghossian, S., Jourdan, D., Veyrat-Durebex, C., Pickering, G., Meynial- Denis, D., et al. (2002). The LOU/c/jall rat as an animal model of healthy aging? *J. Gerontol. A Biol. Sci. Med. Sci.* 57, B312–B320. doi: 10.1093/gerona/57.8.B312

Balschun, D., Manahan-Vaughan, D., Wagner, T., Behnisch, T., Reymann, K. G., and Wetzel, W. (1999). A specific role for group I mGluRs in hippocampal LTP and hippocampus-dependent spatial learning. *Learn. Mem.* 6, 138–152. doi: 10.1101/lm.6.2.138

Barker, G. R., Bashir, Z. I., Brown, M. W., and Warburton, E. C. (2006). A tempo- rally distinct role for group I and group II metabotropic glutamate receptors in object recognition memory. *Learn. Mem.* 13, 178–186. doi: 10.1101/lm.77806

Baudry, M., Bi, X., Gall, C., and Lynch, G. (2011). The biochemistry of memory: the 26year journey of a 'new and specific hypothesis.' *Neurobiol. Learn. Mem.* 95, 125–133. doi: 10.1016/j.nlm.2010.11.015

Bedard, K., Bedard, J., Rocheleau, G., Ferland, G., and Gaudreau, P. (2013). Aging and diets regulate the rat anterior pituitary and hypothalamic transcriptome. *Neuroendocrinology* 97, 146–159. doi: 10.1159/000338411

Bedard, K., Robinette, K., Ferland, G., and Gaudreau, P. (2010). Effects of long-term dietary interventions on pituitary growth hormone-releasing hormone recep- tor in aging rats and potential mechanisms of action. *Mech. Ageing Dev.* 131, 169–178. doi: 10.1016/j.mad.2010.01.003

Beique, J. C., Na, Y., Kuhl, D., Worley, P. F., and Huganir, R. L. (2011). Arc- dependent synapse-specific homeostatic plasticity. *Proc. Natl. Acad. Sci. U.S.A.* 108, 816–821. doi: 10.1073/pnas.1017914108

Benoit, C. E., Rowe, W. B., Menard, C., Sarret, P., and Quirion, R. (2011). Genomic and proteomic strategies to identify novel targets potentially involved in learning and memory. *Trends Pharmacol. Sci.* 32, 43–52. doi: 10.1016/j.tips.2010.10.002

Bilkei-Gorzo, A., Erk, S., Schurmann, B., Mauer, D., Michel, K., Boecker, H., et al. (2012). Dynorphins regulate fear memory: from mice to men. *J. Neurosci.* 32, 9335–9343. doi: 10.1523/JNEUROSCI.1034-12.2012

Bodnoff, S. R., Humphreys, A. G., Lehman, J. C., Diamond, D. M., Rose, G. M., and Meaney, M. J. (1995). Enduring effects of chronic corticosterone treatment on spatial learning, synaptic plasticity, and hippocampal neuropathology in young and mid-aged rats. *J. Neurosci.* 15, 61–69.

Bradbury, M. J., Campbell, U., Giracello, D., Chapman, D., King, C., Tehrani, L., et al. (2005). Metabotropic glutamate receptor mGlu5 is a mediator of appetite and energy balance in rats and mice. *J. Pharmacol. Exp. Ther.* 313, 395–402. doi: 10.1124/jpet.104.076406

Bramham, C. R., Worley, P. F., Moore, M. J., and Guzowski, J. F. (2008). The imme- diate early gene arc/arg3.1: regulation, mechanisms, and function. *J. Neurosci.* 28, 11760–11767. doi: 10.1523/JNEUROSCI.3864-08.2008

Brim, B. L., Haskell, R., Awedikian, R., Ellinwood, N. M., Jin, L., Kumar, A., et al. (2012). Memory in aged mice is rescued by enhanced expression of the GluN2B subunit of the NMDA receptor. *Behav. Brain Res.* 238C, 211–226. doi: 10.1016/j.bbr.2012.10.026

Bunce, D., Batterham, P. J., Mackinnon, A. J., and Christensen, H. (2012). Depression, anxiety and cognition in community-dwelling adults aged 70 years and over. *J. Psychiatr. Res.* 46, 1662–1666. doi: 10.1016/j.jpsychires.2012.08.023

Burke, S. N., Ryan, L., and Barnes, C. A. (2012). Characterizing cognitive aging of recognition memory and related processes in animal models and in humans. *Front. Aging Neurosci.* 4:15. doi: 10.3389/fnagi.2012.00015

Burke, S. N., Wallace, J. L., Hartzell, A. L., Nematollahi, S., Plange, K., and Barnes, C. A. (2011). Age-associated deficits in pattern separation functions of the perirhinal cortex: a cross-species consensus. *Behav. Neurosci.* 125, 836–847. doi: 10.1037/a0026238

Carey, A. N., Lyons, A. M., Shay, C. F., Dunton, O., and McLaughlin, J. P. (2009). Endogenous kappa opioid activation mediates stress-induced deficits in learning and memory. *J. Neurosci.* 29, 4293–4300. doi: 10.1523/JNEUROSCI.6146- 08.2009

Carter, C. S., Leeuwenburgh, C., Daniels, M., and Foster, T. C. (2009). Influence of calorie restriction on measures of age-related cognitive decline: role of increased physical activity. *J. Gerontol. A Biol. Sci. Med. Sci.* 64, 850–859. doi: 10.1093/gerona/glp060

Christoffersen, G. R., Simonyi, A., Schachtman, T. R., Clausen, B., Clement, D., Bjerre, V. K., et al. (2008). MGlu5 antagonism impairs exploration and memory of spatial and non-spatial stimuli in rats. *Behav. Brain Res.* 191, 235–245. doi: 10.1016/j.bbr.2008.03.032

Czerniawski, J., Ree, F., Chia, C., Ramamoorthi, K., Kumata, Y., and Otto, T. A. (2011). The importance of having Arc: expression of the immediate- early gene Arc is required for hippocampus-dependent fear conditioning and blocked by NMDA receptor antagonism. *J. Neurosci.* 31, 11200–11207. doi: 10.1523/JNEUROSCI.2211-11.2011

Fadel, J. R., Jolivalt, C. G., and Reagan, L. P. (2013). Food for thought: the role of appetitive peptides in age-related cognitive decline. *Ageing Res. Rev.* 12, 764–776. doi: 10.1016/j.arr.2013.01.009

Fontan-Lozano, A., Saez-Cassanelli, J. L., Inda, M. C., De Los Santos-Arteaga, M., Sierra-Dominguez, S. A., Lopez-Lluch, G., et al. (2007). Caloric restric- tion increases learning consolidation and facilitates synaptic plasticity through mechanisms dependent on NR2B subunits of the NMDA receptor. *J. Neurosci.* 27, 10185–10195. doi: 10.1523/JNEUROSCI.2757-07.2007

Frankland, P. W., and Bontempi, B. (2005). The organization of recent and remote memories. *Nat. Rev. Neurosci.* 6, 119–130. doi: 10.1038/nrn1607

Geiger, J. R., Melcher, T., Koh, D. S., Sakmann, B., Seeburg, P. H., Jonas, P., et al. (1995). Relative abundance of subunit mRNAs determines gating and Ca2+ per- meability of AMPA receptors in principal neurons and interneurons in rat CNS. *Neuron* 15, 193–204. doi: 10.1016/0896-6273(95)90076-4

Guzowski, J. F., Setlow, B., Wagner, E. K., and McGaugh, J. L. (2001). Experience- dependent gene expression in the rat hippocampus after spatial learning: a comparison of the immediate-early genes Arc, c-fos, and zif268. *J. Neurosci.* 21, 5089–5098.

Harrison, F. E., Hosseini, A. H., and McDonald, M. P. (2009). Endogenous anxi- ety and stress responses in water maze and Barnes maze spatial memory tasks. *Behav. Brain Res.* 198, 247–251. doi: 10.1016/j.bbr.2008.10.015

Holloway, C. M., and McIntyre, C. K. (2011). Post-training disruption of Arc protein expression in the anterior cingulate cortex impairs long-term mem- ory for inhibitory avoidance training. *Neurobiol. Learn. Mem.* 95, 425–432. doi: 10.1016/j.nlm.2011.02.002

Huganir, R. L., and Nicoll, R. A. (2013). AMPARs and synaptic plasticity: the last 25 years. *Neuron* 80, 704–717. doi: 10.1016/j.neuron.2013.10.025

Inoue, N., Nakao, H., Migishima, R., Hino, T., Matsui, M., Hayashi, F., et al. (2009). Requirement of the immediate early gene vesl-1S/homer-1a for fear memory formation. *Mol. Brain* 2, 7. doi: 10.1186/1756-6606-2-7

Inoue, Y., Udo, H., Inokuchi, K., and Sugiyama, H. (2007). Homer1a regulates the activity-induced remodeling of synaptic structures in cultured hippocampal neurons. *Neuroscience* 150, 841–852. doi: 10.1016/j.neuroscience.2007.09.081

Inta, D., Vogt, M. A., Luoni, A., Filipovic, D., Lima-Ojeda, J. M., Pfeiffer, N., et al. (2013). Significant increase in anxiety during aging in mGlu5 receptor knockout mice. *Behav. Brain Res.* 241, 27–31. doi: 10.1016/j.bbr.2012.11.042

Kaja, S., Sumien, N., Borden, P. K., Khullar, N., Iqbal, M., Collins, J. L., et al. (2013). Homer-1a immediate early gene expression correlates with better cognitive performance in aging. *Age* 35, 1799–1808. doi: 10.1007/s11357-012-9479-6

Kammermeier, P. J., and Worley, P. F. (2007). Homer 1a uncouples metabotropicglutamate receptor 5 from postsynaptic effectors. *Proc. Natl. Acad. Sci. U.S.A.* 104, 6055–6060. doi: 10.1073/pnas.0608991104

Kesner, R. P. (2007). Behavioral functions of the CA3 subregion of the hippocam- pus. *Learn. Mem.* 14, 771–781. doi: 10.1101/lm.688207

Kim, E. M., Welch, C. C., Grace, M. K., Billington, C. J., and Levine, A. S. (1996). Chronic food restriction and acute food deprivation decrease mRNA levels of opioid peptides in arcuate nucleus. *Am. J. Physiol.* 270, R1019–R1024.

Klugmann, M., Symes, C. W., Leichtlein, C. B., Klaussner, B. K., Dunning, J., Fong, ., et al. (2005). AAV-mediated hippocampal expression of short and long Homer 1 proteins differentially affect cognition and seizure activity in adult rats. *Mol. Cell. Neurosci.* 28, 347–360. doi: 10.1016/j.mcn.2004.10.002

Kollen, M., Stephan, A., Faivre-Bauman, A., Loudes, C., Sinet, P. M., Alliot, J., et al. (2010). Preserved memory capacities in aged Lou/C/Jall rats. *Neurobiol. Aging* 31, 129–142. doi: 10.1016/j.neurobiolaging.2008.03.010

Kotz, C. M., Weldon, D., Billington, C. J., and Levine, A. S. (2004). Age-related changes in brain proDynorphin gene expression in the rat. *Neurobiol. Aging* 25, 1343–1347. doi: 10.1016/j.neurobiolaging.2004.02.025

Landfield, P. W., Baskin, R. K., and Pitler, T. A. (1981). Brain aging correlates: retar- dation by hormonal-pharmacological treatments. *Science* 214, 581–584. doi: 10.1126/science.6270791

Lee, H. K., Min, S. S., Gallagher, M., and Kirkwood, A. (2005). NMDA receptor- independent long-term depression correlates with successful aging in rats. *Nat. Neurosci.* 8, 1657–1659. doi: 10.1038/nn1586

Levay, E. A., Tammer, A. H., Penman, J., Kent, S., and Paolini, A. G. (2010). Calorie restriction at increasing levels leads to augmented concentrations of corticos- terone and decreasing concentrations of testosterone in rats. *Nutr. Res.* 30, 366–373. doi: 10.1016/j.nutres.2010.05.001

Lu, Y. M., Jia, Z., Janus, C., Henderson, J. T., Gerlai, R., Wojtowicz, J. M., et al. (1997). Mice lacking metabotropic glutamate receptor 5 show impaired learn- ing and reduced CA1 long-term potentiation (LTP) but normal CA3 LTP. *J. Neurosci.* 17, 5196–5205.

Lupien, S. J., Fiocco, A., Wan, N., Maheu, F., Lord, C., Schramek, T., et al. (2005). Stress hormones and human memory function across the lifespan. *Psychoneuroendocrinology* 30, 225–242. doi: 10.1016/j.psyneuen.2004.08.003

Lupien, S. J., McEwen, B. S., Gunnar, M. R., and Heim, C. (2009). Effects of stress throughout the lifespan on the brain, behaviour and cognition. *Nat. Rev. Neurosci.* 10, 434–445. doi: 10.1038/nrn2639

Marissal-Arvy, N., Gaumont, A., Langlois, A., Dabertrand, F., Bouchecareilh, M., Tridon, C., et al. (2007). Strain differences in hypothalamic pituitary adrenocortical axis function and adipogenic effects of corticosterone in rats. *J. Endocrinol.* 195, 473–484. doi: 10.1677/JOE-07-0077

Markowska, A. L., Mooney, M., and Sonntag, W. E. (1998). Insulin-like growth factor-1 ameliorates age-related behavioral deficits. *Neuroscience* 87, 559–569. doi: 10.1016/S0306-4522(98)00143-2

Markowska, A. L., and Savonenko, A. (2002). Retardation of cognitive aging by life-long diet restriction: implications for genetic variance. *Neurobiol. Aging* 23, 75–86. doi: 10.1016/S0197-4580(01)00249-4

Mathus-Vliegen, E. M. (2012). Obesity and the elderly. *J. Clin. Gastroenterol.* 46, 533–544. doi: 10.1097/MCG.0b013e31825692ce

Menard, C., Chartier, E., Patenaude, C., Robinson, P., Cyr, M., Baudry, M., et al. (2007). Calcium-independent phospholipase A(2) influences AMPA-mediated toxicity of hippocampal slices by regulating the GluR1 subunit in synaptic membranes. *Hippocampus* 17, 1109–1120. doi: 10.1002/hipo.20343

Menard, C., Herzog, H., Schwarzer, C., and Quirion, R. (2014). Possible role of dynorphins in Alzheimer's disease and age-related cognitive deficits. *Neurodegener. Dis.* 13, 82–85. doi: 10.1159/000353848

Menard, C., and Quirion, R. (2012a). Group 1 metabotropic glutamate receptor function and its regulation of learning and memory in the aging brain. *Front. Pharmacol.* 3:182. doi: 10.3389/fphar.2012.00182

Menard, C., and Quirion, R. (2012b). Successful cognitive aging in rats: a role for mGluR5 glutamate receptors, homer 1 proteins and downstream signaling pathways. *PLoS ONE* 7:e28666. doi: 10.1371/journal.pone.0028666

Menard, C., Tse, Y. C., Cavanagh, C., Chabot, J. G., Herzog, H., Schwarzer, C., et al. (2013). Knockdown of prodynorphin gene prevents cognitive decline, reduces anxiety, and rescues loss of group 1 metabotropic glutamate receptor function in aging. *J. Neurosci.* 33, 12792–12804. doi: 10.1523/JNEUROSCI.0290-13.2013

Menard, C., Valastro, B., Martel, M. A., Martinoli, M. G., and Massicotte, G. (2004). Strain-related variations of AMPA receptor modulation by calcium-dependent mechanisms in the hippocampus: contribution of lipoxygenase metabolites of arachidonic acid. *Brain Res.* 1010, 134–143. doi: 10.1016/j.brainres.2004.03.012

Moura, P. J., Meirelles, S. T., and Xavier, G. F. (2010). Long-term social recog- nition memory in adult male rats: factor analysis of the social and non- social behaviors. *Braz. J. Med. Biol. Res.* 43, 663–676. doi: 10.1590/S0100-879X2010007500047

Moyse, E., Bedard, K., Segura, S., Mahaut, S., Tardivel, C., Ferland, G., et al. (2012). Effects of aging and caloric restriction on brainstem satiety center signals in rats. *Mech. Ageing Dev.* 133, 83–91. doi: 10.1016/j.mad.2012.01.004

Newmark, R. E., Schon, K., Ross, R. S., and Stern, C. E. (2013). Contributions of the hippocampal subfields and entorhinal cortex to disambiguation during working memory. *Hippocampus* 23, 467–475. doi: 10.1002/hipo.22106

Nguyen, X. V., Masse, J., Kumar, A., Vijitruth, R., Kulik, C., Liu, M., et al. (2005). Prodynorphin knockout mice demonstrate diminished age-associated impair- ment in spatial water maze performance. *Behav. Brain Res.* 161, 254–262. doi: 10.1016/j.bbr.2005.02.010

Nikbakht, N., Zarei, B., Shirani, E., Moshtaghian, J., Esmaeili, A., and Habibian, S. (2012). Experience-dependent expression of rat hippocampal Arc and Homer 1a after spatial learning on 8-arm and 12-arm radial mazes. *Neuroscience* 218, 49–55. doi: 10.1016/j.neuroscience.2012.05.025

O'Donovan, A., Slavich, G. M., Epel, E. S., and Neylan, T. C. (2013). Exaggerated neurobiological sensitivity to threat as a mechanism linking anxiety with increased risk for diseases of aging. *Neurosci. Biobehav. Rev.* 37, 96–108. doi: 10.1016/j.neubiorev.2012.10.013

Paban, V., Billard, J. M., Bouet, V., Freret, T., Boulouard, M., Chambon, C., et al. (2012). Genomic transcriptional profiling in LOU/C/Jall rats identifies genes for successful aging. *Brain Struct. Funct.*. 218, 1501–1512. doi: 10.1007/s00429-012- 0472-8

Penner, M. R., Roth, T. L., Chawla, M. K., Hoang, L. T., Roth, E. D., Lubin, F. D., et al. (2011). Age-related changes in Arc transcription and DNA methylation within the hippocampus. *Neurobiol. Aging* 32, 2198–2210. doi: 10.1016/j.neurobiolaging.2010.01.009

Qiu, G., Spangler, E. L., Wan, R., Miller, M., Mattson, M. P., So, K. F., et al. (2012). Neuroprotection provided by dietary restriction in rats is further enhanced by reducing glucocortocoids. *Neurobiol. Aging* 33, 2398–2410. doi: 10.1016/j.neurobiolaging.2011.11.025

Rossi-Arnaud, C., and Ammassari-Teule, M. (1998). What do comparative stud- ies of inbred mice add to current investigations on the neural basis of spatial behaviors? *Exp. Brain Res.* 123, 36–44. doi: 10.1007/s002210050542

Rowe, W. B., Blalock, E. M., Chen, K. C., Kadish, I., Wang, D., Barrett, J.., et al. (2007). Hippocampal expression analyses reveal selective asso- ciation of immediate-early, neuroenergetic, and myelinogenic pathways with cognitive impairment in aged rats. *J. Neurosci.* 27, 3098–3110. doi: 10.1523/JNEUROSCI.4163-06.2007

Russo, S. J., Murrough, J. W., Han, M. H., Charney, D. S., and Nestler, E. J. (2012). Neurobiology of resilience. *Nat. Neurosci.* 15, 1475–1484. doi: 10.1038/nn.3234

Sandi, C. (2011). Glucocorticoids act on glutamatergic pathways to affect memory processes. *Trends Neurosci.* 34, 165–176. doi: 10.1016/j.tins.2011.01.006

Schwarzer, C. (2009). 30 years of dynorphins–new insights on their func- tions in neuropsychiatric diseases. *Pharmacol. Ther.* 123, 353–370. doi: 10.1016/j.pharmthera.2009.05.006

Shepherd, J. D., and Bear, M. F. (2011). New views of Arc, a master regulator of synaptic plasticity. *Nat. Neurosci.* 14, 279–284. doi: 10.1038/nn.2708

Shukitt-Hale, B., Casadesus, G., Cantuti-Castelvetri, I., and Joseph, J. A. (2001). Effect of age on object exploration, habituation, and response to spatial and nonspatial change. *Behav. Neurosci.* 115, 1059–1064. doi: 10.1037//0735-7044.115.5.1059

Simmons, M. L., Terman, G. W., Drake, C. T., and Chavkin, C. (1994). Inhibition of glutamate release by presynaptic kappa 1-opioid receptors in the guinea pig dentate gyrus. *J. Neurophysiol.* 72, 1697–1705.

Sommer, B., Kohler, M., Sprengel, R., and Seeburg, P. H. (1991). RNA editing in brain controls a determinant of ion flow in glutamate-gated channels. *Cell* 67, 11–19. doi: 10.1016/0092-8674(91)90568-J

Stranahan, A. M., and Mattson, M. P. (2011). Bidirectional metabolic regula- tion of neurocognitive function. *Neurobiol. Learn. Mem.* 96, 507–516. doi: 10.1016/j.nlm.2011.01.004

Traissard, N., Herbeaux, K., Cosquer, B., Jeltsch, H., Ferry, B., Galani, R., et al. (2007). Combined damage to entorhinal cortex and cholinergic basal forebrain neurons, two early neurodegenerative features accompanying Alzheimer's disease: effects on locomotor activity and memory functions in rats. *Neuropsychopharmacology* 32, 851–871. doi: 10.1038/sj.npp.1301116

Tronson, N. C., Guzman, Y. F., Guedea, A. L., Huh, K. H., Gao, C., Schwarz, M. K., et al. (2010). Metabotropic glutamate receptor 5/Homer interac- tions underlie stress effects on fear. *Biol. Psychiatry* 68, 1007–1015. doi: 10.1016/j.biopsych.2010.09.004

Umegaki, H., Hayashi, T., Nomura, H., Yanagawa, M., Nonogaki, Z., Nakshima, H., et al. (2013). Cognitive dysfunction: an emerging concept of a new diabetic complication in the elderly. *Geriatr. Gerontol. Int.* 13, 28–34. doi: 10.1111/j.1447-0594.2012.00922.x

Upchurch, M., and Wehner, J. M. (1988). DBA/2Ibg mice are incapable of cholinergically-based learning in the Morris water task. *Pharmacol. Biochem. Behav.* 29, 325–329. doi: 10.1016/0091-3057(88)90164-5

Upchurch, M., and Wehner, J. M. (1989). Inheritance of spatial learning ability in inbred mice: a classical genetic analysis. *Behav. Neurosci.* 103, 1251–1258. doi:

10.1037/0735-7044.103.6.1251

Vahia, I. V., Chattillion, E., Kavirajan, H., and Depp, C. A. (2011). Psychological protective factors across the lifespan: implications for psychiatry. *Psychiatr. Clin. North Am.* 34, 231–248. doi: 10.1016/j.psc.2010.11.011

Veyrat-Durebex, C., Alliot, J., and Gaudreau, P. (2005). Regulation of the pitu- itary growth hormone-releasing hormone receptor in ageing male and female LOU rats: new insights into healthy ageing. *J. Neuroendocrinol.* 17, 691–700. doi: 10.1111/j.1365-2826.2005.01343.x

Veyrat-Durebex, C., Montet, X., Vinciguerra, M., Gjinovci, A., Meda, P., Foti, M., et al. (2009). The Lou/C rat: a model of spontaneous food restriction associated with improved insulin sensitivity and decreased lipid storage in adipose tissue. *Am. J. Physiol. Endocrinol. Metab.* 296, E1120–E1132. doi: 10.1152/ajpendo.90592.2008

Veyrat-Durebex, C., Poher, A. L., Caillon, A., Somm, E., Vallet, P., Charnay, Y., et al. (2013). Improved leptin sensitivity as a potential candidate responsible for the spontaneous food restriction of the lou/c rat. *PLoS ONE* 8:e73452. doi: 10.1371/journal.pone.0073452

Wagner, J. J., Terman, G. W., and Chavkin, C. (1993). Endogenous dynorphins inhibit excitatory neurotransmission and block LTP induction in the hippocampus. *Nature* 363, 451–454. doi: 10.1038/ 363451a0

Wagner, K. V., Hartmann, J., Mangold, K., Wang, X. D., Labermaier, C., Liebl, C., et al. (2013). Homer1 mediates acute stress-induced cognitive deficits in the dor- sal hippocampus. *J. Neurosci.* 33, 3857–3864. doi: 10.1523/JNEUROSCI.4333- 12.2013

Whittington, R. A., Bretteville, A., Virag, L., Emala, C. W., Maurin, T. O., Marcouiller, F., et al. (2013). Anesthesia-induced hypothermia mediates decreased ARC gene and protein expression through ERK/MAPK inactivation. *Sci. Rep.* 3, 1388. doi: 10.1038/srep01388

Williamson, R., McNeilly, A., and Sutherland, C. (2012). Insulin resistance in the brain: an old-age or new-age problem? *Biochem. Pharmacol.* 84, 737–745. doi: 10.1016/j.bcp.2012.05.007

Wittmann, W., Schunk, E., Rosskothen, I., Gaburro, S., Singewald, N., Herzog, H., et al. (2009). Prodynorphin-derived peptides are critical modulators of anxiety and regulate neurochemistry and corticosterone. *Neuropsychopharmacology* 34, 775–785. doi: 10.1038/npp.2008.142

Xu, J., Zhu, Y., Contractor, A., and Heinemann, S. F. (2009). mGluR5 has a critical role in inhibitory learning. *J. Neurosci.* 29, 3676–3684. doi: 10.1523/JNEUROSCI.5716-08.2009

Yamamoto, Y., Tanahashi, T., Kawai, T., Chikahisa, S., Katsuura, S., Nishida, K., et al. (2009). Changes in behavior and gene expression induced by caloric restriction in C57BL/6 mice. *Physiol. Genomics* 39, 227–235. doi: 10.1152/physiolgenomics.00082.2009

Yang, S., Megill, A., Ardiles, A. O., Ransom, S., Tran, T., Koh, M. T., et al. (2013). Integrity of mGluR-LTD in the Associative/Commissural Inputs to CA3 Correlates with Successful Aging in Rats. *J. Neurosci.* 33, 12670–12678. doi: 10.1523/JNEUROSCI.1086-13.2013

Zhao, X., Rosenke, R., Kronemann, D., Brim, B., Das, S. R., Dunah, A. W., et al. (2009). The effects of aging on N-methyl-D-aspartate receptor subunits in the synaptic membrane and relationships to long-term spatial memory. *Neuroscience* 162, 933–945. doi: 10.1016/j.neuroscience.2009.05.018

Zyzak, D. R., Otto, T., Eichenbaum, H., and Gallagher, M. (1995). Cognitive decline associated with normal aging in rats: a neuropsychological approach. *Learn. Mem.* 2, 1–16. doi: 10.1101/lm.2.1.1

20

Central pathways integrating metabolism and reproduction in teleosts

Md. Shahjahan†, Takashi Kitahashi† and Ishwar S. Parhar *

Brain Research Institute, School of Medicine and Health Sciences, Monash University Malaysia, Petaling Jaya, Malaysia

Edited by:
Rosaria Meccariello, University of Naples Parthenope, Italy

Reviewed by:
Teresa Chioccarelli, Second University of Naples, Italy
Erika Cottone, University of Turin, Italy

***Correspondence:**
Ishwar S. Parhar, Brain Research Institute, School of Medicine and Health Sciences, Monash University Malaysia, Petaling Jaya 46150, Malaysia
e-mail: ishwar@monash.edu

† Md. Shahjahan and Takashi Kitahashi have contributed equally to this work.

Energy balance plays an important role in the control of reproduction. However, the cellular and molecular mechanisms connecting the two systems are not well understood especially in teleosts. The hypothalamus plays a crucial role in the regulation of both energy balance and reproduction, and contains a number of neuropeptides, including gonadotropin-releasing hormone (GnRH), orexin, neuropeptide-Y, ghrelin, pituitary adenylate cyclase-activating polypeptide, α-melanocyte stimulating hormone, melanin-concentrating hormone, cholecystokinin, 26RFamide, nesfatin, kisspeptin, and gonadotropin-inhibitory hormone. These neuropeptides are involved in the control of energy balance and reproduction either directly or indirectly. On the other hand, synthesis and release of these hypothalamic neuropeptides are regulated by metabolic signals from the gut and the adipose tissue. Furthermore, neurons producing these neuropeptides interact with each other, providing neuronal basis of the link between energy balance and reproduction. This review summarizes the advances made in our understanding of the physiological roles of the hypothalamic neuropeptides in energy balance and reproduction in teleosts, and discusses how they interact with GnRH, kisspeptin, and pituitary gonadotropins to control reproduction in teleosts.

Keywords: neuropeptide, metabolism, energy balance, fish, reproduction

INTRODUCTION

A close connection between energy balance and reproduction has been well documented in mammals (1). Energy balance is maintained by a process that controls food consumption, energy expenditure, and energy storage. A number of hypothalamic neuropeptides including orexin, ghrelin, neuropeptide-Y (NPY), melanin-concentrating hormone (MCH), pituitary adenylate cyclase-activating polypeptide (PACAP), proopiomelanocortin (POMC)-derived peptides, cholecystokinin (CCK), chicken gonadotropin-releasing hormone-II (cGnRH-II), 26RFamide (26RFa), galanin (GAL), and cocaine- and amphetamine-regulated transcript (CART) have been implicated in the regulation of feeding behavior and energy balance. On the other hand, peripheral hormones such as leptin and ghrelin provide information about the availability of stored metabolic foods.

Initiation of reproduction is affected by the amount of body energy reserves and is responsive to diverse metabolic factors. The neuroendocrine mechanisms responsible for the association between energy balance and fertility are represented by metabolic hormones and neuropeptides that affect the hypothalamic center controlling the expression and release of gonadotropin-releasing hormone (GnRH) (2, 3). Therefore, adequate body energy stores are crucial for full activation of the hypothalamus–pituitary–gonadal (HPG) axis at puberty and its proper functioning in adulthood (4). Generally high amount of food supply favor reproduction, while low food supply inhibits the reproductive system (1). During energetic challenges, the physiological mechanisms that partition energy into various activities tend to favor the processes for the survival of the individual over the processes for growth, longevity, and reproduction (5). Therefore, the reproductive system is suppressed by energetic challenges. At the same time it is also true that when the reproductive system is highly activated, animal primates reproduction rather than feeding. Many factors such as starvation, eating disorders, excessive exercise, cold exposure, and lactation act on both food intake and reproduction by increasing hunger and/or food ingestion and by suppressing reproductive processes (5, 6).

Most feeding-related neuropeptides in mammals have also been identified in fish species (7), suggesting that the regulatory system of feeding has been well conserved from fish to mammals. On the other hand, as the links between energy balance and reproduction have been demonstrated in several vertebrates (8), this might also exist in teleosts. Indeed, seasonal changes in feeding often coincide with spawning migration and reproduction in fish, suggesting association between nutrition and reproduction (9).

This review focuses on the role of the neuropeptides that regulate feeding and energy balance on reproduction in teleosts, and discusses if the metabolic control of reproduction is conserved from fish to mammals.

REGULATION OF REPRODUCTION IN TELEOSTS

In teleosts, as in other vertebrates, reproduction is coordinated by the HPG axis. The hypothalamus produces GnRH, which regulates the synthesis and release of gonadotropins (GTHs), follicle-stimulating hormone (FSH), and luteinizing hormone (LH), from the pituitary. The GTHs act on the gonads to stimulate gonadal development through the secretion of sex steroid hormones. These steroids, in turn, feedback to the brain and the pituitary to complete the HPG axis and to regulate the reproductive cycle (10, 11). Thus, hypothalamic GnRH is considered as the key player in the regulation of reproduction in teleosts. Furthermore, recent findings of kisspeptin and gonadotropin-inhibitory hormone (GnIH) added new players in the reproductive system, which stimulate and inhibit mostly GnRH neurons, respectively.

GONADOTROPIN-RELEASING HORMONE (GnRH)

In the early 1970s, two research groups simultaneously reported the isolation of a LH-releasing factor from the hypothalamus of pigs and sheep (12, 13), and named it LH-releasing hormone (LHRH). Later, this decapeptide was also found to stimulate FSH release, and accordingly re-named GnRH. The GnRH isolated from mammals is also functional in fish, and stimulates the release of GTH in the carp (14). The first fish GnRH was identified in salmon, and named as salmon GnRH (sGnRH) (15). To date, 15 different forms of GnRH have been identified in vertebrates (13, 15–25), among them 10 original forms in fish species: salmon, sea bream, whitefish, medaka, catfish, herring, dogfish, and lamprey (lamprey I, II, and III). Most vertebrates possess two, and some teleosts have three, forms of GnRH in the brain (23, 25–31). Based on phylogenetic analysis, recent classification defines the species-specific (hypophysiotropic) form as GnRH1, while the most evolutionarily conserved chicken GnRH-II as GnRH2 (32). The third form is GnRH3 (33), which is present only in the brain of certain teleost species (31, 34).

Distribution of three different forms of GnRH in the brain was first reported in a perciform fish, the sea bream (35). GnRH1 neurons are generally present in the region from the ventral forebrain–preoptic area (POA) to basal hypothalamus, whereas GnRH2 neurons are restricted to the dorsal mesencephalon. GnRH3 neurons are located in the caudal-most olfactory bulb as a ganglion and along the terminal nerve in most fish species that possess three GnRH forms (31, 36). On the other hand, in the sea bream and the European sea bass, the distribution of GnRH1 and GnRH3 cells overlap in the olfactory bulbs, ventral telencephalon, and POA (37–40). Similar results were reported in several other fish species (41–45). In the sea bass brain, GnRH1 neuronal fibers are observed in the ventral surface of the forebrain, associated with the ventral telencephalon, POA, and the hypothalamus, whereas GnRH2 and GnRH3 neuronal fibers show profuse distributions throughout the brain (40).

The function of GnRH in the central regulation of LH release has been recognized in all orders of teleosts. Although the assay for FSH peptide is lacking for most fish species, studies in the rainbow trout (46–48) and the Coho salmon (49) show that GnRH also stimulates FSH release in salmonids. However, the different patterns of fiber projections of each GnRH form suggest different physiological function of each GnRH form in the brain (31). GnRH1 neurons are generally present in the ventral forebrain–POA–hypothalamus and send neuronal fibers directly into the pituitary, which represents its primary role in the stimulation of GTH secretion. The physiological significance of GnRH1 as a regulator of GTH secretion and gametogenesis has been established in several teleosts (28, 50–54).

GnRH2 neurons are exclusively present in the midbrain. The absence or low levels of GnRH2 peptide in the pituitary has been demonstrated in several *perciformes* (50, 51, 55–57) and pleuronectiformes species (28, 58), suggesting that GnRH2 is not directly involved in GTH secretion. Rather, its wide fiber projection throughout the brain suggests that GnRH2 has neuromodulatory functions (30). However, in some fish species including the goldfish, GnRH2 seems to act as a hypophysiotropic GnRH together with GnRH3 (59).

GnRH3 has been shown to control reproductive behaviors in several fish species. GnRH3 stimulates nest-building behavior in the male dwarf gourami (60), homing migration in the sockeye salmon (61), and aggressive and nest-building behaviors in the male Nile tilapia (62), which suggests probable neuromodulatory roles of GnRH3. The neuromodulatory role of GnRH3 was confirmed by electrophysiological studies in the retina of goldfish (63, 64) and olfactory receptor cells of the mudpuppy (65). The neuromodulatory function of GnRH3 has also been demonstrated in the rainbow trout (66, 67) and the dwarf gourami [reviewed by Oka (68)]. Fish species such as some salmonids and the zebrafish possess only two forms of GnRH (GnRH2 and GnRH3). In these species, GnRH3 expressed in the basal forebrain acts as a hypophysiotropic GnRH (45, 69–71).

KISSPEPTIN

Kisspeptin is a neuropeptide that plays an important role in reproduction through the stimulation of GnRH neurons by activating GPR54 in mammals (72, 73). In teleosts, two kisspeptin genes, namely *kiss1* and *kiss2*, have been identified in several fish species (74–77), whereas placental mammals possess only the *kiss1* gene. Similarly, two kisspeptin receptor genes, named *kiss1r* and *kiss2r*, were also identified in several fish species (76, 78), suggesting two Kiss/Kissr systems in teleosts. However, this situation is not common among all fish species. Only one kisspeptin gene, *kiss2*, and one receptor, *kiss2r*, are present in some fish species including the Senegalese sole (79), orange-spotted grouper (80), grass puffer (81), and the Atlantic halibut (82), indicating that the *kiss1* and *kiss1r* genes have been lost during evolution in these species (82). Both *kiss1* and *kiss2* mRNAs are expressed in the brain and the gonads in several fish species (74, 76–78, 83). On the other hand, kisspeptin and kisspeptin receptor are also expressed in the fish pituitary, suggesting local actions of kisspeptin in the pituitary (76, 78, 81). In the medaka brain, two populations of *kiss1* neurons are found in the hypothalamus, one in the nucleus ventral tuberis (nVT) and the nucleus posterioris periventricularis (NPPv) (74, 84), while neurons in the dorsal zone of the periventricular hypothalamus (Hd) express *kiss2*. In the zebrafish all hypothalamic populations express *kiss2* mRNA (74). A recent study showed that zebrafish Kiss2 neuronal fibers are found widely in the subpallium, POA, ventral and caudal hypothalamus, and the mesencephalon (85). The fact that all three GnRH neuron types express kisspeptin receptors in the Nile tilapia (86) suggests that the role of Kiss2 neurons in the regulation of the HPG axis is via the activation of the GnRH systems. The *kiss1* neurons are exclusively localized in the habenula in the zebrafish (74), and send fibers only to the ventral part of the interpeduncular nucleus (85, 87). The habenula Kiss1 system is thus implicated in the modulation of serotonergic system rather than the HPG axis in the zebrafish (87).

The role of kisspeptin in the onset of puberty and sexual maturation is conserved among vertebrates including fish. In the zebrafish, both *kiss1* and *kiss2* mRNA levels are increased significantly at the start of the pubertal phase together with GnRH2 and GnRH3 mRNAs (74). Significant positive correlation is observed between the levels of *kiss2* mRNA and those of *gnrh1* mRNA during the spawning period in the grass puffer (81). Kiss2 but not Kiss1 stimulates GTH synthesis and release in the sea bass and the zebrafish (74, 75). Administration of Kiss2–10 peptide increases GnRH1 mRNA levels in the sexually mature female orange-spotted grouper (80), indicating that *Kiss2* most probably plays an important role in the regulation of reproductive functions through the stimulation of GnRH1 secretion.

The information of the interaction between kisspeptin neuronal fibers and GnRH cell bodies had been limited in teleosts due to the lack of specific antibody to kisspeptins. A recent study using an antibody to prepro-Kiss2 proved that Kiss2 neuronal fibers make close contacts with POA GnRH (GnRH3) neurons in the zebrafish (85), suggesting that Kiss2 directly act on GnRH neurons. Moreover, kisspeptin receptor expression in the three GnRH neuronal populations (86) in tilapia suggests that kisspeptin directly stimulates not only GnRH1 neurons to induce LH secretion, but also GnRH2 and GnRH3 neurons to activate other aspects of the reproduction such as sexual behavior.

GONADOTROPIN-INHIBITORY HORMONE (GnIH)

GnIH or RFamide-related peptide (RFRP), which has a characteristic C-terminal LPXRFa motif (X = L or Q), is a hypothalamic neuropeptide that was originally identified from the quail as a neuropeptide that inhibits gonadotropin release from the pituitary (88). Extensive studies revealed that GnIH functions at the level of GnRH neurons and at the level of pituitary gonadotropes to suppress reproduction in avian and mammalian species [see reviews in Ref. (89, 90)]. GnIH in the teleost species has been named LPXRFamide peptide based on the amino acid sequence of the C-terminal motif. All precursors of teleost GnIH identified so far encode three GnIH orthologs (LPXRFa-1, -2, and -3), while only goldfish LPXRFa-3 has been purified as a mature peptide.

As in birds and in mammals, teleost GnIH neurons are located in the hypothalamus, in particular in the NPPv, and send neuronal fibers throughout the brain and to the pituitary (91, 92). The physiological function of teleost GnIH in the control of reproduction is complicated. *In vivo* studies using the goldfish show that GnIH decreases plasma LH levels as in avian and mammalian species (93, 94). On the other hand, GnIH significantly increases pituitary levels of mRNAs for LHβ and FSHβ in a reproductive state-dependent manner *in vivo*, whereas general suppression of LHβ and FSHβ mRNA levels is observed *in vitro* in a study (93). This differential *in vivo* effect of GnIH in different seasons can be explained by the differential action of GnIH on the gonads (95). GnIH does not affect plasma estradiol levels in the female goldfish, but increases plasma testosterone levels in the male goldfish (96). GnIH injections into the female goldfish suppress pituitary LHβ and FSHβ and hypothalamic GnRH mRNA levels (95). In addition, GnIH suppresses GnRH-induced increase in LHβ mRNA levels *in vitro* (95). Therefore, in the goldfish, the inhibition of the HPG axis at the level of hypothalamic GnRH neurons and pituitary gonadotropes appears as an evolutionarily conserved function of GnIH. On the contrary, goldfish GnIH peptides stimulate the synthesis and release of LH and FSH in cultured pituitary cells of the grass puffer and the sockeye salmon, respectively (92, 97). Therefore, as in mammals (98), the stimulatory or inhibitory action of GnIH in fish is probably species dependent or species-specific GnIH peptide might be necessary for an inhibitory action.

More recently, it has been shown that medaka LPXRFa-2 (GnIH-2) peptide decreases the firing frequency of non-hypophsiotropic terminal nerve GnRH3 neurons in the dwarf gourami (99). Since GnRH3 controls nest-building, aggression, and homing migration (60–62), GnIH-2 might negatively regulate reproductive behaviors.

METABOLIC NEUROPEPTIDES INVOLVED IN REPRODUCTION

A number of hypothalamic neuropeptides have been identified in fish species (7), and found to be involved in the control of food intake as well as reproduction (**Table 1**). To understand the overall metabolic control of reproduction, the involvement of metabolic neuropeptides in the regulation of GnRH and GTHs must be taken into consideration. However, compared to mammals, the information related to the role of metabolic neuropeptides in the regulation of reproduction is still limited in fish.

OREXIN

Orexin has two well conserved molecular forms, a 33-amino acid peptide known as orexin A (OXA) and a 28-amino acid peptide known as orexin B (OXB) derived from the same precursor [see review in Ref. (150)]. Orexin was first identified as a ligand of an orphan receptor, and consequently found to stimulate feeding in mammals (151). The orexin's orexigenic action is also observed in teleosts, including the goldfish and the ornate wrasse (101, 152).

In mammals, orexin is known to stimulate the HPG axis via GnRH secretion (153–155). In the goldfish, an interaction between orexin and hypophysiotropic GnRH (GnRH2) has also been proposed. Intracerebroventricular administrations of OXA inhibit spawning behavior and lower GnRH2 mRNA levels, while treatment with GnRH decreases OXA mRNA levels (102). These results suggest that, unlike in mammals, orexins might act as inhibitory agents in the control of GnRH at least in some fish species. In addition, OXA is detected in the pituitary of the medaka (156) and the Japanese sea perch (157), whilst OXB is detected in the pituitary of the Nile tilapia (158), suggesting orexin's local action at the level of pituitary. Thus orexin, an orexigenic neuropeptide, inhibits the HPG axis at the hypothalamus GnRH level and possibly also at the pituitary level, in fish.

NEUROPEPTIDE-Y (NPY)

NPY which is composed of 36 amino acid residues, was first identified in the porcine brain (159), and was found to function as a powerful appetite enhancer in mammals (160). In fish species, NPY also show powerful orexigenic activity in the goldfish (103, 123, 161–164), trout (104), puffer fish (105, 165), and the zebrafish (106).

Centrally or peripherally injected NPY increases plasma LH levels in the goldfish, common carp, rainbow trout, and in the sea bass (107, 109, 111), indicating that NPY stimulates teleost reproduction as was shown in mammals (166).

Table 1 | Neuropeptides and their functions in representative fish species.

Neuropeptide	Species	Function	Reference
Orexin	Goldfish	Increase food intake	(100)
	Ornate wrasse	Increase food intake	(101)
	Goldfish	Inhibit spawning behavior, decrease GnRH2 mRNA level	(102)
NPY	Goldfish	Increase food intake	(103)
	Rainbow trout	Increase food intake	(104)
	Puffer fish	Increase food intake	(105)
	Zebrafish	Increase food intake	(106)
	Goldfish	Stimulate GnRH and LH release	(107, 108)
	Common carp	Increase plasma LH level	(109)
	Sea bream	Stimulate GnRH release	(110)
	Sea bass	Increase plasma LH level	(111)
PACAP	Goldfish	Decrease food intake	(112)
	Goldfish	Stimulate LH release	(113, 114)
	Tilapia	Stimulate GTH subunit mRNA expression	(115)
	Blue gourami	Stimulate FSHβ mRNA expression	(116, 117)
GnRH2	Goldfish	Decrease food intake	(102, 118)
	Zebrafish	Decrease food intake	(119)
	Goldfish	Stimulate LH release	(120)
26RFa	Mouse	Increase food intake	(121)
	Goldfish	Increase plasma LH level	(122)
Galanin	Goldfish	Increase food intake	(123)
	Tench	Increase food intake	(124)
	(Rat)	Stimulate GnRH release	(125)
MCH	Goldfish	Decrease food intake	(126)
	Goldfish	Stimulate LH release	(127)
α-MSH	Goldfish	Decrease food intake	(128)
	Rainbow trout	Decrease food intake	(129)
	(Mouse)	Stimulate GnRH neurons	(130)
CART	Goldfish	Decrease food intake	(131, 132)
	(Rat)	Stimulate GnRH release	(133, 134)
CCK	Goldfish	Decrease food intake	(135)
	Goldfish	Stimulate LH release	(136)
Nesfatin-1	Goldfish	Decrease food intake	(137, 138)
	Goldfish	Decrease plasma LH level	(139)
Leptin	Goldfish	Decrease food intake	(140)
	Rainbow trout	Decrease food intake	(141)
	Sea bass	Stimulate LH release	(142)
	Rainbow trout	Stimulate LH release	(143)
Ghrelin	Goldfish	Increase food intake	(144–146)
	Rainbow trout	Decrease food intake	(147)
	Goldfish	Stimulate LH release	(148)
	Common carp	Stimulate LH release	(149)

(Continued)

In the brown trout (167) and the rainbow trout (168), NPY neuronal fibers project to the areas where hypophysiotropic GnRH neurons exist, particularly in the ventral telencephalon, POA, and in the basal hypothalamus. Furthermore, double immunolabeling reveals close appositions of NPY fibers with GnRH cells in the POA of the ayu (*Plecoglossus altivelis*) (169) and the Siberian sturgeon (170), suggesting the direct action of NPY in the regulation of GnRH neurons. Indeed, NPY stimulates GnRH release *in vitro* in the goldfish (108) and in the sea bream (110).

Neuropeptide-Y also regulates the HPG axis at the level of pituitary. *In vitro* treatment with NPY stimulates LH release from pituitary cells in the goldfish (107) and increases LHβ and GTHα, but not FSHβ mRNA levels in the tilapia pituitary (115). In addition, NPY fibers make close appositions on LH cells in the catfish pituitary (171).

These findings provide strong support for the stimulatory role of NPY in fish reproduction at the levels of hypothalamic GnRH and pituitary LH cells.

26RFamide (QRFP)

26RFamide is a 26-amino acid peptide, and was first isolated from the frog brain (121). In teleosts, 26RFa has been identified only in the goldfish (172). The 26RFa gene is highly expressed in the hypothalamus, and relatively less in the optic tectum-thalamus and in the testis (122). 26RFa and its mammalian homolog QRFP act as an orexigenic hormone in birds, mice (121, 172–174), and probably in fish (122).

The role of 26RFa has been implicated in the integration of metabolism and reproduction in vertebrates, including fish [see review in Ref. (89)]. In mammals, 26RFa stimulates LH and FSH release in rats *in vivo* and *in vitro* (pituitary culture) (175). In teleost, intraperitoneal injections of 26RFa significantly increase plasma LH levels in the goldfish (122). On the other hand, *in vitro* treatment with 26RFa shows no effects on LH release from pituitary cells. These facts indicate that 26RFa might act on the stimulation of the HPG axis through GnRH1 release in fish.

GALANIN (GAL)

GAL is a 29-amino acid peptide, expressed in the central nervous system and in the intestine. GAL stimulates feeding in the goldfish (123) and the doctor fish tench (124), indicating that GAL acts as an orexigenic hormone in fish as in mammals (176, 177).

Involvement of GAL in the control of HPG axis is evidenced in mammals. In rodents and humans, GAL neuronal fibers make close appositions with GnRH1 neurons (178–180), and GnRH neurons express a GAL receptor Gal-R1 in the rat (181). In fact, GAL stimulates *in vitro* GnRH release in rats (125). These data indicate that GAL is involved in the control of reproduction at the level of GnRH neurons.

In fish, there are no studies that demonstrated the role of GAL in the control of reproduction. However, close appositions of GAL fibers with gonadotropes in the proximal pars distalis (PPD) are seen in the sea bass (182). Similarly, fiber projections of GAL neurons in the PPD are observed in the rainbow trout (183), sea bream (184), and Senegalese sole (185), while no GAL fibers are observed in the pituitary of the Siberian sturgeon (170). Therefore, GAL might modulate the HPG axis at the pituitary level at least in some fish species.

GnRH2

As mentioned before, among the different forms of GnRH, neuronal fibers of GnRH2 (also known as chicken GnRH-II) are widely distributed in the vertebrate brain. In an insectivore, the musk shrew, GnRH2 stimulates sexual behavior and seduces food intake (186, 187), indicating that GnRH2 plays a role in connecting reproductive function and feeding regulation.

In fish species, the suppressive effect of GnRH2 on feeding has also been confirmed. Food consumption is significantly decreased by intracerebroventricular injections of GnRH2 but not GnRH3 in a dose dependent manner in the goldfish (102, 118) and the zebrafish (119).

GnRH2 also has effects on sexual behavior of fish. In the goldfish, GnRH2 stimulates reproductive behavior (188). Furthermore, there is a strong positive correlation between spawning behavior and GnRH2 gene expression (189), suggesting stimulatory role of GnRH2 in reproductive behavior. GnRH2 is also detected in the goldfish pituitary (190) and induces LH release *in vitro* (120). Positive correlation between the pituitary GnRH2 levels and gonadal development is also observed in the striped bass (51), suggesting that it also have a hypophysiotropic role in some fish species. In the grass puffer, the amount of GnRH2 mRNA is slightly higher in the post-spawning females compared to spawning female (191). Therefore, GnRH2 may have different physiological roles depending on the physiological conditions of the fish.

PITUITARY ADENYLATE CYCLASE-ACTIVATING POLYPEPTIDE (PACAP)

PACAP was first isolated from the rat hypothalamus (192). PACAP is an anorexigenic factor in various vertebrates, including rodents (193), chicks (194, 195), and fish (196). To date, the role of PACAP in feeding has been studied only in one fish species, the goldfish.

PACAP increases plasma LH levels *in vivo* in the goldfish (197). *In vitro* studies showed that the stimulatory effect of PACAP on LH release is exerted at the level of the pituitary (113, 114). PACAP also stimulates the levels of GTH subunit mRNAs and FSHβ mRNA in the pituitary of tilapia (115) and in the female blue gourami (116, 117), respectively. Dense projection of PACAP nerve terminals is seen in the pars distalis of the pituitary, where gonadotropes are localized, in the goldfish (198) and in the European eel (199). The expression of PACAP receptor in the pituitary is also observed in the goldfish (197). Therefore, PACAP stimulates GTH secretion in fish pituitary.

MELANIN-CONCENTRATING HORMONE (MCH)

MCH is a cyclic peptide, originally isolated from the pituitary of the chum salmon as a hormone involved in body color change (200). In the winter and barfin flounders, fasting stimulates hypothalamic expression of MCH (201, 202), suggesting that MCH acts as an orexigenic hormone as in mammals (203, 204). However, MCH acts as an anorexigenic hormone in the goldfish (105, 126, 205, 206). Therefore, like ghrelin, MCH acts as an orexigenic and anorexigenic neuropeptide depending on the fish species, although its orexigenic action in fish has to be confirmed.

In mammals, MCH modulates LH secretion in an estradiol-dependent manner [see a review in Ref. (207)]. The close appositions between MCH fibers and hypothalamic GnRH neurons (208, 209) and the expression of MCH receptors in GnRH neurons (209) suggest the direct action of MCH on GnRH neurons in mammals. MCH also acts at the pituitary level to modulate the release of LH (210). In teleosts, an *in vitro* study showed that salmon MCH stimulates the release of LH in a dose response manner from dispersed pituitary cells in the goldfish, suggesting a direct action of MCH on LH cells (127). Whether MCH acts on GnRH neurons in fish as in mammals remains unknown.

α-MELANOCYTE STIMULATING HORMONE (α-MSH)

α-MSH is one of melanocortins and derived from a precursor peptide encoded by the POMC gene (211). Among melanocortins and their receptors, α-MSH and melanocortin receptor 4 (MC4R) are involved in the control of food intake in vertebrates including fish. α-MSH or MC4R agonist inhibits food intake in the goldfish (128, 212) and in the rainbow trout (129), suggesting that the α-MSH/MC4R system play a role in the anorexigenic regulation of feeding in fish as in mammals.

Although the α-MSH/MC4R system is known to play a stimulatory role in reproduction at the level of GnRH neurons in mammals [see a review in Ref. (130)], available information is limited in teleost. Projection of α-MSH fibers in the PPD of the pituitary and differential expression of POMC gene between sexually inactive and active fish in the zebrafish suggests that some of POMC-derived products are involved in the stimulation of fish reproduction (213).

COCAINE- AND AMPHETAMINE-REGULATED TRANSCRIPT (CART)

CART is an anorexigenic neuropeptide originally isolated from the rat brain (160, 214). In fish, CART might also act as anorexigenic hormone in the goldfish (131), winter flounder (215), cod (216), channel catfish (217), zebrafish (218), and in the Atlantic salmon (219).

In mammals, CART is involved in the control of GnRH neurons. CART stimulates GnRH pulsatile release in rats (133, 134). The existence of close appositions between CART fibers and hypothalamic GnRH neurons in the Siberian hamster suggests the effect of CART on GnRH neuronal activity is a direct action (220).

In the catfish, the projections of CART fibers are observed in the PPD of the pituitary (221). CART is also expressed in LH cells of the catfish pituitary but only during sexual maturation period (222), suggesting its local function in the sexual maturation process. However, it should be noted that while similar expression of CART in LH cells is observed in the rat pituitary, CART inhibits the release of prolactin but not GTHs (223). Thus, the role of CART in the fish pituitary has to be examined.

CHOLECYSTOKININ (CCK)

CCK is found in the brain and in the gastrointestinal tract of various vertebrates. It has multiple biologically active forms, among which CCK-8 is the most abundant form in the brain (224). As in mammals, CCK has many physiological roles in fish, but functions primarily in the control of food intake as a satiety indicator (135).

In mammals, CCK decreases the pulse interval of GnRH release in goats (225). Furthermore, CCK implants into the POA, where GnRH neurons are located, increase the plasma levels of LH in rats (226). These data suggest that CCK acts at the levels of GnRH and stimulates reproduction. In fish, on the other hand, CCK seems to acts on the pituitary. An immunohistochemical study showed that CCK neurons innervate into the PPD of the pituitary and that CCK stimulates LH release *in vitro* in the goldfish (136).

NESFATIN-1

Nesfatin-1, a nucleobindin-2 (NUCB2) encoded unmodified peptide, was first characterized in rats (227), and was shown to have anorexigenic actions in the goldfish (137, 138).

The number of studies about the function of nesfatin-1 in the control of reproduction is still limited. However, recent studies showed that nesfatin-1 acts as an inhibitory signal in the control of fish reproduction. Although nesfatin-1 plays a stimulatory role in LH secretion in rats (228), an intraperitoneal injection of nesfatin-1 decreases plasma levels of LH in the goldfish (139). At the same time, nesfatin-1 down regulates expression of GnRH, LHβ, and FSHβ genes, suggesting that the inhibitory action of nesfatin-1 takes place at the levels of GnRH neurons. Whether nesfatin-1 also functions at the level of the pituitary remains unclear.

PERIPHERAL HORMONES INVOLVED IN FEEDING, METABOLISM, AND REPRODUCTION

LEPTIN

Leptin is primarily produced by adipocytes of the white adipose tissue (229), and secreted into the blood circulation in proportion to the mass of body fat. The change in plasma leptin levels is detected by the hypothalamus and thereby it acts as a peripheral factor that signals nutritional status to the CNS [see review by Crown et al. (230)]. In teleosts including the goldfish and the rainbow trout, leptin functions as a peripheral signal to inhibit food intake (140, 141, 231, 232) as in mammals (233).

In mammals, leptin stimulates the HPG axis by promoting the synthesis and release of GnRH from the hypothalamus, and LH and FSH from the pituitary (234–236). In teleosts, leptin also stimulates the reproductive axis. Leptin increases *in vitro* LH release from the pituitary culture in the sea bass (142) and the rainbow trout (143). However, it should be noted that the stimulating effect of leptin on LH release is observed only on the pituitary samples from the fish in maturational stages. Furthermore, leptin expression levels increase with the onset of sexual maturation in the Arctic char (237) and the Atlantic salmon (238). Therefore, the role of leptin in sexual maturation seems to be conserved among vertebrate species.

GHRELIN

As in mammals, ghrelin is highly expressed in the stomach and moderately in the brain (144, 239, 240), and is involved in appetite stimulation, energy balance, feeding, and metabolism [see reviews in Ref. (241, 242)]. Interestingly, the role of ghrelin in fish differs in different fish species. It acts as an orexigenic hormone in the goldfish (144–146) and probably in the sea bass (243) and the zebrafish (244). On the other hand, ghrelin acts as an anorexigenic hormone in the rainbow trout (147) and probably in the burbot (245, 246). The opposite effects of ghrelin on food intake can be explained by species-specific neural pathways mediating the effect of ghrelin (247). The variations in the role of ghrelin in feeding may reflect different regulatory mechanisms of feeding in different teleost species.

In fish species, ghrelin acts as a stimulatory factor in the reproduction, although ghrelin inhibits the HPG axis in mammals [reviewed by Tena-Sempere (248)]. Intracerebroventricular injection of ghrelin increases plasma LH levels in the goldfish (148), indicating its stimulatory action on the HPG axis. The increase of plasma LH levels is, however, small and slow compared to the increase of plasma GH levels. This suggests that the stimulatory effect of ghrelin on plasma LH levels is not through the action of ghrelin on hypothalamic GnRH. Actually, the highest levels of ghrelin receptor mRNA are observed in the sea bream and goldfish pituitary (249, 250). *In vitro* treatment with ghrelin stimulates LH release in the goldfish (148, 250) and in the common carp (149), while pituitary levels of mRNA for LHβ subunit is also increased. As no reports show fiber projections of hypothalamic ghrelin neurons into the pituitary in fish, ghrelin released from stomach/intestine might play a role in the LH secretion from the pituitary. Therefore, ghrelin might act as a stimulatory peripheral factor in reproduction at the level of pituitary, whereas its action on GnRH neurons is uncertain.

INTERACTIONS BETWEEN METABOLIC NEUROPEPTIDES AND THE REPRODUCTIVE SYSTEM IN THE CONTROL OF REPRODUCTION

As shown in the above section, many metabolic neuropeptides are involved in the control of reproduction at the level of hypothalamic GnRH neurons and at the level of pituitary gonadotropes (**Figure 1**). Among these metabolic neuropeptides, NPY and nesfatin-1 function as inhibitory factors on GnRH neurons, while orexin stimulates GnRH neurons. It is interesting that NPY and orexin, which possess orexigenic activity, act on the reproductive system in an opposite manner in the goldfish. It suggests that different metabolic neuropeptides might play a role in the control of reproduction under different physiological conditions. It should be noted, however, that the inhibitory role of orexin on spawning behavior and GnRH gene expression might be the result of orexin action on non-hypophysiotropic GnRH system. In the goldfish brain, hypophysiotropic GnRH type is expressed not only in the hypothalamic population but also in the olfactory bulb and midbrain populations (190). Therefore, the inhibitory effect of orexin on the HPG axis need to be confirmed although it is clear that orexin has suppressive role in some aspects of reproduction.

At the pituitary level, it is evident that many metabolic neuropeptides including NPY, MCH, GnRH2, PACAP, and CCK stimulate LH secretion. In addition, peripheral metabolic signals such as ghrelin and leptin also stimulate LH secretion at the pituitary. The fact that most central neuropeptides and peripheral metabolic signals regulate the reproductive system indicates fundamental interaction between energy balance and reproduction, which is evolutionarily conserved from fish to mammal. However, both orexigenic and anorexigenic metabolic signals act as stimulatory factors in the reproductive system in fish. In mammals, feeding and reproduction are two alternatives in general. Therefore, orexigenic factors inhibit reproduction and anorexigenic factors stimulate reproduction [see review in Ref. (251)]. In fish species, on the other hand, a central orexigenic neuropeptide NPY and a peripheral orexigenic peptide ghrelin inhibit LH secretion in the goldfish and other species (**Table 1**). This indicates that metabolic regulation of the reproductive system in teleost is different from that in mammals, at least in some species.

Fish species have a variety of feeding and reproductive behaviors. For example, most salmonids and the winter flounder undergo a period of fasting just before the spawning season as a part of their normal physiology (252), whereas the goldfish do not have such fasting period. The halt of food intake during final maturation might require the differential usage of metabolic signals in these species.

Recently, kisspeptin has been proposed as a mediator of metabolic signals in the mammalian reproductive system, in particular on GnRH neurons [see reviews in Ref. (89, 253)]. In mice (254) and in the sheep (255), kisspeptin neurons in the arcuate nucleus possess leptin receptors, suggesting direct action of leptin on kisspeptin neurons. Furthermore, kisspeptin neurons receive innervations from other neurons that express leptin receptor (255). These facts suggest that leptin controls GnRH neurons through kisspeptin neurons *via* direct and indirect actions. Furthermore, kisspeptin neurons receive fiber projections from NPY and POMC neurons in mammals (255, 256). Therefore kisspeptin neurons might play an important role in the integration of metabolic signals to control the reproductive system. In teleost, fasting induces a significant increase in *kiss2* mRNA levels in the hypothalamus, as well as an increase in LHβ and FSHβ mRNA levels in the pituitary in the Senegalese sole (*Solea senegalensis*) (257), suggesting negative correlation between energy balance and reproduction. However, to our knowledge, there is no information available regarding direct evidence of metabolic regulation of kisspeptin neurons in fish.

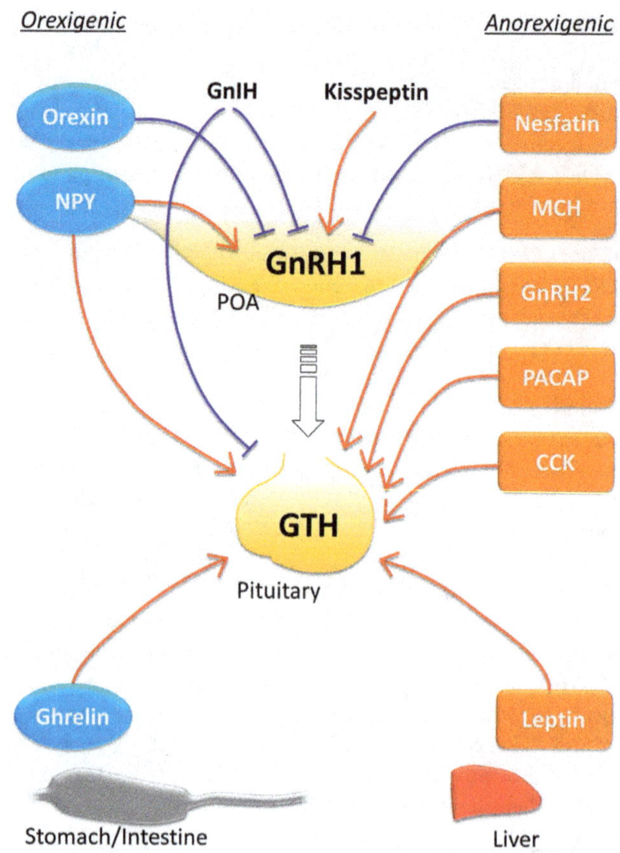

FIGURE 1 | Effects of central and peripheral metabolic hormones on the reproductive system. The hypothalamus–pituitary axis receives many stimulatory and inhibitory inputs from central metabolic neuropeptide neurons and peripheral metabolic signals to control the reproductive system according to the energy status. The hormones indicated with blue circles are orexigenic hormones, while those with orange squares are anorexigenic ones. Red lines indicate stimulatory action and blue lines indicate inhibitory action. Most anorexigenic hormones stimulate gonadotropin secretion at the pituitary level. In the goldfish, NPY and ghrelin, which act as orexigenic hormones, also stimulate the reproductive system at the brain and pituitary levels. It should be noted that this figure is drew primarily based on the information obtained from the goldfish. Function of each metabolic hormone might differ in different species [e.g., Ghrelin functions as an anorexigenic factor in the rainbow trout (147) and GnIH stimulates GTH subunit mRNA expression in the puffer fish (97) and the sockeye salmon (92).]. CCK, cholecystokinin; GnIH, gonadotropin-inhibitory hormone; GnRH, gonadotropin-releasing hormone; MCH, melanin-concentrating hormone; NPY, neuropeptide-Y; PACAP, pituitary adenylate cyclase-activating polypeptide.

In addition to its primary role in reproduction, GnIH stimulates food intake in chickens (258) and in rats (259, 260), suggesting its potential role to switch from reproduction to feeding. Close appositions of GnIH fibers with NPY, orexin, MCH, and POMC neurons in the sheep (261) indicate the involvement of several feeding regulatory pathways. However, there are no studies reporting metabolic regulation of GnIH neurons in vertebrates. On the other hand, GnIH is known to be regulated by stress, photoperiod, and gonadal steroids to suppress the reproductive system (89). Therefore, GnIH neurons might have a role in the modulation of feeding according to the environmental factors in mammals. Whether GnIH plays a similar role in teleosts requires more studies.

INTERACTIONS AMONG NEUROPEPTIDES TO CONTROL FEEDING

To monitor the amount of energy stock, central metabolic neuropeptide neurons receive peripheral signals including leptin and ghrelin. For example, in mammals leptin receptor is expressed in many metabolic neuropeptide neurons including orexin, NPY, GAL, MCH, POMC, CART, and CCK neurons [see reviews in Ref. (262, 263)]. In fish species, leptin also affects several central neuropeptide neurons. Administration of leptin reduces NPY mRNA levels in the goldfish (140), grass carp (264), and in the rainbow trout (141, 265). On the other hand, leptin increases the mRNA levels of CCK and POMC, which are anorexigenic neuropeptides, in the goldfish (140) and the rainbow trout (141, 265), respectively. A recent study showed that leptin receptor knockout medaka exhibit higher levels of NPY mRNA before and after feeding and lower levels of POMC mRNA levels after feeding together with increased food intake (266). Therefore leptin's anorexigenic effect might be mediated by these neuropeptides.

Double immunostaining revealed interactions among orexigenic/anorexigenic neuropeptide neurons in teleosts, in particular in the goldfish (**Figure 2**). Among anorexigenic neuropeptide neurons, MCH neuronal fibers project to α-MSH neurons (206) and α-MSH neuronal fibers project to CRH neurons (267). Furthermore, a study using antagonists against α-MSH receptor and CRH receptor showed that anorexigenic action of MCH is mediated by α-MSH and CRH (268). In addition, GnRH2 mediates anorexigenic effect of α-MSH and CRH (269). These results suggest that the MCH–α-MSH–CRH–GnRH2 pathway suppresses food intake in the goldfish, although it is not known whether CRH directly acts on GnRH2 neurons.

Among orexigenic neuropeptide neurons, NPY and orexin neurons make reciprocal connections in fish as in mammals. NPY neuronal fibers make close appositions with orexin neurons, whereas orexin neuronal fibers make close appositions with NPY neurons in the NPPv in the goldfish (270). Furthermore, co-injections of OXA and NPY result in food intake higher than that observed in fish treated with NPY alone (132). These results indicate that orexins and NPY induce orexigenic actions by mutual signaling pathways in the CNS in teleost. Probably the reciprocal interaction between NPY and orexin functions as a positive-feedback system to maintain food intake.

Moreover, the orexigenic and the anorexigenic circuits are also connected with each other. α-MSH neuronal fibers make close appositions with NPY neurons, whereas NPY neuronal fibers project to α-MSH neurons in the goldfish (271). In addition, MCH neuronal fibers make close appositions with NPY neurons (272). These inhibitory inputs between the orexigenic and anorexigenic neurons might function as an on/off switch to decide whether eat or not eat by activating only one of the two circuits.

Studies using antagonists against of the receptors for metabolic neuropeptides further provided possible interaction among central metabolic neuropeptides in the goldfish. For example, GAL mediates the orexigenic action of orexin, and orexin mediates the orexigenic action of GAL (123). GAL also mediates NPY's action on food intake and *vice versa* (123). Besides, orexin mediates central action of ghrelin in food intake and central ghrelin mediates the action of orexin (273). Furthermore, NPY mediates the orexigenic action of ghrelin (274). These results indicate complex neuronal interactions especially among central orexigenic neuropeptides. This complex neuronal network suggests that many central neuropeptide neurons function in a coordinated manner to regulate food intake. To fully understand the whole circuit that controls food intake, further information on the neuronal interaction among central metabolic neuropeptides have to be obtained.

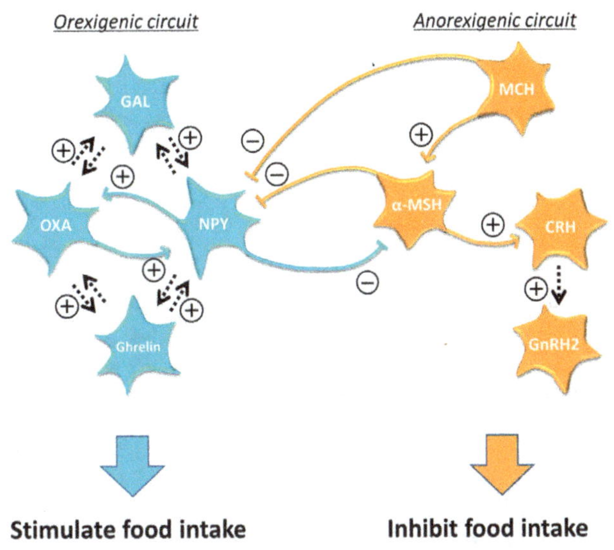

FIGURE 2 | Interaction between the orexigenic circuit and anorexigenic circuit and among neurons in each circuit in the goldfish. Hormones in the orexigenic circuit are shown in blue and those in the anorexigenic circuit are shown in orange. The orexigenic and anorexigenic circuits are connected each other via inhibitory neuronal fiber projections to form an on-off switch. Reciprocal interaction is observed especially between neurons in the orexigenic circuit. Arrows with dotted lines indicate the interactions that have not been confirmed whether direct or indirect. The complex interaction among metabolic neuropeptides suggests that a change in one metabolic signal can affect the reproductive system through the action via other metabolic neuropeptides. Note that in the goldfish ghrelin secreted in the brain also function as an orexigenic signal. α-MSH, alpha-melanocyte stimulating hormone; CRH, corticotropin-releasing hormone; GAL, galanin; GnRH, gonadotropin-releasing hormone; MCH, melanin-concentrating hormone; NPY, neuropeptide-Y; OXA, orexin A; PACAP, pituitary adenylate cyclase-activating polypeptide.

In addition to the evident neuronal interactions in the goldfish, more combinations of neuronal interactions were reported in other fish species. In the masu salmon (275) and the Siberian sturgeon (170), NPY and GAL neurons make reciprocal connections. In the medaka, orexin and MCH neurons send neuronal fibers to each other (156). In the barfin flounder, reciprocal connection between orexin and MCH neurons and between α-MSH and MCH neurons was reported (156). In the rainbow trout, CRH mediates the anorexigenic action of ghrelin (147). These facts suggest that the interaction among central metabolic neuropeptides is really complicated. Therefore, more fiber projection studies together with the localization of the neuropeptide receptors are necessary to understand proper relationships among these neuropeptides that consist of the regulatory circuits of food intake.

PERSPECTIVES

DIRECT INTERACTIONS AMONG CENTRAL METABOLIC NEUROPEPTIDES AND REPRODUCTIVE SYSTEM

Significant amount of information about the relationship among orexigenic and anorexigenic neuropeptides have been accumulated, particularly in the goldfish. However, the knowledge of direct interactions among these neurons is still not enough to draw a complete diagram of the neuronal circuit to control food intake and reproduction in fish. In particular, metabolic regulation of kisspeptin and GnRH neurons are still unknown, while it is suggested from mammalian studies. Further fiber projection studies using double immunostaining and localization of the neuropeptide receptors in certain neuronal cell bodies need to be performed.

SPECIES DIFFERENCES

There are many differences in the regulatory mechanism of food intake and reproduction not only between mammals and fish but also between fish species. The significant difference between fish species might be the result of the adaptation to a wide range of feeding habits and reproductive strategies. Therefore we have to be careful to combine data obtained from different species.

SEX AND MATURATIONAL STAGES

Several studies reported that the responses of the reproductive system to metabolic signals differ depending on the sex and the stage of sexual maturation. In fact, gonadal steroids modulate the effect of NPY on GnRH and LH release in the goldfish (276). Each study should use a particular sex and maturational stage to make comparison easy.

NUTRITIONAL CONDITIONS

Animals might change the metabolic control of reproduction according to the available energy stock. For example, short term food limitation attenuates sexual motivation, while remaining energy stock still maintains activity of the HPG axis. On the other hand, long term food limitation depletes the energy stock and stops the HPG axis to prioritize the energy supply to the survival. Thus, feeding conditions and the timing of experiment might be important to obtain comparable data.

ENDOCANNABINOID SYSTEM

The endocannabinoid system is involved in a variety of physiology including pain-sensation, mood, and memory. Importantly, both energy balance and reproduction are modulated by the endocannabinoid system. Endocannabinoids modulate several hypothalamic metabolic neuropeptides in mammals [see reviews in Ref. (277, 278)]. The endocannabinoid system also regulates food intake in fish (279, 280). In mammalian and non-mammalian vertebrates, the endocannabinoid system regulates hypothalamic GnRH neurons and pituitary LH cells directly and indirectly [see reviews in Ref. (281, 282)]. Interrelation among these systems might be an additional mechanism underlying the interaction between mood, stress, appetite, and reproduction.

CONCLUSION

In summary, the cellular and molecular basis for the integration of feeding and reproduction involves a complex interaction of the reproductive system with metabolic neuropeptides and peripheral fuels. The metabolic neuropeptides, particularly orexin, NPY, PACAP, MCH, nesfatin, GnRH2, and CCK play an important role in the reproduction by either regulating GnRH neurons in the hypothalamus or by stimulating gonadotropes in the pituitary. Peripheral metabolic signals such as ghrelin and leptin also act on the pituitary to stimulate LH secretion. It should be, however, noted that compared to mammals, fishes show a great variety of feeding and reproductive habits. The variations of metabolic control of reproduction in different teleost species may reflect different requirement of energy status for reproduction in different species. Compared to mammals, fish represent a vast phylogenetic group, which shows a significant level of diversity with regards to morphology, ecology, behavior, and genomes (283). Thus, species differences in the neuroendocrine control of reproduction have to be taken into consideration in teleosts. In addition, more detailed studies about the interconnections among metabolic neuropeptide neurons, effects of sexual maturation, and nutritional conditions will provide more precise figure of the metabolic control of reproduction. Furthermore, differential control of multiple GnRH neuronal population by the neuropeptides and metabolic signals should be examined to elucidate their roles in different aspects of metabolic control of reproduction.

ACKNOWLEDGMENTS

This work was supported by grants from Monash University Malaysia, MM-2-5-06, MM-7-07, and MCG006 (to Ishwar S. Parhar), M-3-07 and M-3-08 (to Takashi Kitahashi).

REFERENCES

Schneider JE. Energy balance and reproduction. *Physiol Behav* (2004) 81(2):289–317. doi:10.1016/j.physbeh.2004.02.007

Fernandez-Fernandez R, Martini AC, Navarro VM, Castellano JM, Dieguez C, Aguilar E, et al. Novel signals for the integration of energy balance and reproduction. *Mol Cell Endocrinol* (2006) 254–5:127–32. doi:10.1016/j.mce.2006.04.026

Castellano JM, Roa J, Luque RM, Dieguez C, Aguilar E, Pinilla L, et al. KiSS- 1/kisspeptins and the metabolic control of reproduction: physiologic roles and putative physiopathological implications. *Peptides* (2009) 30(1):139–45. doi:10.1016/j.peptides.2008.06.007

Hill JW, Elmquist JK, Elias CF. Hypothalamic pathways linking energy bal- ance and reproduction. *Am J Physiol Endocrinol Metab* (2008) 294(5):E827–32. doi:10.1152/ajpendo.00670.2007

Schneider JE, Buckley CA, Blum RM, Zhou D, Szymanski L, Day DE, et al. Metabolic signals, hormones and neuropeptides involved in control of energy balance and reproductive success in hamsters. *Eur J Neurosci* (2002) 16(3):377–9. doi:10.1046/j.1460-9568.2002.02118.x

Wade GN, Schneider JE, Li HY. Control of fertility by metabolic cues. *Am J Physiol* (1996) 270(1 Pt 1):E1–19.

Volkoff H, Canosa LF, Unniappan S, Cerda-Reverter JM, Bernier NJ, Kelly SP, et al. Neuropeptides and the control of food intake in fish. *Gen Comp Endocrinol* (2005) 142(1–2):3–19. doi:10.1016/j.ygcen.2004.11.001

Mircea CN, Lujan ME, Pierson RA. Metabolic fuel and clinical implications for female reproduction. *J Obstet Gynaecol Can* (2007) 29(11):887–902.

Volkoff H, Xu M, MacDonald E, Hoskins L. Aspects of the hormonal regulation of appetite in fish with emphasis on goldfish, Atlantic cod and winter flounder: notes on actions and responses to nutritional, environmental and reproduc- tive changes. *Comp Biochem Physiol A Mol Integr Physiol* (2009) 153(1):8–12. doi:10.1016/j.cbpa.2008.12.001

Yaron Z, Gur G, Melamed P, Rosenfeld H, Elizur A, Levavi-Sivan B. Regulation of fish gonadotropins. *Int Rev Cytol* (2003) 225:131–85. doi:10.1016/S0074-7696(05)25004-0

Zohar Y, Munoz-Cueto JA, Elizur A, Kah O. Neuroendocrinology of reproduc- tion in teleost fish. *Gen Comp Endocrinol* (2010) 165(3):438–55. doi:10.1016/ j.ygcen.2009.04.017

Amoss M, Burgus R, Blackwell R, Vale W, Fellows R, Guillemin R. Purification, amino acid composition and N-terminus of the hypothalamic luteinizing hor- mone releasing factor (LRF) of ovine origin. *Biochem Biophys Res Commun* (1971) 44(1):205–10. doi:10.1016/S0006-291X(71)80179-1

Matsuo H, Baba Y, Nair RM, Arimura A, Schally AV. Structure of the porcine LH- and FSH-releasing hormone. I. The proposed amino acid sequence. *Biochem Biophys Res Commun* (1971) 43(6):1334–9. doi:10.1016/S0006-291X(71)80019-0

Breton B, Jalabert B, Billard R, Weil C. In vitro stimulation of the release of pituitary gonadotropic hormone by a hypothalamic factor in the carp *Cypri- nus carpio* L. *C R Acad Sci Hebd Seances Acad Sci D* (1971) 273(25):2591–4.

Sherwood N, Eiden L, Brownstein M, Spiess J, Rivier J, Vale W. Characterization of a teleost gonadotropin-releasing hormone. *Proc Natl Acad Sci U S A* (1983) 80(9):2794–8. doi:10.1073/pnas.80.9.2794

Sherwood NM, Zoeller RT, Moore FL. Multiple forms of gonadotropin- releasing hormone in amphibian brains. *Gen Comp Endocrinol* (1986) 61(2):313–22. doi:10.1016/0016-6480(86)90208-X

Miyamoto K, Hasegawa Y, Minegishi T, Nomura M, Takahashi Y, Igarashi M, et al. Isolation and characterization of chicken hypothalamic luteiniz- ing hormone-releasing hormone. *Biochem Biophys Res Commun* (1982) 107(3):820–7. doi:10.1016/0006-291X(82)90596-4

Miyamoto K, Hasegawa Y, Nomura M, Igarashi M, Kangawa K, Matsuo H. Identification of the second gonadotropin-releasing hormone in chicken hypo- thalamus: evidence that gonadotropin secretion is probably controlled by two distinct gonadotropin-releasing hormones in avian species. *Proc Natl Acad Sci U S A* (1984) 81(12):3874–8. doi:10.1073/pnas.81.12.3874

Lovejoy DA, Stell WK, Sherwood NM. Partial characterization of four forms of immunoreactive gonadotropin-releasing hormone in the brain and termi- nal nerve of the spiny dogfish (Elasmobranchii; *Squalus acanthias*). *Regul Pept* (1992) 37(1):39–48. doi:10.1016/0167-0115(92)90062-Y

Ngamvongchon S, Rivier JE, Sherwood NM. Structure-function studies of five natural, including catfish and dogfish, gonadotropin-releasing hormones and eight analogs on reproduction in Thai catfish (*Clarias macrocephalus*). *Regul Pept* (1992) 42(1–2):63–73. doi:10.1016/0167-0115(92)90024-O

Sower SA, Chiang YC, Lovas S, Conlon JM. Primary structure and biologi- cal activity of a third gonadotropin-releasing hormone from lamprey brain. *Endocrinology* (1993) 132(3):1125–31. doi:10.1210/endo.132.3.8440174

Jimenez-Linan M, Rubin BS, King JC. Examination of guinea pig luteiniz- ing hormone-releasing hormone gene reveals a unique decapeptide and existence of two transcripts in the brain. *Endocrinology* (1997) 138(10):4123–30. doi:10.1210/en.138.10.4123

Carolsfeld J, Powell JF, Park M, Fischer WH, Craig AG, Chang JP, et al. Primary structure and function of three gonadotropin-releasing hormones, includ- ing a novel form, from an ancient teleost, herring. *Endocrinology* (2000) 141(2):505–12. doi:10.1210/endo.141.2.7300

Kavanaugh SI, Nozaki M, Sower SA. Origins of gonadotropin-releasing hor- mone (GnRH) in vertebrates: identification of a novel GnRH in a basal ver- tebrate, the sea lamprey. *Endocrinology* (2008) 149(8):3860–9. doi:10.1210/en.2008-0184

Adams BA, Vickers ED, Warby C, Park M, Fischer WH, Grey Craig A, et al. Three forms of gonadotropin-releasing hormone, including a novel form, in a basal salmonid, *Coregonus clupeaformis*. *Biol Reprod* (2002) 67(1):232–9. doi:10.1095/biolreprod67.1.232

Montaner AD, Mongiat L, Lux-Lantos VA, Park MK, Fischer WH, Craig AG, et al. Structure and biological activity of gonadotropin-releasing hormone isoforms isolated from rat and hamster brains. *Neuroendocrinology* (2001) 74(3):202–12. doi:10.1159/000054687

Mohamed JS, Khan IA. Molecular cloning and differential expression of three GnRH mRNAs in discrete brain areas and lymphocytes in red drum. *J Endocrinol* (2006) 188(3):407–16. doi:10.1677/joe.1.06423

Andersson E, Fjelldal PG, Klenke U, Vikingstad E, Taranger GL, Zohar Y, et al. Three forms of GnRH in the brain and pituitary of the turbot, *Scophthalmus maximus*: immunological characterization and seasonal variation. *Comp Biochem Physiol B Biochem Mol Biol* (2001) 129(2–3):551–8. doi:10.1016/S1096-4959(01)00363-3

Okubo K, Amano M, Yoshiura Y, Suetake H, Aida K. A novel form of gonadotropin-releasing hormone in the medaka, *Oryzias latipes*. *Biochem Bio- phys Res Commun* (2000) 276(1):298–303. doi:10.1006/bbrc.2000.3476

Sherwood NM, von Schalburg KR, Lescheid DW. Origin and evolution of GnRH in vertebrates and invertebrates. In: Parhar IS, Sakuma Y, editors. *GnRH Neurons: From Genes to Behavior*. Tokyo: Brain Shuppan (1997). p. 3–25.

Parhar IS. GnRH in tilapia: three genes, three origins and their roles. In: Parhar IS, Sakuma Y, editors. *GnRH Neurons: Gene to Behavior*. Tokyo: Brain Shuppan (1997). p. 99–122.

Parhar IS. Cell migration and evolutionary significance of GnRH subtypes. *Prog Brain Res* (2002) 141:3–17. doi:10.1016/S0079-6123(02)41080-1

Millar RP, Lu ZL, Pawson AJ, Flanagan CA, Morgan K, Maudsley SR. Gonadotropin-releasing hormone receptors. *Endocr Rev* (2004) 25(2):235–75. doi:10.1210/er.2003-0002

Karigo T, Oka Y. Neurobiological study of fish brains gives insights into the nature of gonadotropin-releasing hormone 1-3 neurons. *Front Endocrinol* (2013) 4:177. doi:10.3389/fendo.2013.00177

Powell JF, Zohar Y, Elizur A, Park M, Fischer WH, Craig AG, et al. Three forms of gonadotropin-releasing hormone characterized from brains of one species. *Proc Natl Acad Sci U S A* (1994) 91(25):12081–5. doi:10.1073/pnas.91.25.12081

Okubo K, Nagahama Y. Structural and functional evolution of gonadotropin- releasing hormone in vertebrates. *Acta Physiol* (2008) 193(1):3–15. doi:10. 1111/j.1748-1716.2008.01832.x

White SA, Kasten TL, Bond CT, Adelman JP, Fernald RD. Three gonadotropin- releasing hormone genes in one organism suggest novel roles for an ancient peptide. *Proc Natl Acad Sci U S A* (1995) 92(18):8363–7. doi:10.1073/pnas.92. 18.8363

Gothilf Y, Munoz-Cueto JA, Sagrillo CA, Selmanoff M, Chen TT, Kah O, et al. Three forms of gonadotropin-releasing hormone in a perciform fish (*Sparus aurata*): complementary deoxyribonucleic acid characterization and brain localization. *Biol Reprod* (1996) 55(3):636–45. doi:10.1095/biolreprod55.3.636

Gonzalez-Martinez D, Madigou T, Zmora N, Anglade I, Zanuy S, Zohar Y, et al. Differential expression of three different prepro-GnRH (gonadotropin- releasing hormone) messengers in the brain of the European sea bass (*Dicen- trarchus labrax*). *J Comp Neurol* (2001) 429(1):144–55. doi:10.1002/1096-9861(20000101)429:1<144::AID-CNE11>3.0.CO;2-B

Gonzalez-Martinez D, Zmora N, Mananos E, Saligaut D, Zanuy S, Zohar Y, et al. Immunohistochemical localization of three different prepro-GnRHs in the brain and pituitary of the European sea bass (*Dicentrarchus labrax*) using antibodies to the corresponding GnRH-associated peptides. *J Comp Neurol* (2002) 446(2):95–113. doi:10.1002/cne.10190

Palevitch O, Kight K, Abraham E, Wray S, Zohar Y, Gothilf Y. Ontogeny of the GnRH systems in zebrafish brain: in situ hybridization and promoter-reporter expression analyses in intact animals. *Cell Tissue Res* (2007) 327(2):313–22. doi:10.1007/s00441-006-0279-0

Vickers ED, Laberge F, Adams BA, Hara TJ, Sherwood NM. Cloning and local- ization of three forms of gonadotropin-releasing hormone, including the novel whitefish form, in a salmonid, *Coregonus clupeaformis*. *Biol Reprod* (2004) 70(4):1136–46. doi:10.1095/biolreprod.103.023846

Pandolfi M, Munoz-Cueto JA, Lo Nostro FL, Downs JL, Paz DA, Maggese MC, et al. GnRH systems of *Cichlasoma dimerus* (*Perciformes, Cichlidae*) revisited: a localization study with antibodies and riboprobes to GnRH-associated peptides. *Cell Tissue Res* (2005) 321(2):219–32. doi:10.1007/s00441-004-1055-7

Mohamed JS, Thomas P, Khan IA. Isolation, cloning, and expression of three prepro-GnRH mRNAs in Atlantic croaker brain and pituitary. *J Comp Neurol* (2005) 488(4):384–95. doi:10.1002/cne.20596

Parhar IS, Iwata M. Gonadotropin releasing hormone (GnRH) neurons project to growth hormone and somatolactin cells in the steelhead trout. *Histochemistry* (1994) 102(3):195–203. doi:10.1007/BF00268896

Breton B, Govoroun M, Mikolajczyk T. GTH I and GTH II secretion profiles during the reproductive cycle in female rainbow trout: relationship with pitu- itary responsiveness to GnRH-A stimulation. *Gen Comp Endocrinol* (1998) 111(1):38–50. doi:10.1006/gcen.1998.7088

Mananos EL, Anglade I, Chyb J, Saligaut C, Breton B, Kah O. Involvement of gamma-aminobutyric acid in the control of GTH-1 and GTH-2 secretion in male and female rainbow trout. *Neuroendocrinology* (1999) 69(4):269–80. doi:10.1159/000054428

Weil C, Carre F, Blaise O, Breton B, Le Bail PY. Differential effect of insulin- like growth factor I on in vitro gonadotropin (I and II) and growth hormone secretions in rainbow trout (*Oncorhynchus mykiss*) at different stages of the reproductive cycle. *Endocrinology* (1999) 140(5):2054–62. doi:10.1210/endo. 140.5.6747

Dickey JT, Swanson P. Effects of sex steroids on gonadotropin (FSH and LH) regulation in Coho salmon (*Oncorhynchus kisutch*). *J Mol Endocrinol* (1998) 21(3):291–306. doi:10.1677/jme.0.0210291

Senthilkumaran B, Okuzawa K, Gen K, Ookura T, Kagawa H. Distribution and seasonal variations in levels of three native GnRHs in the brain and pituitary of perciform fish. *J Neuroendocrinol* (1999) 11(3):181–6. doi:10.1046/j.1365-2826.1999.00304.x

Holland MC, Hassin S, Zohar Y. Seasonal fluctuations in pituitary levels of the three forms of gonadotropin-releasing hormone in striped bass, *Morone saxatilis* (*Teleostei*), during juvenile and pubertal development. *J Endocrinol* (2001) 169(3):527–38. doi:10.1677/joe.0.1690527

Amano M, Okubo K, Yamanome T, Yamada H, Aida K, Yamamori K. Changes in brain GnRH mRNA and pituitary GnRH peptide during testicular matu- ration in barfin flounder. *Comp Biochem Physiol B Biochem Mol Biol* (2004) 138(4):435–43. doi:10.1016/j.cbpc.2004.05.005

Amano M, Pham KX, Amiya N, Yamanome T, Yamamori K. Changes in brain seabream GnRH mRNA and pituitary seabream GnRH peptide levels during ovarian maturation in female barfin flounder. *Gen Comp Endocrinol* (2008) 158(2):168–72. doi:10.1016/j.ygcen.2008.06.008

Okuzawa K, Gen K, Bruysters M, Bogerd J, Gothilf Y, Zohar Y, et al. Sea- sonal variation of the three native gonadotropin-releasing hormone messen- ger ribonucleic acids levels in the brain of female red seabream. *Gen Comp Endocrinol* (2003) 130(3):324–32. doi:10.1016/S0016-6480(02)00629-9

Okubo K, Sakai F, Lau EL, Yoshizaki G, Takeuchi Y, Naruse K, et al. Forebrain gonadotropin-releasing hormone neuronal development: insights from trans- genic medaka and the relevance to X-linked Kallmann syndrome. *Endocrinol- ogy* (2006) 147(3):1076–84. doi:10.1210/en.2005-0468

Holland MC, Gothilf Y, Meiri I, King JA, Okuzawa K, Elizur A, et al. Lev- els of the native forms of GnRH in the pituitary of the gilthead seabream, *Sparus aurata*, at several characteristic stages of the gonadal cycle. *Gen Comp Endocrinol* (1998) 112(3):394–405. doi:10.1006/gcen.1998.7138

Zandbergen MA, Kah O, Bogerd J, Peute J, Goos HJ. Expression and distrib- ution of two gonadotropin-releasing hormones in the catfish brain. *Neuroen- docrinology* (1995) 62(6):571–8. doi:10.1159/000127052

Amano M, Oka Y, Yamanome T, Okuzawa K, Yamamori K. Three GnRH sys- tems in the brain and pituitary of a pleuronectiform fish, the barfin flounder *Verasper moseri*. *Cell Tissue Res* (2002) 309(2):323–9. doi:10.1007/s00441-002- 0594-z

Lethimonier C, Madigou T, Munoz-Cueto JA, Lareyre JJ, Kah O. Evolutionary aspects of GnRHs, GnRH neuronal systems and GnRH receptors in teleost fish. *Gen Comp Endocrinol* (2004) 135(1):1–16. doi:10.1016/j.ygcen.2003.10.007

Yamamoto N, Oka Y, Kawashima S. Lesions of gonadotropin-releasing hormone-immunoreactive terminal nerve cells: effects on the reproductive behavior of male dwarf gouramis. *Neuroendocrinology* (1997) 65(6):403–12. doi:10.1159/000127203

Kitahashi T, Sato A, Alok D, Kaeriyama M, Zohar Y, Yamauchi K, et al. Gonadotropin-releasing hormone analog and sex steroids shorten homing duration of sockeye salmon in Lake Shikotsu. *Zoolog Sci* (1998) 15(5):767–71. doi:10.2108/zsj.15.767

Ogawa S, Akiyama G, Kato S, Soga T, Sakuma Y, Parhar IS. Immunoneutraliza- tion of gonadotropin-releasing hormone type-III suppresses male reproductive behavior of cichlids. *Neurosci Lett* (2006) 403(3):201–5. doi:10.1016/j.neulet. 2006.02.041

Umino O, Dowling JE. Dopamine release from interplexiform cells in the retina: effects of GnRH, FMRFamide, bicuculline, and enkephalin on horizontal cell activity. *J Neurosci* (1991) 11(10):3034–46.

Walker SE, Stell WK. Gonadotropin-releasing hormone (GnRF), molluscan cardioexcitatory peptide (FMRFamide), enkephalin and related neuropeptides affect goldfish retinal ganglion cell activity. *Brain Res* (1986) 384(2):262–73. doi:10.1016/0006-8993(86)91162-5

Eisthen HL, Delay RJ, Wirsig-Wiechmann CR, Dionne VE. Neuromodula- tory effects of gonadotropin releasing hormone on olfactory receptor neurons. *J Neurosci* (2000) 20(11):3947–55.

Saito D, Hasegawa Y, Urano A. Gonadotropin-releasing hormones modulate electrical activity of vasotocin and isotocin neurons in the brain of rainbow trout. *Neurosci Lett* (2003) 351(2):107–10. doi:10.1016/j.neulet.2003.08.017

Kinoshita M, Kobayashi S, Urano A, Ito E. Neuromodulatory effects of gonadotropin-releasing hormone on retinotectal synaptic transmission in the optic tectum of rainbow trout. *Eur J Neurosci* (2007) 25(2):480–4. doi:10.1111/j.1460-9568.2006.05294.x

Oka Y. Three types of gonadotrophin-releasing hormone neurones and steroid- sensitive sexually dimorphic kisspeptin neurones in teleosts. *J Neuroendocrinol* (2009) 21(4):334–8. doi:10.1111/j.1365-2826.2009.01850.x

Amano M, Urano A, Aida K. Distribution and function of gonadotropin- releasing hormone (GnRH) in the teleost brain. *Zoolog Sci* (1997) 14(1):1–11. doi:10.2108/zsj.14.1

Abraham E, Palevitch O, Gothilf Y, Zohar Y. The zebrafish as a model sys- tem for forebrain GnRH neuronal development. *Gen Comp Endocrinol* (2009) 164(2–3):151–60. doi:10.1016/j.ygcen.2009.01.012

Parhar IS, Tosaki H, Sakuma Y, Kobayashi M. Sex differences in the brain of goldfish: gonadotropin-releasing hormone and vasotocinergic neurons. *Neuroscience* (2001) 104(4):1099–110. doi:10.1016/S0306-4522(01)00153-1

Oakley AE, Clifton DK, Steiner RA. Kisspeptin signaling in the brain. *Endocr Rev* (2009) 30(6):713–43. doi:10.1210/er.2009-0005

Kotani M, Detheux M, Vandenbogaerde A, Communi D, Vanderwinden JM, Le Poul E, et al. The metastasis suppressor gene KiSS-1 encodes kisspeptins, the natural ligands of the orphan G protein-coupled receptor GPR54. *J Biol Chem* (2001) 276(37):34631–6. doi:10.1074/jbc.M104847200

Kitahashi T, Ogawa S, Parhar IS. Cloning and expression of kiss2 in the zebrafish and medaka. *Endocrinology* (2009) 150(2):821–31. doi:10.1210/en.2008-0940

Felip A, Zanuy S, Pineda R, Pinilla L, Carrillo M, Tena-Sempere M, et al. Evidence for two distinct KiSS genes in non-placental vertebrates that encode kisspeptins with different gonadotropin-releasing activities in fish and mammals. *Mol Cell Endocrinol* (2009) 312(1–2):61–71. doi:10.1016/j.mce. 2008.11.017

Li S, Zhang Y, Liu Y, Huang X, Huang W, Lu D, et al. Structural and functional multiplicity of the kisspeptin/GPR54 system in goldfish (*Carassius auratus*). *J Endocrinol* (2009) 201(3):407–18. doi:10.1677/joe-09-0016

Lee YR, Tsunekawa K, Moon MJ, Um HN, Hwang JI, Osugi T, et al. Molecular evolution of multiple forms of kisspeptins and GPR54 receptors in vertebrates. *Endocrinology* (2009) 150(6):2837–46. doi:10.1210/en.2008-1679

Biran J, Ben-Dor S, Levavi-Sivan B. Molecular identification and functional characterization of the kisspeptin/kisspeptin receptor system in lower verte- brates. *Biol Reprod* (2008) 79(4):776–86. doi:10.1095/biolreprod.107.066266

Mechaly AS, Vinas J, Piferrer F. Identification of two isoforms of the Kisspeptin- 1 receptor (kiss1r) generated by alternative splicing in a modern teleost, the Senegalese sole (*Solea senegalensis*). *Biol Reprod* (2009) 80(1):60–9. doi:10.1095/biolreprod.108.072173

Shi Y, Zhang Y, Li S, Liu Q, Lu D, Liu M, et al. Molecular identifica- tion of the Kiss2/Kiss1ra system and its potential function during 17alpha- methyltestosterone-induced sex reversal in the orange-spotted grouper, *Epi- nephelus coioides*1 . *Biol Reprod* (2010) 83(1):63–74. doi:10.1095/biolreprod.109.080044

Shahjahan M, Motohashi E, Doi H, Ando H. Elevation of Kiss2 and its receptor gene expression in the brain and pituitary of grass puffer during the spawning season. *Gen Comp Endocrinol* (2010) 169(1):48–57. doi:10.1016/j.ygcen.2010. 07.008

Mechaly AS, Vinas J, Murphy C, Reith M, Piferrer F. Gene structure of the Kiss1 receptor-2 (Kiss1r-2) in the Atlantic halibut: insights into the evolution and regulation of Kiss1r genes. *Mol Cell Endocrinol* (2010) 317(1–2):78–89. doi:10.1016/j.mce.2009.11.005

Yang B, Jiang Q, Chan T, Ko WKW, Wong AOL. Goldfish kisspeptin: molecular cloning, tissue distribution of transcript expression, and stimulatory effects on prolactin, growth hormone and luteinizing hormone secretion and gene expression via direct actions at the pituitary level. *Gen Comp Endocrinol* (2010) 165(1):60–71. doi:10.1016/j.ygcen.2009.06.001

Kanda S, Akazome Y, Matsunaga T, Yamamoto N, Yamada S, Tsukamura H, et al. Identification of KiSS-1 product kisspeptin and steroid-sensitive sexu- ally dimorphic kisspeptin neurons in medaka (*Oryzias latipes*). *Endocrinology* (2008) 149(5):2467–76. doi:10.1210/en.2007-1503

Servili A, Le Page Y, Leprince J, Caraty A, Escobar S, Parhar IS, et al. Organiza- tion of two independent kisspeptin systems derived from evolutionary-ancient kiss genes in the brain of zebrafish. *Endocrinology* (2011) 152(4):1527–40. doi:10.1210/en.2010-0948

Parhar IS, Ogawa S, Sakuma Y. Laser-captured single digoxigenin-labeled neu- rons of gonadotropin-releasing hormone types reveal a novel G protein- coupled receptor (Gpr54) during maturation in cichlid fish. *Endocrinology* (2004) 145(8):3613–8. doi:10.1210/en.2004-0395

Ogawa S, Ng KW, Ramadasan PN, Nathan FM, Parhar IS. Habenular Kiss1 neu- rons modulate the serotonergic system in the brain of zebrafish. *Endocrinology* (2012) 153(5):2398–407. doi:10.1210/en.2012-1062

Tsutsui K, Saigoh E, Ukena K, Teranishi H, Fujisawa Y, Kikuchi M, et al. A novel avian hypothalamic peptide inhibiting gonadotropin release. *Biochem Biophys Res Commun* (2000) 275(2):661–7. doi:10.1006/bbrc.2000.3350

Parhar I, Ogawa S, Kitahashi T. RFamide peptides as mediators in envi- ronmental control of GnRH neurons. *Prog Neurobiol* (2012) 98(2):176–96. doi:10.1016/j.pneurobio.2012.05.011

Tsutsui K, Ubuka T, Bentley GE, Kriegsfeld LJ. Gonadotropin-inhibitory hor- mone (GnIH): discovery, progress and prospect. *Gen Comp Endocrinol* (2012) 177(3):305–14. doi:10.1016/j.ygcen.2012.02.013

Sawada K, Ukena K, Satake H, Iwakoshi E, Minakata H, Tsutsui K. Novel fish hypothalamic neuropeptide. *Eur J Biochem* (2002) 269(24):6000–8. doi:10.1046/j.1432-1033.2002.03351.x

Amano M, Moriyama S, Iigo M, Kitamura S, Amiya N, Yamamori K, et al. Novel fish hypothalamic neuropeptides stimulate the release of gonadotrophins and growth hormone from the pituitary of sockeye salmon. *J Endocrinol* (2006) 188(3):417–23. doi:10.1677/joe.1.06494

Moussavi M, Wlasichuk M, Chang JP, Habibi HR. Seasonal effect of GnIH on gonadotrope functions in the pituitary of goldfish. *Mol Cell Endocrinol* (2012) 350(1):53–60. doi:10.1016/j.mce.2011.11.020

Zhang Y, Li S, Liu Y, Lu D, Chen H, Huang X, et al. Structural diversity of the GnIH/GnIH receptor system in teleost: its involvement in early develop- ment and the negative control of LH release. *Peptides* (2010) 31(6):1034–43. doi:10.1016/j.peptides.2010.03.003

Qi X, Zhou W, Li S, Lu D, Yi S, Xie R, et al. Evidences for the regulation of GnRH and GTH expression by GnIH in the goldfish, *Carassius auratus*. *Mol Cell Endocrinol* (2013) 366(1):9–20. doi:10.1016/j.mce.2012.11.001

Qi X, Zhou W, Lu D, Wang Q, Zhang H, Li S, et al. Sexual dimorphism of steroidogenesis regulated by GnIH in the goldfish, *Carassius auratus*. *Biol Reprod* (2013) 88(4):89. doi:10.1095/biolreprod.112.105114

Shahjahan M, Ikegami T, Osugi T, Ukena K, Doi H, Hattori A, et al. Synchro- nised expressions of LPXRFamide peptide and its receptor genes: seasonal, diurnal and circadian changes during spawning period in grass puffer. *J Neu- roendocrinol* (2011) 23(1):39–51. doi:10.1111/j.1365-2826.2010.02081.x

Ubuka T, Inoue K, Fukuda Y, Mizuno T, Ukena K, Kriegsfeld LJ, et al. Identification, expression, and physiological functions of Siberian hamster gonadotropin-inhibitory hormone. *Endocrinology* (2012) 153(1):373–85. doi:10.1210/en.2011-1110

Umatani C, Abe H, Oka Y. Neuropeptide RFRP inhibits the pacemaker activ- ity of terminal nerve GnRH neurons. *J Neurophysiol* (2013) 109(9):2354–63. doi:10.1152/jn.00712.2012

Yokobori E, Kojima K, Azuma M, Kang KS, Maejima S, Uchiyama M, et al. Stimulatory effect of intracerebroventricular administration of orexin A on food intake in the zebrafish, *Danio rerio*. *Peptides* (2011) 32(7):1357–62. doi:10.1016/j.peptides.2011.05.010

Facciolo RM, Crudo M, Giusi G, Alo R, Canonaco M. Light- and dark-dependent orexinergic neuronal signals promote neurodegenerative phenom- ena accounting for distinct behavioral responses in the teleost *Thalassoma pavo*. *J Neurosci Res* (2009) 87(3):748–57. doi:10.1002/jnr.21886

Hoskins LJ, Xu M, Volkoff H. Interactions between gonadotropin-releasing hormone (GnRH) and orexin in the regulation of feeding and reproduction in goldfish (*Carassius auratus*). *Horm Behav* (2008) 54(3):379–85. doi:10.1016/j. yhbeh.2008.04.011

Lopez-Patino MA, Guijarro AI, Isorna E, Delgado MJ, Alonso-Bedate M, de Pedro N. Neuropeptide Y has a stimulatory action on feeding behavior in goldfish (*Carassius auratus*). *Eur J Pharmacol* (1999) 377(2–3):147–53. doi:10.1016/S0014-2999(99)00408-2

Aldegunde M, Mancebo M. Effects of neuropeptide Y on food intake and brain biogenic amines in the rainbow trout (*Oncorhynchus mykiss*). *Peptides* (2006) 27(4):719–27. doi:10.1016/j.peptides.2005.09.014

Matsuda K. Recent advances in the regulation of feeding behavior by neu- ropeptides in fish. *Ann N Y Acad Sci* (2009) 1163:241–50. doi:10.1111/j.1749-6632.2008.03619.x

Yokobori E, Azuma M, Nishiguchi R, Kang KS, Kamijo M, Uchiyama M, et al. Neuropeptide Y stimulates food intake in the zebrafish, *Danio rerio*. *J Neuroendocrinol* (2012) 24(5):766–73. doi:10.1111/j.1365-2826.2012.02281.x

Peng C, Humphries S, Peter RE, Rivier JE, Blomqvist AG, Larhammar D. Actions of goldfish neuropeptide Y on the secretion of growth hor- mone and gonadotropin-II in female goldfish. *Gen Comp Endocrinol* (1993) 90(3):306–17. doi:10.1006/gcen.1993.1086

Peng C, Chang JP, Yu KL, Wong AO, Van Goor F, Peter RE, et al. Neuropeptide-Y stimulates growth hormone and gonadotropin-II secretion in the goldfish pitu- itary: involvement of both presynaptic and pituitary cell actions. *Endocrinology* (1993) 132(4):1820–9. doi:10.1210/endo.132.4.8462479

Breton B, Mikolajczyk T, Popek W, Bieniarz K, Epler P. Neuropeptide Y stim ulates in vivo gonadotropin secretion in teleost fish. *Gen Comp Endocrinol* (1991) 84(2):277–83. doi:10.1016/0016-6480(91)90050-G

Senthilkumaran B, Okuzawa K, Gen K, Kagawa H. Effects of serotonin, GABA and neuropeptide Y on seabream gonadotropin releasing hormone release in vitro from preoptic-anterior hypothalamus and pituitary of red seabream, *Pagrus major*. *J Neuroendocrinol* (2001) 13(5):395–400. doi:10.1046/j.1365-2826.2001.00645.x

Cerda-Reverter JM, Sorbera LA, Carrillo M, Zanuy S. Energetic dependence of NPY-induced LH secretion in a teleost fish (*Dicentrarchus labrax*). *Am J Physiol* (1999) 277(6 Pt 2):R1627–34.

Matsuda K, Maruyama K, Nakamachi T, Miura T, Uchiyama M, Shioda S. Inhibitory effects of pituitary adenylate cyclase-activating polypeptide (PACAP) and vasoactive intestinal peptide (VIP) on food intake in the goldfish, *Carassius auratus. Peptides* (2005) 26(9):1611–6. doi:10.1016/j.peptides.2005. 02.022

Sawisky GR, Chang JP. Intracellular calcium involvement in pituitary adeny- late cyclase-activating polypeptide stimulation of growth hormone and gonadotrophin secretion in goldfish pituitary cells. *J Neuroendocrinol* (2005) 17(6):353–71. doi:10.1111/j.1365-2826.2005.01312.x

Chang JP, Wirachowsky NR, Kwong P, Johnson JD. Pacap stimulation of gonadotropin-II secretion in goldfish pituitary cells: mechanisms of action and interaction with gonadotropin releasing hormone signalling. *J Neuroendocrinol* (2001) 13(6):540–50. doi:10.1046/j.1365-2826.2001.00667.x

Yaron Z, Gur G, Melamed P, Rosenfeld H, Levavi-Sivan B, Elizur A. Reg- ulation of gonadotropin subunit genes in tilapia. *Comp Biochem Physiol B Biochem Mol Biol* (2001) 129(2–3):489–502. doi:10.1016/S1096-4959(01) 00345-1

Levy G, Jackson K, Degani G. Association between pituitary adenylate cyclase- activating polypeptide and reproduction in the blue gourami. *Gen Comp Endocrinol* (2010) 166(1):83–93. doi:10.1016/j.ygcen.2009.09.015

Levy G, Degani G. Involvement of GnRH, PACAP and PRP in the reproduc- tion of blue gourami females (*Trichogaster trichopterus*). *J Mol Neurosci* (2012) 48(3):603–16. doi:10.1007/s12031-012-9730-8

Matsuda K, Nakamura K, Shimakura S, Miura T, Kageyama H, Uchiyama M, et al. Inhibitory effect of chicken gonadotropin-releasing hormone II on food intake in the goldfish, *Carassius auratus. Horm Behav* (2008) 54(1):83–9. doi:10.1016/j.yhbeh.2008.01.011

Nishiguchi R, Azuma M, Yokobori E, Uchiyama M, Matsuda K. Gonadotropin- releasing hormone 2 suppresses food intake in the zebrafish, *Danio rerio. Front Endocrinol* (2012) 3:122. doi:10.3389/fendo.2012.00122

Chang JP, Freedman GL, de Leeuw R. Use of a pituitary cell dispersion method and primary culture system for the studies of gonadotropin-releasing hormone action in the goldfish, *Carassius auratus*. II. Extracellular calcium dependence and dopaminergic inhibition of gonadotropin responses. *Gen Comp Endocrinol* (1990) 77(2):274–82. doi:10.1016/0016-6480(90)90311-9

Chartrel N, Dujardin C, Anouar Y, Leprince J, Decker A, Clerens S, et al. Identi- fication of 26RFa, a hypothalamic neuropeptide of the RFamide peptide family with orexigenic activity. *Proc Natl Acad Sci U S A* (2003) 100(25):15247–52. doi:10.1073/pnas.2434676100

Liu Y, Zhang Y, Li S, Huang W, Liu X, Lu D, et al. Molecular cloning and func- tional characterization of the first non-mammalian 26RFa/QRFP orthologue in goldfish, *Carassius auratus. Mol Cell Endocrinol* (2009) 303(1–2):82–90. doi:10.1016/j.mce.2009.01.009

Volkoff H, Peter RE. Interactions between orexin A, NPY and galanin in the control of food intake of the goldfish, *Carassius auratus. Regul Pept* (2001) 101(1–3):59–72. doi:10.1016/S0167-0115(01)00261-0

Guijarro AI, Delgado MJ, Pinillos ML, López-Patiño MA, Alonso-Bedate M, De Pedro N. Galanin and β-endorphin as feeding regulators in cyprinids: effect of temperature. *Aquac Res* (1999) 30(7):483–9. doi:10.1046/j.1365-2109.1999.00360.x

Merchenthaler I, Lopez FJ, Negro-Vilar A. Colocalization of galanin and luteinizing hormone-releasing hormone in a subset of preoptic hypothalamic neurons: anatomical and functional correlates. *Proc Natl Acad Sci U S A* (1990) 87(16):6326–30. doi:10.1073/pnas.87.16.6326

Matsuda K, Shimakura S, Maruyama K, Miura T, Uchiyama M, Kawauchi H, et al. Central administration of melanin-concentrating hormone (MCH) suppresses food intake, but not locomotor activity, in the goldfish, *Carassius auratus. Neurosci Lett* (2006) 399(3):259–63. doi:10.1016/j.neulet.2006.02.005

Cerda-Reverter JM, Canosa LF, Peter RE. Regulation of the hypothalamic melanin-concentrating hormone neurons by sex steroids in the goldfish: possi- ble role in the modulation of luteinizing hormone secretion. *Neuroendocrinol- ogy* (2006) 84(6):364–77. doi:10.1159/000098334

Cerda-Reverter JM, Schioth HB, Peter RE. The central melanocortin sys- tem regulates food intake in goldfish. *Regul Pept* (2003) 115(2):101–13. doi:10.1016/S0167-0115(03)00144-7

Schjolden J, Schioth HB, Larhammar D, Winberg S, Larson ET. Melanocortin peptides affect the motivation to feed in rainbow trout (*Oncorhynchus mykiss*). *Gen Comp Endocrinol* (2009) 160(2):134–8. doi:10.1016/j.ygcen.2008.11.003

Roa J. Role of GnRH neurons and their neuronal afferents as key integrators between food intake regulatory signals and the control of reproduction. *Int J Endocrinol* (2013) 2013:518046. doi:10.1155/2013/518046

Volkoff H, Peter RE. Effects of CART peptides on food consumption, feeding and associated behaviors in the goldfish, *Carassius auratus*: actions on neuropeptide Y- and orexin A-induced feeding. *Brain Res* (2000) 887(1):125–33. doi:10.1016/S0006-8993(00)03001-8

Volkoff H, Peter RE. Characterization of two forms of cocaine- and amphetamine-regulated transcript (CART) peptide precursors in goldfish: molecular cloning and distribution, modulation of expression by nutritional status, and interactions with leptin. *Endocrinology* (2001) 142(12):5076–88. doi:10.1210/en.142.12.5076

Lebrethon MC, Vandersmissen E, Gerard A, Parent AS, Bourguignon JP. Cocaine and amphetamine-regulated-transcript peptide mediation of leptin stimulatory effect on the rat gonadotropin-releasing hormone pulse generator in vitro. *J Neuroendocrinol* (2000) 12(5):383–5. doi:10.1046/j.1365-2826.2000.00497.x

Parent AS, Lebrethon MC, Gerard A, Vandersmissen E, Bourguignon JP. Lep- tin effects on pulsatile gonadotropin releasing hormone secretion from the adult rat hypothalamus and interaction with cocaine and amphetamine regulated transcript peptide and neuropeptide Y. *Regul Pept* (2000) 92(1–3):17–24. doi:10.1016/S0167-0115(00)00144-0

Himick BA, Peter RE. CCK/gastrin-like immunoreactivity in brain and gut, and CCK suppression of feeding in goldfish. *Am J Physiol* (1994) 267(3 Pt 2):R841–51.

Himick BA, Golosinski AA, Jonsson AC, Peter RE. CCK/gastrin-like immunore- activity in the goldfish pituitary: regulation of pituitary hormone secretion by CCK-like peptides in vitro. *Gen Comp Endocrinol* (1993) 92(1):88–103. doi:10.1006/gcen.1993.1146

Gonzalez R, Kerbel B, Chun A, Unniappan S. Molecular, cellular and physio- logical evidences for the anorexigenic actions of nesfatin-1 in goldfish. *PLoS One* (2010) 5(12):e15201. doi:10.1371/journal.pone.0015201

Kerbel B, Unniappan S. Nesfatin-1 suppresses energy intake, co-localises ghre- lin in the brain and gut, and alters ghrelin, cholecystokinin and orexin mRNA expression in goldfish. *J Neuroendocrinol* (2012) 24(2):366–77. doi:10.1111/j.1365-2826.2011.02246.x

Gonzalez R, Shepperd E, Thiruppugazh V, Lohan S, Grey CL, Chang JP, et al. Nesfatin-1 regulates the hypothalamo-pituitary-ovarian axis of fish. *Biol Reprod* (2012) 87(4):84. doi:10.1095/biolreprod.112.099630

Volkoff H, Eykelbosh AJ, Peter RE. Role of leptin in the control of feeding of goldfish *Carassius auratus*: interactions with cholecystokinin, neuropeptide Y and orexin A, and modulation by fasting. *Brain Res* (2003) 972(1–2):90–109. doi:10.1016/S0006-8993(03)02507-1

Murashita K, Uji S, Yamamoto T, Ronnestad I, Kurokawa T. Production of recombinant leptin and its effects on food intake in rainbow trout (*Oncorhynchus mykiss*). *Comp Biochem Physiol B Biochem Mol Biol* (2008) 150(4):377–84. doi:10.1016/j.cbpb.2008.04.007

Peyon P, Zanuy S, Carrillo M. Action of leptin on in vitro luteinizing hormone release in the European sea bass (*Dicentrarchus labrax*). *Biol Reprod* (2001) 65(5):1573–8. doi:10.1095/biolreprod65.5.1573

Weil C, Le Bail PY, Sabin N, Le Gac F. In vitro action of leptin on FSH and LH production in rainbow trout (*Onchorynchus mykiss*) at different stages of the sexual cycle. *Gen Comp Endocrinol* (2003) 130(1):2–12. doi:10.1016/S0016-6480(02)00504-X

Unniappan S, Lin X, Cervini L, Rivier J, Kaiya H, Kangawa K, et al. Goldfish ghrelin: molecular characterization of the complementary deoxyribonucleic acid, partial gene structure and evidence for its stimulatory role in food intake. *Endocrinology* (2002) 143(10):4143–6. doi:10.1210/en.2002-220644

Matsuda K, Miura T, Kaiya H, Maruyama K, Shimakura S, Uchiyama M, et al. Regulation of food intake by acyl and des-acyl ghrelins in the goldfish. *Peptides* (2006) 27(9):2321–5. doi:10.1016/j.peptides.2006.03.028

Miura T, Maruyama K, Kaiya H, Miyazato M, Kangawa K, Uchiyama M, et al. Purification and properties of ghrelin from the intestine of the goldfish, *Car- as- sius auratus. Peptides* (2009) 30(4):758–65. doi:10.1016/j.peptides.2008.12.016

Jonsson E, Kaiya H, Bjornsson BT. Ghrelin decreases food intake in juve- nile rainbow trout (*Oncorhynchus mykiss*) through the central anorexi- genic corticotropin-releasing factor system. *Gen Comp Endocrinol* (2010) 166(1):39–46. doi:10.1016/j.ygcen.2009.11.001

Unniappan S, Peter RE. In vitro and in vivo effects of ghrelin on luteinizing hormone and growth hormone release in goldfish. *Am J Physiol Regul Integr Comp Physiol* (2004) 286(6):R1093–101. doi:10.1152/ajpregu.00669.2003

Sokolowska-Mikolajczyk M, Socha M, Szczerbik P, Epler P. The effects of ghre- lin on the in vitro spontaneous and sGnRH-A stimulated luteinizing hor- mone (LH) release from the pituitary cells of common carp (*Cyprinus car- pio* L.). *Comp Biochem Physiol A Mol Integr Physiol* (2009) 153(4):386–90. doi:10.1016/j.cbpa.2009.03.012

Wong KK, Ng SY, Lee LT, Ng HK, Chow BK. Orexins and their receptors from fish to mammals: a comparative approach. *Gen Comp Endocrinol* (2011) 171(2):124–30. doi:10.1016/j.ygcen.2011.01.001

Sakurai T, Amemiya A, Ishii M, Matsuzaki I, Chemelli RM, Tanaka H, et al. Orexins and orexin receptors: a family of hypothalamic neuropeptides and G protein-coupled receptors that regulate feeding behavior. *Cell* (1998) 92(4):573–85. doi:10.1016/S0092-8674(02)09256-5

Nakamachi T, Matsuda K, Maruyama K, Miura T, Uchiyama M, Funahashi H, et al. Regulation by orexin of feeding behaviour and locomotor activity in the goldfish. *J Neuroendocrinol* (2006) 18(4):290–7. doi:10.1111/j.1365-2826.2006.01415.x

Sasson R, Dearth RK, White RS, Chappell PE, Mellon PL. Orexin A induces GnRH gene expression and secretion from GT1-7 hypothalamic GnRH neu- rons. *Neuroendocrinology* (2006) 84(6):353–63. doi:10.1159/000098333

Russell SH, Small CJ, Kennedy AR, Stanley SA, Seth A, Murphy KG, et al. Orexin A interactions in the hypothalamo-pituitary gonadal axis. *Endocrinol- ogy* (2001) 142(12):5294–302. doi:10.1210/endo.142.12.8558

Campbell RE, Grove KL, Smith MS. Gonadotropin-releasing hormone neu- rons coexpress orexin 1 receptor immunoreactivity and receive direct contacts by orexin fibers. *Endocrinology* (2003) 144(4):1542–8. doi:10.1210/en.2002- 220958

Amiya N, Amano M, Oka Y, Iigo M, Takahashi A, Yamamori K. Immuno- histochemical localization of orexin/hypocretin-like immunoreactive peptides and melanin-concentrating hormone in the brain and pituitary of medaka. *Neurosci Lett* (2007) 427(1):16–21. doi:10.1016/j.neulet.2007.07.043

Suzuki H, Miyoshi Y, Yamamoto T. Orexin-A (hypocretin 1)-like immunore- activity in growth hormone-containing cells of the Japanese seaperch (*Late- olabrax japonicus*) pituitary. *Gen Comp Endocrinol* (2007) 150(2):205–11. doi:10.1016/j.ygcen.2006.08.008

Suzuki H, Matsumoto A, Yamamoto T. Orexin-B-like immunoreactivity localized in both luteinizing hormone- and thyroid-stimulating hormone- containing cells in the Nile tilapia (*Oreochromis niloticus*) pituitary. *Tissue Cell* (2009) 41(1):75–8. doi:10.1016/j.tice.2008.06.001

Tatemoto K, Carlquist M, Mutt V. Neuropeptide Y – a novel brain peptide with structural similarities to peptide YY and pancreatic polypeptide. *Nature* (1982) 296(5858):659–60. doi:10.1038/296659a0

Valassi E, Scacchi M, Cavagnini F. Neuroendocrine control of food intake. *Nutr Metab Cardiovasc Dis* (2008) 18(2):158–68. doi:10.1016/j.numecd.2007.06.004

de Pedro N, Lopez-Patino MA, Guijarro AI, Pinillos ML, Delgado MJ, Alonso- Bedate M. NPY receptors and opioidergic system are involved in NPY-induced feeding in goldfish. *Peptides* (2000) 21(10):1495–502. doi:10.1016/S0196- 9781(00)00303-X

Narnaware YK, Peyon PP, Lin X, Peter RE. Regulation of food intake by neuropeptide Y in goldfish. *Am J Physiol Regul Integr Comp Physiol* (2000) 279(3):R1025–34.

Narnaware YK, Peter RE. Effects of food deprivation and refeeding on neu- ropeptide Y (NPY) mRNA levels in goldfish. *Comp Biochem Physiol B Biochem Mol Biol* (2001) 129(2–3):633–7. doi:10.1016/S1096-4959(01)00359-1

Narnaware YK, Peter RE. Neuropeptide Y stimulates food consumption through multiple receptors in goldfish. *Physiol Behav* (2001) 74(1–2):185–90. doi:10.1016/S0031-9384(01)00556-X

Kamijo M, Kojima K, Maruyama K, Konno N, Motohashi E, Ikegami T, et al. Neuropeptide Y in tiger puffer (*Takifugu rubripes*): distribution, cloning, char- acterization, and mRNA expression responses to prandial condition. *Zoolog Sci* (2011) 28(12):882–90. doi:10.2108/zsj.28.882

Wojcik-Gladysz A, Polkowska J. Neuropeptide Y – a neuromodulatory link between nutrition and reproduction at the central nervous system level. *Reprod Biol* (2006) 6(Suppl 2):21–8.

Breton B, Motin A, Billard R, Kah O, Geoffre S, Precigoux G. Immunoreac- tive gonadotropin-releasing hormone-like material in the brain and the pitu- itary gland during the periovulatory period in the brown trout (*Salmo trutta* L.): relationships with the plasma and pituitary gonadotropin. *Gen Comp Endocrinol* (1986) 61(1):109–19. doi:10.1016/0016-6480(86)90255-8

Danger JM, Breton B, Vallarino M, Fournier A, Pelletier G, Vaudry H. Neuropeptide-Y in the trout brain and pituitary: localization, characteriza- tion, and action on gonadotropin release. *Endocrinology* (1991) 128(5):2360–8. doi:10.1210/endo-128-5-2360

Chiba A, Sohn YC, Honma Y. Distribution of neuropeptide Y and gonadotropin-releasing hormone immunoreactivities in the brain and hypophysis of the ayu, *Plecoglossus altivelis* (*Teleostei*). *Arch Histol Cytol* (1996) 59(2):137–48. doi:10.1679/aohc.59.137

Amiya N, Amano M, Tabuchi A, Oka Y. Anatomical relations between neu- ropeptide Y, galanin, and gonadotropin-releasing hormone in the brain of chondrostean, the Siberian sturgeon *Acipenser baeri*. *Neurosci Lett* (2011) 503(2):87–92. doi:10.1016/j.neulet.2011.08.008

Gaikwad A, Biju KC, Subhedar N. GnRH-LH secreting cells axis in the pitu- itary of the teleost *Clarias batrachus* responds to neuropeptide Y treatment: an immunocytochemical study. *Gen Comp Endocrinol* (2003) 131(2):126–33. doi:10.1016/S0016-6480(02)00631-7

Ukena K, Tachibana T, Iwakoshi-Ukena E, Saito Y, Minakata H, Kawaguchi R, et al. Identification, localization, and function of a novel avian hypothala- mic neuropeptide, 26RFa, and its cognate receptor, G protein-coupled receptor- 103. *Endocrinology* (2010) 151(5):2255–64. doi:10.1210/en.2009-1478

Primeaux SD. QRFP in female rats: effects on high fat food intake and hypothal- amic gene expression across the estrous cycle. *Peptides* (2011) 32(6):1270–5. doi:10.1016/j.peptides.2011.03.022

Takayasu S, Sakurai T, Iwasaki S, Teranishi H, Yamanaka A, Williams SC, et al. A neuropeptide ligand of the G protein-coupled receptor GPR103 regulates feeding, behavioral arousal, and blood pressure in mice. *Proc Natl Acad Sci U S A* (2006) 103(19):7438–43. doi:10.1073/pnas.0602371103

Navarro VM, Fernandez-Fernandez R, Nogueiras R, Vigo E, Tovar S, Chartrel N, et al. Novel role of 26RFa, a hypothalamic RFamide orexigenic peptide, as putative regulator of the gonadotropic axis. *J Physiol* (2006) 573(Pt 1):237–49. doi:10.1113/jphysiol.2006.106856

Gundlach AL. Galanin/GALP and galanin receptors: role in central control of feeding, body weight/obesity and reproduction? *Eur J Pharmacol* (2002) 440(2–3):255–68. doi:10.1016/S0014-2999(02)01433-4

Vrontakis ME. Galanin: a biologically active peptide. *Curr Drug Targets CNS Neurol Disord* (2002) 1(6):531–41. doi:10.2174/1568007023338914

Rajendren G, Li X. Galanin synaptic input to gonadotropin-releasing hormone perikarya in juvenile and adult female mice: implications for sexual maturity. *Brain Res Dev Brain Res* (2001) 131(1–2):161–5. doi:10.1016/S0165-3806(01) 00257-7

Merchenthaler I, Lopez FJ, Lennard DE, Negro-Vilar A. Sexual differences in the distribution of neurons coexpressing galanin and luteinizing hormone- releasing hormone in the rat brain. *Endocrinology* (1991) 129(4):1977–86. doi:10.1210/endo-129-4-1977

Dudas B, Merchenthaler I. Bi-directional associations between galanin and luteinizing hormone-releasing hormone neuronal systems in the human diencephalon. *Neuroscience* (2004) 127(3):695–707. doi:10.1016/j.neuroscience. 2004.05.018

Mitchell V, Bouret S, Prevot V, Jennes L, Beauvillain JC. Evidence for expression of galanin receptor Gal-R1 mRNA in certain gonadotropin releasing hormone neurones of the rostral preoptic area. *J Neuroendocrinol* (1999) 11(10):805–12. doi:10.1046/j.1365-2826.1999.00399.x

Batten TF, Moons L, Cambre M, Vandesande F. Anatomical distribution of galanin-like immunoreactivity in the brain and pituitary of teleost fishes. *Neu- rosci Lett* (1990) 111(1–2):12–7. doi:10.1016/0304-3940(90)90336-8

Anglade I, Wang Y, Jensen J, Tramu G, Kah O, Conlon JM. Characterization of trout galanin and its distribution in trout brain and pituitary. *J Comp Neurol* (1994) 350(1):63–74. doi:10.1002/cne.903500105

Power DM, Canario AV, Ingleton PM. Somatotropin release-inhibiting factor and galanin innervation in the hypothalamus and pituitary of seabream (*Sparus aurata*). *Gen Comp Endocrinol* (1996) 101(3):264–74. doi:10.1006/gcen.1996. 0029

Rodriguez-Gomez FJ, Rendon-Unceta MC, Sarasquete C, Munoz-Cueto JA. Localization of galanin-like immunoreactive structures in the brain of the Senegalese sole, *Solea senegalensis. Histochem J* (2000) 32(2):123–31. doi:10. 1023/A:1004074430973

Kauffman AS, Rissman EF. The evolutionarily conserved gonadotropin- releasing hormone II modifies food intake. *Endocrinology* (2004) 145(2):686–91. doi:10.1210/en.2003-1150

Kauffman AS, Wills A, Millar RP, Rissman EF. Evidence that the type-2 gonadotrophin-releasing hormone (GnRH) receptor mediates the behavioural effects of GnRH-II on feeding and reproduction in musk shrews. *J Neuroen- docrinol* (2005) 17(8):489–97. doi:10.1111/j.1365-2826.2005.01334.x

Volkoff H, Peter RE. Actions of two forms of gonadotropin releasing hormone and a GnRH antagonist on spawning behavior of the goldfish *Caras- sius auratus. Gen Comp Endocrinol* (1999) 116(3):347–55. doi:10.1006/gcen.1999.7377

Canosa LF, Stacey N, Peter RE. Changes in brain mRNA levels of gonadotropin- releasing hormone, pituitary adenylate cyclase activating polypeptide, and somatostatin during ovulatory luteinizing hormone and growth hor- mone surges in goldfish. *Am J Physiol Regul Integr Comp Physiol* (2008) 295(6):R1815–21. doi:10.1152/ajpregu.00166.2008

Kim MH, Oka Y, Amano M, Kobayashi M, Okuzawa K, Hasegawa Y, et al. Immunocytochemical localization of sGnRH and cGnRH-II in the brain of goldfish, *Carassius auratus. J Comp Neurol* (1995) 356(1):72–82. doi:10.1002/cne.903560105

Shahjahan M, Hamabata T, Motohashi E, Doi H, Ando H. Differential expres- sion of three types of gonadotropin-releasing hormone genes during the spawning season in grass puffer, *Takifugu niphobles. Gen Comp Endocrinol* (2010) 167(1):153–63. doi:10.1016/j.ygcen.2010.01.018

Miyata A, Arimura A, Dahl RR, Minamino N, Uehara A, Jiang L, et al. Isolation of a novel 38 residue-hypothalamic polypeptide which stimulates adenylate cyclase in pituitary cells. *Biochem Biophys Res Commun* (1989) 164(1):567–74. doi:10.1016/0006-291X(89)91757-9

Morley JE, Horowitz M, Morley PM, Flood JF. Pituitary adenylate cyclase activating polypeptide (PACAP) reduces food intake in mice. *Peptides* (1992) 13(6):1133–5. doi:10.1016/0196-9781(92)90019-Y

Tachibana T, Saito S, Tomonaga S, Takagi T, Saito ES, Boswell T, et al. Intracere- broventricular injection of vasoactive intestinal peptide and pituitary adenylate cyclase-activating polypeptide inhibits feeding in chicks. *Neurosci Lett* (2003) 339(3):203–6. doi:10.1016/S0304-3940(03)00017-X

Tachibana T, Tomonaga S, Oikawa D, Saito S, Takagi T, Saito ES, et al. Pitu- itary adenylate cyclase activating polypeptide and vasoactive intestinal peptide inhibit feeding in the chick brain by different mechanisms. *Neurosci Lett* (2003) 348(1):25–8. doi:10.1016/S0304-3940(03)00646-3

Matsuda K, Kang KS, Sakashita A, Yahashi S, Vaudry H. Behavioral effect of neuropeptides related to feeding regulation in fish. *Ann N Y Acad Sci* (2011) 1220:117–26. doi:10.1111/j.1749-6632.2010.05884.x

Wong AO, Li WS, Lee EK, Leung MY, Tse LY, Chow BK, et al. Pituitary adeny- late cyclase activating polypeptide as a novel hypophysiotropic factor in fish. *Biochem Cell Biol* (2000) 78(3):329–43. doi:10.1139/o00-055

Wong AO, Leung MY, Shea WL, Tse LY, Chang JP, Chow BK. Hypophys- iotropic action of pituitary adenylate cyclase-activating polypeptide (PACAP) in the goldfish: immunohistochemical demonstration of PACAP in the pitu- itary, PACAP stimulation of growth hormone release from pituitary cells, and molecular cloning of pituitary type I PACAP receptor. *Endocrinology* (1998) 139(8):3465–79. doi:10.1210/endo.139.8.6145

Montero M, Yon L, Rousseau K, Arimura A, Fournier A, Dufour S, et al. Distribution, characterization, and growth hormone-releasing activity of pituitary adenylate cyclase-activating polypeptide in the European eel, *Anguilla anguilla. Endocrinology* (1998) 139(10):4300–10. doi:10.1210/endo. 139.10.6239

Kawauchi H, Kawazoe I, Tsubokawa M, Kishida M, Baker BI. Characterization of melanin-concentrating hormone in chum salmon pituitaries. *Nature* (1983) 305(5932):321–3. doi:10.1038/305321a0

Takahashi A, Tsuchiya K, Yamanome T, Amano M, Yasuda A, Yamamori K, et al. Possible involvement of melanin-concentrating hormone in food intake in a teleost fish, barfin flounder. *Peptides* (2004) 25(10):1613–22. doi:10.1016/j.peptides.2004.02.022

Tuziak SM, Volkoff H. A preliminary investigation of the role of melanin- concentrating hormone (MCH) and its receptors in appetite regulation of winter flounder (*Pseudopleuronectes americanus*). *Mol Cell Endocrinol* (2012) 348(1):281–96. doi:10.1016/j.mce.2011.09.015

Qu D, Ludwig DS, Gammeltoft S, Piper M, Pelleymounter MA, Cullen MJ, et al. A role for melanin-concentrating hormone in the central regulation of feeding behaviour. *Nature* (1996) 380(6571):243–7. doi:10.1038/380243a0

Pissios P, Bradley RL, Maratos-Flier E. Expanding the scales: the multiple roles of MCH in regulating energy balance and other biological functions. *Endocr Rev* (2006) 27(6):606–20. doi:10.1210/er.2006-0021

Matsuda K, Kojima K, Shimakura S, Takahashi A. Regulation of food intake by melanin-concentrating hormone in goldfish. *Peptides* (2009) 30(11):2060–5. doi:10.1016/j.peptides.2009.02.015

Shimakura S, Kojima K, Nakamachi T, Kageyama H, Uchiyama M, Shioda S, et al. Neuronal interaction between melanin-concentrating hormone- and alpha-melanocyte-stimulating hormone-containing neurons in the goldfish hypothalamus. *Peptides* (2008) 29(8):1432–40. doi:10.1016/j.peptides.2008.04.009

Naufahu J, Cunliffe AD, Murray JF. The roles of melanin-concentrating hor- mone in energy balance and reproductive function: are they connected? *Repro- duction* (2013) 146(5):R141–50. doi:10.1530/REP-12-0385

Smith MS, Grove KL. Integration of the regulation of reproductive func- tion and energy balance: lactation as a model. *Front Neuroendocrinol* (2002) 23(3):225–56. doi:10.1016/S0091-3022(02)00002-X

Williamson-Hughes PS, Grove KL, Smith MS. Melanin concentrating hormone (MCH): a novel neural pathway for regulation of GnRH neurons. *Brain Res* (2005) 1041(2):117–24. doi:10.1016/j.brainres.2004.11.066

Chiocchio SR, Gallardo MG, Louzan P, Gutnisky V, Tramezzani JH. Melanin- concentrating hormone stimulates the release of luteinizing hormone-releasing hormone and gonadotropins in the female rat acting at both median emi- nence and pituitary levels. *Biol Reprod* (2001) 64(5):1466–72. doi:10.1095/ biolreprod64.5.1466

Schauer E, Trautinger F, Kock A, Schwarz A, Bhardwaj R, Simon M, et al. Proopiomelanocortin-derived peptides are synthesized and released by human keratinocytes. *J Clin Invest* (1994) 93(5):2258–62. doi:10.1172/JCI117224

Cerda-Reverter JM, Ringholm A, Schioth HB, Peter RE. Molecular cloning, pharmacological characterization, and brain mapping of the melanocortin 4 receptor in the goldfish: involvement in the control of food intake. *Endocrinol- ogy* (2003) 144(6):2336–49. doi:10.1210/en.2002-0213

Salbert G, Chauveau I, Bonnec G, Valotaire Y, Jego P. One of the two trout proopiomelanocortin messenger RNAs potentially encodes new peptides. *Mol Endocrinol* (1992) 6(10):1605–13. doi:10.1210/mend.6.10.1448114

Kuhar MJ, Adams S, Dominguez G, Jaworski J, Balkan B. CART peptides. *Neu- ropeptides* (2002) 36(1):1–8. doi:10.1054/npep.2002.0887

Sakata I, Nakamura K, Yamazaki M, Matsubara M, Hayashi Y, Kangawa K, et al. Ghrelin-producing cells exist as two types of cells, closed- and opened-type cells, in the rat gastrointestinal tract. *Peptides* (2002) 23(3):531–6. doi:10.1016/S0196-9781(01)00633-7

Kehoe AS, Volkoff H. Cloning and characterization of neuropeptide Y (NPY) and cocaine and amphetamine regulated transcript (CART) in Atlantic cod (*Gadus morhua*). *Comp Biochem Physiol A Mol Integr Physiol* (2007) 146(3):451–61. doi:10.1016/j.cbpa.2006.12.026

Kobayashi Y, Peterson BC, Waldbieser GC. Association of cocaine- and amphetamine-regulated transcript (CART) messenger RNA level, food intake, and growth in channel catfish. *Comp Biochem Physiol A Mol Integr Physiol* (2008) 151(2):219–25. doi:10.1016/j.cbpa.2008.06.029

Nishio S, Gibert Y, Berekelya L, Bernard L, Brunet F, Guillot E, et al. Fasting induces CART down-regulation in the zebrafish nervous system in a cannabi- noid receptor 1-dependent manner. *Mol Endocrinol* (2012) 26(8):1316–26. doi:10.1210/me.2011-1180

Murashita K, Kurokawa T, Ebbesson LO, Stefansson SO, Ronnestad I. Charac- terization, tissue distribution, and regulation of agouti-related protein (AgRP), cocaine- and amphetamine-regulated transcript (CART) and neuropeptide Y (NPY) in Atlantic salmon (*Salmo salar*). *Gen Comp Endocrinol* (2009) 162(2):160–71. doi:10.1016/j.ygcen.2009.03.015

Leslie RA, Sanders SJ, Anderson SI, Schuhler S, Horan TL, Ebling FJ. Apposi- tions between cocaine and amphetamine-related transcript- and gonadotropin releasing hormone-immunoreactive neurons in the hypothalamus of the Siber- ian hamster. *Neurosci Lett* (2001) 314(3):111–4. doi:10.1016/S0304-3940(01)02291-1

Singru PS, Mazumdar M, Sakharkar AJ, Lechan RM, Thim L, Clausen JT, et al. Immunohistochemical localization of cocaine- and amphetamine-regulated transcript peptide in the brain of the catfish, *Clarias batrachus* (Linn.). *J Comp Neurol* (2007) 502(2):215–35. doi:10.1002/cne.21295

Barsagade VG, Mazumdar M, Singru PS, Thim L, Clausen JT, Subhedar N. Reproductive phase-related variations in cocaine- and amphetamine-regulated transcript (CART) in the olfactory system, forebrain, and pituitary of the female catfish, *Clarias batrachus* (Linn.). *J Comp Neurol* (2010) 518(13):2503–24. doi:10.1002/cne.22349

Kuriyama G, Takekoshi S, Tojo K, Nakai Y, Kuhar MJ, Osamura RY. Cocaine- and amphetamine-regulated transcript peptide in the rat anterior pituitary gland is localized in gonadotrophs and suppresses prolactin secretion. *Endocrinology* (2004) 145(5):2542–50. doi:10.1210/en.2003-0845

Moran TH, Kinzig KP. Gastrointestinal satiety signals II. Cholecystokinin. *Am J Physiol Gastrointest Liver Physiol* (2004) 286(2):G183–8. doi:10.1152/ajpgi. 00434.2003

Ichimaru T, Matsuyama S, Ohkura S, Mori Y, Okamura H. Central cholecystokinin-octapeptide accelerates the activity of the hypothalamic gonadotropin-releasing hormone pulse generator in goats. *J Neuroendocrinol* (2003) 15(1):80–6. doi:10.1046/j.1365-2826.2003.00965.x

Kimura F, Hashimoto R, Kawakami M. The stimulatory effect of cholecys- tokinin implanted in the medial preoptic area on luteinizing hormone secretion in the ovariectomized estrogen-primed rat. *Endocrinol Jpn* (1983) 30(3):305–9. doi:10.1507/endocrj1954.30.305

Oh IS, Shimizu H, Satoh T, Okada S, Adachi S, Inoue K, et al. Identifica- tion of nesfatin-1 as a satiety molecule in the hypothalamus. *Nature* (2006) 443(7112):709–12. doi:10.1038/nature05162

Garcia-Galiano D, Navarro VM, Roa J, Ruiz-Pino F, Sanchez-Garrido MA, Pineda R, et al. The anorexigenic neuropeptide, nesfatin-1, is indispensable for normal puberty onset in the female rat. *J Neurosci* (2010) 30(23):7783–92. doi:10.1523/JNEUROSCI.5828-09.2010

Zhang Y, Proenca R, Maffei M, Barone M, Leopold L, Friedman JM. Positional cloning of the mouse obese gene and its human homologue. *Nature* (1994) 372(6505):425–32. doi:10.1038/372425a0

Crown A, Clifton DK, Steiner RA. Neuropeptide signaling in the integration of metabolism and reproduction. *Neuroendocrinology* (2007) 86(3):175–82. doi:10.1159/000109095

de Pedro N, Martinez-Alvarez R, Delgado MJ. Acute and chronic leptin reduces food intake and body weight in goldfish (*Carassius auratus*). *J Endocrinol* (2006) 188(3):513–20. doi:10.1677/joe.1.06349

Aguilar AJ, Conde-Sieira M, Polakof S, Miguez JM, Soengas JL. Central lep- tin treatment modulates brain glucosensing function and peripheral energy metabolism of rainbow trout. *Peptides* (2010) 31(6):1044–54. doi:10.1016/j.peptides.2010.02.026

Maffei M, Halaas J, Ravussin E, Pratley RE, Lee GH, Zhang Y, et al. Lep- tin levels in human and rodent: measurement of plasma leptin and ob RNA in obese and weight-reduced subjects. *Nat Med* (1995) 1(11):1155–61. doi:10.1038/nm1195-1155

Watanobe H. Leptin directly acts within the hypothalamus to stimulate gonadotropin-releasing hormone secretion in vivo in rats. *J Physiol* (2002) 545(Pt 1):255–68. doi:10.1113/jphysiol.2002.023895

Smith GD, Jackson LM, Foster DL. Leptin regulation of reproductive function and fertility. *Theriogenology* (2002) 57(1):73–86. doi:10.1016/S0093-691X(01)00658-6

Barb CR, Hausman GJ, Czaja K. Leptin: a metabolic signal affecting cen- tral regulation of reproduction in the pig. *Domest Anim Endocrinol* (2005) 29(1):186–92. doi:10.1016/j.domaniend.2005.02.024

Froiland E, Murashita K, Jorgensen EH, Kurokawa T. Leptin and ghrelin in anadromous arctic charr: cloning and change in expressions dur- ing a seasonal feeding cycle. *Gen Comp Endocrinol* (2010) 165(1):136–43. doi:10.1016/j.ygcen.2009.06.010

Trombley S, Schmitz M. Leptin in fish: possible role in sexual matura- tion in male Atlantic salmon. *Fish Physiol Biochem* (2013) 39(1):103–6. doi:10.1007/s10695-012-9731-0

Kaiya H, Kojima M, Hosoda H, Riley LG, Hirano T, Grau EG, et al. Amidated fish ghrelin: purification, cDNA cloning in the Japanese eel and its biological activity. *J Endocrinol* (2003) 176(3):415–23. doi:10.1677/joe.0.1760415

Kaiya H, Kojima M, Hosoda H, Moriyama S, Takahashi A, Kawauchi H, et al. Peptide purification, complementary deoxyribonucleic acid (DNA) and genomic DNA cloning, and functional characterization of ghrelin in rainbow trout. *Endocrinology* (2003) 144(12):5215–26. doi:10.1210/en.2003-1085

Kaiya H, Miyazato M, Kangawa K, Peter RE, Unniappan S. Ghrelin: a multi- functional hormone in non-mammalian vertebrates. *Comp Biochem Physiol A Mol Integr Physiol* (2008) 149(2):109–28. doi:10.1016/j.cbpa.2007.12.004

Kang KS, Yahashi S, Matsuda K. Central and peripheral effects of ghrelin on energy balance, food intake and lipid metabolism in teleost fish. *Peptides* (2011) 32(11):2242–7. doi:10.1016/j.peptides.2011.05.006

Terova G, Rimoldi S, Bernardini G, Gornati R, Saroglia M. Sea bass ghrelin: molecular cloning and mRNA quantification during fasting and refeeding. *Gen Comp Endocrinol* (2008) 155(2):341–51. doi:10.1016/j.ygcen.2007.05.028

Amole N, Unniappan S. Fasting induces preproghrelin mRNA expression in the brain and gut of zebrafish, *Danio rerio*. *Gen Comp Endocrinol* (2009) 161(1):133–7. doi:10.1016/j.ygcen.2008.11.002

Jonsson E, Forsman A, Einarsdottir IE, Kaiya H, Ruohonen K, Bjornsson BT. Plasma ghrelin levels in rainbow trout in response to fasting, feeding and food composition, and effects of ghrelin on voluntary food intake. *Comp Biochem Physiol A Mol Integr Physiol* (2007) 147(4):1116–24. doi:10.1016/j.cbpa.2007. 03.024

Nieminen P, Mustonen AM, Hyvarinen H. Fasting reduces plasma leptin- and ghrelin-immunoreactive peptide concentrations of the burbot (*Lota lota*) at 2 degrees C but not at 10 degrees C. *Zoolog Sci* (2003) 20(9):1109–15. doi:10.2108/zsj.20.1109

Jonsson E. The role of ghrelin in energy balance regulation in fish. *Gen Comp Endocrinol* (2013) 187:79–85. doi:10.1016/j.ygcen.2013.03.013

Tena-Sempere M. Ghrelin as a pleotrophic modulator of gonadal function and reproduction. *Nat Clin Pract Endocrinol Metab* (2008) 4(12):666–74. doi:10.1038/ncpendmet1003

Chan CB, Cheng CH. Identification and functional characterization of two alternatively spliced growth hormone secretagogue receptor transcripts from the pituitary of black seabream *Acanthopagrus schlegeli*. *Mol Cell Endocrinol* (2004) 214(1–2):81–95. doi:10.1016/j.mce.2003.11.020

Grey CL, Grayfer L, Belosevic M, Chang JP. Ghrelin stimulation of gonadotropin (LH) release from goldfish pituitary cells: presence of the growth hormone secretagogue receptor (GHS-R1a) and involvement of voltage- sensitive Ca2+ channels. *Mol Cell Endocrinol* (2010) 317(1–2):64–77. doi:10. 1016/j.mce.2009.12.024

Schneider JE, Wise JD, Benton NA, Brozek JM, Keen-Rhinehart E. When do we eat? Ingestive behavior, survival, and reproductive success. *Horm Behav* (2013) 64(4):702–28. doi:10.1016/j.yhbeh.2013.07.005

Milla S, Wang N, Mandiki SN, Kestemont P. Corticosteroids: friends or foes of teleost fish reproduction? *Comp Biochem Physiol A Mol Integr Physiol* (2009) 153(3):242–51. doi:10.1016/j.cbpa.2009.02.027

Castellano JM, Bentsen AH, Mikkelsen JD, Tena-Sempere M. Kisspeptins: bridging energy homeostasis and reproduction. *Brain Res* (2010) 1364:129–38. doi:10.1016/j.brainres.2010.08.057

Smith JT, Acohido BV, Clifton DK, Steiner RA. KiSS-1 neurones are direct tar- gets for leptin in the ob/ob mouse. *J Neuroendocrinol* (2006) 18(4):298–303. doi:10.1111/j.1365-2826.2006.01417.x

Backholer K, Smith JT, Rao A, Pereira A, Iqbal J, Ogawa S, et al. Kisspeptin cells in the ewe brain respond to leptin and communicate with neuropep- tide Y and proopiomelanocortin cells. *Endocrinology* (2010) 151(5):2233–43. doi:10.1210/en.2009-1190

Fu LY, van den Pol AN. Kisspeptin directly excites anorexigenic proopiome- lanocortin neurons but inhibits orexigenic neuropeptide Y cells by an indi- rect synaptic mechanism. *J Neurosci* (2010) 30(30):10205–19. doi:10.1523/JNEUROSCI.2098-10.2010

Mechaly AS, Vinas J, Piferrer F. Gene structure analysis of kisspeptin-2 (Kiss2) in the Senegalese sole (*Solea senegalensis*): characterization of two splice vari- ants of Kiss2, and novel evidence for metabolic regulation of kisspeptin signal- ing in non-mammalian species. *Mol Cell Endocrinol* (2011) 339(1–2):14–24. doi:10.1016/j.mce.2011.03.004

Tachibana T, Sato M, Takahashi H, Ukena K, Tsutsui K, Furuse M. Gonadotropin-inhibiting hormone stimulates feeding behavior in chicks. *Brain Res* (2005) 1050(1–2):94–100. doi:10.1016/j.brainres.2005.05.035

Johnson MA, Tsutsui K, Fraley GS. Rat RFamide-related peptide-3 stimulates GH secretion, inhibits LH secretion, and has variable effects on sex behavior in the adult male rat. *Horm Behav* (2007) 51(1):171–80. doi:10.1016/j.yhbeh. 2006.09.009

Murakami M, Matsuzaki T, Iwasa T, Yasui T, Irahara M, Osugi T, et al. Hypophysiotropic role of RFamide-related peptide-3 in the inhibition of LH secretion in female rats. *J Endocrinol* (2008) 199(1):105–12. doi:10.1677/JOE-08-0197

Qi Y, Oldfield BJ, Clarke IJ. Projections of RFamide-related peptide-3 neu- rones in the ovine hypothalamus, with special reference to regions regulat- ing energy balance and reproduction. *J Neuroendocrinol* (2009) 21(8):690–7. doi:10.1111/j.1365-2826.2009.01886.x

Ahima RS, Saper CB, Flier JS, Elmquist JK. Leptin regulation of neuroendocrine systems. *Front Neuroendocrinol* (2000) 21(3):263–307. doi:10.1006/frne.2000. 0197

Williams G, Bing C, Cai XJ, Harrold JA, King PJ, Liu XH. The hypothala- mus and the control of energy homeostasis: different circuits, different pur- poses. *Physiol Behav* (2001) 74(4–5):683–701. doi:10.1016/S0031-9384(01)00612-6

Li GG, Liang XF, Xie Q, Li G, Yu Y, Lai K. Gene structure, recombinant expres- sion and functional characterization of grass carp leptin. *Gen Comp Endocrinol* (2010) 166(1):117–27. doi:10.1016/j.ygcen.2009.10.009

Aguilar AJ, Conde-Sieira M, Lopez-Patino MA, Miguez JM, Soengas JL. In vitro leptin treatment of rainbow trout hypothalamus and hindbrain affects glucosensing and gene expression of neuropeptides involved in food intake regulation. *Peptides* (2011) 32(2):232–40. doi:10.1016/j.peptides.2010. 11.007

Chisada S-I, Kurokawa T, Murashita K, Rønnestad I, Taniguchi Y, Toyoda A, et al. Leptin receptor-deficient (knockout) medaka, *Oryzias latipes*, show chronical up-regulated levels of orexigenic neuropeptides, elevated food intake and stage specific effects on growth and fat allocation. *Gen Comp Endocrinol* (2014) 195:9–20. doi:10.1016/j.ygcen.2013.10.008

Matsuda K, Kojima K, Shimakura S, Wada K, Maruyama K, Uchiyama M, et al. Corticotropin-releasing hormone mediates alpha-melanocyte- stimulating hormone-induced anorexigenic action in goldfish. *Peptides* (2008) 29(11):1930–6. doi:10.1016/j.peptides.2008.06.028

Shimakura S, Miura T, Maruyama K, Nakamachi T, Uchiyama M, Kageyama H, et al. Alpha-melanocyte-stimulating hormone mediates melanin-concentrating hormone-induced anorexigenic action in goldfish. *Horm Behav* (2008) 53(2):323–8. doi:10.1016/j.yhbeh.2007.10.009

Kang KS, Shimizu K, Azuma M, Ui Y, Nakamura K, Uchiyama M, et al. Gonadotropin-releasing hormone II (GnRH II) mediates the anorex- igenic actions of alpha-melanocyte-stimulating hormone (alpha-MSH) and corticotropin-releasing hormone (CRH) in goldfish. *Peptides* (2011) 32(1):31–5. doi:10.1016/j.peptides.2010.10.013

Kojima K, Kamijo M, Kageyama H, Uchiyama M, Shioda S, Matsuda K. Neu- ronal relationship between orexin-A- and neuropeptide Y-induced orexigenic actions in goldfish. *Neuropeptides* (2009) 43(2):63–71. doi:10.1016/j.npep.2009.01.004

Kojima K, Amiya N, Kamijo M, Kageyama H, Uchiyama M, Shioda S, et al. Relationship between alpha-melanocyte-stimulating hormone- and neuropep- tide Y-containing neurons in the goldfish hypothalamus. *Gen Comp Endocrinol* (2010) 167(3):366–72. doi:10.1016/j.ygcen.2009.12.004

Matsuda K, Kojima K, Shimakura S, Miura T, Uchiyama M, Shioda S, et al. Relationship between melanin-concentrating hormone- and neuropeptide Y- containing neurons in the goldfish hypothalamus. *Comp Biochem Physiol A Mol Integr Physiol* (2009) 153(1):3–7. doi:10.1016/j.cbpa.2008.10.002

Miura T, Maruyama K, Shimakura S, Kaiya H, Uchiyama M, Kangawa K, et al. Regulation of food intake in the goldfish by interaction between ghrelin and orexin. *Peptides* (2007) 28(6):1207–13. doi:10.1016/j.peptides.2007.03.023

Miura T, Maruyama K, Shimakura S, Kaiya H, Uchiyama M, Kangawa K, et al. Neuropeptide Y mediates ghrelin-induced feeding in the goldfish, *Carassius auratus*. *Neurosci Lett* (2006) 407(3):279–83. doi:10.1016/j.neulet.2006.08.071

Amano M, Amiya N, Hiramatsu M, Tomioka T, Oka Y. Interaction between neuropeptide Y immunoreactive neurons and galanin immunoreactive neu- rons in the brain of the masu salmon, *Oncorhynchus masou*. *Neurosci Lett* (2009) 462(1):33–8. doi:10.1016/j.neulet.2009.06.067

Peng C, Trudeau VL, Peter RE. Seasonal variation of neuropeptide Y actions on growth hormone and gonadotropin-II secretion in the goldfish: effects of sex steroids. *J Neuroendocrinol* (1993) 5(3):273–80. doi:10.1111/j.1365-2826.1993.tb00483.x

Flores A, Maldonado R, Berrendero F. Cannabinoid-hypocretin cross-talk in the central nervous system: what we know so far. *Front Neurosci* (2013) 7:256. doi:10.3389/fnins.2013.00256

Bermudez-Silva FJ, Cardinal P, Cota D. The role of the endocannabinoid system in the neuroendocrine regulation of energy balance. *J Psychopharmacol* (2012) 26(1):114–24. doi:10.1177/0269881111408458

Piccinetti CC, Migliarini B, Petrosino S, Di Marzo V, Carnevali O. Anandamide and AM251, via water, modulate food intake at central and peripheral level in fish. *Gen Comp Endocrinol* (2010) 166(2):259–67. doi:10.1016/j.ygcen.2009. 09.017

Valenti M, Cottone E, Martinez R, De Pedro N, Rubio M, Viveros MP, et al. The endocannabinoid system in the brain of *Carassius auratus* and its pos- sible role in the control of food intake. *J Neurochem* (2005) 95(3):662–72. doi:10.1111/j.1471-4159.2005.03406.x

Cottone E, Pomatto V, Bovolin P. Role of the endocannabinoid system in the central regulation of nonmammalian vertebrate reproduction. *Int J Endocrinol* (2013) 2013:941237. doi:10.1155/2013/941237

Battista N, Meccariello R, Cobellis G, Fasano S, Di Tommaso M, Pirazzi V, et al. The role of endocannabinoids in gonadal function and fertility along the evolutionary axis. *Mol Cell Endocrinol* (2012) 355(1):1–14. doi:10.1016/j.mce.2012.01.014

Volff JN. Genome evolution and biodiversity in teleost fish. *Heredity* (2004) 94(3):280–94. doi:10.1038/sj.hdy.6800635

21

Regulation of neurosteroid biosynthesis by neurotransmitters and neuropeptides

Jean Luc Do Rego[1,2,3], Jae Young Seong[4], Delphine Burel[1,2,3,5], Jerôme Leprince[1,2,3,5], David Vaudry[1,2,3,5], Van Luu-The[6], Marie-Christine Tonon[1,2,3,5], Kazuyoshi Tsutsui[7,8], Georges Pelletier[6] and Hubert Vaudry[1,2,3,5] *

[1] INSERM, Mont-Saint-Aignan, France
[2] European Institute for Peptide Research, IFRMP 23, Regional Platform for Cell Imaging, PRIMACEN, University of Rouen, Mont-Saint-Aignan, France
[3] International Associated Laboratory Samuel de Champlain, Mont-Saint-Aignan, France
[4] Laboratory of G Protein-Coupled Receptors, Graduate School of Medicine, Korea University College of Medicine, Seoul, Korea
[5] Laboratory of Neuronal and Neuroendocrine Differentiation and Communication, INSERM U982, University of Rouen, Mont-Saint-Aignan, France
[6] Research Center in Molecular Endocrinology, Oncology and Genetics, Laval University Hospital Center, Québec, QC, Canada
[7] Laboratory of Integrative Brain Sciences, Department of Biology, Waseda University, Tokyo, Japan
[8] Center for Medical Life Science of Waseda University, Tokyo, Japan

Edited by:
Olivier Kah, CNRS UMR 6026, France

Reviewed by:
Gustavo M. Somoza, Instituto de Investigaciones Biotecnologicas-Instituto Tecnologico de Chascomus, Argentina
James A. Carr, Texas Tech University, USA

***Correspondence:**
Hubert Vaudry, INSERM U982, European Institute for Peptide Research, IFRMP 23, University of Rouen, 76821 Mont-Saint-Aignan, France.
e-mail: hubert.vaudry@univ-rouen.fr

The enzymatic pathways leading to the synthesis of bioactive steroids in the brain are now almost completely elucidated in various groups of vertebrates and, during the last decade, the neuronal mechanisms involved in the regulation of neurosteroid production have received increasing attention. This report reviews the current knowledge concerning the effects of neurotransmitters, peptide hormones, and neuropeptides on the biosynthesis of neurosteroids. Anatomical studies have been carried out to visualize the neurotransmitter- or neuropeptide-containing fibers contacting steroid-synthesizing neurons as well as the neurotransmitter, peptide hormones, or neuropeptide receptors expressed in these neurons. Biochemical experiments have been conducted to investigate the effects of neurotransmitters, peptide hormones, or neuropeptides on neurosteroid biosynthesis, and to characterize the type of receptors involved. Thus, it has been found that glutamate, acting through kainate and/or AMPA receptors, rapidly inactivates P450arom, and that melatonin produced by the pineal gland and eye inhibits the biosynthesis of 7α-hydroxypregnenolone (7α-OH-Δ^5P), while prolactin produced by the adenohypophysis enhances the formation of 7α-OH-Δ^5P. It has also been demonstrated that the biosynthesis of neurosteroids is inhibited by GABA, acting through $GABA_A$ receptors, and neuropeptide Y, acting through Y1 receptors. In contrast, it has been shown that the octadecaneuropetide ODN, acting through central-type benzodiazepine receptors, the triakontatetraneuropeptide TTN, acting though peripheral-type benzodiazepine receptors, and vasotocin, acting through V1a-like receptors, stimulate the production of neurosteroids. Since neurosteroids are implicated in the control of various neurophysiological and behavioral processes, these data suggest that some of the neurophysiological effects exerted by neurotransmitters and neuropeptides may be mediated via the regulation of neurosteroid production.

Keywords: neurosteroids, glutamate, GABA, melatonin, prolactin, endozepines, vasopressin, neuropeptide Y

INTRODUCTION

The regulatory effects of steroid hormones in the central nervous system (CNS) have long been recognized (McEwen, 1994; Baulieu et al., 1999; Dubrovsky, 2005; Leskiewicz et al., 2006). Steroids acting on the CNS originate from two sources: (1) steroids produced by peripheral endocrine glands, i.e., gonads, adrenal, and placenta, that have to cross the blood–brain barrier to act on the brain, are usually designated as *neuroactive steroids*; (2) steroids directly synthesized within the CNS, either *de novo* from cholesterol or by *in situ* metabolism of circulating steroid precursors, are designated by the generic term *neurosteroids* (Robel and Baulieu, 1985, 1994; Baulieu, 1997, 1998). The capability of the nervous system to synthesize steroids was originally discovered in mammals (Corpéchot et al., 1981, 1983; Lanthier and Patwardhan, 1986) and was subsequently generalized in other vertebrates including birds, amphibians, and fish (Mensah-Nyagan et al., 1999; Mellon and Vaudry, 2001; Tsutsui et al., 2003, 2009; Do Rego et al., 2009; Diotel et al., 2010) indicating that *de novo* neurosteroidogenesis is a conserved property in the vertebrate phylum.

There is growing evidence that neurosteroids play an important role as endogenous modulators of neuronal functions and behavioral processes, and that alterations of neurosteroid concentrations may contribute to the pathophysiology of neuronal disorders (Majewska, 1992; Robel et al., 1999; Rupprecht and Holsboer, 1999; Lapchak et al., 2000; Lapchak and Araujo, 2001; Rupprecht et al., 2001; Dubrovsky, 2005; Belelli et al., 2006; Strous et al., 2006). For instance, in rat, infusion of pregnenolone sulfate (Δ^5PS) and dehydroepiandrosterone sulfate (DHEAS) into the nucleus basalis magnocellularis enhances learning and memory (Mayo et al., 1993; Robel et al., 1995). Reciprocally, deficit in cognitive performances in aged rats and mice is correlated with low Δ^5PS and DHEAS levels in the hippocampus (Flood et al., 1988, 1992; Vallée et al., 1997, 2001; Ladurelle et al., 2000). In chickens, administration of DHEA and DHEAS enhances learning and memory (Migues et al., 2002). In humans, DHEA and DHEAS are considered to play a role in memory both in normal subjects and aging patients (Sunderland et al., 1989; Nasman et al., 1991; Strous et al., 2006). More specifically, with regards to Alzheimer's disease, decreased levels of several neurosteroids have been observed in the frontal cortex, hippocampus, amygdala, striatum, hypothalamus, and cerebellum (Sunderland et al., 1989; Nasman et al., 1991; Weill-Engerer et al., 2002; Schumacher et al., 2003). The best known role of neurosteroids is their involvement in the control of mood disorders. Numerous behavioral investigations have shown that neurosteroids exert anxiolytic (Hodge et al., 2002; Strous et al., 2003), anti-depressant (Uzunova et al., 2003; van Broekhoven and Verkes, 2003), anti-aggressive (Kavaliers and Kinsella, 1995; Pinna et al., 2008), hypnotic (Lancel et al., 1997; Damianisch et al., 2001), anti-convulsive (Landgren et al., 1987; Belelli et al., 1989), and anti-stress actions (Patchev et al., 1996; Hu et al., 2000). In animal models, an effect of neurosteroids in eating disorders has been reported (Reddy and Kulkarni, 1998, 1999; Strous et al., 2006). In particular, DHEA decreases food intake (Svec and Porter, 1996; Svec et al., 1998), reduces insulin resistance (Svec and Porter, 1998a,b), and lowers adiposity (Svec and Porter, 1998a,b; Pham et al., 2000). DHEAS has also been found to induce a significant decrease in food intake and body weight (Reddy and Kulkarni, 1999; Kaur and Kulkarni, 2001). In contrast, allopregnanolone causes hyperphagia in male and female rats (Reddy and Kulkarni, 1999). The dose-dependent effects of Δ^5PS on locomotion of mice placed in a novel environment show the existence of a possible role of neurosteroids in adaptation to novelty (Fahey et al., 1995a). Neurosteroids are also involved in the regulation of excitotoxic and apoptotic processes (Kimonides et al., 1999; Frank and Sagratella, 2000; Manji et al., 2003; Charalampopoulos et al., 2004; Wojtal et al., 2006). *In vivo* studies indicate that progesterone, allopregnanolone, and DHEA exert neuroprotective effects in models of traumatic brain injury (Stein, 2001; Malik et al., 2003; Djebaili et al., 2004; He et al., 2004) and in focal cerebral ischemia (Malik et al., 2003; Sayeed et al., 2006). *In vitro* data also point to the neuroprotective effects of neurosteroids in models of neuronal injury against neurotoxic insults inflicted by excitatory amino acids (Kimonides et al., 1999; Gursoy et al., 2001) and β-amyloid peptides (Kimonides et al., 1998, 1999; Frank and Sagratella, 2000; Lockhart et al., 2002; Xilouri and Papazafiri, 2006). It has been demonstrated that neurosteroids play important functions in neurodevelopment and neuronal remodeling, including neurogenesis (Roberts, 1986; Weaver et al., 1997; Schumacher et al., 2000; Magnaghi et al., 2001; Young, 2002), axonal and dendritic growth, and synaptic connectivity (Jones, 1994; Compagnone and Mellon, 1998). In addition to their protective effects on the brain, neurosteroids can regulate myelin formation and increase expression of myelin proteins in the sciatic nerve (Koenig et al., 1995; Murakami et al., 2000; Plassart-Schiess and Baulieu, 2001; Laurine et al., 2003; Melcangi et al., 2003; Iwata et al., 2005).

The effects of neurosteroids on neuronal activity are mediated through several distinct categories of receptors. Neurosteroids, like other steroid hormones, can act at the transcriptional level through interaction with nuclear receptors (McEwen, 1994; Rupprecht, 1997; Mo et al., 2004). Neurosteroids may also interact with plasma membrane G protein-coupled receptors either directly (Schiess and Partridge, 2005; Tasker et al., 2006) or indirectly by modulating the binding of neuropeptides to their receptors (Grazzini et al., 1998; Zwain et al., 2002; Torres and Ortega, 2003). In addition, neurosteroids can stimulate tubulin polymerization in cultured neurons by binding to the microtubule-associated protein-2 (Murakami et al., 2000; Plassart-Schiess and Baulieu, 2001; Laurine et al., 2003; Iwata et al., 2005). However, most of the actions of neurosteroids are mediated via allosteric modulation of neurotransmitter receptors, including the $GABA_A$/central-type benzodiazepine receptor (CBR) complex (Belelli and Lambert, 2005; Belelli et al., 2006; Zheng, 2009), *N*-methyl-D-aspartate (NMDA; Mameli et al., 2005; Monnet and Maurice, 2006), kainate (Costa et al., 2000; Dubrovsky, 2005), α-amino-3-hydroxy-5-methyl-4-isoxazole-propionic acid (AMPA; Rupprecht and Holsboer, 2001; Dubrovsky, 2005), glycine (Jiang et al., 2006; Mitchell et al., 2007), sigma (Monnet et al., 1995; Maurice et al., 2006), serotonergic (Kostowski and Bienkowski, 1999; Shannon et al., 2005a,b), nicotinic (Valera et al., 1992; Bullock et al., 1997), and muscarinic receptors (Horishita et al., 2005; Steffensen et al., 2006). For example, the effects of GABA on the $GABA_A$ receptor are allosterically potentiated by progesterone and deoxycorticosterone metabolites such as allopregnanolone, pregnanolone, and tetrahydrodeoxycorticosterone (Majewska et al., 1986; Majewska, 1992; Paul and Purdy, 1992; Bergeron et al., 1996). On the other hand, Δ^5PS and DHEA have been reported to inhibit $GABA_A$ receptor activity (Majewska and Schwartz, 1987; Park-Chung et al., 1999). Allopregnanolone is a negative modulator of the NMDA receptors (Wu et al., 1991; Bowlby, 1993). In contrast, Δ^5PS and DHEA potentiate several NMDA-receptor-mediated responses, and thus act as excitatory neurosteroids (Wu et al., 1991; Irwin et al., 1992; Fahey et al., 1995b; Compagnone and Mellon, 1998). At the AMPA and kainate receptors, Δ^5PS behaves as a negative modulator (Rupprecht, 1997; Mellon and Griffin, 2002). It has also been demonstrated that DHEAS acts as a sigma receptor agonist, Δ^5PS as a sigma receptor inverse agonist, and progesterone as a sigma receptor antagonist (Monnet et al., 1995).

The biochemical pathways leading to the synthesis of steroids in the nervous system of vertebrates have now been almost completely elucidated (Tsutsui and Yamazaki, 1995; Tsutsui et al., 1999; Compagnone and Mellon, 2000; Do Rego et al., 2009; Diotel et al., 2011; Vaudry et al., 2011) and it is now firmly established that neurosteroids regulate neuronal activity (Reddy, 2003, 2010; Dubrovsky, 2005; Belelli et al., 2006; Strous et al., 2006). Over the last decade, a number of studies have thus been undertaken to decipher the neuronal mechanisms involved in the regulation of neurosteroid production. In the present report, we review the current knowledge regarding the effects and mode of action of neurotransmitters, peptide hormones, and neuropeptides on the biosynthesis of neurosteroids in the CNS of vertebrates. Remarkably, most of these studies have been conducted in the brain of amphibians and birds. In fact, since the rate of steroid synthesis is relatively high in the CNS of frog, quail, and zebra finch (Mensah-Nyagan et al., 1994, 1996; Tsutsui et al., 2006, 2009; Do Rego et al., 2007a; Schlinger and Remage-Healey, 2011), these animals have proved to be suitable models in which to investigate the neuronal mechanisms regulating neurosteroid production.

EFFECT OF GLUTAMATE ON NEUROSTEROID BIOSYNTHESIS

In the quail forebrain, all classes of ionotropic glutamate receptors, i.e., NMDA, AMPA, and kainate receptors, are expressed in the medial preoptic nucleus, a region which is enriched with P450arom-containing cell bodies (Cornil et al., 2000), suggesting that these neurons may be regulated by glutamate. Consistent with this hypothesis, incubation of quail hypothalamic fragments with AMPA and kainate, and to a certain extent NMDA, inhibits P450arom activity (Balthazart et al., 2001a). In mice, administration of NMDA or glutamate within the nidopallium provokes a substantial decrease in the local concentration of estradiol (Remage-Healey et al., 2008; Cornil, 2009). These observations indicate that, in birds and mammals, glutamate exerts an inhibitory action on the formation of neuroestrogens. In the quail brain, the inhibitory effects of AMPA and kainate are mimicked by ATP, Ca^{2+} and Mg^{2+}, and the Ca^{2+} response is abrogated by PKA, PKC, and CAMK (Balthazart et al., 2001b, 2003). Since P450arom possesses several concensus phosphorylation sites in its sequence (Harada, 1988; Balthazart et al., 2003), it appears that the rapid inhibitory effect of AMPA, kainate, or NMDA on P450arom activity can be ascribed to Ca^{2+}-dependent phosphorylation of the P450arom protein (Balthazart et al., 2001c, 2003).

EFFECT OF MELATONIN ON NEUROSTEROID BIOSYNTHESIS

Measurement of neurosteroid content and/or biosynthesis in the brain of vertebrates has revealed that marked changes in Δ^5P, 7α-hydroxypregnenolone (7α-OH-Δ^5P), P, THP, and Δ^5PS occur during circadian and seasonal cycles (Jo et al., 1990; Takase et al., 1999; Inai et al., 2003; Matsunaga et al., 2004; Tsutsui et al., 2008). These changes often parallel or mirror variations in plasma melatonin concentrations (Hau and Gwinner, 1994; Warren and Cassone, 1995; Marumoto et al., 1996; Murakami et al., 2001). It has been shown that melatonin regulates locomotor activity in house sparrow, Japanese quail, red-bellied newt, ural owl, rock pigeon, and Sprague Dawley rat (Hau and Gwinner, 1994; Warren and Cassone, 1995; Murakami et al., 2001). 7α-OH-Δ^5P, in very much the same as melatonin, regulates locomotor activity in Japanese quail and red-bellied newt (Matsunaga et al., 2004; Tsutsui et al., 2008), suggesting that melatonin may control 7α-OH-Δ^5P production. In support of this notion, male quails which exhibit marked diurnal variations in locomotor activity also show substantial changes in brain level of 7α-OH-Δ^5P while female quails which do not show locomotor rhythms have low level of 7α-OH-Δ^5P (Tsutsui et al., 2008). Similarly, it has been found that the synthesis of 7α-OH-Δ^5P in the brain of male newts undergoes marked diurnal changes with higher levels during the dark phase when locomotor activity of males is high. In contrast, 7α-OH-Δ^5P production in female newts does not change (Haraguchi et al., 2009, 2010; Koyama et al., 2009; Tsutsui et al., 2010). In male quail, suppression of endogenous melatonin through pinealectomy (Px) and orbital enucleation (Ex) causes a significant increase of the expression of CYP7B mRNA and biosynthesis of 7α-OH-Δ^5P (Tsutsui et al., 2008). ICV injection of melatonin suppresses the effects of Px and Ex on CYP7B gene transcription and 7α-OH-Δ^5P production. Finally, the melatonin receptor antagonist luzindole abrogates the inhibitory effect of melatonin on 7α-OH-Δ^5P formation (Tsutsui et al., 2008). Collectively, these data support the contention that, in male birds, melatonin inhibits the expression of CYP7B and that the subsequent decrease of 7α-OH-Δ^5P in the brain is responsible for the nocturnal reduction of locomotor activity.

EFFECT OF PROLACTIN ON NEUROSTEROID BIOSYNTHESIS

In male newts, as in many other wild animals, locomotor activity increases during the breeding season (Iwata et al., 2000). This hyperlocomotor response is associated with a concomitant increase in 7α-OH-Δ^5P in the newt brain (Haraguchi et al., 2009, 2010). The pituitary hormone prolactin (PRL) exerts pleiotropic functions in the control of reproduction in urodeles (Polzonetti-Magni et al., 1995; Kikuyama et al., 2003). In particular, PRL is involved in migration to water at the breeding season (Chadwick, 1941) and stimulates expression of courtship behavior with rapid tail vibration by male newts (Toyoda et al., 1993). Indeed, in male newts, plasma PRL concentration increases during the breeding season (Matsuda et al., 1990; Mosconi et al., 1994) and it has been shown that PRL acts centrally to activate courtship behavior (Toyoda et al., 2005), suggesting that PRL may be involved in the control of 7α-OH-Δ^5P synthesis in the brain to increase locomotor activity during the reproductive period. In support of this hypothesis, PRL receptor immunoreactivity is observed in CYP7B-expressing neurons in the anterior preoptic area (Poa) and the magnocellular preoptic nucleus (Mg) of the newt brain (Haraguchi et al., 2010). Hypophysectomy markedly reduces brain concentration and biosynthesis of 7α-OH-Δ^5P in breeding male newts and these effects are suppressed by ICV injection of PRL (Haraguchi et al., 2010). Reciprocally, ICV administration of newt PRL antiserum dose-dependently decreases 7α-OH-Δ^5P synthesis (Haraguchi et al., 2010). Taken together, these observations indicate that PRL directly acts on Mg neurons expressing CYP7B to enhance the biosynthesis of 7α-OH-Δ^5P which in turn mediates the stimulatory effect of PRL on locomotion.

EFFECT OF GABA ON NEUROSTEROID BIOSYNTHESIS

Gamma-aminobutyric acid (GABA) is the major neurotransmitter in the CNS (Krnjevic and Schwartz, 1966; Meldrum, 1982; Paredes and Agmo, 1992). In mammals, brain nuclei that express steroidogenic enzymes (Tsutsui et al., 1999; Do Rego et al., 2009) are innervated by GABAergic nerve fibers (Tappaz et al., 1983; Sakaue et al., 1988) and are also enriched with $GABA_A$ receptors (De Montis et al., 1981; McDonald and Mascagni, 1996; Bäckberg et al., 2004), suggesting that GABA may regulate the activity of steroidogenic nerve cells. As a matter of fact, pharmacological studies have shown that administration of the GABA synthesis inhibitor isoniazid induces an increase of endogenous Δ^5P and P in the rat brain (Barbaccia et al., 1996). In contrast, in rat retinal ganglion cells, GABA, acting through $GABA_A$ receptors, stimulates the biosynthesis of Δ^5P (Guarneri et al., 1995).

The effect and mechanism of action of GABA in the control of neurosteroidogenesis has been mainly investigated in non-mammalian vertebrate models. Indeed, in amphibians as in mammals, a rich GABAergic innervation (Franzoni and Morino, 1989; Hollis and Boyd, 2005) and a dense accumulation of $GABA_A$ receptor subunits (Aller et al., 1997) have been observed in hypothalamic regions which contain steroidogenic neurons (Mensah-Nyagan et al., 1994, 1999; Tsutsui et al., 1999; Do Rego et al., 2009). In the frog *Rana esculenta*, double labeling experiments have shown the presence of $GABA_A$ receptor $\alpha 3$ and β_2/β_3 subunit-like immunoreactivity in 3β-HSD-expressing cell bodies (**Figure 1A**) in the Poa, the posterior tuberculum, the nucleus of the periventricular organ, and the ventral and dorsal hypothalamic nuclei of the hypothalamus (Do Rego et al., 2000) suggesting that, in amphibians as in mammals, GABA may play a role in the control of neurosteroid biosynthesis. In agreement with this hypothesis, GABA has been shown to inhibit in a dose-dependent manner *de novo* biosynthesis of various neurosteroids including 17OH-Δ^5P, P, 17OH-P, and DHEA, by frog hypothalamic explants (Do Rego et al., 2000). The inhibitory effect of GABA on neurosteroid production is mimicked by the $GABA_A$ receptor agonist muscimol and is blocked by the selective $GABA_A$ receptor antagonists bicuculline and SR95531, but is not affected by the $GABA_B$ receptor agonist baclofen (Do Rego et al., 2000). The observation that bicuculline and SR95531 induce on their own a significant stimulation of steroid formation suggests that endogenous GABA exerts a tonic inhibitory control on neurosteroid-producing neurons (Do Rego et al., 2000). These data indicate that GABA inhibits the biosynthesis of neurosteroids through activation of $GABA_A$ receptors (**Figure 1D**). Since several neuroactive steroids are potent allosteric regulators of $GABA_A$ receptor function in amphibians (Le Foll et al., 1997a,b; Hollis et al., 2004) as in mammals (Majewska, 1992; Belelli and Lambert, 2005; Belelli et al., 2006), these observations reveal the existence of an ultrashort feedback loop through which certain neurosteroids may regulate their own production via modulation of $GABA_A$ receptor activity (**Figure 1D**).

EFFECT OF ENDOZEPINES ON NEUROSTEROID BIOSYNTHESIS

The term endozepines designates a family of endogenous peptides that act as natural ligands of CBRs and peripheral-type benzodiazepine receptors also called translocator protein (TSPO; Tonon et al., 2006). The occurrence of endozepines has been reported in the CNS of all classes of vertebrates including fish (Malagon et al., 1992b; Matsuda et al., 2007), amphibians (Malagon et al., 1992a; Lihrmann et al., 1994), birds (Todaro et al., 1991; Rose et al., 1992), and mammals (Alho et al., 1989; Tonon et al., 1990; Tong et al., 1991; Malagon et al., 1993). The endozepine family encompasses diazepam-binding inhibitor (DBI), an 86-amino acid polypeptide (Guidotti et al., 1983), and its processing products the triakontatetraneuropeptide (TTN) and the octadecaneuropeptide (ODN; Ferrero et al., 1984; Slobodyansky et al., 1989). TTN is a selective ligand of TSPO (Slobodyansky et al., 1989; Papadopoulos et al., 2006) while ODN acts as an inverse agonist of CBRs

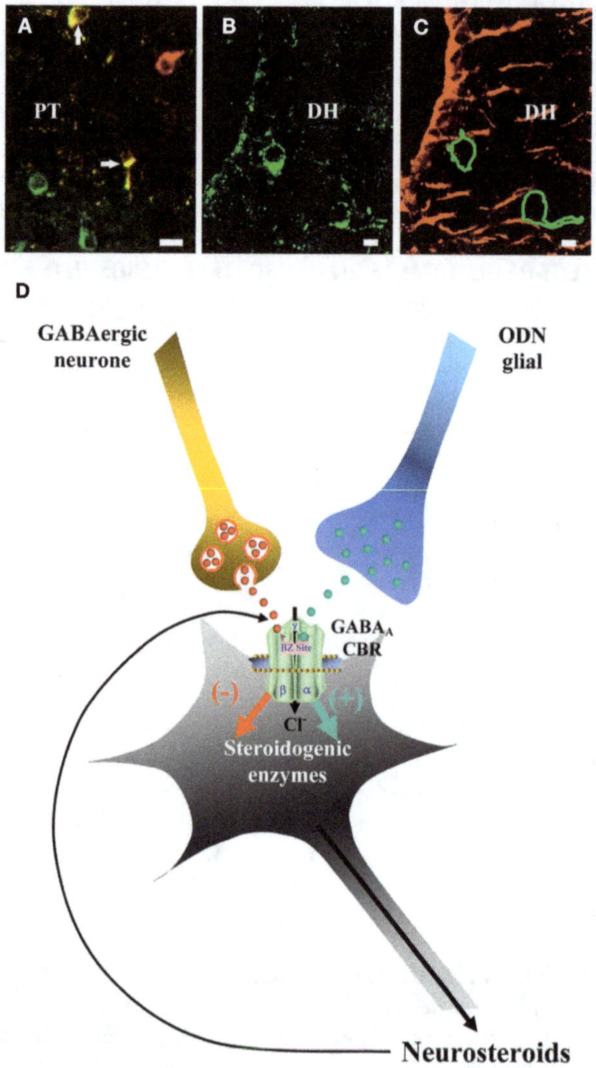

FIGURE 1 | Effect of GABA and the octadecaneuropeptide ODN on neurosteroid biosynthesis. (A) Immunohistochemical localization of 3β-HSD-like immunoreactivity (red) and $GABA_A$ receptor β_2/β_3 subunit-like immunoreactivity (green) in the posterior tuberculum (PT) of the frog brain. 3β-HSD-positive neurons that possess $GABA_A$ receptor β_2/β_3 subunits appear in yellow. **(B)** Immunohistochemical localization of 3β-HSD-like immunoreactivity in the dorsal hypothalamic nucleus (DH; green). **(C)** Consecutive section to B showing the immunohistochemical localization of ODN-like immunoreactivity in glial cells bordering the third ventricle (red). The contours of two 3β-HSD-positive neurons labeled in B are shown. For details regarding antibodies and immunohistochemical procedures, see references by Malagon et al. (1992a) and Do Rego et al. (2000, 2001). In brief, polyclonal antibodies raised in rabbit were used to label 3β-HSD-containing neurons, a mouse monoclonal antibody was used to label $GABA_A$ receptor β_2/β_3 subunit-expressing cells, and polyclonal antibodies raised in rabbit were used to label ODN-immunoreactive glial cells. Scale bars: 10 μm. **(D)** Schematic drawing depicting the effects of GABA and ODN on steroidogenic neurons. GABA acting through $GABA_A$ receptors, inhibits the biosynthesis of neurosteroids, while the endozepine ODN, released by glial fibers, acting as an inverse agonist on central-type benzodiazepine receptors (CBR), stimulates the biosynthesis of 17OH-Δ^5P, DHEA, 17OH-P, and P. Neurosteroids, released by these neurons, may in turn modulate allosterically the activity of the $GABA_A$ receptor and thus control their own biosynthesis.

(Ferrero et al., 1984). Endozepines have been shown to regulate steroid secretion by adrenocortical cells (Yanagibashi et al., 1989; Papadopoulos, 1993; Lesouhaitier et al., 1996, 1998) and Leydig cells (Papadopoulos et al., 1990, 1991a,b; Garnier et al., 1993, 1994; Duparc et al., 2003). Concurrently, it has been found that TTN stimulates Δ^5P biosynthesis by isolated mitochondria from C6 glioma cells (Papadopoulos et al., 1992) indicating that endozepines may be involved in the regulation of neurosteroid production.

The distribution of endozepines has been investigated in the brain of mammals and amphibians by *in situ* hybridization and immunohistochemistry. In the rat brain, DBI mRNA is expressed in various glial cell populations of the ependyma, area postrema, and cerebellum (Alho et al., 1988; Tong et al., 1991; Bürgi et al., 1999). In rat, monkey, and human, endozepine immunoreactivity is found in astrocytes in the arcuate nucleus of the hypothalamus, ependymocytes bordering the third ventricle, tanycytes in the median eminence, pituicytes in the neurohypophysis, and Bergman cells in the cerebellum (Slobodyansky et al., 1992; Malagon et al., 1993; Alho et al., 1995; Yanase et al., 2002). In the frog *R. esculenta*, DBI mRNA and ODN-like immunoreactivity are present in radial glial cells of the periventricular systems of the diencephalon and rhombencephalon (Malagon et al., 1992a; Lihrmann et al., 1994). Immunolabeling of consecutive sections revealed that, in the Poa, the dorsal and ventral hypothalamic nuclei, the nucleus of the periventricular organ, and the posterior tuberculum of the frog brain, ODN-immunoreactive ependymocytes project toward 3β-HSD-positive perikarya (Do Rego et al., 2001; **Figures 1B,C**). These neuroanatomical observations led us to investigate the possible effects of endozepines on neurosteroid biosynthesis in the diencephalon of amphibians.

Incubation of frog hypothalamic slices with graded concentrations of human and rat ODN induces a dose-dependent stimulation of the conversion of $[^3H]\Delta^5$P into Δ^4-3-ketosteroids and Δ^5-3β-hydroxysteroids *in vitro* (Do Rego et al., 2001). The biological activity of ODN is borne by the C-terminal portion of the peptide (Do Rego et al., 2007b) whose sequence has been strongly preserved across vertebrate species (Mocchetti et al., 1986; Lihrmann et al., 1994; Tonon et al., 2006). The stimulatory action of ODN on neurosteroid biosynthesis is mimicked by β-carbolines that act as inverse agonists of CBR, and is blocked by the CBR antagonist flumazenil (Do Rego et al., 2001). The fact that flumazenil alone inhibits the formation of neurosteroids supports the view that ODN plays a physiological role as an endogenous positive modulator of CBR (Do Rego et al., 2001; **Figure 1D**).

In intact mammalian endocrine cells, TTN stimulates the secretion of glucocorticoids (Yanagibashi et al., 1989; Papadopoulos et al., 1991a) and testosterone (Garnier et al., 1993; Duparc et al., 2003). TTN also stimulates steroidogenesis by mitochondria isolated from adrenocortical and testicular Leydig cells (Besman et al., 1989; Yanagibashi et al., 1989; Papadopoulos et al., 1991a). In frog adrenal tissue, TTN stimulates corticosterone and aldosterone secretion *in vitro* (Lesouhaitier et al., 1996, 1998). Since TSPO is expressed not only in peripheral organs but also in the CNS (Braestrup and Squires, 1977; Benavides et al., 1983a,b; Anholt et al., 1984; Richards and Möhler, 1984; Gehlert et al., 1985), these observations suggest that TTN may be involved in the regulation of neurosteroidogenesis. To test this hypothesis, we have investigated the effect of TTN on the biosynthesis of steroids in the brain of amphibians.

Double labeling experiments have shown the presence of TSPO-like immunoreactivity in steroidogenic neurons of the frog Poa and dorsal hypothalamus (Do Rego et al., 1998; **Figure 2A**). Exposure of frog hypothalamic fragments to synthetic human TTN causes a concentration-dependent stimulation of the conversion of $[^3H]\Delta^5$P into 17OH-Δ^5P and 17OH-P (Do Rego et al., 1998). The TSPO agonist Ro5-4864 mimics the stimulatory effect of TTN while the TSPO antagonist PK11195 inhibits TTN-induced steroid production. In contrast, the action of TTN is not impaired by flumazenil, indicating that TTN acts specifically through TSPO to activate neurosteroid biosynthesis (Do Rego et al., 1998; **Figure 2B**).

The fact that ODN and TTN, acting via CBR and TSPO, respectively, stimulate the formation of a number of neurosteroids suggests that endozepines should play multiple functions. Indeed, *in vivo* studies indicate that endozepines, like neurosteroids, exert numerous behavioral effects. In particular, endozepines induce anxiety (Guidotti, 1991; Garcia de Mateos-Verchere et al., 1999), increase aggressivity (Guidotti et al., 1983; Ferrero et al., 1984; Kavaliers and Hirst, 1986; Guidotti, 1991), and possess anticonvulsant properties (Garcia de Mateos-Verchere et al., 1999). In addition, endozepines are potent anorexigenic neuropeptides (Garcia de Mateos-Verchere et al., 2001; Do Rego et al., 2007). Since endozepines and neurosteroids are involved in the control of the same behavioral processes, it is conceivable that neurosteroids can mediate some of the neurobiological effects of endozepines.

EFFECTS OF VASOTOCIN AND MESOTOCIN ON NEUROSTEROID BIOSYNTHESIS

Anatomical studies support the existence of neurochemical communication between steroidogenic neurons on the one hand, and neurons producing either arginine vasopressin (AVP) and oxytocin (OXT) in mammals or their orthologs arginine vasotocin (AVT) and mesotocin (MT) in submammalian vertebrates on the other hand. For instance, in birds, AVT-immunoreactive fibers innervate aromatase-expressing neurons in the preoptic nucleus and the lateral septum (Viglietti-Panzica et al., 1994; Balthazart, 1997). In the brain of amphibians, AVT- and/or MT-containing fibers project in the vicinity of 3β-HSD- and $P450_{C17}$-positive neurons (Do Rego et al., 2006; **Figure 3A**). In addition, the Poa, the dorsal and ventral hypothalamic nuclei, the suprachiasmatic nucleus, the posterior tuberculum, the nucleus of the periventricular organ, and the ventral part of the magnocellular preoptic nucleus of the frog diencephalon that contain the major populations of steroidogenic neurons are also enriched with AVP and MT receptor mRNAs. These close neuroanatomical relationships led us to investigate the possible effects of AVT and MT on neurosteroid biosynthesis in amphibians.

Static incubation of frog hypothalamic explants with AVT or MT stimulates the biosynthesis of 17OH-Δ^5P, P, 17OH-P, and DHEA in a concentration-dependent manner (Do Rego et al., 2006). This stimulatory effect is observed within the first 30-min, indicating that AVT and MT act at the post-translational level, possibly by activating phosphorylation of steroidogenic enzymes.

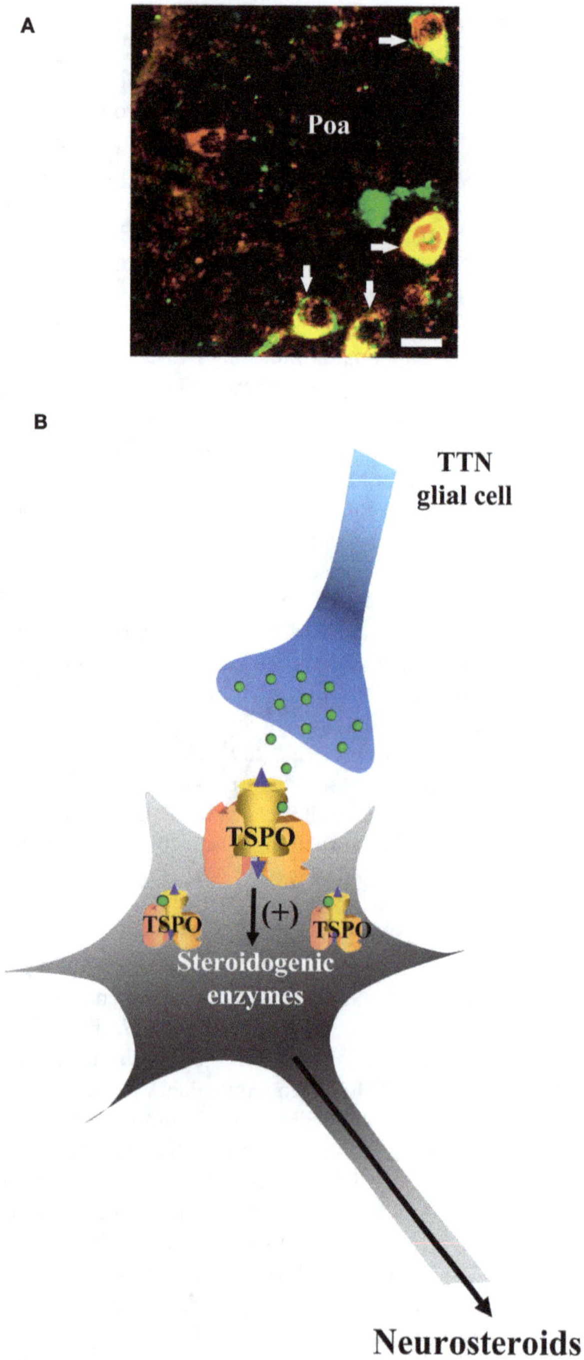

FIGURE 2 | Effect of the triakontatetraneuropeptide (TTN) on neurosteroid biosynthesis. (A) Immunohistochemical localization of 3β-HSD-like immunoreactivity (red) and translocator protein (TSPO)-like immunoreactivity (green) in the anterior preoptic area (Poa) of the frog brain. 3β-HSD-positive neurons that possess TSPO appear in yellow. For details regarding antibodies and immunohistochemical procedures, see reference by Do Rego et al. (1998). In brief, polyclonal antibodies raised in rabbit were used to label 3β-HSD-containing neurons, and polyclonal antibodies raised in chicken were used to label the TSPO-expressing cells. Scale bars: 10 μm. **(B)** Schematic drawing depicting the effect of TTN on steroidogenic neurons. TTN, acting through TSPO, stimulates the biosynthesis of 17OH-Δ^5P, DHEA, and 17OH-P.

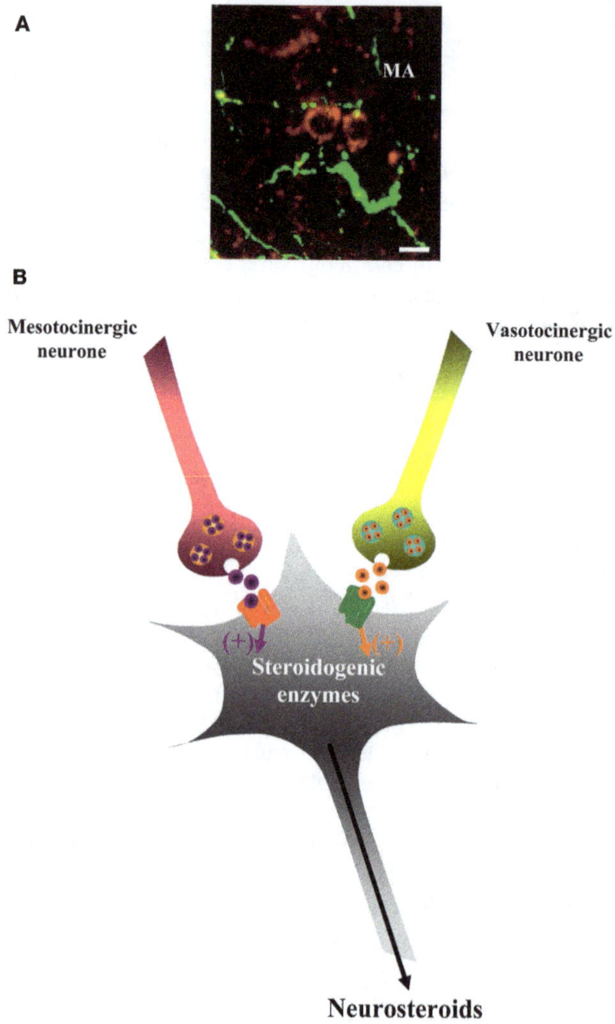

FIGURE 3 | Effect of vasotocin (AVT) and mesotocin (MT) on neurosteroid biosynthesis. (A) Immunohistochemical localization of $P450_{C17}$-like immunoreactivity (red) and AVT-like immunoreactivity (green) in the medial amygdala (MA) of the frog brain. AVT-containing nerve endings are located in close proximity of $P450_{C17}$-expressing neurons. For details regarding antibodies and immunohistochemical procedures, see reference by Do Rego et al. (2006). In brief, polyclonal antibodies raised in rabbit were used to label 3β-HSD-or $P450_{C17}$-containing neurons, and a mouse monoclonal antibody was used to label AVT-immunoreactive fibers. Scale bars: 10 μm. **(B)** Schematic drawing depicting the effects of AVT and MT on steroidogenic neurons. AVT acting through a V1a-like receptor, and MT acting through an MT receptor, stimulate the biosynthesis of 17OH-Δ^5P, DHEA, 17OH-P, and P.

The mammalian peptides AVP and OXT also induce a dose-related stimulation of neurosteroid biosynthesis (Do Rego et al., 2006). Pharmacological studies conducted with specific AVT and MT agonists and antagonists revealed that the effect of AVT and MT are mediated through V1a and MT receptors, respectively (Do Rego et al., 2006; **Figure 3B**). These observations are in agreement with the intense expression of V1a and MT receptor mRNAs in the hypothalamic nuclei that contain neurosteroidogenic neurons (Do Rego et al., 2006). Interestingly, in frog adrenocortical cells, AVT is also a potent stimulator of corticosteroid secretion although, in this latter case, AVT acts via V2 receptors (Larcher et al., 1989, 1992).

In vertebrates, AVP and related peptides exert a vast array of biological effects in the CNS (De Wied et al., 1993; Reghunandanan et al., 1998). For instance, in mammals, AVP enhances learning and memory (Alescio-Lautier and Soumireu-Mourat, 1998; Croiset et al., 2000; Engelmann et al., 2000; Engelmann, 2008) and increases aggressivity and anxiety-like behaviors (Ferris et al., 1997; Everts and Koolhaas, 1999; Heinrichs and Domes, 2008; Amikishieva et al., 2011; Mak et al., 2011; Meyer-Lindenberg et al., 2011). In birds, depending of the species, AVT increases or attenuates aggressive behavior (Goodson et al., 2004, 2009; Dewan et al., 2011). In amphibians, AVT stimulates vocalization and courtship behavior (Woolley et al., 2004; Moore et al., 2005; Thompson et al., 2008; Kikuyama et al., 2009). Certain neurosteroids also affect cognitive and mnemonic functions, aggressiveness and sexual activity (Frye, 2001; Vallée et al., 2001; Darnaudery et al., 2002; MacKenzie et al., 2007; Morrow, 2007). It thus appears that some of the behavioral effects of AVP/AVT may be ascribed to their stimulatory action on neurosteroid biosynthesis.

EFFECT OF NEUROPEPTIDE Y ON NEUROSTEROID BIOSYNTHESIS

Hydroxysteroid sulfotransferase (HST) catalyzes the transfer of a sulfate moiety from 3′-phosphoadenosine 5′-phosphosulfate (PAPS, a universal donor of sulfate radical) on the 3-hydroxyl group of steroids (Klaassen and Boles, 1997; Strott, 2002). While the presence of HST-containing neurons has been clearly demonstrated in the amphibian hypothalamus (Beaujean et al., 1999; Vaudry et al., 2011), the existence of HST in the brain of mammals is still a matter of debate (Geese and Raftogianis, 2001; Shimada et al., 2001; Shimizu et al., 2003; Kohjitani et al., 2006). Neuropeptide Y (NPY) is one of the most widely distributed biologically active peptides in the CNS of vertebrates (Allen et al., 1983; De Quidt and Emson, 1986; Bons et al., 1990; Danger et al., 1990, 1991; Aste et al., 1991; Hendry, 1993) and NPY, like sulfated neurosteroids, exerts a wide range of neurobiological activities (Dumont and Quirion, 2006).

In frog, the Poa and the magnocellular preoptic nucleus where HST-positive cell bodies are located (Beaujean et al., 1999; Do Rego et al., 2009) are abundantly innervated by NPY-immunoreactive fibers (Danger et al., 1985), suggesting that NPY could play a role in the regulation of HST-expressing neurons. In support of this hypothesis, double labeling experiments revealed that, in the frog diencephalon, numerous NPYergic axon terminals are apposed onto HST-containing perikarya (Beaujean et al., 2002; **Figure 4A**). In addition, the mRNAs encoding the Y_1 and Y_5 NPY receptor subtypes are expressed in the Poa and the magnocellular preoptic nucleus (Beaujean et al., 2002). Incubation of frog hypothalamic tissue with $[^3H]\Delta^5P$ or $[^3H]$DHEA as steroid precursors and $[^{35}S]$PAPS as a sulfate donor leads to the biosynthesis of $[^3H, ^{35}S]\Delta^5PS$ or $[^3H, ^{35}S]$DHEAS, respectively, confirming the existence of a biologically active form of HST in the amphibian brain (Beaujean et al., 1999). Synthetic frog NPY (Chartrel et al., 1991) causes a concentration-dependent inhibition of the *de novo* formation of Δ^5PS and DHEAS (Beaujean et al., 2002). The

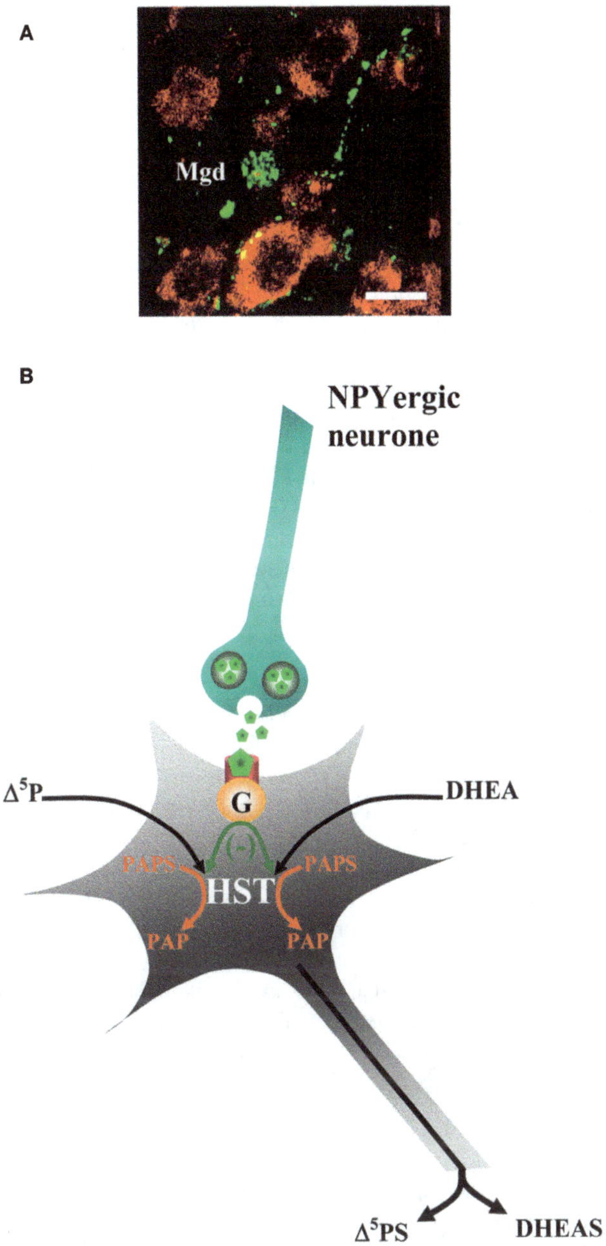

FIGURE 4 | Effect of neuropeptide Y (NPY) on neurosteroid biosynthesis. (A) Immunohistochemical localization of hydroxysteroid sulfotransferase (HST)-like immunoreactivity (red) and NPY-like immunoreactivity (green) in the dorsal part of the magnocellular preoptic nucleus (Mgd) of the frog brain. NPY-containing nerve endings are located in close proximity of HST-expressing neurons. For details regarding antibodies and immunohistochemical procedures, see reference by Beaujean et al. (2002). In brief, polyclonal antibodies raised in rabbit were used to label HST-containing neurons, and polyclonal antibodies raised in sheep were used to label NPY-immunoreactive fibers. Scale bars: 20 μm. **(B)** Schematic drawing depicting the effect of NPY on steroidogenic neurons. NPY acting through Y_1 receptors negatively coupled to adenylyl cyclase, inhibits the biosynthesis of Δ^5PS and DHEAS.

inhibitory effect of NPY is suppressed by the Y_1 receptor antagonist BIBP3226 while the Y_2 receptor antagonist $NPY_{(13-36)}$ is totally inactive (Beaujean et al., 2002). The fact that the Y_1 receptor antagonist *per se* slightly increases the biosynthesis of Δ^5PS and DHEAS reveals that endogenous NPY likely acts as a physiological modulator of the formation of sulfated neurosteroids (Beaujean et al., 2002). These data, together with the observation that Y_1 receptor mRNA is expressed in the Poa and the dorsal magnocellular nucleus, provide strong evidence for a Y_1-mediated inhibitory action of NPY on the biosynthesis of sulfated neurosteroids (**Figure 4B**).

Neuropeptide Y and sulfated neurosteroids are known to regulate the same behavioral activities including response to novelty (von Horsten et al., 1998; Tasan et al., 2009), feeding and satiety (Kalra and Kalra, 2004a,b; Ramos et al., 2005; Beck, 2006; Ueno et al., 2008), and reproductive behavior (Wehrenberg et al., 1989). NPY and sulfated neurosteroids are also implicated in the physiopathology of cognitive disorders, pain, epilepsy, anxiety, and depression (Engel and Grant, 2001; Rupprecht and Holsboer, 2001; Dumont and Quirion, 2006; Gibbs et al., 2006; Reddy, 2010; Thorsell, 2010; Nguyen et al., 2011). The fact that NPY reduces the biosynthesis of sulfated neurosteroids would thus indicate that some of the neurophysiological activities of NPY could be attributed to inhibition of HST activity.

CONCLUDING REMARKS

Studies conducted over the last decade have shown that the biosynthesis of neurosteroids is finely regulated by neurotransmitters (melatonin, GABA), pituitary hormones (prolactin), and various neuropeptides (ODN, TTN, AVT, MT, NPY). Several projects are currently in progress and there is little doubt that additional factors involved in the control of neurosteroid formation will be identified in the near future. As illustrated in the present report, most of the studies aimed at identifying the neurochemical regulation of neurosteroid biosynthesis have been conducted in non-mammalian models, mainly birds and amphibians. It will be now essential to examine whether the same mechanisms are operating in the brain of mammals and to look for their potential physiopathological significance. Little is currently known regarding the molecular mechanisms implicated in the regulation of neurosteroid biosynthesis. In particular, it has to be determined whether the neuroendocrine factors controlling neurosteroid production act at the transcriptional level to regulate the expression of the genes encoding the steroidogenic enzymes or at the post-translational level, e.g., to modulate the phosphorylation and thus the activity of these enzymes. The fact that neurosteroids are usually implicated in the same biological processes as the neuroendocrine factors which regulate their biosynthesis strongly suggests that some of the neurophysiological and behavioral activities of these latter factors could be mediated by neurosteroids. To test this hypothesis, it will be necessary to investigate whether specific activities of these regulatory factors are impaired in conditional KO mice lacking selectively expression of steroidogenic enzymes in the brain. The neuroendocrine regulation of neurosteroid biosynthesis by neurotransmitters, neuropeptides, and hormonal factors is currently an emerging theme that will undoubtedly flourish in the years to come.

ACKNOWLEDGMENTS

This work was supported by grants from the Institut National de la Santé et de la Recherche Médical (INSERM U413/U982), the Ministère des Affaires Etrangères (France–Québec exchange program to Georges Pelletier and Hubert Vaudry), a France–Québec exchange program (INSERM-Fonds de la Recherche en Santé du Québec, FRSQ, to Georges Pelletier and Hubert Vaudry), France–Korean exchange programs (INSERM-Korea Science and Engineering Foundation, KOSEF, to Jae Young Seong and Hubert Vaudry; and Science and Technology Amicable Relationships, STAR, to Jean Luc Do Rego, Jae Young Seong, and Hubert Vaudry), a France–Japan exchange program (INSERM-Japan Society for the Promotion of Science, JSPS, to Kazuyoshi Tsutsui, Hubert Vaudry, and Jean Luc Do Rego), the Plate-Forme Régionale de Recherche en Imagerie Cellulaire de Haute-Normandie (PRIMACEN), and the Région Haute-Normandie. Hubert Vaudry is Associated Researcher at the Research Center in Molecular Endocrinology, Oncology and Genetics, Laval University, Québec.

REFERENCES

Alescio-Lautier, B., and Soumireu-Mourat, B. (1998). Role of vasopressin in learning and memory in the hippocampus. *Prog. Brain Res.* 119, 501–521.

Alho, H., Bovolin, P., Jenkins, D., Guidotti, A., and Costa, E. (1989). Cellular and subcellular localization of an octadecaneuropeptide derived from diazepam binding inhibitor: immunohistochemical studies in the rat brain. *J. Chem. Neuroanat.* 2, 301–318.

Alho, H., Fremeau, R. T. Jr., Tiedge, H., Wilcox, J., Bovolin, P., Broslus, J., Roberts, J. L., and Costa, E. (1988). Diazepam binding inhibitor gene expression: location in brain and peripheral tissues of rat. *Proc. Natl. Acad. Sci. U.S.A.* 85, 7018–7022.

Alho, H., Kolmer, M., Harjuntausta, T., and Helen, P. (1995). Increased expression of diazepam binding inhibitor in human brain tumors. *Cell Growth Differ.* 6, 309–314.

Allen, Y. S., Adrian, T. E., Allen, J. M., Tatemoto, K., Crow, T. J., Bloom, S. R., and Polak, J. M. (1983). Neuropeptide Y distribution in the rat brain. *Science* 221, 877–879.

Aller, M. I., Janusonis, S., Fite, K. V., and Fernández-López, A. (1997). Distribution of the $GABA_A$ receptor complex β2/3 subunits in the brain of the frog *Rana pipiens*. *Neurosci. Lett.* 225, 65–68.

Amikishieva, A. V., Ilnitskaya, S. I., Nikolin, V. P., and Popova, N. A. (2011). Effect of vasopressin V1B receptor antagonist, SSR149415, on anxiety-like behavior and Lewis lung carcinoma metastasis in mice. *Exp. Oncol.* 33, 126–129.

Anholt, R. R., Murphy, K. M., Mack, G. E., and Snyder, S. H. (1984). Peripheral-type benzodiazepine receptors in the central nervous system: localization to olfactory nerves. *J. Neurosci.* 4, 593–603.

Aste, N., Viglietti-Panzica, C., Fasolo, A., Andreone, C., Vaudry, H., Pelletier, G., and Panzica, G. C. (1991). Localization of neuropeptide Y-immunoreactive cells and fibres in the brain of the Japanese quail. *Cell Tissue Res.* 265, 219–230.

Bäckberg, M., Ultenius, C., Fritschy, J. M., and Meister, B. (2004). Cellular localization of GABA receptor α subunit immunoreactivity in the rat hypothalamus: relationship with neurons containing orexigenic or anorexigenic peptides. *J. Neuroendocrinol.* 16, 589–604.

Balthazart, J. (1997). Steroid control and sexual differentiation of brain aromatase. *J. Steroid Biochem. Mol. Biol.* 61, 323–339.

Balthazart, J., Baillien, M., and Ball, G. F. (2001a). Rapid and reversible inhibition of brain aromatase activity. *J. Neuroendocrinol.* 13, 63–73.

Balthazart, J., Baillien, M., and Ball, G. F. (2001b). Phosphorylation processes mediate rapid changes of brain aromatase activity. *J. Steroid Biochem. Mol. Biol.* 79, 261–277.

Balthazart, J., Baillien, M., Charlier, T. D., Cornil, C. A., and Ball, G. F. (2001c). Multiple mechanisms control brain aromatase activity at the genomic and non-genomic level. *J. Steroid Biochem. Mol. Biol.* 86, 367–379.

Balthazart, J., Baillien, M., Charlier, T. D., and Ball, G. F. (2003). Calcium-dependent phosphorylation processes control brain aromatase in quail. *Eur. J. Neurosci.* 17, 1591–1606.

Barbaccia, M. L., Roscetti, G., Trabucchi, M., Purdy, R. H., Mostallino, M. C., Perra, C., Concas, A., and Biggio, G. (1996). Isoniazid-induced inhibition of GABAergic transmission enhances neurosteroid content in the rat brain. *Neuropharmacology* 35, 1299–1305.

Baulieu, E. E. (1997). Neurosteroids: of the nervous system by the nervous system, for the nervous system. *Recent Prog. Horm. Res.* 52, 1–32.

Baulieu, E. E. (1998). Neurosteroids: a novel function of the brain. *Psychoneuroendocrinology* 23, 963–987.

Baulieu, E. E., Robel, P., and Schumacher, M. (1999). "Neurosteroids: a new regulatory function in the nervous system," eds E. E. Baulieu, P. Robel, and M. Schumacher (Totowa, NJ: Humana Press), 1–26.

Beaujean, D., Do Rego, J. L., Galas, L., Mensah-Nyagan, A. G., Fredriksson, R., Larhammar, D., Fournier, A., Luu-The, V., Pelletier, G., and Vaudry, H. (2002). Neuropeptide Y inhibits the biosynthesis of sulfated neurosteroids in the hypothalamus through activation of Y1 receptors. *Endocrinology* 143, 1950–1963.

Beaujean, D., Mensah-Nyagan, A. G., Do Rego, J. L., Luu-The, V., Pelletier, G., and Vaudry, H. (1999). Immunocytochemical localization and biological activity of hydroxysteroid sulfotransferase in the frog brain. *J. Neurochem.* 72, 848–857.

Beck, B. (2006). Neuropeptide Y in normal eating and in genetic and dietary-induced obesity. *Philos. Trans. R. Soc. Lond. B Biol. Sci.* 361, 1159–1185.

Belelli, D., Bolger, M. B., and Gee, K. W. (1989). Anticonvulsant profile of the progesterone metabolite 3α-hydroxy 5α-pregnan-20-one. *Eur. J. Pharmacol.* 166, 325–329.

Belelli, D., Herd, M. B., Mitchell, E. A., Peden, D. R., Vardy, A. W., Gentet, L., and Lambert, J. J. (2006). Neuroactive steroids and inhibitory neurotransmission: mechanisms of action and physiological relevance. *Neuroscience* 138, 821–829.

Belelli, D., and Lambert, J. J. (2005). Neurosteroids: endogenous regulators of the $GABA_A$ receptor. *Nat. Rev. Neurosci.* 6, 565–575.

Benavides, J., Quarteronet, D., Imbault, F., Malgouris, C., Uzan, A., Renault, C., Dubroeucq, M. C., Gueremy, C., and Le Fur, G. (1983a). Labelling of "peripheral-type" benzodiazepine binding sites in the rat brain by using $[^3H]$PK 11195, an isoquinoline carboxamide derivative: kinetic studies and autoradiographic localization. *J. Neurochem.* 41, 1744–1750.

Benavides, J., Malgouris, C., Imbault, F., Begassat, F., Uzan, A., Renault, C., Dubroeucq, M. C., Gueremy, C., and Le Fur, G. (1983b). "Peripheral type" benzodiazepine binding sites in rat adrenals: binding studies with $[^3H]$PK 11195 and autoradiographic localization. *Arch. Int. Pharmacodyn. Ther.* 266, 38–49.

Bergeron, R., de Montigny, C., and Debonnel, G. (1996). Potentiation of neuronal NMDA response induced by dehydroepiandrosterone and its suppression by progesterone: effects mediated via sigma receptors. *J. Neurosci.* 16, 1193–1202.

Besman, M. J., Yanagibashi, K., Lee, T. D., Kawamura, M., Hall, P. F., and Shively, J. E. (1989). Identification of des-(Gly-Ile)-endozepine as an effector of corticotropin-dependent adrenal steroidogenesis: stimulation of cholesterol delivery is mediated by the peripheral benzodiazepine receptor. *Proc. Natl. Acad. Sci. U.S.A.* 86, 4897–4901.

Bons, N., Mestre, N., Petter, A., Danger, J. M., Pelletier, G., and Vaudry, H. (1990). Localization and characterization of neuropeptide Y in the brain of *Microcebus murinus* (Primate, Lemurian). *J. Comp. Neurol.* 298, 343–361.

Bowlby, M. R. (1993). Pregnenolone sulfate potentiation of N-methyl-D-aspartate receptor channels in hippocampal neurons. *Mol. Pharmacol.* 43, 813–819.

Braestrup, C., and Squires, R. F. (1977). Specific benzodiazepine receptors in rat brain characterized by high-affinity (^3H)diazepam binding. *Proc. Natl. Acad. Sci. U.S.A.* 74, 3805–3809.

Bullock, A. E., Clark, A. L., Grady, S. R., Robinson, S. F., Slobe, B. S., Marks, M. J., and Collins, A. C. (1997). Neurosteroids modulate nicotinic receptor function in mouse striatal and thalamic synaptosomes. *J. Neurochem.* 68, 2412–2423.

Bürgi, B., Lichtensteiger, W., Lauber, M. E., and Schlumpf, M. (1999). Ontogeny of diazepam binding inhibitor/acyl-CoA binding protein mRNA and peripheral benzodiazepine receptor mRNA expression in the rat. *J. Neuroendocrinol.* 11, 85–100.

Chadwick, C. S. (1941). Identity of prolactin with water drive factor in *Triturus viridescens*. *Proc. Soc. Exp. Biol. Med.* 45, 335–337.

Charalampopoulos, I., Tsatsanis, C., Dermitzaki, E., Alexaki, V. I., Castanas, E., Margioris, A. N., and Gravanis, A. (2004). Dehydroepiandrosterone and allopregnanolone protect sympathoadrenal medulla cells against apoptosis via antiapoptotic Bcl-2 proteins. *Proc. Natl. Acad. Sci. U.S.A.* 101, 8209–8214.

Chartrel, N., Conlon, J. M., Danger, J. M., Fournier, A., Tonon, M. C., and Vaudry, H. (1991). Characterization of melanotropin-release-inhibiting factor (melanostatin) from frog brain: homology with human neuropeptide Y. *Proc. Natl. Acad. Sci. U.S.A.* 88, 3862–3866.

Compagnone, N. A., and Mellon, S. H. (1998). Dehydroepiandrosterone: a potential signalling molecule for neocortical organization during development. *Proc. Natl. Acad. Sci. U.S.A.* 95, 4678–4683.

Compagnone, N. A., and Mellon, S. H. (2000). Neurosteroids: biosynthesis and function of these novel neuromodulators. *Front. Neuroendocrinol.* 21, 1–56.

Cornil, C., Foidart, A., Minet, A., and Balthazart, J. (2000). Immunocytochemical localization of ionotropic glutamate receptors subunits in the adult quail forebrain. *J. Comp. Neurol.* 428, 577–608.

Cornil, C. A. (2009). Rapid regulation of brain oestrogen synthesis: the behavioural roles of oestrogens and their fates. *J. Neuroendocrinol.* 21, 217–226.

Corpéchot, C., Robel, P., Axelson, M., Sjövall, J., and Baulieu, E. E. (1981). Characterization and measurement of dehydroepiandrosterone sulfate in rat brain. *Proc. Natl. Acad. Sci. U.S.A.* 78, 4704–4707.

Corpéchot, C., Synguelakis, M., Talha, S., Axelson, M., Sjövall, J., Vihko, R., Baulieu, E. E., and Robel, P. (1983). Pregnenolone and its sulfate ester in the rat brain. *Brain Res.* 270, 119–125.

Costa, E. T., Soto, E. E., Cardoso, R. A., Olivera, D. S., and Valenzuela, C. F. (2000). Acute effects of ethanol on kainate receptors in cultured hippocampal neurons. *Alcohol. Clin. Exp. Res.* 24, 220–225.

Croiset, G., Nijsen, M. J. M. A., and Kamphuis, P. J. G. H. (2000). Role of corticotrophin-releasing factor, vasopressin and autonomic nervous system in learning and memory. *Eur. J. Pharmacol.* 405, 225–234.

Damianisch, K., Rupprecht, R., and Lancel, M. (2001). The influence of subchronic administration of the neurosteroid allopregnanolone on sleep in the rat. *Neuropsychopharmacology* 25, 576–584.

Danger, J. M., Breton, B., Vallarino, M., Fournier, A., Pelletier, G., and Vaudry, H. (1991). Neuropeptide-Y in the trout brain and pituitary: localization, characterization, and action on gonadotropin release. *Endocrinology* 128, 2360–2368.

Danger, J. M., Guy, J., Benyamina, J., Jégou, S., Leboulenger, F., Coté, J., Tonon, M. C., Pelletier, G., and Vaudry, H. (1985). Localization and identification of neuropeptide Y (NPY)-like immunoreactivity in the frog brain. *Peptides* 6, 1225–1236.

Danger, J. M., Tonon, M. C., Jenks, B. G., Saint-Pierre, S., Martel, J. C., Fasolo, A., Breton, B., Quirion, R., Pelletier, G., and Vaudry, H. (1990). Neuropeptide Y: localization in the central nervous system and neuroendocrine functions. *Fundam. Clin. Pharmacol.* 4, 307–340.

Darnaudery, M., Pallarès, M., Piazza, P. V., Le Moal, M., and Mayo, W. (2002). The neurosteroid pregnenolone sulfate infused into the medial septum nucleus increases hippocampal acetylcholine and spatial memory in rats. *Brain Res.* 95, 237–242.

De Montis, G. M., Olianas, M. C., Mulas, G., Lloyd, K. G., and Tagliamonte, A. (1981). GABA receptors distribution in rat substantia nigra. *Neurosci. Lett.* 23, 257–261.

De Quidt, M. E., and Emson, P. C. (1986). Distribution of neuropeptide Y-like immunoreactivity in the rat central nervous system II. Immunohistochemical analysis. *Neuroscience* 18, 545–618.

De Wied, D., Diamant, M., and Fodor, M. (1993). Central nervous system effects of the neurohypophyseal hormones and related peptides. *Front. Neuroendocrinol.* 14, 251–302.

Dewan, A. K., Ramey, M. L., and Tricas, T. C. (2011). Arginine vasotocin neuronal phenotypes, telencephalic fiber varicosities, and social behavior in butterflyfishes (Chaetodontidae): potential similarities to birds and mammals. *Horm. Behav.* 59, 56–66.

Diotel, N., Do Rego, J. L., Anglade, I., Vaillant, C., Pellegrini, E., Gueguen, M. M., Mironov, S., Vaudry, H., and Kah, O. (2011). Activity and expression of steroidogenic enzymes in the brain of adult zebrafish. *Eur. J. Neurosci.* 34, 45–56.

Diotel, N., Le Page, Y., Mouriec, K., Tong, S. K., Pellegrini, E., Vaillant, C., Anglade, I., Brion, F., Pakdel, F., Chung, B. C., and Kah, O. (2010). Aromatase in the brain of teleost fish: expression, regulation and putative functions. *Front. Neuroendocrinol.* 31, 172–192.

Djebaili, M., Hoffman, S. W., and Stein, D. G. (2004). Allopregnanolone and progesterone decrease cell death and cognitive deficits after a contusion of the rat pre-frontal cortex. *Neuroscience* 123, 349–359.

Do Rego, J. C., Orta, M. H., Leprince, J., Tonon, M. C., Vaudry, H., and Costentin, J. (2007). Pharmacological characterization of the receptor mediating the anorexigenic action of the octadecaneuropeptide: evidence for an endozepinergic tone regulating food intake. *Neuropsychopharmacology* 32, 1641–1648.

Do Rego, J. L., Acharjee, S., Seong, J. Y., Galas, L., Alexandre, D., Bizet, P., Burlet, A., Kwon, H. B., Luu-The, V., Pelletier, G., and Vaudry, H. (2006). Vasotocin and mesotocin stimulate the biosynthesis of neurosteroids in the frog brain. *J. Neurosci.* 26, 6749–6760.

Do Rego, J. L., Mensah-Nyagan, A. G., Beaujean, D., Leprince, J., Tonon, M. C., Luu-The, V., Pelletier, G., and Vaudry, H. (2001). The octadecaneuropeptide ODN stimulates neurosteroid biosynthesis through activation of central-type benzodiazepine receptors. *J. Neurochem.* 76, 128–138.

Do Rego, J. L., Mensah-Nyagan, A. G., Beaujean, D., Vaudry, D., Sieghart, W., Luu-The, V., Pelletier, G., and Vaudry, H. (2000). GABA, acting through $GABA_A$ receptors, inhibits biosynthesis of neurosteroids in the frog hypothalamus. *Proc. Natl. Acad. Sci. U.S.A.* 97, 13925–13930.

Do Rego, J. L., Mensah-Nyagan, A. G., Feuilloley, M., Ferrara, P., Pelletier, G., and Vaudry, H. (1998). The endozepine triakontatetraneuropeptide diazepam-binding inhibitor [17-50] stimulates neurosteroid biosynthesis in the frog hypothalamus. *Neuroscience* 83, 555–570.

Do Rego, J. L., Seong, J. Y., Burel, D., Leprince, J., Luu-The, V., Tsutsui, K., Tonon, M. C., Pelletier, G., and Vaudry, H. (2009). Neurosteroid biosynthesis: enzymatic pathways and neuroendocrine regulation by neurotransmitters and neuropeptides. *Front. Neuroendocrinol.* 30, 259–301.

Do Rego, J. L., Tremblay, Y., Luu-The, V., Repetto, E., Castel, H., Vallarino, M., Bélanger, A., Pelletier, G., and Vaudry, H. (2007a). Immunohistochemical localization and biological activity of the steroidogenic enzyme cytochrome P450 17α-hydroxylase/C17, 20-lyase ($P450_{C17}$) in the frog brain and pituitary. *J. Neurochem.* 100, 251–268.

Do Rego, J. L., Leprince, J., Luu-The, V., Pelletier, G., Tonon, M. C., and Vaudry, H. (2007b). Structure-activity relationships of a series of analogs of the endozepine octadecaneuropeptide (ODN_{11-18}) on neurosteroid biosynthesis by hypothalamic explants. *J. Med. Chem.* 50, 3070–3076.

Dubrovsky, B. O. (2005). Steroids, neuroactive steroids and neurosteroids in psychopathology. *Prog. Neuropsychopharmacol. Biol. Psychiatry* 29, 169–192.

Dumont, Y., and Quirion, R. (2006). "Neuropeptide Y," in *Handbook of Biologically Active Peptides*, ed. A. J. Kastin (New York: Academic Press), 683–688.

Duparc, C., Lefebvre, H., Tonon, M. C., Vaudry, H., and Kuhn, J. M. (2003). Characterization of endozepines in the human testicular tissue: effect of triakontatetraneuropeptide on testosterone secretion. *J. Clin. Endocrinol. Metab.* 88, 5521–5528.

Engel, S. R., and Grant, K. A. (2001). Neurosteroids and behavior. *Int. Rev. Neurobiol.* 46, 321–348.

Engelmann, M. (2008). Vasopressin in the septum: not important versus causally involved in learning and memory – two faces of the same coin? *Prog. Brain Res.* 170, 389–395.

Engelmann, M., Wotjak, C. T., Ebner, K., and Landgraf, R. (2000). Behavioral impact of intraseptally released vasopressin and oxytocin in rats. *Exp. Physiol.* 85, 125S–130S.

Everts, H. G. J., and Koolhaas, J. M. (1999). Differential modulation of lateral septal vasopressin receptor blockade in spatial learning, social recognition, and anxiety-related behaviors in rats. *Behav. Brain Res.* 99, 7–16.

Fahey, J. M., Miller, L. G., and Isaacson, R. L. (1995a). Neurosteroid modulation of locomotor activity in mice. *Neurosci. Res. Commun.* 17, 159–167.

Fahey, J. M., Lindquist, D. G., Pritchard, G. A., and Miller, L. G. (1995b). Pregnenolone sulfate potentiation of NMDA-mediated increases in intracellular calcium in cultured chick cortical neurons. *Brain Res.* 669, 183–188.

Ferrero, P., Guidotti, A., and Conti-Tronconi, B. (1984). A brain octadecaneuropeptide generated by tryptic digestion of DBI (diazepam binding inhibitor) functions as a proconflict ligand of benzodiazepine recognition sites. *Neuropharmacology* 23, 1359–1362.

Ferris, C. F., Melloni, R. H. Jr., Koppel, G., Perry, K. W., Fuller, R. W., and Delville, Y. (1997). Vasopressin/serotonin interactions in the anterior hypothalamus control aggressive behavior in golden hamsters. *J. Neurosci.* 17, 4331–4340.

Flood, J. F., Morley, J. E., and Roberts, E. (1992). Memory-enhancing effects in male mice of pregnenolone and steroids metabolically derived from it. *Proc. Natl. Acad. Sci. U.S.A.* 89, 1567–1571.

Flood, J. F., Smith, G. E., and Roberts, E. (1988). Dehydroepiandrosterone and its sulfate enhance memory retention in mice. *Brain Res.* 447, 269–278.

Frank, C., and Sagratella, S. (2000). Neuroprotective effects of allopregnenolone on hippocampal irreversible neurotoxicity in vitro. *Prog. Neuropsychopharmacol. Biol. Psychiatry* 24, 1117–1126.

Franzoni, M. F., and Morino, P. (1989). The distribution of GABA-like-immunoreactive neurons in the brain of the newt, *Tritucus cristatus carnifex*, and the green frog *Rana esculenta*. *Cell Tissue Res.* 255, 155–166.

Frye, C. A. (2001). The role of neurosteroids and non-genomic effects of progestins and androgens in mediating sexual receptivity of rodents. *Brain Res. Rev.* 37, 201–222.

Garcia de Mateos-Verchere, J., Leprince, J., Tonon, M. C., Vaudry, H., and Costentin, J. (1999). Reduction of pentylenetetrazol-induced convulsions by the octadecaneuropeptide ODN. *Peptides* 20, 1431–1436.

Garcia de Mateos-Verchere, J., Leprince, J., Tonon, M. C., Vaudry, H., and Costentin, J. (2001). The octadecaneuropeptide [diazepam-binding inhibitor (33-50)] exerts potent anorexigenic effects in rodents. *Eur. J. Pharmacol.* 414, 225–231.

Garnier, M., Boujrad, N., Ogwuegbu, S. O., Hudson, J. R. Jr., and Papadopoulos, V. (1994). The polypeptide diazepam-binding inhibitor and a higher affinity mitochondrial peripheral-type benzodiazepine receptor sustain constitutive steroidogenesis in the R2C Leydig tumor cell line. *J. Biol. Chem.* 269, 22105–22112.

Garnier, M., Boujrad, N., Oke, B. O., Brown, A. S., Riond, J., Ferrara, P., Shoyab, M., Suarez-Quian, C. A., and Papadopoulos, V. (1993). Diazepam binding inhibitor is a paracrine/autocrine regulator of Leydig cell proliferation and steroidogenesis: action via peripheral-type benzodiazepine receptor and independent mechanisms. *Endocrinology* 132, 444–458.

Geese, W. J., and Raftogianis, R. B. (2001). Biochemical characterization and tissue distribution of human SULT2B1. *Biochem. Biophys. Res. Commun.* 288, 280–289.

Gehlert, D. R., Yamamura, H. I., and Wamsley, J. K. (1985). Autoradiographic localization of "peripheral-type" benzodiazepine binding sites in the rat brain, heart and kidney. *Naunyn Schmiedebergs Arch. Pharmacol.* 328, 454–460.

Gibbs, J. L., Flores, C. M., and Hargreaves, K. M. (2006). Attenuation of capsaicin-evoked mechanical allodynia by peripheral neuropeptide Y Y1 receptors. *Pain* 124, 167–174.

Goodson, J. L., Kabelik, D., and Schrock, S. E. (2009). Dynamic neuromodulation of aggression by vasotocin: influence of social context and social phenotype in territorial songbirds. *Biol. Lett.* 5, 554–556.

Goodson, J. L., Lindberg, L., and Johnson, P. (2004). Effects of central vasotocin and mesotocin manipulations on social behavior in male and female zebra finches. *Horm. Behav.* 45, 136–143.

Grazzini, E., Guillon, G., Mouillac, B., and Zingg, H. H. (1998). Inhibition of oxytocin receptor function by direct binding of progesterone. *Nature* 392, 509–512.

Guarneri, P., Guarneri, R., Cascio, C., Piccoli, F., and Papadopoulos, V. (1995). γ-aminobutyric acid type A/benzodiazepine receptors regulate rat retina neurosteroidogenesis. *Brain Res.* 683, 65–72.

Guidotti, A. (1991). Role of DBI in brain and its posttranslational processing products in normal and abnormal behavior. *Neuropharmacology* 30, 1425–1433.

Guidotti, A., Forchetti, C. M., Corda, M. G., Kondel, D., Bennett, C. D., and Costa, E. (1983). Isolation, characterization and purification to homogeneity of an endogenous polypeptide with agonistic action on benzodiazepine receptors. *Proc. Natl. Acad. Sci. U.S.A.* 80, 3531–3535.

Gursoy, E., Cardounel, A., and Kalimi, A. (2001). Pregnenolone protects mouse hippocampal (HT-22) cells against glutamate and amyloid beta protein toxicity. *Neurochem. Res.* 26, 15–21.

Harada, N. (1988). Novel properties of human placental aromatase as cytochrome P-450: purification and characterization of a unique form of aromatase. *J. Biochem.* 103, 106–113.

Haraguchi, S., Koyama, T., Do Rego, J. L., and Tsutsui, K. (2009). Seasonal changes in the synthesis of 7α-hydroxypregnenolone stimulating locomotor activity in newts. *Ann. N. Y. Acad. Sci.* 1163, 410–413.

Haraguchi, S., Koyama, T., Hasunuma, I., Vaudry, H., and Tsutsui, K. (2010). Prolactin increases the synthesis of 7α-hydroxypregnenolone, a key factor for induction of locomotor activity, in breeding male newts. *Endocrinology* 151, 2211–2222.

Hau, M., and Gwinner, E. (1994). Melatonin facilitates synchronization of sparrow circadian rhythms to light. *J. Comp. Physiol. A* 175, 343–347.

He, J., Hoffman, S. W., and Stein, D. G. (2004). Allopregnanolone, a progesterone metabolite, enhances behavioral recovery and decreases neuronal loss after traumatic brain injury. *Restor. Neurol. Neurosci.* 22, 19–31.

Heinrichs, M., and Domes, G. (2008). Neuropeptides and social behavious: effect of oxytocin and vasopressin in humans. *Prog. Brain Res.* 170, 337–350.

Hendry, S. H. (1993). "Organization of neuropeptide Y neurons in the mammalian central nervous system," in *The Biology of Neuropeptide Y and Related Peptides*, eds W. F. Colmers and C. Wahlested (Totowa, NJ: Humana Press), 65–156.

Hodge, C. W., Raber, J., McMahon, T., Walter, H., Sanchez-Perez, A. M., Olive, M. F., Mehmert, K., Morrow, A. L., and Messing, R. O. (2002). Decreased anxiety-like behavior, reduced stress hormones, and neurosteroid supersensitivity in mice lacking protein kinase Cepsilon. *J. Clin. Invest.* 110, 1003–1010.

Hollis, D. M., and Boyd, S. K. (2005). Distribution of GABA-like immunoreactive cell bodies in the brains of two amphibians, *Rana catesbeiana* and *Xenopus laevis*. *Brain Behav. Evol.* 65, 127–142.

Hollis, D. M., Goetz, F. W., Roberts, S. B., and Boyd, S. K. (2004). Acute neurosteroid modulation and subunit isolation of the gamma-aminobutyric $acid_A$ receptor in the bullfrog, *Rana catesbeina*. *J. Mol. Endocrinol.* 32, 921–934.

Horishita, T., Minami, K., Uezono, Y., Shiraishi, M., Ogata, J., Okamoto, T., Terada, T., and Sata, T. (2005). The effects of the neurosteroids: pregnenolone, progesterone and dehydroepiandrosterone on muscarinic receptor-induced responses in *Xenopus* oocytes expressing M1 and M3 receptors. *Naunyn Schmiedebergs Arch. Pharmacol.* 371, 221–228.

Hu, Y., Cardounel, A., Gursoy, E., Anderson, P., and Kalimi, M. (2000). Anti-stress effects of dehydroepiandrosterone: protection of rats against repeated immobilization stress-induced weight loss, glucocorticoid receptor production, and lipid peroxidation. *Biochem. Pharmacol.* 59, 753–762.

Inai, Y., Nagai, K., Ukena, K., Oishi, T., and Tsutsui, K. (2003). Seasonal changes in neurosteroid concentrations in the amphibian brain and environmental factors regulating their changes. *Brain Res.* 959, 214–225.

Irwin, R. P., Maragakis, N. J., Rogawski, M. A., Purdy, R. H., Farb, D. H., and Paul, S. M. (1992). Pregnenolone sulfate augments NMDA receptor mediated increases in intracellular Ca^{2+} in cultured rat hippocampal neurons. *Neurosci. Lett.* 141, 30–34.

Iwata, M., Muneoka, K. T., Shirayama, Y., Yamamoto, A., and Kawahara, R. (2005). A study of a dendritic marker, microtubule-associated protein 2 (MAP-2), in rats neonatally treated neurosteroids, pregnenolone and dehydroepiandrosterone (DHEA). *Neurosci. Lett.* 386, 145–149.

Iwata, T., Toyoda, F., Yamamoto, K., and Kikuyama, S. (2000). Hormonal control of urodele reproductive behavior. *Comp. Biochem. Physiol. B. Biochem. Mol. Biol.* 126, 221–229.

Jiang, P., Yang, C. X., Wang, Y. T., and Xu, T. L. (2006). Mechanisms of modulation of pregnanolone on glycinergic response in cultured spinal dorsal horn neurons of rat. *Neuroscience* 141, 2041–2050.

Jo, D. H., Sánchez de la Peña, S., Halberg, F., Ungar, F., Baulieu, E. E., and Robel, P. (1990). Circadian-infradian rhythmic variation of brain neurosteroids in the female rat. *Prog. Clin. Biol. Res.* 341B, 125–134.

Jones, K. (1994). Androgenic enhancement of motor neuron regeneration. *Ann. N. Y. Acad. Sci.* 743, 141–164.

Kalra, S. P., and Kalra, P. S. (2004a). NPY and cohorts in regulating appetite, obesity and metabolic syndrome: beneficial effects of gene therapy. *Neuropeptides* 38, 201–211.

Kalra, S. P., and Kalra, P. S. (2004b). NPY: an endearing journey in search of a neurochemical on/off switch for appetite, sex and reproduction. *Peptides* 25, 465–471.

Kaur, G., and Kulkarni, S. K. (2001). Subchronic studies on modulation of feeding behavior and body weight by neurosteroids in female mice. *Methods Find. Exp. Clin. Pharmacol.* 23, 115–119.

Kavaliers, M., and Hirst, M. (1986). An octadecaneuropeptide (ODN) derived from diazepam binding inhibitor increases aggressive interactions in mice. *Brain Res.* 383, 343–349.

Kavaliers, M., and Kinsella, D. M. (1995). Male preference for the odors of estrous female mice is reduced by the neurosteroid pregnenolone sulfate. *Brain Res.* 682, 222–226.

Kikuyama, S., Hasunuma, I., Toyoda, F., Haraguchi, S., and Tsutsui, K. (2009). Hormone-mediated reproductive behavior in the red-bellied newt. *Ann. N. Y. Acad. Sci.* 1163, 79–86.

Kikuyama, S., Tanaka, S., and Moore, F. L. (2003). "Reproductive biology and phylogeny of urodela," in *Endocrinology of Reproduction*, ed. D. M. Sever (Enfield, NH: Science Publishers), 275–321.

Kimonides, V. G., Khatibi, N. H., Svendsen, C. N., Sofroniew, M. V., and Herbert, J. (1998). Dehydroepiandrosterone (DHEA) and DHEA-sulfate (DHEAS) protect hippocampal neurons against excitatory amino acid-induced neurotoxicity. *Proc. Natl. Acad. Sci. U.S.A.* 95, 1852–1857.

Kimonides, V. G., Spillantini, M. G., Sofroniew, M. V., fawcett, J. W., and Herbert, J. (1999). Dehydroepiandrosterone antagonizes the neurotoxic effects of corticosterone and translocation of stress-activated protein kinase 3 in hippocampal primary cultures. *Neuroscience* 89, 429–436.

Klaassen, C. D., and Boles, J. W. (1997). Sulfation and sulfotransferases 5: the importance of 3′-phosphoadenosine 5′-phosphosulfate (PAPS) in the regulation of sulfation. *FASEB J.* 11, 404–418.

Koenig, H. L., Schumacher, M., Ferzaz, B., Do, T. A. N., Ressouches, A., Guennoun, R., Jung-Testas, I., Robel, P., Akwa, Y., and Baulieu, E. E. (1995). Progesterone synthesis and myelin formation by Schwann cells. *Science* 268, 1500–1503.

Kohjitani, A., Fuda, H., Hanyu, O., and Strott, C. A. (2006). Cloning, characterization and tissue expression of rat SULT2B1a and SULT2B1b steroid/sterol sulfotransferase isoforms: divergence of the rat SULT2B1 gene structure from orthologous human and mouse genes. *Gene* 367, 66–73.

Kostowski, W., and Bienkowski, P. (1999). Discriminative stimulus effects of ethanol: neuropharmacological characterization. *Alcohol* 17, 63–80.

Koyama, T., Haraguchi, S., Vaudry, H., and Tsutsui, K. (2009). Diurnal changes in the synthesis of 7α-hydroxypregnenolone stimulating locomotor activity in newts. *Ann. N. Y. Acad. Sci.* 1163, 444–447.

Krnjevic, K., and Schwartz, S. (1966). Is gamma-aminobutyric acid an inhibitory transmitter? *Nature* 211, 1372–1374.

Ladurelle, N., Eychenne, B., Denton, D., Blair-West, J., Schumacher, M., and Baulieu, E. E. (2000). Prolonged intracerebroventricular infusion of neurosteroids affects cognitive performances in the mouse. *Brain Res.* 858, 371–379.

Lancel, M., Faulhaber, J., Schiffelholz, T., Romeo, E., di Michele, F., Holsboer, F., and Rupprecht, R. (1997). Allopregnanolone affects sleep in a benzodiazepine-like fashion. *J. Pharmacol. Exp. Ther.* 282, 1213–1218.

Landgren, S., Backstrom, T., and Dubrovsky, B. (1987). The effect of progesterone and its metabolites on the interictal epileptiform discharge in the cat's cerebral cortex. *Acta Physiol. Scand.* 131, 33–42.

Lanthier, A., and Patwardhan, V. V. (1986). Sex steroids and 5-en-3β-hydroxysteroids in specific regions of the human brain and cranial nerves. *J. Steroid Biochem.* 25, 445–449.

Lapchak, P. A., and Araujo, D. M. (2001). Preclinical development of neurosteroids as neuroprotective agents for the treatment of neurodegenerative diseases. *Int. Rev. Neurobiol.* 46, 379–397.

Lapchak, P. A., Chapman, D. F., Nunez, S. Y., and Zivin, J. A. (2000). Dehydroepiandrosterone sulfate is neuroprotective in a reversible spinal cord ischemia model. *Stroke* 31, 1953–1957.

Larcher, A., Delarue, C., Homo-Delarche, F., Kikuyama, S., Kupryszewski, G., and Vaudry, H. (1992). Pharmacological characterization of vasotocin stimulation of phosphoinositide turnover in frog adrenal gland. *Endocrinology* 130, 475–483.

Larcher, A., Delarue, C., Idres, S., Lefebvre, H., Feuilloley, M., Vandesande, F., Pelletier, G., and Vaudry, H. (1989). Identification of VT-like immunoreactivity in chromaffin cells of the frog adrenal gland: effect of VT on corticosteroid secretion. *Endocrinology* 125, 2691–2700.

Laurine, E., Lafitte, D., Grégoire, C., Sérée, E., Loret, E., Douillard, S., Michel, B., Briand, C., and Verdier, J. M. (2003). Specific binding of dehydroepiandrosterone to the N terminus of the microtubule-associated protein MAP2. *J. Biol. Chem.* 278, 29979–29986.

Le Foll, F., Louiset, E., Castel, H., Vaudry, H., and Cazin, L. (1997a). Electrophysiological effects of various neuroactive steroids on the GABAA receptor in pituitary melanotrope cells. *Eur. J. Pharmacol.* 331, 303–311.

Le Foll, F., Castel, H., Louiset, E., Vaudry, H., and Cazin, L. (1997b). Multiple modulatory effects of the neuroactive steroid pregnanolone on GABAA receptor in frog pituitary melanotrophs. *J. Physiol.* 504, 387–400.

Leskiewicz, M., Budziszewska, B., Basta-Kaim, A., Zajac, A., Kacinski, M., and Lason, W. (2006). Effects of neurosteroids on neuronal survival: molecular basis and clinical perspectives. *Acta Neurobiol. Exp. (Wars.)* 66, 359–367.

Lesouhaitier, O., Feuilloley, M., Lihrmann, I., Ugo, I., Fasolo, A., Tonon, M. C., and Vaudry, H. (1996). Localization of diazepam-binding inhibitor-related peptides and peripheral type benzodiazepine receptors in the frog adrenal gland. *Cell Tissue Res.* 283, 403–412.

Lesouhaitier, O., Feuilloley, M., and Vaudry, H. (1998). Effect of the triakontatetraneuropeptide (TTN) on corticosteroid secretion by the frog adrenal gland. *J. Mol. Endocrinol.* 20, 45–53.

Lihrmann, I., Plaquevent, J. C., Tostivint, H., Raijmakers, R., Tonon, M. C., Conlon, J. M., and Vaudry, H. (1994). Frog diazepam-binding inhibitor: peptide sequence, cDNA cloning, and expression in the brain. *Proc. Natl. Acad. Sci. U.S.A.* 91, 6899–6903.

Lockhart, E. M., Warner, D. S., Pearlstein, R. D., Penning, D. H., Mehrabani, S., and Boustany, R. M. (2002). Allopregnanolone attenuates N-methyl-D-aspartate-induced excitotoxicity and apoptosis in human NT2 cell line in culture. *Neurosci. Lett.* 328, 33–36.

MacKenzie, E. M., Odontiadis, J., Le Melledo, J. M., Prior, T. I., and Baker, G. B. (2007). The relevance of neuroactive steroids in schizophrenia, depression, and anxiety disorders. *Cell. Mol. Neurobiol.* 27, 541–574.

Magnaghi, V., Cavarretta, I., Galbiati, M., Martini, L., and Melcangi, R. C. (2001). Neuroactive steroids and peripheral myelin proteins. *Brain Res. Rev.* 37, 360–371.

Majewska, M. D. (1992). Neurosteroids: endogenous bimodal modulators of the GABAA receptor. Mechanism of action and physiological significance. *Prog. Neurobiol.* 38, 379–395.

Majewska, M. D., Harrison, N. L., Schwartz, R. D., Barker, J. L., and Paul, S. M. (1986). Steroid hormone metabolites are barbiturate-like modulators of the GABA receptor. *Science* 232, 1004–1007.

Majewska, M. D., and Schwartz, R. D. (1987). Pregnenolone-sulfate: an endogenous antagonist of the gamma-aminobutyric acid receptor complex in brain? *Brain Res.* 404, 355–360.

Mak, P., Broussard, C., Vacy, K., and Broadbear, J. H. (2011). Modulation of anxiety behavior in the elevated plus maze using peptidic oxytocin and vasopressin receptor ligands in the rat. *J. Psychopharmacol.* (in press).

Malagon, M., Vaudry, H., Vallarino, M., Gracia-Navarro, F., and Tonon, M. C. (1992a). Distribution and characterization of endozepine-like immunoreactivity in the central nervous system of the frog *Rana ridibunda*. *Peptides* 13, 99–107.

Malagon, M., Vallarino, M., Tonon, M. C., and Vaudry, H. (1992b). Localization and characterization of diazepam-binding inhibitor (DBI)-like peptides in the brain and pituitary of the trout (*Salmo gairdneri*). *Brain Res.* 576, 208–214.

Malagon, M., Vaudry, H., Van Strien, F., Pelletier, G., Gracia-Navarro, F., and Tonon, M. C. (1993). Ontogeny of diazepam-binding inhibitor-related peptides (endozepines) in the rat brain. *Neuroscience* 57, 777–786.

Malik, A. S., Narayan, R. K., and Wendling, W. W. (2003). A novel dehydroepiandrosterone analog improves functional recovery in a rat traumatic brain injury model. *J. Neurotrauma* 20, 463–476.

Mameli, M., Carta, M., Partridge, L. D., and Valenzuela, C. F. (2005). Neurosteroid-induced plasticity of immature synapses via retrograde modulation of presynaptic NMDA receptors. *J. Neurosci.* 25, 2285–2294.

Manji, H. K., Quiroz, J. A., Sporn, J., Payne, J. L., Denicoff, K., and Gray, M. (2003). Enhancing neuronal plasticity and cellular resilience to develop novel, improved therapeutics for difficult-to-treat depression. *Biol. Psychiatry* 53, 707–742.

Marumoto, N., Murakami, N., Katayama, T., Kuroda, H., and Murakami, T. (1996). Effects of daily injections of melatonin on locomotor activity rhythms in rats maintained under constant bright or dim light. *Physiol. Behav.* 60, 767–773.

Matsuda, K., Tanaka, S., Yamamoto, K., and Kikuyama, S. (1990). Annual changes of plasma prolactin levels in the newt, *Cynops pyrrhogaster*. *Zool. Sci.* 7, 1143.

Matsuda, K., Wada, K., Miura, T., Maruyama, K., Shimakura, S. I., Uchiyama, M., Leprince, J., Tonon, M. C., and Vaudry, H. (2007). Effect of the diazepam-binding inhibitor-derived peptide, octadecaneuropeptide, on food intake in goldfish. *Neuroscience* 150, 425–432.

Matsunaga, M., Ukena, K., Baulieu, E. E., and Tsutsui, K. (2004). 7α-Hydroxypregnenolone acts as a neuronal activator to stimulate locomotor activity of breeding newts by means of the dopaminergic system. *Proc. Natl. Acad. Sci. U.S.A.* 101, 17282–17287.

Maurice, T., Grégoire, C., and Espallergues, J. (2006). Neuro(active)steroids actions at the neuromodulatory sigma1 (σ1) receptor: biochemical and physiological evidences, consequences in neuroprotection. *Pharmacol. Biochem. Behav.* 84, 581–597.

Mayo, W., Dellu, F., Robel, P., Cherkaoui, J., Le Moal, M., Baulieu, E. E., and Simon, H. (1993). Infusion of neurosteroids into the nucleus basalis magnocellularis affects cognitive processes in the rat. *Brain Res.* 607, 324–328.

McDonald, A. J., and Mascagni, F. (1996). Immunohistochemical localization of the β2 and β3 subunits of the $GABA_A$ receptor in the basolateral amygdala of the rat and monkey. *Neuroscience* 75, 407–419.

McEwen, B. S. (1994). Steroid hormone actions on the brain: when is the genome involved? *Horm. Behav.* 28, 396–405.

Melcangi, R. C., Azcoitia, I., Ballabio, M., Cavarretta, I., Gonzalez, L. C., Leonelli, E., Magnaghi, V., Veiga, S., and Garcia-Segura, L. M. (2003). Neuroactive steroids influence peripheral myelination: a promising opportunity for preventing or treating age-dependent dysfunctions of peripheral nerves. *Prog. Neurobiol.* 71, 57–66.

Meldrum, B. (1982). Pharmacology of GABA. *Clin. Neuropharmacol.* 5, 293–316.

Mellon, S., and Vaudry, H. (2001). Biosynthesis of neurosteroids and regulation of their synthesis. *Int. Rev. Neurobiol.* 46, 33–78.

Mellon, S. H., and Griffin, L. D. (2002). Neurosteroids: biochemistry and clinical significance. *Trends Endocrinol. Metab.* 13, 35–43.

Mensah-Nyagan, A. G., Do Rego, J. L., Beaujean, D., Luu-The, V., Pelletier, G., and Vaudry, H. (1999). Neurosteroids: expression of steroidogenic enzymes and regulation of steroid biosynthesis in the central nervous system. *Pharmacol. Rev.* 51, 63–81.

Mensah-Nyagan, A. G., Feuilloley, M., Do Rego, J. L., Marcual, A., Lange, C., Tonon, M. C., Pelletier, G., and Vaudry, H. (1996). Localization of 17β-hydroxysteroid dehydrogenase and characterization of testosterone in the brain of the male frog. *Proc. Natl. Acad. Sci. U.S.A.* 93, 1423–1428.

Mensah-Nyagan, A. G., Feuilloley, M., Dupont, E., Do Rego, J. L., Leboulenger, F., Pelletier, G., and Vaudry, H. (1994). Immunocytochemical localization and biological activity of 3β-hydroxysteroid dehydrogenase in the central nervous system of the frog. *J. Neurosci.* 14, 7306–7318.

Meyer-Lindenberg, A., Domes, G., Kirsch, P., and Heinrichs, M. (2011). Oxytocin and vasopressin in the human brain: social neuropeptides for translational medicine. *Nat. Rev. Neurosci.* 12, 524–538.

Migues, P. V., Johnston, A. N., and Rose, S. P. (2002). Dehydroepiandrosterone and its sulphate enhance memory retention in day-old chicks. *Neuroscience* 109, 243–251.

Mitchell, E. A., Gentet, L. J., Dempster, J., and Belelli, D. (2007). $GABA_A$ and glycine receptor-mediated transmission in rat lamina II neurones: relevance to the analgesic actions of neuroactive steroids. *J. Physiol.* 583, 1021–1040.

Mo, Q., Lu, S. F., Hu, S., and Simon, N. G. (2004). DHEA and DHEA sulfate differentially regulate neural androgen receptor and its transcriptional activity. *Brain Res. Mol. Brain Res.* 126, 165–172.

Mocchetti, I., Einstein, R., and Brosius, J. (1986). Putative diazepam binding inhibitor peptide: cDNA clones from rat. *Proc. Natl. Acad. Sci. U.S.A.* 83, 7221–7225.

Monnet, F. P., Mahe, V., Robel, P., and Baulieu, E. E. (1995). Neurosteroids, via σ receptors, modulate the $[^3H]$norepinephrine release evoked by N-methyl-D-aspartate in the rat hippocampus. *Proc. Natl. Acad. Sci. U.S.A.* 92, 3774–3778.

Monnet, F. P., and Maurice, T. (2006). The sigma1 protein as a target for the non-genomic effects of neuro(active)steroids: molecular, physiological, and behavioral aspects. *J. Pharmacol. Sci.* 100, 93–118.

Moore, F. L., Boyd, S. K., and Kelley, D. B. (2005). Historical perspective: hormonal regulation of behaviors in amphibians. *Horm. Behav.* 48, 373–383.

Morrow, A. L. (2007). Recent developments in the significance and therapeutic relevance of neuroactive steroids – introduction to the special issue. *Pharmacol. Ther.* 116, 1–6.

Mosconi, G., Yamamoto, K., Kikuyama, S., Carnevali, O., Mancuso, A., and Vellano, C. (1994). Seasonal changes of plasma prolactin concentration in the reproduction of the crested newt (*Triturus carnifex* Laur). *Gen. Comp. Endocrinol.* 95, 342–349.

Murakami, K., Fellous, A., Baulieu, E. E., and Robel, P. (2000). Pregnenolone binds to microtubule-associated protein 2 and stimulates microtubule assembly. *Proc. Natl. Acad. Sci. U.S.A.* 97, 3579–3584.

Murakami, N., Kawano, T., Nakahara, K., Nasu, T., and Shiota, K. (2001). Effect of melatonin on circadian rhythm, locomotor activity and body temperature in the intact house sparrow, Japanese quail and owl. *Brain Res.* 889, 220–224.

Nasman, B., Olsson, T., Backstrom, T., Eriksson, S., Grankvist, K., Vitanen, M., and Bucht, G. (1991). Serum dehydroepiandrosterone sulfate in Alzeimer's disease and in multi-infarct dementia. *Biol. Psychiatry* 30, 684–690.

Nguyen, A. D., Herzog, H., and Sainsbury, A. (2011). Neuropeptide Y and peptide YY. Important regulators of energy metabolism. *Curr. Opin. Endocrinol. Diabetes Obes.* 18, 56–60.

Papadopoulos, V. (1993). Peripheral-type benzodiazepine/diazepam binding inhibitor receptor: biological role in steroidogenic cell function. *Endocr. Rev.* 14, 222–240.

Papadopoulos, V., Baraldi, M., Guilarte, T. R., Knudsen, T. B., Lacapère, J. J., Lindemann, P., Norenberg, M. D., Nutt, D., Weizman, A., Zhang, M. R., and Gavish, M. (2006). Translocator protein (18kDa): new nomenclature for the peripheral-type benzodiazepine receptor based on its structure and molecular function. *Trends Pharmacol. Sci.* 27, 402–409.

Papadopoulos, V., Berkovich, A., and Krueger, K. E. (1991a). The role of diazepam binding inhibitor and its processing products at mitochondrial benzodiazepine receptors: regulation of steroid biosynthesis. *Neuropharmacology* 30, 1417–1423.

Papadopoulos, V., Berkovich, A., Krueger, K. E., Costa, E., and Guidotti, A. (1991b). Diazepam binding inhibitor and its processing products stimulate mitochondrial steroid biosynthesis via an interaction with mitochondrial benzodiazepine receptors. *Endocrinology* 129, 1481–1488.

Papadopoulos, V., Guarneri, P., Krueger, K. E., Guidotti, A., and Costa, E. (1992). Pregnenolone biosynthesis in C6-2B glioma cell mitochondria: regulation by a mitochondrial diazepam binding inhibitor receptor. *Proc. Natl. Acad. Sci. U.S.A.* 89, 5113–5117.

Papadopoulos, V., Mukhin, A. G., Costa, E., and Krueger, K. E. (1990). The peripheral-type benzodiazepine receptor is functionally linked to Leydig cell steroidogenesis. *J. Biol. Chem.* 265, 3772–3779.

Paredes, R. G., and Agmo, A. (1992). GABA and behavior: the role of receptor subtypes. *Neurosci. Biobehav. Rev.* 16, 145–170.

Park-Chung, M., Malayev, A., Purdy, R. H., Gibbs, T. T., and Farb, D. H. (1999). Sulfated and unsulfated steroids modulate gamma-aminobutyric acid A receptor function through distinct sites. *Brain Res.* 830, 72–87.

Patchev, V. K., Hassan, A. H. S., Holsboer, F., and Almeida, O. F. X. (1996). The neurosteroid tetrahydroprogesterone attenuates the endocrine response to stress and exerts glucocorticoid-like effects on vasopressin gene transcription in the rat hypothalamus. *Neuropsychopharmacology* 15, 533–540.

Paul, S. M., and Purdy, S. H. (1992). Neuroactive steroids. *FASEB J.* 6, 2311–2322.

Pham, J., Porter, J., Svec, D., Eiswirth, C., and Svec, F. (2000). The effect of dehydroepiandrosterone on Zucker rats selected for fat food preference. *Physiol. Behav.* 70, 431–441.

Pinna, G., Agis-Balboa, R. C., Pibiri, F., Nelson, M., Guidotti, A., and Costa, E. (2008). Neurosteroid biosynthesis regulates sexually dimorphic fear and aggressive behavior in mice. *Neurochem. Res.* 33, 1990–2007.

Plassart-Schiess, E., and Baulieu, E. E. (2001). Neurosteroids: recent findings. *Brain Res. Rev.* 37, 133–140.

Polzonetti-Magni, A., Carnevali, O., Yamamoto, K., and Kikuyama, S. (1995). Growth hormone and prolactin in amphibian reproduction. *Zool. Sci.* 12, 683–694.

Ramos, E. J., Meguid, M. M., Campos, A. C., and Coelho, J. C. (2005). Neuropeptide Y, α-melanocyte-stimulating hormone, and monoamines in food intake regulation. *Nutrition* 21, 269–279.

Reddy, D. S. (2003). Pharmacology of endogenous neuroactive steroids. *Crit. Rev. Neurobiol.* 15, 197–234.

Reddy, D. S. (2010). Neurosteroids: endogenous role in the human brain and therapeutic potentials. *Prog. Brain Res.* 186, 113–137.

Reddy, D. S., and Kulkarni, S. K. (1998). The role of the GABA-A and mitochondrial diazepam-binding inhibitor receptors on the effects of neurosteroids on food intake in mice. *Psychopharmacology (Berl.)* 137, 391–400.

Reddy, D. S., and Kulkarni, S. K. (1999). Sex and estrous cycle-dependent changes in neurosteroid and benzodiazepine effects on food consumption and plus-maze learning behaviors in rats. *Pharmacol. Biochem. Behav.* 62, 53–60.

Reghunandanan, V., Reghunandanan, R., and Mahajan, K. K. (1998). Arginine vasopressin as a neurotransmitter in brain. *Indian J. Exp. Biol.* 36, 635–643.

Remage-Healey, L., Maidment, N. T., and Schlinger, B. A. (2008). Forebrain steroid levels fluctuate rapidly during social interactions. *Nat. Neurosci.* 11, 1327–1334.

Richards, J. G., and Möhler, H. (1984). Benzodiazepine receptors. *Neuropharmacology* 23, 233–242.

Robel, P., and Baulieu, E. E. (1985). Neurosteroids, 3β-hydroxy-Δ5-derivatives in the rodent brain. *Neurochem. Int.* 7, 953–958.

Robel, P., and Baulieu, E. E. (1994). Neurosteroids: biosynthesis and function. *Trends Endocrinol. Metab.* 5, 1–8.

Robel, P., Schumacher, M., and Baulieu, E. E. (1999). "Neurosteroids: from definition and biochemistry to physiopathologic function," in *Contemporary Endocrinology*, eds E. E. Baulieu, P. Robel, and M. Schumacher (Totowa: Humana Press), 1–26.

Robel, P., Young, J., Corpéchot, C., Mayo, W., Perche, F., Haug, M., Simon, H., and Baulieu, E. E. (1995). Biosynthesis and assay of neurosteroids in rats and mice: functional correlates. *J. Steroid Biochem. Mol. Biol.* 53, 355–360.

Roberts, E. (1986). "Guides through the labyrinth of AD: dehydroepiandrosterone, potassium channels and the C4 component of complement," in *Treatment Development Strategies for Alzheimer's Disease* eds T. Crook, R. T. Bartus, S. Ferris, and S. Gershon (Madison, CT: Prowley), 173–219.

Rose, T. M., Schultz, E. R., and Todaro, G. J. (1992). Molecular cloning of the gene for the yeast homolog (ACB) of diazepam binding inhibitor/endozepine/acyl-CoA-binding protein. *Proc. Natl. Acad. Sci. U.S.A.* 89, 11287–11291.

Rupprecht, R. (1997). The neuropsychopharmacological potential of neuroactive steroids. *J. Psychiatr. Res.* 31, 297–314.

Rupprecht, R., di Michele, F., Hermann, B., Ströhle, A., Lancel, M., Romeo, E., and Holsboer, F. (2001). Neuroactive steroids: molecular mechanisms of action and implications for neuropsychopharmacology. *Brain Res. Rev.* 37, 59–67.

Rupprecht, R., and Holsboer, F. (1999). Neuroactive steroids: mechanisms of action and neuropsychopharmacological perspectives. *Trends Neurosci.* 22, 410–416.

Rupprecht, R., and Holsboer, F. (2001). Neuroactive steroids in neuropsychopharmacology. *Int. Rev. Neurobiol.* 46, 461–477.

Sakaue, M., Saito, N., Taniguchi, H., Baba, S., and Tanaka, C. (1988). Immunohistochemical localization of γ-aminobutyric acid in the rat pituitary gland and related hypothalamic regions. *Brain Res.* 446, 343–353.

Sayeed, I., Guo, Q., Hoffman, S. W., and Stein, D. G. (2006). Allopregnanolone, a progesterone metabolite, is more effective than progesterone in reducing cortical infarct volume after transient middle cerebral artery occlusion. *Ann. Emerg. Med.* 47, 381–389.

Schiess, A. R., and Partridge, L. D. (2005). Pregnenolone sulfate acts through a G-protein-coupled sigma1-like receptor to enhance short term facilitation in adult hippocampal neurons. *Eur. J. Pharmacol.* 25, 22–29.

Schlinger, B. A., and Remage-Healey, L. (2011). Neurosteroidogenesis: insights from studies of songbirds. *J. Neuroendocrinol.* 24, 16–21.

Schumacher, M., Akwa, Y., Guennoun, R., Robert, F., Labombarda, F., Desarnaud, F., Robel, P., De Nicola, A. F., and Baulieu, E. E. (2000). Steroid synthesis and metabolism in the nervous system: trophic and protective effects. *J. Neurocytol.* 29, 307–326.

Schumacher, M., Weill-Engerer, S., Liere, P., Robert, F., Franklin, R. J., Garcia-Segura, L. M., Lambert, J. J., Mayo, W., Melcangi, R. C., Parducz, A., Suter, U., Carelli, C., Baulieu, E. E., and Akwa, Y. (2003). Steroid hormones and neurosteroids in normal and pathological aging of the nervous system. *Prog. Neurobiol.* 71, 3–29.

Shannon, E. E., Purdy, R. H., and Grant, K. A. (2005a). Discriminative stimulus effects of 5.6 mg/kg pregnanolone in DBA/2J and C57BL/6J inbred mice. *Alcohol* 37, 35–45.

Shannon, E. E., Porcu, P., Purdy, R. H., and Grant, K. A. (2005b). Characterization of the discriminative stimulus effects of the neuroactive steroid pregnanolone in DBA/2J and C57BL/6J inbred mice. *J. Pharmacol. Exp. Ther.* 314, 675–685.

Shimada, M., Yoshinari, K., Tanabe, E., Shimakawa, E., Kobashi, M., Nagata, K., and Yamazoe, Y. (2001). Identification of ST2A1 as a rat brain neurosteroid sulfotransferase mRNA. *Brain Res.* 920, 222–225.

Shimizu, C., Fuda, H., Yanai, H., and Strott, C. A. (2003). Conservation of the hydroxysteroid sulfotransferase SULT2B1 gene structure in the mouse: pre- and postnatal expression, kinetic analysis of isoforms, and comparison with prototypical SULT2A1. *Endocrinology* 144, 1186–1193.

Slobodyansky, E., Guidotti, A., Wambebe, C., Berkovich, A., and Costa, E. (1989). Isolation and characterization of a triakontatetraneuropeptide (TTN) a posttranslational product of diazepam binding inhibitor: specific action at the Ro5-4864 recognition sites. *J. Neurochem.* 53, 1276–1284.

Slobodyansky, E., Kurriger, G., and Kultas-Llinsky, K. (1992). Diazepam binding inhibitor processing in the rhesus monkey brain: an immunocytochemical study. *J. Chem. Neuroanat.* 5, 169–180.

Steffensen, S. C., Jones, M. D., Hales, K., and Allison, D. W. (2006). Dehydroepiandrosterone sulfate and estrone sulfate reduce GABA-recurrent inhibition in the hippocampus via muscarinic acetylcholine receptors. *Hippocampus* 16, 1080–1090.

Stein, D. G. (2001). Brain damage, sex hormones and recovery: a new role for progesterone and estrogen? *Trends Neurosci.* 24, 386–391.

Strott, C. A. (2002). Sulfonation and molecular action. *Endocr. Rev.* 23, 703–732.

Strous, R. D., Maayan, R., Lapidus, R., Stryjer, R., Lustig, M., Kotler, M., and Weizman, A. (2003). Value of dehydroepiandrosterone (DHEA) augmentation in the management of negative symptoms in schizophrenia. *Arch. Gen. Psychiatry* 60, 133–141.

Strous, R. D., Maayan, R., and Weizman, A. (2006). The relevance of neurosteroids to clinical psychiatry: from the laboratory to the bedside. *Eur. Neuropsychopharmacol.* 16, 155–169.

Sunderland, T., Merril, C. R., Harrington, M. G., Lawlor, B. A., Molchan, S. E., Martinez, R., and Murphy, D. L. (1989). Reduced plasma dehydroepiandrosterone concentrations in Alzheimer's disease. *Lancet* 2, 570.

Svec, F., and Porter, J. (1996). Effect of DHEA on macronutrient selection by Zucker rats. *Physiol. Behav.* 59, 721–727.

Svec, F., and Porter, J. (1998a). Dehydroepiandrosterone: a nutritional supplement with actions in the central nervous system. *Nutr. Neurosci.* 1, 9–19.

Svec, F., and Porter, J. (1998b). The actions of exogenous dehydroepiandrosterone in experimental animals and humans. *Proc. Soc. Exp. Biol. Med.* 218, 174–191.

Svec, F., Richards, R. J., and Porter, J. R. (1998). Investigating the debate: does DHEA alter food intake? *Nutr. Neurosci.* 1, 93–101.

Takase, M., Ukena, K., Yamazaki, T., Kominami, S., and Tsutsui, K. (1999). Pregnenolone, pregnenolone sulfate, and cytochrome P450 side-chain cleavage enzyme in the amphibian brain and their seasonal changes. *Endocrinology* 140, 1936–1944.

Tappaz, M. L., Wassef, M., Oertel, W. H., Paut, L., and Pujol, J. F. (1983). Light- and electron-microscopic immunocytochemistry of glutamic acid decarboxylase (GAD) in the basal hypothalamus: morphological evidence for neuroendocrine γ-aminobutyrate (GABA). *Neuroscience* 9, 271–287.

Tasan, R. O., Lin, S., Hetzenauer, A., Singewald, N., Herzog, H., and Sperk, G. (2009). Increased novelty-induced motor activity and reduced depression-like behavior in neuropeptide Y (NPY)-Y4 receptor knockout mice. *Neuroscience* 158, 1717–1730.

Tasker, J. G., Di, S., and Malcher-Lopes, R. (2006). Minireview: rapid glucocorticoid signaling via membrane-associated receptors. *Endocrinology* 147, 5549–5556.

Thompson, R. R., Dickinson, P. S., Rose, J. D., Dakin, K. A., Civiello, G. M., Segerdahl, A., and Bartlett, R. (2008). Pheromones enhance somatosensory processing in newt brains through a vasotocin-dependent mechanism. *Proc. Biol. Sci.* 275, 1685–1693.

Thorsell, A. (2010). Brain neuropeptide Y and corticotropin-releasing hormone in mediating stress and anxiety. *Exp. Biol. Med.* 235, 1163–1167.

Todaro, G. J., Rose, T. M., and Shoyab, M. (1991). Human DBI (endozepine): relationship to a homologous membrane associated protein (MA-DBI). *Neuropharmacology* 30, 1373–1380.

Tong, Y., Toranzo, D., and Pelletier, G. (1991). Localization of diazepam-binding inhibitor (DBI) mRNA in the rat brain by high resolution in situ hybridization. *Neuropeptides* 20, 33–40.

Tonon, M. C., Désy, L., Nicolas, P., Vaudry, H., and Pelletier, G. (1990). Immunocytochemical localization of the endogenous benzodiazepine ligand octadecaneuropeptide (ODN) in the rat brain. *Neuropeptides* 15, 17–24.

Tonon, M. C., Leprince, J., Gandolfo, P., Compère, V., Pelletier, G., Malagon, M. M., and Vaudry, H. (2006). "Endozepines," in *Handbook of Biologically Active Peptides*, ed. A. J. Kastin (New York: Elsevier), 813–819.

Torres, J. M., and Ortega, E. (2003). DHEA, PREG and their sulfate derivatives on plasma and brain after CRH and ACTH administration. *Neurochem. Res.* 28, 1187–1191.

Toyoda, F., Hasunuma, I., Yamamoto, K., Yamashita, M., and Kikuyama, S. (2005). Prolactin acts centrally to enhance newt courtship behavior. *Gen. Comp. Endocrinol.* 141, 172–177.

Toyoda, F., Ito, M., Tanaka, S., and Kikuyama, S. (1993). Hormonal induction of male courtship behavior in the Japanese newt, *Cynops pyrrhogaster*. *Horm. Behav.* 27, 511–522.

Tsutsui, K., Haraguchi, S., Matsunaga, M., Koyama, T., Do Rego, J. L., and Vaudry, H. (2010). Identification of 7α-hydroxypregnenolone, a novel bioactive amphibian neurosteroid stimulating locomotor activity, and its physiological roles in the regulation of locomotion. *Gen. Comp. Endocrinol.* 168, 275–279.

Tsutsui, K., Inoue, K., Miyabara, H., Suzuki, S., Ogura, Y., and Tobari, Y. And Haraguchi, S. (2009). Discovery of a novel avian neurosteroid, 7α-hydroxypregnenolone, and its role in the regulation of the diurnal rhythm of locomotor activity in Japanese quail. *Gen. Comp. Endocrinol.* 163, 117–122.

Tsutsui, K., Inoue, K., Miyabara, H., Suzuki, S., Ogura, Y.,and Haraguchi, S. (2008). 7α-Hydroxypregnenolone mediates melatonin action underlying diurnal locomotor rhythms. *J. Neurosci.* 28, 2158–2167.

Tsutsui, K., Matsunaga, M., Miyabara, H., and Ukena, K. (2006). Neurosteroid biosynthesis in the quail brain: a review. *J. Exp. Zoolog. Part A Comp. Exp. Biol.* 305, 733–742.

Tsutsui, K., Matsunaga, M., and Ukena, K. (2003). Review: biosynthesis and biological actions of neurosteroids in the avian brain. *Avian Poultry Biol. Rev.* 14, 63–78.

Tsutsui, K., Ukena, K., Takase, M., Kohchi, C., and Lea, R. W. (1999). Neurosteroid biosynthesis in vertebrate brains. *Comp. Biochem. Physiol. C Pharmacol. Toxicol. Endocrinol.* 124, 121–129.

Tsutsui, K., and Yamazaki, T. (1995). Avian neurosteroids I. Pregnenolone biosynthesis in the quail brain. *Brain Res.* 678, 1–9.

Ueno, H., Yamaguchi, H., Mizuta, M., and Nakazato, M. (2008). The role of PYY in feeding regulation. *Regul. Pept.* 145, 12–16.

Uzunova, V., Ceci, M., Kohler, C., Uzunov, D. P., and Wrynn, A. S. (2003). Region-specific dysregulation of allopregnanolone brain content in the olfactory bulbectomized rat model of depression. *Brain Res.* 976, 1–8.

Valera, S., Ballivet, M., and Bertrand, D. (1992). Progesterone modulates a neuronal nicotinic acetylcholine receptor. *Proc. Natl. Acad. Sci. U.S.A.* 89, 9949–9953.

Vallée, M., Mayo, W., Darnaudery, M., Corpéchot, C., Young, J., Koehl, M., Le Moal, M., Baulieu, E. E., Robel, P., and Simon, H. (1997). Neurosteroids: deficient cognitive performance in aged rats depends on low pregnenolone sulfate levels in the hippocampus. *Proc. Natl. Acad. Sci. U.S.A.* 94, 14865–14870.

Vallée, M., Mayo, W., and Le Moal, M. (2001). Role of pregnenolone, dehydroepiandrosterone and their sulfate esters on learning and memory in cognitive ageing. *Brain Res. Rev.* 37, 301–312.

van Broekhoven, F., and Verkes, R. J. (2003). Neurosteroids in depression: a review. *Psychopharmacology (Berl.)* 165, 97–110.

Vaudry, H., Do Rego, J. L., Burel, D., Luu-The, V., Pelletier, G., and Tsutsui, K. (2011). Neurosteroid biosynthesis in the brain of amphibians. *Front. Neuroendocr. Sci.* 2:79. doi:10.3389/fendo.2011.00079

Viglietti-Panzica, C., Aste, N., Balthazart, J., and Panzica, G. C. (1994). Vasotocinergic innervation of sexually dimorphic medial preoptic nucleus of the male Japanese quail:

influence of testosterone. *Brain Res.* 657, 171–184.

von Horsten, S., Exton, N. G., Exton, M. S., Helfritz, F., Nave, H., Ballof, J., Stalp, M., and Pabst, R. (1998). Brain NPY Y1 receptors rapidly mediate the behavioral response to novelty and a compartment-specific modulation of granulocyte function in blood and spleen. *Brain Res.* 806, 282–286.

Warren, W. S., and Cassone, V. M. (1995). The pineal gland: photoreception and coupling of behavioral, metabolic, and cardiovascular circadian outputs. *J. Biol. Rhythms* 10, 64–79.

Weaver, Jr. C. E., Marek, P., Park-Chung, M., Tam, S. W., and Farb, D. H. (1997). Neuroprotective activity of a new class of steroidal inhibitors of the N-methyl-D-aspartate receptor. *Proc. Natl. Acad. Sci. U.S.A.* 94, 10450–10454.

Wehrenberg, W. B., Corder, R., and Gaillard, R. C. (1989). A physiological role for neuropeptide Y in regulating the estrogen/progesterone induced luteinizing hormone surge in ovariectomized rats. *Neuroendocrinology* 49, 680–682.

Weill-Engerer, S., David, J. P., Sazdovitch, V., Liere, P., Eychenne, B., Pianos, A., Schumacher, M., Delacourte, A., Baulieu, E. E., and Akwa, Y. (2002). Neurosteroid quantification in human brain regions: comparison between Alzheimer's and nondemented patients. *J. Clin. Endocrinol. Metab.* 87, 5138–5143.

Wojtal, K., Trojnar, M. K., and Czuczwar, S. J. (2006). Endogenous neuroprotective factors: neurosteroids. *Pharmacol. Rep.* 58, 335–340.

Woolley, S. C., Sakata, J. T., and Crews, D. (2004). Evolutionary insights into the regulation of courtship behavior in male amphibians and reptiles. *Physiol. Behav.* 83, 347–360.

Wu, F. S., Gibbs, T. T., and Farb, D. H. (1991). Pregnenolone sulfate: a positive allosteric modulator at the N-methyl-D-aspartate receptor. *Mol. Pharmacol.* 40, 333–336.

Xilouri, M., and Papazafiri, P. (2006). Anti-apoptotic effects of allopregnanolone on P19 neurons. *Eur. J. Neurosci.* 23, 43–54.

Yanagibashi, K., Ohno, Y., Nakamichi, N., Matsui, T., Hayashida, K., Takamura, M., Yamada, K., Tou, S., and Kawamura, M. (1989). Peripheral-type benzodiazepine receptors are involved in the regulation of cholesterol side chain cleavage in adrenocortical mitochondria. *J. Biochem.* 106, 1026–1029.

Yanase, H., Shimizu, H., Yamada, K., and Iwanaga, T. (2002). Cellular localization of the diazepam binding inhibitor in glial cells with special reference to its coexistence with brain-type fatty acid binding protein. *Arch. Histol. Cytol.* 65, 27–36.

Young, L. T. (2002). Neuroprotective effects of antidepressant and mood stabilizing drugs. *J. Psychiatry Neurosci.* 27, 8–9.

Zheng, P. (2009). Neuroactive steroid regulation of neurotransmitter release in the CNS: action, mechanism and possible significance. *Prog. Neurobiol.* 89, 134–152.

Zwain, I. H., Arroyo, A., Amato, P., and Yen, S. S. (2002). A role for hypothalamic astrocytes in dehydroepiandrosterone and estradiol regulation of gonadotropin-releasing hormone (GnRH) release by GnRH neurons. *Neuroendocrinology* 75, 375–383.

22

Biological significance of GPCR heteromerization in the neuroendocrine system

Maud Kamal[1,2,3] and Ralf Jockers[1,2,3]*

[1] Department of Endocrinology, Metabolism and Cancer, INSERM U1016, Institut Cochin, Paris, France
[2] CNRS UMR 8104, Paris, France
[3] University Paris Descartes, Paris, France

Edited by:
Regina Pekelmann Markus, University of São Paulo, Brazil

Reviewed by:
Regina Pekelmann Markus, University of São Paulo, Brazil
Krystyna Skwarlo-Sonta, University of Warsaw, Poland
Sandra Helena Poliselli Farsky, University of São Paulo, Brazil

*Correspondence:
Ralf Jockers, Institut Cochin, 22 rue Méchain, 75014 Paris, France.
e-mail: ralf.jockers@inserm.fr

Clustering of proteins in higher order complexes is a common theme in biology and profoundly influences protein function. The idea that seven-transmembrane spanning G protein-coupled receptors (GPCRs) might form dimers or higher order oligomeric complexes has been formulated more than 20 years ago. Since then, this phenomenon has been investigated with many different biochemical and biophysical techniques. The more recent notion of GPCR heteromerization describes the specific association of two different GPCRs. GPCR heteromerization may be of primary importance in neuroendocrinology, as this may explain at least some of the functional crosstalks described between different hormonal systems. Importantly, many GPCR heteromers have distinct functional properties compared to their corresponding homomers. Heteromer-specific pharmacological profiles might be exploited for drug design and open new therapeutic options. GPCR heteromerization has been first studied in heterologous expression systems. Today, increasing evidence for the existence of GPCR heteromers in endogenous systems is emerging providing crucial evidence for the physiological function of GPCR heteromerization.

Keywords: GPCR, heterodimers, direct physical interaction, functional crosstalk, endocrinology

INTRODUCTION

The seven-transmembrane spanning G protein-coupled receptor (GPCR) family represent in humans, with more than 800 members, the largest family of cell surface proteins corresponding to about 3% of all genes. Although generally expressed at relatively low levels, every cell typically expresses at least one and in most cases several GPCRs at their cell surface. Not surprisingly, GPCRs are involved in all major biological processes ranging form cell migration, proliferation, inflammation, immunity, etc… GPCRs respond to a remarkable diversity of ligands ranging from photons, to ions, metabolites, amino acids, lipids, peptides, and proteins. Over the last 20 years, GPCRs have been among the most tractable targets for the development of therapeutic small molecule drugs.

The canonical signaling pathway of GPCRs involves monomeric receptors, heterotrimeric G proteins, and various effector systems. Subsequently, several features have been added to this basic concept. Notably, addition of GPCR interacting proteins other than G proteins opened the possibility of fine-tuning of signaling in a receptor subtype- and tissue-specific manner. Moreover, alternative, G protein-independent, i.e., β-arrestin-dependent, signaling pathways have been described. Further diversity has been introduced by the notion that GPCRs might not only exist as monomeric peptides but can also cluster in dimeric or oligomeric structures. The current review gives a short overview of the proposed functions of GPCR oligomers and discusses the biological relevance and participation of such complexes in functional crosstalk. In the second part, examples of GPCR oligomers in the neuro-endocrine system will be critically assessed.

GPCR OLIGOMERS, WHAT ARE THEY GOOD FOR?

The concept of GPCR di(oligo)merization has raised considerable interest over the last 20 years. Supporting evidence comes form numerous reports using biochemical, biophysical, and functional assays (see Bouvier, 2001; Angers et al., 2002 for review). Whereas the first pioneering studies considered the clustering of one specific GPCR into homomers, it become rapidly evident that different types of GPCRs might also assemble into heteromers, thus broadening the potential impact of GPCR oligomerization considerably (see Prinster et al., 2005; Milligan, 2009 for review). Having accepted that GPCR dimers exist, the question of the functional significance of these dimers arises.

In the case of obligatory dimers, the functional significance of GPCR dimers is obvious. Indeed, early studies showed that co-expression of $GABA_{B1}$ and $GABA_{B2}$ subunits is necessary for the functional expression of the $GABA_B$ receptor (Jones et al., 1998; White et al., 1998). Subsequently, it was shown that the $GABA_{B1}$ subunit binds the natural ligand whereas the $GABA_{B2}$ subunit is necessary for G protein coupling and cell surface expression of the heteromeric complex. Similar observations have been made for sweet and umami taste receptors (Nelson et al., 2001, 2002). The issue is however more complex for non-obligatory dimers. The major difficulty resides in preparing pure monomeric and dimeric GPCR samples rather than measuring their biological function. An elegant way to determine the function of monomeric GPCRs was achieved by the reconstitution of purified β2AR in high-density lipoprotein phospholipid bilayer particles. Importantly, the geometry of these particles allows only integration of monomeric receptor protomers. Addition of purified heterotrimeric G proteins showed that G protein activation was as efficient as in intact cells (Whorton et al., 2007). Similar conclusions were drawn by two further studies using rhodopsin as model receptor (Bayburt et al., 2007; Ernst et al., 2007). These studies show that monomeric GPCRs are sufficient for G protein activation leaving the question of the function of GPCR dimers unanswered.

The role of GPCR dimer formation is clear in non-obligatory heteromers with distinct functional properties (Prinster et al., 2005; Milligan, 2009). GPCR heteromerization between orphan GPCRs for which no natural ligand is known and non-orphan GPCRs with known ligand is very interesting in the sense that it might define the function of orphan GPCRs. The existence of ligand-independent functions of some of the more than 100 still orphan GPCRs has indeed been determined in several heteromers containing non-orphan GPCRs (Levoye et al., 2006).

A number of studies have suggested that GPCR oligomerization may be important in cell surface delivery implying that oligomerization occurs early in the biosynthetic pathway (Bulenger et al., 2005). According to this model, successful oligomerization is part of the quality control process. A prominent example is the $GABA_B$ receptors, where the $GABA_{B2}$ subunit controls the proper cell surface expression of $GABA_{B1}$.

Formation of functional dimers offers the possibility for allosteric regulation of one protomer by the other. Several reports confirmed indeed the existence of allosteric interactions between the two orthosteric binding sites within a dimer. Negative and positive allosteric effects have been reported (Durroux, 2005).

Allosteric interactions between the protomers of GPCR dimers imply asymmetry within the GPCR cluster. The concept of asymmetric dimers on the level of the ligand binding site can be further extended toward G protein coupling or binding of GPCR interacting proteins (GIPs) in general. Assymetric binding of G proteins to only one of the two protomers was shown for several GPCRs. In the case of $GABA_B$ receptors, ligand binding to the GB1 subunit *trans*-activates the GB2 subunit that binds to the G proteins (Galvez et al., 2001). In contrast, in the leukotriene B4 BLT1 receptor the same protomer binds the ligand and activates the G protein in a *cis* manner, therefore questioning the function of the second protomer (Baneres and Parello, 2003). Recent studies on the melatonin MT_1 receptor complex with G_i proteins and the regulator of G protein (RGS) 20 suggest that one protomer binds to the G protein whereas the second protomer binds to other GIPs, RGS20 in the present case. These results provide an additional justification for dimer formations and for the fine-tuning of GPCR signaling through GIPs.

FUNCTIONAL CROSSTALK BETWEEN GPCRs WITH OR WITHOUT DIMERIZATION

Signal integration between different hormones is a common feature of the endocrine system. Indeed, each cell expresses typically several GPCR subtypes that integrate different hormonal signals in time and space to produce an adequate cellular response. The ability of one hormone, acting on a specific GPCR, to modulate the function of a second GPCR does not inherently imply heteromerization between these two GPCRs. Indeed receptor heteromerization represent only one out of several ways of functional crosstalk at the cellular level (**Figure 1**). Heterologous sensitization and desensitization, i.e., through activation of protein kinase A or C, are often involved in the integration of cellular signals (Jockers et al., 1998). Crosstalk may also occur at receptor-proximal levels through competition for a common and limited G protein pool as indicated in a recent study on the virally encoded BILF1 receptor (Nijmeijer et al., 2010). Clustering of this G_i-coupled constitutively active receptor with either the chemokine CXCR4 or the histamine H_4 receptor appears to sequester G_i proteins away from the two latter receptors impairing their G_i-dependent signal transduction. Furthermore, potentiation of cellular signals at the level of $G\beta\gamma$ subunits has been reported in a number of studies (see Prezeau et al., 2010 for review). Stimulation of G_i-coupled $GABA_B$ receptor is known to potentiate Ca^{2+} signaling of the G_q-coupled $mGlu_{1a}$ receptor, in cortical neurons co-expressing both receptors (Hirono et al., 2001). Studies in transfected HEK293 cells confirmed this functional crosstalk and indicated that $G\beta\gamma$ subunits, liberated upon activation of $GABA_B$ receptor, are responsible for the Ca^{2+} potentiation in the absence of any evidence of receptor heteromerization (Rives et al., 2009). Importantly, similar potentiating effects can be seen between other G_i- and G_q-coupled GPCRs suggesting a general mechanism of signal integration.

A further mechanism of cellular crosstalk was recently suggested for the corticotropin-releasing factor receptor 1 (CRF_1) and serotonin 5-HT_2 receptors (Magalhaes et al., 2010) Cellular 5-HT_2 responses and serotonin-dependent anxiety were sensitized by CRF stimulation. Sensitization of 5-HT_2 responses correlated with increased cell surface expression of 5-HT_2 receptors, which are known to constitutively internalize. Interestingly this effect was dependent on the presence of functional PDZ domain binding motifs of the CRF_1 and 5-HT_2 receptors and intact endocytotic and recycling pathways suggesting a putative scaffolding function of multi-PDZ domain-containing proteins to facilitate recycling of 5-HT_2 and CRF_1 receptors.

Crosstalk at the level of GPCR oligomers has been demonstrated in several cases. For example, discovery of heteromer-specific signaling pathways (Rashid et al., 2007) and heteromer-selective ligands strongly suggest the importance of opioid receptor (OR) heteromers in physiology (Waldhoer et al., 2005). Unique heteromer-specific cellular responses have been also associated with the 5-HT_{2A}/$mGlu_2$ heteromer, which has been implicated in psychosis (Gonzalez-Maeso et al., 2008). By constructing chimeric receptors between $mGlu_2$, which interacts with 5-HT_{2A} receptors and $mGlu_3$, which does not interact with 5-HT_{2A}, the authors convincingly showed that the cellular responses were exclusively dependent on the formation of 5-HT_{2A}/$mGlu_2$ heteromers.

Collectively, these data show that functional crosstalk may occur at different levels of cellular signaling and trafficking that may or may not depend on GPCR heteromerization. The examples presented in the chapter "Examples in the neuro-endocrine system" will be analyzed in respect of the molecular level of crosstalk.

BIOLOGICAL SIGNIFICANCE OF GPCR HETEROMERIZATION – CRITERIA

Evidence for the formation of GPCR heteromers is mostly based on observations made in transfected cell lines raising the question of the biological significance of these complexes. Nevertheless, an increasing number of articles provide evidence of GPCR heter-

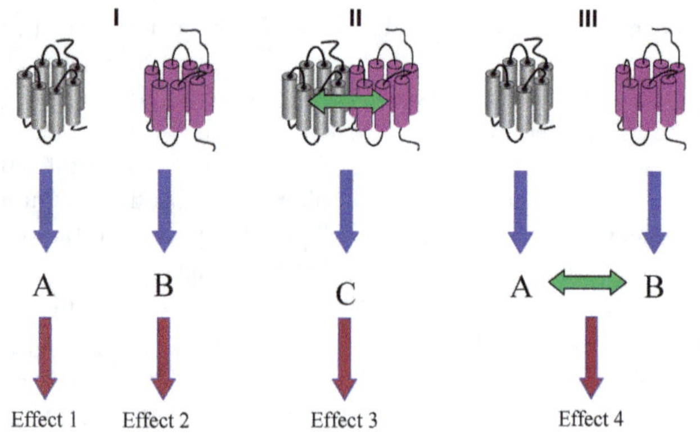

FIGURE 1 | Functional versus physical interaction of GPCRs. (I) In the absence of any physical or functional interaction, the activation of two different GPCRs induces two independent signaling pathways A and B, which consequently result in two independent effects 1 and 2. **(II)** Physical interaction of two different GPCRs results in the activation of the heteromer-specific signaling pathway C that will be responsible of a downstream effect 3. **(III)** In the absence of physical interaction, a functional interaction can be observed when signaling pathways A and B crosstalk to produce effect 4.

omerization in endogenous tissues, some of which will be discussed in the next chapter. To provide some guidance in defining the physiological relevance of GPCR heterodimers, the International Union of Basic and Clinical Pharmacology (IUPHAR) released some recommendations in 2007 (Pin et al., 2007). The first criterion concerned the evidence for physical interaction (or proximity) of both receptors in native tissues or primary cells. This may be achieved by performing co-immunoprecipitation experiments with selective antibodies or energy transfer techniques between labeled ligands or antibodies. The second criterion requests evidence for heteromer-specific properties such as heteromer-specific signaling properties, the identification of heteromer-selective ligands and the presence of allosteric ligand binding properties. The third criterion recommends supporting evidence from knockout animals or RNAi technologies to further validate the possible functional role of heteromers *in vivo*. Obviously, none of these criteria alone provides conclusive evidence for the existence and functional significance of GPCR heteromers. The comity therefore proposes that at least two of the three criteria have to be fulfilled for the acceptance of GPCR heteromers.

EXAMPLES IN THE NEURO-ENDOCRINE SYSTEM

G protein-coupled receptor oligomerization has become an extensively studied field. The current chapter will focus on the description of GPCR heteromers relevant in neuroendocrinology. A more extensive list of GPCR heteromers is provided in **Table 1**. Complementary information on GPCR heteromerization may be also found in other recent expert reviews (Birdsall, 2010; Ferre et al., 2010; Rozenfeld and Devi, 2010).

GPCR HETEROMERS IN THE CENTRAL NERVOUS SYSTEM

G protein-coupled receptors are widely distributed in the nervous system, and mediate key physiological processes including cognition, mood, appetite, pain, and synaptic transmission. The important role of GPCRs in central nervous system (CNS) disorders is outlined by the great quest of pharmaceutical companies for drug discovery. Several GPCRs, in particular the metabotropic glutamate, adenosine, dopamine as well as serotonin receptor, and cannabinoid receptors, were shown to be implicated in CNS disorders such as Parkinson, Alzheimer, schizophrenia, depression, and psychosis. Despite the lack of direct evidence for the implication of GPCR heteromers in neuropathologies, several examples in the literature show the importance of heteromerization in receptor functions suggesting that alterations in GPCR crosstalk can directly impact health.

Opioid and Cannabinoid receptor heteromers

Opioid receptors bind endogenous peptides with effects resembling those of opiate drugs and are very well known for their roles in pain, analgesia and reward. Heteromerization between the different OR subtypes was extensively studied over the last 20 years (see van Rijn et al., 2010 for review) with some evidence *in vivo*. For example, the δ/κ OR selective ligand, the 6′-guanidinonaltrindole (6′-GNTI), is an analgesic and has the unique property of preferentially activating OR heterodimers over the corresponding homomers, indicating that OR heteromers are functionally relevant *in vivo* (Waldhoer et al., 2005). In the current review we will address only examples of OR heteromerization with other GPCRs.

Opiates and exogenous cannabinoids are analgesics used for the treatment of patients with neuropathic pain. Considerable behavioral, anatomical, and biochemical evidence describe similarities between the OR and the cannabinoid receptor systems. The first study to suggest direct physical interactions between the cannabinoid CB_1 receptor and κOR and δOR (CB_1/κOR and CB_1/δOR) was conducted in transfected cells by Rios et al. (2006). The authors identified a reciprocal antagonistic relationship between the two receptors in transfected cells and in native tissues exposed to increasing concentrations of an agonist for one receptor along with non-activating concentrations of an agonist for the other receptor. Another study showed, in 2008, a direct interaction between CB_1 and μOR using FRET and co-immunoprecipitation experiments in CHO cells exogenously expressing both receptors (Hojo et al., 2008). *In vivo*, functional interaction of these receptors is very well exemplified by 9-tetrahydrocannabinol, the major psychoactive constituent of marijuana, which enhances the potency of opioids such as morphine in animal models (Cichewicz, 2004). Moreover, anatomical studies confirmed the co-localization of μOR and CB_1 in common somatodendritic compartments of catecholaminergic neurons in the *locus coeruleus*, the center of opiate addiction and withdrawal, and also revealed CB_1-positive axon terminals forming synaptic contact with μOR-containing dendrites (Scavone et al., 2010).

Recently, ORs were shown to interact functionally with chemokine receptors (Salanga et al., 2009). CXCR4 is able to cross-desensitize the chemotaxis and calcium mobilization response as well as analgesia associated with κOR. Activation of CXCR4 with CXCL12 induces desensitization of κOR and this leads to an impairment of analgesic activity *in vivo* (Finley et al., 2008). Using FRET, CXCR4 was shown to form heteromeric complexes with δOR. Intriguingly, simultaneous application of δOR and CXCR4 agonists to human monocytes (MM-1 cells) expressing both

Table 1 | Non-exhaustive list of GPCR heteromers in the neuro-endocrine system.

Heterodimer	Physical interaction		Functional interaction *in vivo*	References
	In vitro	*In vivo*		
β_2AR/EP$_1$	BRET and co-IP	–	–	McGraw et al. (2006)
β_2AR/κOR	co-IP	–	–	Jordan et al. (2001)
β_2AR/μOR	co-IP	–	–	Jordan et al. (2001)
5- HT$_{2A}$/D$_2$	FRET	–	–	Lukasiewicz et al. (2010)
5-HT$_{1A}$/Gal$_1$	FRET	–	S and BP	Borroto-Escuela et al. (2010), Kehr et al. (2002)
5-HT$_{2A}$/mGlu$_2$	co-IP and BRET	co-IP frontal cortex samples	S and B	Gonzalez-Maeso et al. (2008)
5-HT$_4$/5-HT$_{2(A,B)}$	–	–	S	Derangeon et al. (2010)
A$_1$/A$_{2A}$	BRET and co-IP	co-IP rat striatum	B and S	Ciruela et al. (2006)
A$_1$/mGlu$_{1\alpha}$	co-IP	co-IP rat cerebellar synaptosomes	S	Ciruela et al. (2001)
A$_1$/P2Y$_1$R	co-IP	co-IP rat brain, hippocampus and human astroglial cells	S	Yoshioka et al. (2002), Tonazzini et al. (2008)
A$_2$/mGlu$_5$	co-IP	–	S and BP	Ferre et al. (2002), Kachroo et al. (2005), Adams et al. (2008)
A$_2$/mGlu$_5$/D$_2$	BRET and FRET	co-IP rat striatum	S	Cabello et al. (2009)
A$_{2A}$/D$_2$	FRET and co-IP	co-IP rat striatum and neuroblastoma	S and BP	Canals et al. (2003), Tanganelli et al. (2004)
AT$_1$/β_2AR	co-IP		S	Barki-Harrington et al. (2003)
AT$_1$/APJ	BRET and FRET and co-IP	–	–	Chun et al. (2008)
AT$_1$/B$_2$	Not clear	Not clear	S	AbdAlla et al. (2005), Hansen et al. (2009)
CB$_1$/A$_{2A}$	BRET	co-IP rat striatum	S and BP	Andersson et al. (2005), Carriba et al. (2007), Tebano et al. (2009)
CB$_1$/D$_2$	FRET	–	B	Marcellino et al. (2008), Kearn et al. (2005), Glass and Felder (1997)
CB$_1$/δOR	BRET	–	S	Rios et al. (2006)
CB$_1$/κOR	BRET	–	S	Rios et al. (2006)
CB$_1$/μOR	FRET and co-IP	–	S	Rios et al. (2006), Hojo et al. (2008), Cichewicz (2004)
CB$_1$/OX$_1$	FRET	–	–	Hilairet et al. (2003), Ellis et al. (2006)
CCR5/μOR	co-IP	–	–	Chen et al. (2004)
CRF$_1$/5-HT$_2$	–	–	S and T	Magalhaes et al. (2010)
CXCR4/δOR	FRET	–	S	Pello et al. (2008)
CXCR4/κOR	–	–	S and BP	Finley et al. (2008)
D$_1$/D$_2$	co-IP	co-IP and new Gq coupling	S	Lee et al. (2004), Rashid et al. (2007)
D$_1$/H$_3$	BRET	–	S and BP	Ferrada et al. (2008)
D$_1$/μOR	BRET	–	S and E	Tien et al. (2010), Becker et al. (2001)
D$_2$/H$_3$	BRET	–	S and BP	Ferrada et al. (2008)
D$_2$/SST$_2$	FRET	photo-bleaching FRET in rat striatum	Bivalent ligands and S	Baragli et al. (2007), Jaquet et al. (2005)
D$_2$/SST$_5$	photo-bleaching FRET		S	Rocheville et al. (2000)
D$_5$/D$_2$	BRET	–	S	So et al. (2009)
EP$_1$/D$_1$	–	–	S	Kitaoka et al. (2007)
EP$_1$/D$_2$	–	–	S	Kitaoka et al. (2007)
ET$_A$/ET$_B$	FRET	–	–	Evans and Walker (2008)
GABA$_{B1}$/CaS	co-IP	co-IP brain lysates	S and E	Chang et al. (2007)
GABA$_{B2}$/M$_2$	FRET and TIRF	co-IP cortex	–	Boyer et al. (2009)
GHSR/D$_1$	–	–	–	Chow et al. (2008)
GHSR/EP$_1$	BRET and co-IP	–	–	Chow et al. (2008)
GHSR/IP	BRET and co-IP	–	–	Chow et al. (2008)

(Continued)

Table 1 | Continued

Heterodimer	Physical interaction		Functional interaction *in vivo*	References
	In vitro	*In vivo*		
GHSR/MC_3	FRET and ELISA	–	–	Rediger et al. (2009)
GHSR/NTS_1	co-IP	–	S	Takahashi et al. (2006)
GHSR/TP	BRET and co-IP	–	–	Chow et al. (2008)
IP/TP	co-IP	–	–	Wilson et al. (2004)
MC_4/GPR7	FRET and ELISA	–	–	Rediger et al. (2009)
MC_4/MC_4 D90N	FRET and ELISA	–	S	Biebermann et al. (2003)
NK_1/μOR	BRET and co-IP	–	S and BP	Ripley et al. (2002), Pfeiffer et al. (2003)
T1R1/T1R3	co-IP and ligand binding	Rescue of T1R3 KO mice	S	Nelson et al. (2001, 2002), Xu et al. (2004)
T1R2/T1R3	co-IP and Ligand binding		S	Nelson et al. (2001, 2002), Xu et al. (2004)
V_{1A}/OT	co-IP and BRET	–	–	Terrillon et al. (2003)
V_2/OT	co-IP and BRET	–	–	Terrillon et al. (2003)
β_1AR/β_2AR	co-IP	–	S	Zhu et al. (2005)

This table enumerates the major GPCR heteromers and details the, in vitro and in vivo, evidence for physical interaction, if present. S, signaling modulation; T, trafficking modulation; B, binding modulation; E, expression modulation; BP, Behavioral or pain modulation in mice; BRET, bioluminescence resonance energy transfer; FRET, fluorescence resonance energy transfer; co-IP, co-immunoprecipitation; βAR, beta adrenergic receptor; EP_1, prostanoid receptor 1; κOR, kappa opioid receptor; μOR, mu opioid receptor; δOR, delta opioid receptor; 5-HT_2, serotonin receptor 2; D_2, dopamine receptor 2; 5-HT_1, serotonin receptor 1; 5-HT_4, serotonin receptor 4; Gal, galanin receptor; mGlu, mGlutamate receptor; A, adenosine receptor; P2YR, purinergic P2Y receptors; AT, angiotensin receptor; APJ, apelin receptor; B, Bradikinin receptor; CB, canabinoid receptor; OX, orexin receptor; CCR5, C-C chemokine receptor type 5; CXCR4, C-X-C chemokine receptor type 4; CRF_1, corticotrophin releasing factor receptor subtype 1; H_3, histamine receptor 3; SST, somatostatin receptor; ET, endothelin receptor; $GABA_B$, γ-aminobutyric acid; CaS, calcium-sensing receptor; M_2, muscarinic receptor 2; GHSR, ghrelin receptor; IP, prostaglandin (prostacyclin) receptor; MC, melanocortin receptor; NTS, neurotensin receptor; TP, thromboxane receptor; NK_1, substance P receptor; T1R, taste receptor 1; V, vasopressin receptor; OT, oxytocin receptor.

receptors endogenously, abolished functional effects observed upon treatment of these cells with either agonist alone (Pello et al., 2008).

CCR5 was reported to interact physically, *in vitro*, with μOR using co-immunoprecipitation assays inducing cross desensitization of the receptor without modulation of receptor internalization. DAMGO (μOR agonist) and RANTES induced chemotaxis in CHO cells co-expressing both receptors. Preincubation with either DAMGO or RANTES inhibited chemotaxis caused by the other ligand. Moreover, DAMGO pretreatment enhanced phosphorylation of CCR5 and reduced RANTES-promoted GTPγS binding suggesting heterologous desensitization (Chen et al., 2004).

Several different GPCRs are implicated in the regulation of striatal functions. Notably, *in vivo* functional crosstalks have been reported between dopamine and ORs. As an example, methamphetamine-induced *zif*268 (transcription factor also known as Egr1, Early Growth Response Protein 1) expression was abolished in μOR-knockout mice in which dopamine receptors were blocked by haloperidol. However, the expression of zif268 mRNA was not altered in μOR knockout mice without blockade of dopamine receptors or in wild-type mice with blockade of dopamine receptors (Tien et al., 2010). These results suggest a crosstalk between the μ-opioid system and the dopamine system in the modulation of the expression of *zif*268 induced by methamphetamine. D_1 knockout mice were shown to have a reduced μOR expression in striatal patches without alterations in κOR and δOR expression patterns (Becker et al., 2001). Co-localization of these receptors was shown in rat striatal and cortical neurons, however direct interactions were only reported in transfected cells using the BRET assay (Juhasz et al., 2008).

Another example is the μOR and the substance P (NK_1) receptor, which is highly expressed in brain regions implicated in depression, anxiety, and stress. They are also present in the *nucleus accumbens*, which mediates the motivational properties of drugs of abuse including opioids. The rewarding effects of morphine are absent in mice lacking NK_1 suggesting that these receptors are critical for the reinforcing properties of morphine, and for adaptive responses elicited by repeated opiate administration (Ripley et al., 2002). Direct interaction between NK_1 and μOR was reported *in vitro* and functional characterization of cells expressing both receptors revealed cross-modulation of receptor internalization and desensitization (Pfeiffer et al., 2003).

Cannabinoid receptors family remain one of the most important GPCR drug discovery targets due to the intense interest in CB_1 receptor antagonists for treating obesity and the metabolic syndrome. Heteromerization of CB_1 in the context of metabolism will be discussed later. The literature reports many examples of functional interaction between cannabinoid and dopamine receptors. Functional antagonism was shown in rat brain where the CB_1 agonist CP55,940 reduced the affinity of D_2 agonist binding sites in the dorsal and ventral striatum. Similarly, *in vivo* administration of CP55,940 inhibited D_2-promoted locomotor activity (Marcellino et al., 2008). *In vitro*, heteromer formation was demonstrated using FRET (Marcellino et al., 2008). Co-expression of both receptors in HEK293 cells showed that co-stimulation of D_2 and CB_1 results in a switch of G protein coupling preference of these $G_{i/o}$-coupled receptors toward the pertussis toxin-insensitive $G_{\alpha s}$ protein (Kearn et al., 2005). Similar observations have been reported in primary striatal neuron cultures (Glass and Felder, 1997) supporting the physiological relevance of D_2/CB_1 heteromer formation.

In the last few years, it has been suggested that A_{2A} receptors could exert a permissive role on CB_1 function in a way that a basal adenosinergic tone would be important for cannabinoid-mediated effects. Specifically, it has been demonstrated that the ability of a CB_1 agonist to inhibit motor activity requires the presence and the activation of A_{2A} (Andersson et al., 2005; Carriba et al., 2007). The activation state of A_{2A} seems also to regulate synaptic effects of CB_1, which is partly dependent on $mGlu_5$ (Tebano et al., 2009). Heteromer formation between CB_1 and A_{2A} was shown *in vitro*, in cells exogenously expressing both receptors using BRET and, *in vivo*, by immunoprecipitation assays in rat striatum suggesting that heteromer formation may participate in the functional crosstalk between these two receptors (Carriba et al., 2007).

Adenosine, Dopamine, and Glutamate receptor heteromers

Adenosine activates four GPCRs, A_1, A_{2A}, A_{2B}, and A_3, which are widespread throughout the body. They are involved in a variety of physiological processes and pathologies including neurological, cardiovascular, inflammatory diseases, and cancer (see Trincavelli et al., 2010 for review).

Heteromerization between the different adenosine receptor subtypes is exemplified by the A_1/A_{2A} heteromer, which was reported *in vitro* and *in vivo* in 2006 by Ciruela et al. (2006). Immunogold detection and co-immunoprecipitation experiments confirmed the heteromer formation in rat striatal glutamatergic nerve terminals. The authors showed that A_{2A} activation reduces the affinity of A_1 for agonists, which might explain the stimulatory effect of adenosine on glutamatergic neurotransmission at higher ligand concentrations. Moreover, the authors speculate about a possible role of A_1/A_{2A} heteromers in the tolerance to the psychostimulant effects of caffeine (Ciruela et al., 2006).

Using co-immunoprecipitation assays Ciruela et al. (2001) showed a subtype-specific interaction between $mGlu_{1\alpha}$ and A_1 receptors in both rat cerebellar synaptosomes and co-transfected HEK293 cells. This heteromer was reported to be implicated in neuroprotection suggesting a potential role in neurodegenerative diseases such as Alzheimer. Importantly, the timing of $mGlu_{1\alpha}$ and A_1 receptor activation is very important to achieve a maximal effect in adenosine- and glutamate-mediated neuroprotection/neurodegeneration (Ciruela et al., 2001).

Purinergic P2Y receptors are involved in neuromodulation and neuron–glia interactions and respond to a wider range of agonists, including di- or tri-phosphates of nucleosides, and uridine diphosphate-glucose. The $P2Y_1$ subtype has been reported to form heteromers with the A_1 receptor *in vivo* as determined by co-localization and co-immunoprecipitation experiments in rat brain (Yoshioka et al., 2002), rat hippocampus (Tonazzini et al., 2007), and in human astroglial cells (Tonazzini et al., 2008). $P2Y_1$ stimulation impaired the potency of A_1 coupling to G proteins, whereas the stimulation of A_1 increased the functional responsiveness of $P2Y_1$, indicating a functional interaction between these receptors in rat hippocampus (Tonazzini et al., 2007).

Several reports highlight the physical and functional interaction between A_2 and D_2 receptors. BRET and FRET assays as well as co-immunoprecipitation in neuroblastoma cells and striatum indicate formation of A_2/D_2 heteromers (Canals et al., 2003). It was also reported that A_{2A} receptor antagonists increase locomotion in reserpinized (dopamine-depleted) mice and produce contralateral rotational behavior in rats only after the treatment with sub-threshold doses of the D_2-like receptor agonist quinpirole (Tanganelli et al., 2004).

A physical interaction between A_2 and $mGlu_5$ was shown *in vitro* by co-immunoprecipitation. Simultaneous stimulation of cells co-expressing both receptors led to a synergistic increase in ERK phosphorylation (Ferre et al., 2002). *In vivo*, the anti-Parkinsonian effects of $mGlu_5$ antagonists, known to increase motor control, were potentiated by an A_{2A} antagonist confirming a functional interaction between these two receptors (Kachroo et al., 2005). A combination of a sub-threshold dose of SCH 58261 (A_{2A} antagonist) with a sub-threshold dose of MTEP ($mGlu_5$ antagonist) reduced alcohol self-administration (Adams et al., 2008). In addition, A_{2A} and $mGlu_5$ seem to form higher order oligomeric complexes with D2. Cabello et al. (2009) were able to show *in vitro* using BRET and FRET assays as well as co-immunoprecipitation the presence of the latter three receptors in the same complex. Similar results were obtained in rat striatum homogenates (Cabello et al., 2009).

Dopamine is a neurotransmitter in many brain regions, and regarding Parkinson disease – the most important is the striatum. In addition, relevant studies regarding receptor oligomerization are described in nucleus accumbens, i.e., a nucleus of the striatum. Dopamine binds and activates five types of receptors, D_1, D_2, D_3, D_4, and D_5. The literature reports many examples of dopamine subtype heteromerization and postulate their implication in neuropathologies such as Parkinson and dyskinesia (Missale et al., 2010). D_1/D_2 heteromers are convincingly demonstrated *in vivo* by co-immunoprecipitation (Lee et al., 2004). Whereas D_1 and D_2 homomers are coupled to G_s and G_i proteins, respectively, D_1/D_2 heteromers are coupled to $G_{q/11}$ when both protomers are activated. Activation of this heteromer-specific $G_{q/11}$ pathway increases levels of calcium/calmodulin-dependent protein kinase IIα in the nucleus accumbens, unlike activation of the G_s-coupled D_1 receptors, indicating a mechanism by which D_1/D_2 may contribute to synaptic plasticity (Rashid et al., 2007).

Recently, D_1 and D_2 were reported to form heteromeric complexes with histamine H_3 (but not H_4) receptors *in vitro* using BRET. Functional interaction in mice is suggested in light of the important role of postsynaptic H_3 receptors in the modulation of dopaminergic transmission by means of a negative modulation of D_2 receptor function. Indeed, selective H_3 receptor agonists inhibit D_1- and D_2-promoted locomotor activity and the H_3 receptor antagonist thioperamide has a potentiating effect. Moreover, radioligand binding experiments in striatal membrane preparations showed that activation of H_3 decreased the binding affinity of D_2 (Ferrada et al., 2008).

Pituitary tumors express both somatostatin and dopamine receptors (Colao et al., 2007). D_2 and somatostatin SST_2 receptors are co-localized in three different brain regions including the cerebral cortex, striatum, and substantia nigra. *In vivo*, D_2/SST_2 heteromer formation was confirmed in rat striatal neurons using photo-bleaching FRET (Baragli et al., 2007). Another evidence supporting D_2/SST_2 formation comes from the high efficacy of bivalent ligands, designed to target somatostatin and dopamine receptors, on the inhibition of growth hormone (GH) and prolactin secretion from GH-secreting pituitary adenomas, which are partially responsive to somatostatin analog therapy (Jaquet et al., 2005).

The literature reports several studies pinpointing a functional crosstalk between the prostanoid receptor EP_1 as well as D_1 and D_2 receptors without evidences for physical interactions. EP_1 is expressed in more than one-half of medium spiny neurons in the striatum, and its ligand, prostaglandin E_2 (PGE_2) is produced in the striatum in response to stimulation with a D_1 or D_2 agonist. The PGE_2–EP_1 pathway facilitates both D_1 and D_2 signaling as indicated by the Thr34 phosphorylation of the dopamine- and cAMP-Regulated PhosphoProtein 32 (DARPP-32) *in vitro* in striatal slices. EP_1-knock out mice exhibit a significant suppression of hyperlocomotion induced by cocaine or SKF81297, a D_1 agonist, and significant attenuation of catalepsy induced by raclopride, a D_2 antagonist (Kitaoka et al., 2007).

GABA receptor heteromers

$GABA_B$ are critical receptors in the CNS, where their function is mainly the suppression of neuronal activity. The $GABA_{B1}/GABA_{B2}$ heteromer, is one of the best characterized examples of GPCR heteromerization as detailed above. There is also some evidence for the formation of heteromers between $GABA_{B1}$ and the calcium-sensing receptor (CaS) *in vitro* and in hippocampal neurons. CaS receptors control systemic calcium balance *via* the regulation of parathyroid hormone secretion and renal calcium excretion. Heteromer formation seems to modulate the expression of CaS as expression of the CaS is increased in brain lysates of $GABA_{B1}$ knockout mice and in cultured hippocampal neurons (Chang et al., 2007).

$GABA_{B2}$ was recently shown to interact functionally and physically with muscarinic M_2 receptors. *In vitro*, a combination of FRET and TIRF microscopy detected the heteromers at the cell surface. $GABA_{B2}$ and M_2 are both localized in the somatosensory cortex and are shown to interact *in vivo* by co-immunoprecipitation. In PC12 cells, $GABA_{B2}$ expression rescues M_2 surface expression, M_2-induced activation of GIRKs, and inhibition of cAMP production (Boyer et al., 2009).

Serotonin receptor heteromers

Serotonin (5-HT) receptors represent one of the largest subfamilies of GPCRs. There are 14 different 5-HT receptor subtypes widely distributed throughout the peripheral and CNS, representing therapeutic targets for drugs used to treat anxiety, depression, schizophrenia, obesity, and other disorders (Millan et al., 2008).

Alterations in either serotonin or dopamine neurotransmission seems to be implicated in many human neurological and psychiatric disorders, including depression, anxiety, and schizophrenia (de Almeida et al., 2008). Recently, formation of $5\text{-}HT_{2A}/D_2$ heteromers was reported *in vitro* using FRET but the functional properties of this complex are not known. Nevertheless, $5\text{-}HT_{2A}$ and D_2 receptors are co-localized in the medial prefrontal cortex as well as in the pars reticulate of the substantia nigra in rat, suggesting, at least, the possibility of functional crosstalk between these two receptors *in vivo* (Lukasiewicz et al., 2010).

The $5\text{-}HT_{2A}/mGlu_2$ heteromer plays a role in anxiety and constitutes one of the most interesting examples of GPCR heteromerization reported so far. Compelling pharmacological and biochemical evidence *in vivo* confirmed the physical interaction between $5\text{-}HT_{2A}$ and $mGlu_2$. Moreover, the metabotropic glutamate agonist, LY379268 increases the affinity of different hallucinogens for the $5\text{-}HT_{2A}$ receptor-binding site but also, a selective $5\text{-}HT_{2A}$ receptor agonist decreases the affinity of different agonists for the $mGlu_2$ receptor-binding site (Gonzalez-Maeso et al., 2008).

Galanin is co-expressed with and modulates serotonin and noradrenaline release, two neurotransmitters implicated in depression. Stimulation of galanin GAL_1 and/or GAL_3 receptors results in a depression-like phenotype, while activation of the GAL_2 receptor attenuates depression-like behavior (Kuteeva et al., 2008). $5\text{-}HT_{1A}$ and GAL_1 interact with each other *in vitro* as demonstrated by FRET. After simultaneous activation of both receptors, G_i and MAPK signaling did not show any additive or synergistic effects indicating that activation of each receptor alone is sufficient to reach maximal signaling capacity for these specific pathways (Borroto-Escuela et al., 2010). However, an antagonistic effect of GAL_1 activation on $5\text{-}HT_{1A}$-induced hippocampal serotonin release and hypothermia and locomotor activity were shown in the rat brain (Kehr et al., 2002).

Another example of functional crosstalk with no evidence, at least for now, of physical interaction has been described for CRF_1 and $5HT_2$ receptors involved in anxiety as detailed above (Magalhaes et al., 2010).

GPCR HETEROMERS IN THE CARDIOVASCULAR–RENAL SYSTEM

The most commonly studied and clinically targeted cardiac GPCRs include adrenergic, angiotensin, endothelin, and adenosine receptors. Drugs, targeting adrenergic, and angiotensin receptor signaling pathways alone, account for the majority of prescriptions for cardiovascular diseases (Salazar et al., 2007).

Angiotensin II (AngII) causes vasoconstriction both by a direct action on smooth muscle cells and, indirectly, through the facilitation of noradrenaline release from postganglionic sympathetic neurons. AngII binds to two main receptors, AT_1 and AT_2. *Via* stimulation of AT_1 receptors, AngII causes virtually all of its physiological actions, namely the cardiovascular, neuronal, renal, endocrine, and hepatic effect see (Guimaraes and Pinheiro, 2005) for review. Bradykinin (BK), an endogenous vasoactive peptide mainly produced from plasma with a physiological role in inflammation and nociception, binds two main receptors, B_1 and B_2 (Fincham et al., 2009). AbdAlla et al. (2000) reported functional and physical interaction between AT_1 and B_2 receptors with major implications in pre-eclampsia and hypertensions. In the cortical thick ascending limb in the kidney, BK exerts negative modulatory effects on AngII-induced calcium responses dependent on tyrosine kinase and MAPK pathways. In the presence of BK AngII-induced sodium transport is suppressed (Hus-Citharel et al., 2010). The AT_1/B_2 heteromer has also been suggested to contribute to AngII hyper-responsiveness of mesangial cells in experimental hypertension (AbdAlla et al., 2005). However, the existence of AT_1/B_2 heteromers has been questioned by several groups suggesting that the documented *in vivo* crosstalk between these two hormones is most likely based on a functional rather than physical interactions (Hansen et al., 2009).

AT_1/β_2AR heteromers were described in mouse cardiac myocytes transfected with the corresponding cDNAs. The main functional consequence of this interaction is the enhancement of agonist-induced β_2AR signaling and the silencing of the spontaneous activation of β_2AR, suggesting that heteromerization mutually stabilizes both receptor subtypes in their respective inactive conformations in the absence of agonist. *In vivo*, selective blockade of β_2AR in mouse cardiomyocytes inhibits angiotensin-induced contractility and administration of the AT_1 antagonist valsartan reduces the maximal response to catecholamine-induced elevation of heart rate (Barki-Harrington et al., 2003), further supporting the physiological relevance of heteromerization.

Another heteromeric partner described for AT_1 is the apelin receptor (APJ). Apelin seems to be an important factor in the regulation of vascular tone and cardiovascular function (Kalea and Batlle, 2010). AT_1 was shown to physically interact with APJ *in vitro* by BRET, FRET, and co-immunoprecipitation assays. Whereas *in vivo* evidence for AT_1/APJ heteromer formation is still lacking, many examples support an *in vivo* functional crosstalk. In apelin knockout mice, exogenous Ang II induces atherosclerosis and abdominal aortic aneurysm formation while co-infusion of apelin abrogated these effects. Moreover, in a vein graft mode, apelin treatment rescued AngII-mediated increase in neointimal formation and vascular remodeling (Chun et al., 2008).

Adrenergic receptors are responsible for translating chemical messages from the sympathetic nervous system into cardiovascular responses. Three β-adrenergic receptor subtypes are found in the mammalian heart β_1, β_2, and β_3-AR (Salazar et al., 2007). Heteromerization between the different subtypes has been described and is implicated in many cardiovascular functions. For example, alterations in receptor pharmacology and function were seen in intact adult mouse cardiomyocytes lacking β_1AR and β_2AR, where heteromerization reduced spontaneous receptor activity and enhanced responsiveness to catecholamines (Zhu et al., 2005).

Another key player in the regulation of the cardiovascular systems are endothelin receptors. Endothelins are composed of a family of 21 amino acid peptides (ET-1, ET-2, and ET-3). ET-1 is the predominant endothelin in the cardiovascular system binding to endothelin A (ET_A) and B (ET_B) receptors (Sakurai et al., 1990). ET_A and ET_B have been reported to form heteromers, which induce sustained calcium signaling as compared to the corresponding homomers, known to induce a more transient calcium release in transfected HEK293 cells (Evans and Walker, 2008).

Serotonin was found in multiple cardiovascular tissues, including heart, blood vessels, brain, platelets, adrenal gland, and kidney. 5-HT_4 (mainly 5-HT_{4b}), 5-HT_{2A}, and 5-HT_{2B} receptors coexist in auricular myocytes of newborn rats. 5-HT_4 and 5-HT_2 receptors appear to regulate intercellular communication at rat cardiac myocyte gap junctions. Unexpectedly, 5-HT_4 activation reduces cAMP, L-type calcium currents, and intercellular coupling while 5-HT_{2A} or 5-HT_{2B} activation enhances gap junctional intercellular communication (Derangeon et al., 2010). These results suggest receptor heteromerization, which are still to be assessed.

Prostacyclin (PGI_2) and Thromboxane A2 (TxA_2) are biological opposites: PGI_2 is a vasodilator and inhibitor of platelet aggregation, which limits the deleterious actions of TxA_2, a vasoconstrictor, and platelet activator. The molecular mechanisms involved in the counter-regulation of PGI_2 and TxA_2 promoted signaling are unclear. Physical and functional interaction between the PGI_2 receptor (IP_1) and TxA_2 receptor (TP) were reported *in vitro* in HEK293 cells. IP_1 seems to facilitate TP-mediated generation of cAMP in a manner independent of IP_1-induced cAMP formation (Wilson et al., 2004).

Opioid receptors and β_2ARs have been shown to coexist and functionally interact in cardiac myocyte sarcolemma. Low doses of selective opioids are known to inhibit norepinephrine-mediated functions (Pepe et al., 1997). Physical interaction was reported by co-immunoprecipitation studies in CHO cells exogenously expressing both receptors. *In vitro*, heteromerization results in an alteration of trafficking properties with no significant alterations in ligand binding. Moreover, opioid-selective agonists alter β_2AR internalization, thus providing a possible molecular mechanism for the lack of β_2AR agonist-mediated effects after OR activation (Jordan et al., 2001).

Prostanoids EP_1 receptors and β_2AR form heteromers *in vitro* (BRET, co-immunoprecipitation). EP_1 and β_2AR colocalize in airway smooth muscle cells, where activation of EP_1 was reported to reduce β_2AR-stimulated cAMP without affecting β_2AR phosphorylation or trafficking. EP_1/β_2AR heteromers might be implicated in asthma (McGraw et al., 2006).

P2Y receptors play various physiological roles, including mediation of vasodilatation in the endothelium, vasoconstriction of smooth muscles, and control of mitogenic actions and secretory processes. A_{2A}/$P2Y_1$ and A_{2A}/$P2Y_{12}$ heteromers were detected in human platelet membranes by co-immunoprecipitation techniques, and seem to have a crucial role in the physiology of platelet aggregation (Nakata et al., 2010).

GPCR HETEROMERS IN TASTE

Taste, or gustation, is mediated by a specialized anatomically and physiologically defined chemosensory gustatory system. The gustatory system in mammals includes taste receptor cells (TRC) organized in taste buds located within the gustatory papillae, located mainly, but not exclusively in the tongue. Reception of taste qualities that humans describe as sweet, umami, and bitter involves GPCRs from the T1R and T2R subfamilies (Bachmanov and Beauchamp, 2007). Whereas T1R are typical class C GPCRs with a large N-terminal "Venus fly trap" (VFT) domain, T2R belong to rhodopsin-like class A GPCRs with small N-terminal domains. The T1R family is composed of three subtypes T1R1, T1R2, and T1R3 that have been shown to form obligatory T1R1/T1R3 and T1R2/T1R3 heteromers (Nelson et al., 2001, 2002). Binding of sweet stimuli such as sucrose or aspartame to the VFT of T1R2 and umami taste stimuli such as L-glutamate to the orthosteric binding site of the VFT of T1R1 activate T1R2/T1R3 and T1R1/T1R3 heterodimers, respectively (Nelson et al., 2001, 2002; Xu et al., 2004). Several molecules binding to allosteric binding site within the VFT domain or the TM domain of taste receptors have been characterized.

For example, IMP and GMP bind near the opening of the orthosteric glutamate binding site of T1R1 thus further stabilize the closed conformation of the VFT (Zhang et al., 2008). Newly developed enhancers of sweet taste bind to a similar site in the T1R2 stabilize the sucrose-promoted closure of the VFT (Zhang et al., 2010). Such compounds could help reduce the caloric content in food and beverages. Other compounds such as lactisole and cyclamate have been proposed to bind to allosteric binding site located in the TM domain of T1R3 and thus regulate orthosteric ligand binding to the VFT of T1R1 and T1R2 in the respective heterodimers.

Much less is known about the T2R subfamily that comprises approximately 40 members in humans (Bachmanov and Beauchamp, 2007). T1R and T2R are expressed in distinct subsets of TRC excluding any functional crosstalk at the cellular level. However, nearly all T2R members are typically co-expressed within individual TRCs suggesting signal integration at the cellular level. The existence and potential functional importance of T2R heteromers remains to be studied.

GPCR HETEROMERS IN REPRODUCTION

Different GPCRs participate in reproductive functions at the level of the hypothalamic–pituitary axes and reproductive organs. Oxytocin is a hypothalamic hormone stored in the posterior pituitary, which has uterine-contracting and milk-releasing actions. The receptor for oxytocin, OT, has been shown to cluster into homomers but also into heteromers with closely related vasopressin V_{1A} and V_2 receptors in transfected HEK293 cells (Terrillon et al., 2003). The existence of OT homomers has been recently confirmed in mammary gland tissue using classical radioligand binding assays and a newly developed time-resolved FRET assay between two fluorescently labeled OT ligands (Albizu et al., 2010). In contrast to previous energy transfer assays that require expression of modified receptors fused to energy donors and acceptors, this novel assay can be applied to unmodified wild-type receptors and is thus likely to boost research on GPCR homo- and heteromerization in native tissues (**Figure 2**).

The luteinizing hormone (LH) is produced by the anterior pituitary gland. Whereas LH stimulates testosterone production in Leydig cells in males, it triggers ovulation in females. LH constitutes together with the follicle-stimulating hormone (FSH) and the thyroid-stimulating hormone (TSH) the glycoprotein hormone family. Their respective receptors LHR belong to a distinct subgroup of GPCRs that are characterized by a large N-terminal ligand binding domain-containing leucine-rich repeats and the typical heptahelical transmembrane domain. Biophysical and pharmacological assays were employed to show the formation of LHR homomers that display negative cooperativity between the ligand binding sites of receptor protomers (Urizar et al., 2005). More recently, the existence and functional relevance of LHR homomers was shown *in vivo* by using an elegant trans-complementation assay (Rivero-Muller et al., 2010). By generating transgenic mice co-expressing signaling deficient and ligand binding deficient forms of the LHR with targeted deletion of the wild-type LHR, the authors succeeded in completely restoring normal gonadal and genital function. This study provides compelling *in vivo* evidence for GPCR oligomerization by intermolecular functional complementation of two mutant receptors (**Figure 3**).

Follicle-stimulating hormone, another hormone produced by the anterior pituitary gland, acts synergistically with LH to regulate pubertal maturation and reproductive processes. Based on the recent resolution of the crystal structure of FSH together with ectodomain of its receptor (FSHR) suggested formation of a tetrameric complex composed of a FSH dimer that bridges two FSHR ectodomains (Fan and Hendrickson, 2005). Such complexes were observed in the crystals and in solution, at high concentrations (μM range), suggesting the possible stabilization of FSHR oligomers in the presence of FSH. Subsequent studies did not confirm a major role of FSH binding and/or the ectodomain in oligomerization of the FSHR but pointed rather to the central role of the TM domain in stabilizing constitutive oligomers (Guan et al., 2010).

The existence of FSHR dimers inspired chemists to synthesize FSHR antagonist composed of two pharmacophores connected through ethylene glycol spacers (Bonger et al., 2009). These antagonists were indeed more potent than dimeric compounds in which one of the pharmacophores was replaced by an inactive confomer.

The gonadotropin-releasing hormone (GnRH) is produced in the hypothalamus and responsible for the release of FSH and LH from the anterior pituitary. Oligomerization of human GnRH

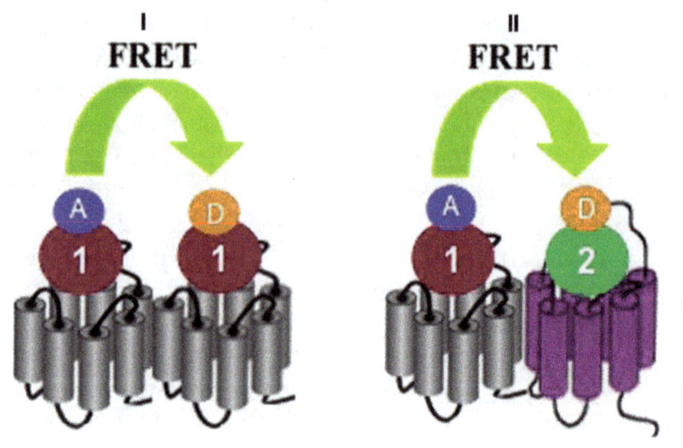

FIGURE 2 | Detection of homo/heteromer formation by FRET using fluorescent ligands. **(I)** In the case of homomer formation a FRET signal can be detected between a selective donor (D) ligand I that binds the first protomer and a selective acceptor (A) ligand 1 that binds the second protomer The donor and acceptor ligands can be the same molecule but labeled differently. **(II)** In the case of heteromer formation, a FRET signal can be detected between a selective donor ligand 1 that binds the first protomer and a selective acceptor ligand 2 that binds the second protomer. In this case, donor and acceptor ligands are different molecules.

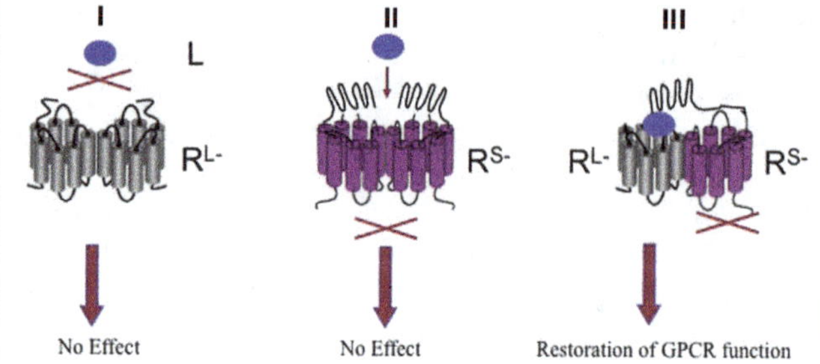

FIGURE 3 | G protein-coupled receptors oligomerization by intermolecular functional complementation of mo mutant receptors. **(I)** Oligomerization of ligand binding deficient receptor mutant (R^{L-}) does not trigger GPCR function. **(II)** Oligomerization of signaling deficient receptor mutant (R^{s-}) does not trigger GPCR function. **(III)** Co-expression of R^{L-} and R^{s-} restores GPCR function. L; ligand.

receptors has been documented in transfected cells but remain still controversial *in vivo* (Pfleger et al., 2004). Convincing evidence for GnRH receptor heteromerization has been gathered in the protochordate *Ciona intestinalis*, which expresses six GnRH isoforms (tGnRH-3 to -8) and four GnRH receptor subtypes (R1-4). Heteromerization between R1, which binds to tGnRH-6, and the orphan R4 has been demonstrated in *Ciona* ovaries in co-immunoprecipitation experiments (Sakai et al., 2009). Importantly, tGnRH-6-induced ERK1/2 activation of R1 was robustly potentiated in the presence of R4 most likely originating from R1/R4 heteromerization.

GPCR HETEROMERS IN METABOLISM

The increasing prevalence of obesity is responsible for the dramatic increase in the number of scientific and clinical studies on the control of energy homeostasis. Regulation of energy balance relies on a well-orchestrated communication between the CNS and peripheral organs. Many GPCRs, including cannabinoid, ghrelin, and melanocortin (MC) receptors, play a central role in the regulation of lipid metabolism and are therefore of major interest for drug development. In the current chapter, we will discuss some examples of GPCR heteromerization, which might be implicated in energy metabolism and related diseases as type 2 diabetes and obesity.

The endocannabinoid system comprises the enzymatic machinery for endocannabinoid synthesis and degradation, and cannabinoid CB_1 and CB_2 receptors. The endocannabinoid system controls energy balance and lipid metabolism centrally, in the hypothalamus and mesolimbic pathways, and peripherally, in adipocytes, liver, skeletal muscle, and pancreatic islet cells, acting through numerous anorexigenic and orexigenic pathways. Obese people display an increased endocannabinoid tone, driving CB_1 in a feed-forward dysfunction. Several CB_1 antagonists/inverse agonists were developed for the treatment of obesity. However, beside their efficiency in reducing food intake, these drugs were not devoid of side effects like psychiatric disorders and suicide (Bermudez-Silva et al., 2010). Orexins are orexigenic mediators selectively expressed in the hypothalamus, within neurons of the lateral hypothalamic area. Orexin A is involved in food intake in satiated rats but also in the regulation of drinking behavior. Co-expression of CB_1 and the orexin OX_1 receptor in CHO cells enhances the potency of orexin A to stimulate ERK kinase phosphorylation, and this effect was blocked by addition of SR-141716A, a CB_1 antagonist (Hilairet et al., 2003). FRET assays indicate that CB_1 and OX_1 can form heteromers *in vitro* in CHO cells exogenously expressing these receptors. Heteromer formation was shown to modulate receptor distribution *in vitro* (Ellis et al., 2006).

Ghrelin plays an important role in energy homeostasis (Castaneda et al., 2010). It is synthesized by the stomach and is believed to exert the majority of its actions through the ghrelin receptor (GHSR), which is present in high density in both the hypothalamus and the pituitary gland. Neurotensin is a 13-amino acid neurohormone, located in the synaptic vesicles and released from the neuronal terminals in a calcium-dependent manner. It plays an important role in the physiology of pain-induction, central blood pressure control, and inflammation. There are three known neurotensin receptors, NTS_1, NTS_2, NTS_3 but only NTS_1 and NTS_2 belong to the GPCR family (Stolakis et al., 2010). GHSR and NTS_1 are shown to physically interact *in vitro* and neuromedin U was described as ligand for this heteromer. GHSR/NTS_1 heteromers have been suggested to play a role for an autocrine growth-promoting pathway in non–small cell lung cancers by modulating the transcription of downstream target genes including the Forkhead box protein M1 (FOXM1; Takahashi et al., 2006).

Jiang et al. (2006) identified neurons co-expressing GHSR and D_1 in *GHSR-IRES-tauGFP* mice, suggesting at least a functional interaction between these two receptors. *In vitro*, the activation of GHSR by ghrelin amplifies dopamine/D_1-induced cAMP accumulation (Jiang et al., 2006). *In vivo*, ghrelin and dopamine crosstalk was suggested based on the observation in rats that ghrelin administration increased dopamine-related hyperactivity (Wellman et al., 2005). Till date, there is no direct evidence *in vitro* or *in vivo* confirming GHSR/D_1 heteromerization. GHSR can constitutively hetero-oligomerize with members of the prostanoid receptor family. GHSR is reported to heteromerize with EP_{3-I}, IP_1, and TPα receptors *in vitro* using BRET and co-immmunoprecipitation. The constitutive activation of phospholipase C by GHSR was significantly decreased in HEK 293 cells co-transfected with EP_{3-I}, IP, or TPα. Moreover, cell surface expression of GHSR was reduced in presence of the prostanoids receptors (Chow et al., 2008). Despite lack of direct evidence, the expression of GHSR and prostanoid receptors in atherosclerotic plaques suggests heteromer implication in this pathology (Gomez-Hernandez et al., 2006).

Melanocortin receptors have a diverse range of physiological functions; MC_1 controls skin pigmentation, MC_2, the receptor for the adrenocorticotropic hormone (ACTH), plays a critical role in the hypothalamic–pituitary–adrenal axis, whereas MC_3 and MC_4 have essential roles in energy homeostasis and MC_5 is believed to be involved in exocrine function (Cone, 2006). Mutations in the *MC4R* gene are the most frequent monogenic cause of severe obesity. Biebermann et al. present an interesting mechanistic explanation why a particular heterozygous inactivating MC_4 mutation leads to the development of extreme obesity by a dominant-negative effect. This dominant-negative effect of the D90N mutation is caused by a functionally altered wild-type MC_4/D90N receptor heteromer. MC_4 can actually form heteromers, at least *in vitro*, with a mutant MC_4 D90N resulting in functional alterations as exemplified by the complete loss of activation of the G_s/adenylyl cyclase pathways (Biebermann et al., 2003). In addition, MC_4 can physically interact, *in vitro*, with GPR7. MC_3 was shown to heteromerize with GHSR resulting in the modulation of MC_3 trafficking (Rediger et al., 2009).

CONCLUSIONS AND PERSPECTIVES

G protein-coupled receptor oligomerization has been an intensely studied field of research over the last 20 years. There is a broad consensus that GPCR oligomerization is not necessary for efficient activation of heterotrimeric G proteins as monomeric receptors are sufficient to ascertain this basic function. In contrast, GPCR oligomerization appears to be important for allosteric regulation and fine-tuning of signaling and receptor trafficking. It is furthermore admitted that most if not all GPCRs can form oligomers in intact cells. The detailed knowledge of the dimerization interface of some receptors (Guo et al., 2003; Wu et al., 2010) will undoubtedly guide the development of such tools. The lack of adequate tools (specific high-affinity antibodies, specific ligands, etc.) to study GPCR oligomerization *in vivo* or tissues expressing endogenous receptors has hampered faster progress for a long time. However, by employing original methods and developing new pharmacological tools more and more convincing evidence for the existence of GPCR oligomers is now increasingly gathered. GPCR oligomers, in particular heteromers provide new opportunities for specific pharmacological intervention. Based on the restricted expression profile of heteromers compared to the corresponding homomers, heteromer-specific drugs are expected to be very specific and to have fewer side effects. However, the great potential of heteromers is only beginning to be exploited as only very few heteromer-selective compounds are known today. Identification of such compounds will not only be important for future drug development but will also be indispensable tools for the identification and characterization of these heteromers *in vivo*. GPCR oligomers do not exist as isolated functional entities. It is now well established that GPCRs are integral part of protein networks composed of GPCRs and GPCR-associated protein complexes (Daulat et al., 2007, 2009; Bockaert et al., 2010). Learning more about the dynamics and tissue-specific composition of these clusters will undoubtedly provide new insights into the function of GPCR involved in neuroendocrinology.

ACKNOWLEDGMENTS

This work was supported by grants from SERVIER, the Fondation Recherche Médicale ("Equipe FRM"), Institut National de la Santé et de la Recherche Médicale (INSERM), Centre National de la Recherche Scientifique (CNRS). We thank Jean-Luc Guillaume and Dr. Nathalie Clement for critical reading of the manuscript.

REFERENCES

AbdAlla, S., Abdel-Baset, A., Lother, H., el Massiery, A., and Quitterer, U. (2005). Mesangial AT1/B2 receptor heterodimers contribute to angiotensin II hyperresponsiveness in experimental hypertension. *J. Mol. Neurosci.* 26, 185–192.

AbdAlla, S., Lother, H., and Quitterer, U. (2000). AT(1)-receptor heterodimers show enhanced G-protein activation and altered receptor sequestration. *Nature* 407, 94–98.

Adams, C. L., Cowen, M. S., Short, J. L., and Lawrence, A. J. (2008). Combined antagonism of glutamate mGlu5 and adenosine A2A receptors interact to regulate alcohol-seeking in rats. *Int. J. Neuropsychopharmacol.* 11, 229–241.

Albizu, L., Cottet, M., Kralikova, M., Stoev, S., Seyer, R., Brabet, I., Roux, T., Bazin, H., Bourrier, E., Lamarque, L., Breton, C., Rives, M. L., Newman, A., Javitch, J., Trinquet, E., Manning, M., Pin, J. P., Mouillac, B., and Durroux, T. (2010). Time-resolved FRET between GPCR ligands reveals oligomers in native tissues. *Nat. Chem. Biol.* 6, 587–594.

Andersson, M., Usiello, A., Borgkvist, A., Pozzi, L., Dominguez, C., Fienberg, A. A., Svenningsson, P., Fredholm, B. B., Borrelli, E., Greengard, P., and Fisone, G. (2005). Cannabinoid action depends on phosphorylation of dopamine- and cAMP-regulated phosphoprotein of 32 kDa at the protein kinase A site in striatal projection neurons. *J. Neurosci.* 25, 8432–8438.

Angers, S., Salahpour, A., and Bouvier, M. (2002). Dimerization: an emerging concept for G protein-coupled receptor ontogeny and function. *Annu. Rev. Pharmacol. Toxicol.* 42, 409–435.

Bachmanov, A. A., and Beauchamp, G. K. (2007). Taste receptor genes. *Annu. Rev. Nutr.* 27, 389–414.

Baneres, J. L., and Parello, J. (2003). Structure-based analysis of GPCR function: evidence for a novel pentameric assembly between the dimeric leukotriene B4 receptor BLT1 and the G-protein. *J. Mol. Biol.* 329, 815–829.

Baragli, A., Alturaihi, H., Watt, H. L., Abdallah, A., and Kumar, U. (2007). Heterooligomerization of human dopamine receptor 2 and somatostatin receptor 2 Co-immunoprecipitation and fluorescence resonance energy transfer analysis. *Cell. Signal.* 19, 2304–2316.

Barki-Harrington, L., Luttrell, L. M., and Rockman, H. A. (2003). Dual inhibition of beta-adrenergic and angiotensin II receptors by a single antagonist: a functional role for receptor–receptor interaction in vivo. *Circulation* 108, 1611–1618.

Bayburt, T. H., Leitz, A. J., Xie, G., Oprian, D. D., and Sligar, S. G. (2007). Transducin activation by nanoscale lipid bilayers containing one and two rhodopsins. *J. Biol. Chem.* 282, 14875–14881.

Becker, A., Grecksch, G., Kraus, J., Peters, B., Schroeder, H., Schulz, S., and Hollt, V. (2001). Loss of locomotor sensitisation in response to morphine in D1 receptor deficient mice. *Naunyn Schmiedebergs Arch. Pharmacol.* 363, 562–568.

Bermudez-Silva, F. J., Viveros, M. P., McPartland, J. M., and Rodriguez de Fonseca, F. (2010). The endocannabinoid system, eating behavior and energy homeostasis: the end or a new beginning? *Pharmacol. Biochem. Behav.* 95, 375–382.

Biebermann, H., Krude, H., Elsner, A., Chubanov, V., Gudermann, T., and Gruters, A. (2003). Autosomal-dominant mode of inheritance of a melanocortin-4 receptor mutation in a patient with severe early-onset obesity is due to a dominant-negative effect caused by receptor dimerization. *Diabetes* 52, 2984–2988.

Birdsall, N. J. (2010). Class A GPCR heterodimers: evidence from binding studies. *Trends Pharmacol. Sci.* 31, 499–508.

Bockaert, J., Perroy, J., Becamel, C., Marin, P., and Fagni, L. (2010). GPCR interacting proteins (GIPs) in the nervous system: roles in physiology and pathologies. *Annu. Rev. Pharmacol. Toxicol.* 50, 89–109.

Bonger, K. M., Hoogendoorn, S., van Koppen, C. J., Timmers, C. M., Overkleeft, H. S., and van der Marel, G. A. (2009). Synthesis and pharmacological evaluation of dimeric follicle-stimulating hormone receptor antagonists. *ChemMedChem* 4, 2098–2102.

Borroto-Escuela, D. O., Narvaez, M., Marcellino, D., Parrado, C., Narvaez, J. A., Tarakanov, A. O., Agnati, L. F., Diaz-Cabiale, Z., and Fuxe, K. (2010). Galanin receptor-1 modulates 5-hydroxtryptamine-1A signaling via heterodimerization. *Biochem. Biophys. Res. Commun.* 393, 767–772.

Bouvier, M. (2001). Oligomerization of G-protein-coupled transmitter receptors. *Nat. Rev. Neurosci.* 2, 274–286.

Boyer, S. B., Clancy, S. M., Terunuma, M., Revilla-Sanchez, R., Thomas, S. M., Moss, S. J., and Slesinger, P. A. (2009). Direct interaction of GABAB receptors with M2 muscarinic receptors enhances muscarinic signaling. *J. Neurosci.* 29, 15796–15809.

Bulenger, S., Marullo, S., and Bouvier, M. (2005). Emerging role of homo- and heterodimerization in G-protein-coupled receptor biosynthesis and maturation. *Trends Pharmacol. Sci.* 26, 131–137.

Cabello, N., Gandia, J., Bertarelli, D. C., Watanabe, M., Lluis, C., Franco, R., Ferre, S., Lujan, R., and Ciruela, F. (2009). Metabotropic glutamate type 5, dopamine D2 and adenosine A2a receptors form higher-order oligomers in living cells. *J. Neurochem.* 109, 1497–1507.

Canals, M., Marcellino, D., Fanelli, F., Ciruela, F., de Benedetti, P., Goldberg, S. R., Neve, K., Fuxe, K., Agnati, L. F., Woods, A. S., Ferre, S., Lluis, C., Bouvier, M., and Franco, R. (2003). Adenosine A2A-dopamine D2 receptor–receptor heteromerization: qualitative and quantitative assessment by fluorescence and bioluminescence energy transfer. *J. Biol. Chem.* 278, 46741–46749.

Carriba, P., Ortiz, O., Patkar, K., Justinova, Z., Stroik, J., Themann, A., Muller, C., Woods, A. S., Hope, B. T., Ciruela, F., Casado, V., Canela, E. I., Lluis, C., Goldberg, S. R., Moratalla, R., Franco, R., and Ferre, S. (2007). Striatal adenosine A2A and cannabinoid CB1 receptors form functional heteromeric complexes that mediate the motor effects of cannabinoids. *Neuropsychopharmacology* 32, 2249–2259.

Castaneda, T. R., Tong, J., Datta, R., Culler, M., and Tschop, M. H. (2010). Ghrelin in the regulation of body weight and metabolism. *Front. Neuroendocrinol.* 31:1. doi: 10.1016/j.yfrne.2009.10.008

Chang, W., Tu, C., Cheng, Z., Rodriguez, L., Chen, T. H., Gassmann, M., Bettler, B., Margeta, M., Jan, L. Y., and Shoback, D. (2007). Complex formation with the Type B gamma-aminobutyric acid receptor affects the expression and signal transduction of the extracellular calcium-sensing receptor. Studies with HEK-293 cells and neurons. *J. Biol. Chem.* 282, 25030–25040.

Chen, C., Li, J., Bot, G., Szabo, I., Rogers, T. J., and Liu-Chen, L. Y. (2004). Heterodimerization and cross-desensitization between the mu-opioid receptor and the chemokine CCR5 receptor. *Eur. J. Pharmacol.* 483, 175–186.

Chow, K. B., Leung, P. K., Cheng, C. H., Cheung, W. T., and Wise, H. (2008). The constitutive activity of ghrelin receptors is decreased by co-expression with vasoactive prostanoid receptors when over-expressed in human embryonic kidney 293 cells. *Int. J. Biochem. Cell Biol.* 40, 2627–2637.

Chun, H. J., Ali, Z. A., Kojima, Y., Kundu, R. K., Sheikh, A. Y., Agrawal, R., Zheng, L., Leeper, N. J., Pearl, N. E., Patterson, A. J., Anderson, J. P., Tsao, P. S., Lenardo, M. J., Ashley, E. A., and Quertermous, T. (2008). Apelin signaling antagonizes Ang II effects in mouse models of atherosclerosis. *J. Clin. Invest.* 118, 3343–3354.

Cichewicz, D. L. (2004). Synergistic interactions between cannabinoid and opioid analgesics. *Life Sci.* 74, 1317–1324.

Ciruela, F., Casado, V., Rodrigues, R. J., Lujan, R., Burgueno, J., Canals, M., Borycz, J., Rebola, N., Goldberg, S. R., Mallol, J., Cortes, A., Canela, E. I., Lopez-Gimenez, J. F., Milligan, G., Lluis, C., Cunha, R. A., Ferre, S., and Franco, R. (2006). Presynaptic control of striatal glutamatergic neurotransmission by adenosine A1-A2A receptor heteromers. *J. Neurosci.* 26, 2080–2087.

Ciruela, F., Escriche, M., Burgueno, J., Angulo, E., Casado, V., Soloviev, M. M., Canela, E. I., Mallol, J., Chan, W. Y., Lluis, C., McIlhinney, R. A., and Franco, R. (2001). Metabotropic glutamate 1alpha and adenosine A1 receptors assemble into functionally interacting complexes. *J. Biol. Chem.* 276, 18345–18351.

Colao, A., Filippella, M., Pivonello, R., Di Somma, C., Faggiano, A., and Lombardi, G. (2007). Combined therapy of somatostatin analogues and dopamine agonists in the treatment of pituitary tumours. *Eur. J. Endocrinol.* 156(Suppl. 1), S57–S63.

Cone, R. D. (2006). Studies on the physiological functions of the melanocortin system. *Endocr. Rev.* 27, 736–749.

Daulat, A. M., Maurice, P., Froment, C., Guillaume, J. L., Broussard, C., Monsarrat, B., Delagrange, P., and Jockers, R. (2007). Purification and identification of G protein-coupled receptor protein complexes under native conditions. *Mol. Cell Proteomics* 6, 835–844.

Daulat, A. M., Maurice, P., and Jockers, R. (2009). Recent methodological advances in the discovery of GPCR-associated protein complexes. *Trends Pharmacol. Sci.* 30, 72–78.

de Almeida, J., Palacios, J. M., and Mengod, G. (2008). Distribution of 5-HT and DA receptors in primate prefrontal cortex: implications for pathophysiology and treatment. *Prog. Brain Res.* 172, 101–115.

Derangeon, M., Bozon, V., Defamie, N., Peineau, N., Bourmeyster, N., Sarrouilhe, D., Argibay, J. A., and Herve, J. C. (2010). 5-HT4 and 5-HT2 receptors antagonistically influence gap junctional coupling between rat auricular myocytes. *J. Mol. Cell. Cardiol.* 48, 220–229.

Durroux, T. (2005). Principles: a model for the allosteric interactions between ligand binding sites within a dimeric GPCR. *Trends Pharmacol. Sci.* 26, 376–384.

Ellis, J., Pediani, J. D., Canals, M., Milasta, S., and Milligan, G. (2006). Orexin-1 receptor-cannabinoid CB1 receptor heterodimerization results in both ligand-dependent and -independent coordinated alterations of receptor localization and function. *J. Biol. Chem.* 281, 38812–38824.

Ernst, O. P., Gramse, V., Kolbe, M., Hofmann, K. P., and Heck, M. (2007). Monomeric G protein-coupled receptor rhodopsin in solution activates its G protein transducin at the diffusion limit. *Proc. Natl. Acad. Sci. U.S.A.* 104, 10859–10864.

Evans, N. J., and Walker, J. W. (2008). Endothelin receptor dimers evaluated by FRET, ligand binding, and calcium mobilization. *Biophys. J.* 95, 483–492.

Fan, Q. R., and Hendrickson, W. A. (2005). Structure of human follicle-stimulating hormone in complex with its receptor. *Nature* 433, 269–277.

Ferrada, C., Ferre, S., Casado, V., Cortes, A., Justinova, Z., Barnes, C., Canela, E. I., Goldberg, S. R., Leurs, R., Lluis, C., and Franco, R. (2008). Interactions between histamine H3 and dopamine D2 receptors and the implications for striatal function. *Neuropharmacology* 55, 190–197.

Ferre, S., Karcz-Kubicha, M., Hope, B. T., Popoli, P., Burgueno, J., Gutierrez, M. A., Casado, V., Fuxe, K., Goldberg, S. R., Lluis, C., Franco, R., and Ciruela, F. (2002). Synergistic interaction between adenosine A2A and glutamate mGlu5 receptors: implications for striatal neuronal function. *Proc. Natl. Acad. Sci. U.S.A.* 99, 11940–11945.

Ferre, S., Navarro, G., Casado, V., Cortes, A., Mallol, J., Canela, E. I., Lluis, C., and Franco, R. (2010). G protein-coupled receptor heteromers as new targets for drug development. *Prog. Mol. Biol. Transl. Sci.* 91, 41–52.

Fincham, C. I., Bressan, A., Paris, M., Rossi, C., and Fattori, D. (2009). Bradykinin receptor antagonists – a review of the patent literature 2005–2008. *Expert Opin. Ther. Pat.* 19, 919–941.

Finley, M. J., Chen, X., Bardi, G., Davey, P., Geller, E. B., Zhang, L., Adler, M. W., and Rogers, T. J. (2008). Bi-directional heterologous desensitization between the major HIV-1 co-receptor CXCR4 and the kappa-opioid receptor. *J. Neuroimmunol.* 197, 114–123.

Galvez, T., Duthey, B., Kniazeff, J., Blahos, J., Rovelli, G., Bettler, B., Prezeau, L., and Pin, J. P. (2001). Allosteric interactions between GB1 and GB2 subunits are required for optimal GABA(B) receptor function. *EMBO J.* 20, 2152–2159.

Glass, M., and Felder, C. C. (1997). Concurrent stimulation of cannabinoid CB1 and dopamine D2 receptors augments cAMP accumulation in striatal neurons: evidence for a Gs linkage to the CB1 receptor. *J. Neurosci.* 17, 5327–5333.

Gomez-Hernandez, A., Martin-Ventura, J. L., Sanchez-Galan, E., Vidal, C., Ortego, M., Blanco-Colio, L. M., Ortega, L., Tunon, J., and Egido, J. (2006). Overexpression of COX-2, Prostaglandin E synthase-1 and prostaglandin E receptors in blood mononuclear cells and plaque of patients with carotid atherosclerosis: regulation by nuclear factor-kappaB. *Atherosclerosis* 187, 139–149.

Gonzalez-Maeso, J., Ang, R. L., Yuen, T., Chan, P., Weisstaub, N. V., Lopez-Gimenez, J. F., Zhou, M., Okawa, Y., Callado, L. F., Milligan, G., Gingrich, J. A., Filizola, M., Meana, J. J., and Sealfon, S. C. (2008). Identification of a serotonin/glutamate receptor complex implicated in psychosis. *Nature* 452, 93–97.

Guan, R., Wu, X., Feng, X., Zhang, M., Hebert, T. E., and Segaloff, D. L. (2010). Structural determinants underlying constitutive dimerization of unoccupied human follitropin receptors. *Cell. Signal.* 22, 247–256.

Guimaraes, S., and Pinheiro, H. (2005). Functional evidence that in the cardiovascular system AT1 angiotensin II receptors are AT1B prejunctionally and AT1A postjunctionally. *Cardiovasc. Res.* 67, 208–215.

Guo, W., Shi, L., and Javitch, J. A. (2003). The fourth transmembrane segment forms the interface of the dopamine D2 receptor homodimer. *J. Biol. Chem.* 278, 4385–4388.

Hansen, J. L., Hansen, J. T., Speerschneider, T., Lyngso, C., Erikstrup, N., Burstein, E. S., Weiner, D. M., Walther, T., Makita, N., Iiri, T., Merten, N., Kostenis, E., and Sheikh, S. P. (2009). Lack of evidence for AT1R/B2R heterodimerization in COS-7, HEK293, and NIH3T3 cells: how common is the AT1R/B2R heterodimer? *J. Biol. Chem.* 284, 1831–1839.

Hilairet, S., Bouaboula, M., Carriere, D., Le Fur, G., and Casellas, P. (2003). Hypersensitization of the Orexin 1 receptor by the CB1 receptor: evidence for cross-talk blocked by the specific CB1 antagonist, SR141716. *J. Biol. Chem.* 278, 23731–23737.

Hirono, M., Yoshioka, T., and Konishi, S. (2001). GABA(B) receptor activation enhances mGluR-mediated responses at cerebellar excitatory synapses. *Nat. Neurosci.* 4, 1207–1216.

Hojo, M., Sudo, Y., Ando, Y., Minami, K., Takada, M., Matsubara, T., Kanaide, M., Taniyama, K., Sumikawa, K., and Uezono, Y. (2008). mu-Opioid receptor forms a functional heterodimer with cannabinoid CB1 receptor: electrophysiological and FRET assay analysis. *J. Pharmacol. Sci.* 108, 308–319.

Hus-Citharel, A., Bouby, N., Iturrioz, X., and Llorens-Cortes, C. (2010). Multiple cross talk between angiotensin II, bradykinin, and insulin signaling in the cortical thick ascending limb of rat kidney. *Endocrinology* 151, 3181–3194.

Jaquet, P., Gunz, G., Saveanu, A., Dufour, H., Taylor, J., Dong, J., Kim, S., Moreau, J. P., Enjalbert, A., and Culler, M. D. (2005). Efficacy of chimeric molecules directed towards multiple somatostatin and dopamine receptors on inhibition of GH and prolactin secretion from GH-secreting pituitary adenomas classified as partially responsive to somatostatin analog therapy. *Eur. J. Endocrinol.* 153, 135–141.

Jiang, H., Betancourt, L., and Smith, R. G. (2006). Ghrelin amplifies dopamine signaling by cross talk involving formation of growth hormone secretagogue receptor/dopamine receptor subtype 1 heterodimers. *Mol. Endocrinol.* 20, 1772–1785.

Jockers, R., Issad, T., Zilberfarb, V., de Coppet, P., Marullo, S., and Strosberg, A. D. (1998). Desensitization of the beta-adrenergic response in human brown adipocytes. *Endocrinology* 139, 2676–2684.

Jones, K. A., Borowsky, B., Tamm, J. A., and Gerald, C. (1998). GABAb receptors function as a heterotrimeric assembly of the subunits GABAbR1 and GAGbR2. *Nature* 396, 674–679.

Jordan, B. A., Trapaidze, N., Gomes, I., Nivarthi, R., and Devi, L. A. (2001). Oligomerization of opioid receptors with beta 2-adrenergic receptors: a role in trafficking and mitogen-activated protein kinase activation. *Proc. Natl. Acad. Sci. U.S.A.* 98, 343–348.

Juhasz, J. R., Hasbi, A., Rashid, A. J., So, C. H., George, S. R., and O'Dowd, B. F.

(2008). Mu-opioid receptor heterooligomer formation with the dopamine D1 receptor as directly visualized in living cells. *Eur. J. Pharmacol.* 581, 235–243.

Kachroo, A., Orlando, L. R., Grandy, D. K., Chen, J. F., Young, A. B., and Schwarzschild, M. A. (2005). Interactions between metabotropic glutamate 5 and adenosine A2A receptors in normal and parkinsonian mice. *J. Neurosci.* 25, 10414–10419.

Kalea, A. Z., and Batlle, D. (2010). Apelin and ACE2 in cardiovascular disease. *Curr. Opin. Investig. Drugs* 11, 273–282.

Kearn, C. S., Blake-Palmer, K., Daniel, E., Mackie, K., and Glass, M. (2005). Concurrent stimulation of cannabinoid CB1 and dopamine D2 receptors enhances heterodimer formation: a mechanism for receptor cross-talk? *Mol. Pharmacol.* 67, 1697–1704.

Kehr, J., Yoshitake, T., Wang, F. H., Razani, H., Gimenez-Llort, L., Jansson, A., Yamaguchi, M., and Ogren, S. O. (2002). Galanin is a potent in vivo modulator of mesencephalic serotonergic neurotransmission. *Neuropsychopharmacology* 27, 341–356.

Kitaoka, S., Furuyashiki, T., Nishi, A., Shuto, T., Koyasu, S., Matsuoka, T., Miyasaka, M., Greengard, P., and Narumiya, S. (2007). Prostaglandin E2 acts on EP1 receptor and amplifies both dopamine D1 and D2 receptor signaling in the striatum. *J. Neurosci.* 27, 12900–12907.

Kuteeva, E., Hokfelt, T., Wardi, T., and Ogren, S. O. (2008). Galanin, galanin receptor subtypes and depression-like behaviour. *Cell. Mol. Life Sci.* 65, 1854–1863.

Lee, S. P., So, C. H., Rashid, A. J., Varghese, G., Cheng, R., Lanca, A. J., O'Dowd, B. F., and George, S. R. (2004). Dopamine D1 and D2 receptor Co-activation generates a novel phospholipase C-mediated calcium signal. *J. Biol. Chem.* 279, 35671–35678.

Levoye, A., Dam, J., Ayoub, M. A., Guillaume, J. L., and Jockers, R. (2006). Do orphan G-protein-coupled receptors have ligand-independent functions? New insights from receptor heterodimers. *EMBO Rep.* 7, 1094–1098.

Lukasiewicz, S., Polit, A., Kedracka-Krok, S., Wedzony, K., Mackowiak, M., and Dziedzicka-Wasylewska, M. (2010). Hetero-dimerization of serotonin 5-HT(2A) and dopamine D(2) receptors. *Biochim. Biophys. Acta* 1803, 1347–1358.

Magalhaes, A. C., Holmes, K. D., Dale, L. B., Comps-Agrar, L., Lee, D., Yadav, P. N., Drysdale, L., Poulter, M. O., Roth, B. L., Pin, J. P., Anisman, H., and Ferguson, S. S. (2010). CRF receptor 1 regulates anxiety behavior via sensitization of 5-HT2 receptor signaling. *Nat. Neurosci.* 13, 622–629.

Marcellino, D., Carriba, P., Filip, M., Borgkvist, A., Frankowska, M., Bellido, I., Tanganelli, S., Muller, C. E., Fisone, G., Lluis, C., Agnati, L. F., Franco, R., and Fuxe, K. (2008). Antagonistic cannabinoid CB1/dopamine D2 receptor interactions in striatal CB1/D2 heteromers. A combined neurochemical and behavioral analysis. *Neuropharmacology* 54, 815–823.

McGraw, D. W., Mihlbachler, K. A., Schwarb, M. R., Rahman, F. F., Small, K. M., Almoosa, K. F., and Liggett, S. B. (2006). Airway smooth muscle prostaglandin-EP1 receptors directly modulate beta2-adrenergic receptors within a unique heterodimeric complex. *J. Clin. Invest.* 116, 1400–1409.

Millan, M. J., Marin, P., Bockaert, J., and Mannoury la Cour, C. (2008). Signaling at G-protein-coupled serotonin receptors: recent advances and future research directions. *Trends Pharmacol. Sci.* 29, 454–464.

Milligan, G. (2009). G protein-coupled receptor hetero-dimerization: contribution to pharmacology and function. *Br. J. Pharmacol.* 158, 5–14.

Missale, C., Fiorentini, C., Collo, G., and Spano, P. (2010). The neurobiology of dopamine receptors: evolution from the dual concept to heterodimer complexes. *J. Recept. Signal Transduct. Res.* 30, 347–354.

Nakata, H., Suzuki, T., Namba, K., and Oyanagi, K. (2010). Dimerization of G protein-coupled purinergic receptors: increasing the diversity of purinergic receptor signal responses and receptor functions. *J. Recept. Signal Transduct. Res.* 30, 337–346.

Nelson, G., Chandrashekar, J., Hoon, M. A., Feng, L., Zhao, G., Ryba, N. J., and Zuker, C. S. (2002). An amino-acid taste receptor. *Nature* 416, 199–202.

Nelson, G., Hoon, M. A., Chandrashekar, J., Zhang, Y., Ryba, N. J., and Zuker, C. S. (2001). Mammalian sweet taste receptors. *Cell* 106, 381–390.

Nijmeijer, S., Leurs, R., Smit, M. J., and Vischer, H. F. (2010). The Epstein–Barr virus-encoded G protein-coupled receptor BILF1 hetero-oligomerizes with human CXCR4, scavenges Galphai proteins, and constitutively impairs CXCR4 functioning. *J. Biol. Chem.* 285, 29632–29641.

Pello, O. M., Martinez-Munoz, L., Parrillas, V., Serrano, A., Rodriguez-Frade, J. M., Toro, M. J., Lucas, P., Monterrubio, M., Martinez, A. C., and Mellado, M. (2008). Ligand stabilization of CXCR4/delta-opioid receptor heterodimers reveals a mechanism for immune response regulation. *Eur. J. Immunol.* 38, 537–549.

Pepe, S., Xiao, R. P., Hohl, C., Altschuld, R., and Lakatta, E. G. (1997). "Cross talk" between opioid peptide and adrenergic receptor signaling in isolated rat heart. *Circulation* 95, 2122–2129.

Pfeiffer, M., Kirscht, S., Stumm, R., Koch, T., Wu, D., Laugsch, M., Schroder, H., Hollt, V., and Schulz, S. (2003). Heterodimerization of substance P and mu-opioid receptors regulates receptor trafficking and resensitization. *J. Biol. Chem.* 278, 51630–51637.

Pfleger, K. D., Kroeger, K. M., and Eidne, K. A. (2004). Receptors for hypothalamic releasing hormones TRH and GnRH: oligomerization and interactions with intracellular proteins. *Semin. Cell Dev. Biol.* 15, 269–280.

Pin, J. P., Neubig, R., Bouvier, M., Devi, L., Filizola, M., Javitch, J. A., Lohse, M. J., Milligan, G., Palczewski, K., Parmentier, M., and Spedding, M. (2007). International union of basic and clinical pharmacology. LXVII. recommendations for the recognition and nomenclature of G protein-coupled receptor heteromultimers. *Pharmacol. Rev.* 59, 5–13.

Prezeau, L., Rives, M. L., Comps-Agrar, L., Maurel, D., Kniazeff, J., and Pin, J. P. (2010). Functional crosstalk between GPCRs: with or without oligomerization. *Curr. Opin. Pharmacol.* 10, 6–13.

Prinster, S. C., Hague, C., and Hall, R. A. (2005). Heterodimerization of g protein-coupled receptors: specificity and functional significance. *Pharmacol. Rev.* 57, 289–298.

Rashid, A. J., So, C. H., Kong, M. M., Furtak, T., El-Ghundi, M., Cheng, R., O'Dowd, B. F., and George, S. R. (2007). D1–D2 dopamine receptor heterooligomers with unique pharmacology are coupled to rapid activation of Gq/11 in the striatum. *Proc. Natl. Acad. Sci. U.S.A.* 104, 654–659.

Rediger, A., Tarnow, P., Bickenbach, A., Schaefer, M., Krude, H., Gruters, A., and Biebermann, H. (2009). Heterodimerization of hypothalamic G-protein-coupled receptors involved in weight regulation. *Obes. Facts* 2, 80–86.

Rios, C., Gomes, I., and Devi, L. A. (2006). mu opioid and CB1 cannabinoid receptor interactions: reciprocal inhibition of receptor signaling and neuritogenesis. *Br. J. Pharmacol.* 148, 387–395.

Ripley, T. L., Gadd, C. A., De Felipe, C., Hunt, S. P., and Stephens, D. N. (2002). Lack of self-administration and behavioural sensitisation to morphine, but not cocaine, in mice lacking NK1 receptors. *Neuropharmacology* 43, 1258–1268.

Rivero-Muller, A., Chou, Y. Y., Ji, I., Lajic, S., Hanyaloglu, A. C., Jonas, K., Rahman, N., Ji, T. H., and Huhtaniemi, I. (2010). Rescue of defective G protein-coupled receptor function in vivo by intermolecular cooperation. *Proc. Natl. Acad. Sci. U.S.A.* 107, 2319–2324.

Rives, M. L., Vol, C., Fukazawa, Y., Tinel, N., Trinquet, E., Ayoub, M. A., Shigemoto, R., Pin, J. P., and Prezeau, L. (2009). Crosstalk between GABAB and mGlu1a receptors reveals new insight into GPCR signal integration. *EMBO J.* 28, 2195–2208.

Rocheville, M., Lange, D. C., Kumar, U., Patel, S. C., Patel, R. C., and Patel, Y. C. (2000). Receptors for dopamine and somatostatin: formation of hetero-oligomers with enhanced functional activity. *Science* 288, 154–157.

Rozenfeld, R., and Devi, L. A. (2010). Receptor heteromerization and drug discovery. *Trends Pharmacol. Sci.* 31, 124–130.

Sakai, T., Aoyama, M., Kusakabe, T., Tsuda, M., and Satake, H. (2009). Functional diversity of signaling pathways through G protein-coupled receptor heterodimerization with a species-specific orphan receptor subtype. *Mol. Biol. Evol.* 27, 1097–1106.

Sakurai, T., Yanagisawa, M., Takuwa, Y., Miyazaki, H., Kimura, S., Goto, K., and Masaki, T. (1990). Cloning of a cDNA encoding a non-isopeptide-selective subtype of the endothelin receptor. *Nature* 348, 732–735.

Salanga, C. L., O'Hayre, M., and Handel, T. (2009). Modulation of chemokine receptor activity through dimerization and crosstalk. *Cell. Mol. Life Sci.* 66, 1370–1386.

Salazar, N. C., Chen, J., and Rockman, H. A. (2007). Cardiac GPCRs: GPCR signaling in healthy and failing hearts. *Biochim. Biophys. Acta* 1768, 1006–1018.

Scavone, J. L., Mackie, K., and Van Bockstaele, E. J. (2010). Characterization of cannabinoid-1 receptors in the locus coeruleus: relationship with mu-opioid receptors. *Brain Res.* 1312, 18–31.

So, C. H., Verma, V., Alijaniaram, M., Cheng, R., Rashid, A. J., O'Dowd, B. F., and George, S. R. (2009). Calcium signaling by dopamine D5 receptor and D5-D2 receptor hetero-oligomers occurs by a mechanism distinct from that for dopamine D1-D2 receptor hetero-oligomers. *Mol. Pharmacol.* 75, 843–854.

Stolakis, V., Kalafatakis, K., Botis, J., Zarros, A., and Liapi, C. (2010). The regulatory role of neurotensin on the hypothalamic-anterior pituitary axons: emphasis on the control of thyroid-related functions. *Neuropeptides* 44, 1–7.

Takahashi, K., Furukawa, C., Takano, A., Ishikawa, N., Kato, T., Hayama, S., Suzuki, C., Yasui, W., Inai, K., Sone, S., Ito, T., Nishimura, H., Tsuchiya, E., Nakamura, Y., and Daigo, Y. (2006). The neuromedin U-growth hormone secretagogue receptor 1b/neurotensin receptor 1 oncogenic signaling pathway as a therapeutic target for lung cancer. *Cancer Res.* 66, 9408–9419.

Tanganelli, S., Sandager Nielsen, K., Ferraro, L., Antonelli, T., Kehr, J., Franco, R., Ferre, S., Agnati, L. F., Fuxe, K., and Scheel-Kruger, J. (2004). Striatal plasticity at the network level. Focus on adenosine A2A and D2 interactions in models of Parkinson's disease. *Parkinsonism Relat. Disord.* 10, 273–280.

Tebano, M. T., Martire, A., Chiodi, V., Pepponi, R., Ferrante, A., Domenici, M. R., Frank, C., Chen, J. F., Ledent, C., and Popoli, P. (2009). Adenosine A2A receptors enable the synaptic effects of cannabinoid CB1 receptors in the rodent striatum. *J. Neurochem.* 110, 1921–1930.

Terrillon, S., Durroux, T., Mouillac, B., Breit, A., Ayoub, M. A., Taulan, M., Jockers, R., Barberis, C., and Bouvier, M. (2003). Oxytocin and vasopressin V1a and V2 receptors form constitutive homo- and heterodimers during biosynthesis. *Mol. Endocrinol.* 17, 677–691.

Tien, L. T., Ho, I. K., and Ma, T. (2010). Methamphetamine-induced expression of zif268 mRNA is prevented by haloperidol in mice lacking mu-opioid receptor. *Neurotoxicology* 31, 326–330.

Tonazzini, I., Trincavelli, M. L., Montali, M., and Martini, C. (2008). Regulation of A1 adenosine receptor functioning induced by P2Y1 purinergic receptor activation in human astroglial cells. *J. Neurosci. Res.* 86, 2857–2866.

Tonazzini, I., Trincavelli, M. L., Storm-Mathisen, J., Martini, C., and Bergersen, L. H. (2007). Co-localization and functional cross-talk between A1 and P2Y1 purine receptors in rat hippocampus. *Eur. J. Neurosci.* 26, 890–902.

Trincavelli, M. L., Daniele, S., and Martini, C. (2010). Adenosine receptors: what we know and what we are learning. *Curr. Top. Med. Chem.* 10, 860–877.

Urizar, E., Montanelli, L., Loy, T., Bonomi, M., Swillens, S., Gales, C., Bouvier, M., Smits, G., Vassart, G., and Costagliola, S. (2005). Glycoprotein hormone receptors: link between receptor homodimerization and negative cooperativity. *EMBO J.* 24, 1954–1964.

van Rijn, R. M., Whistler, J. L., and Waldhoer, M. (2010). Opioid-receptor-heteromer-specific trafficking and pharmacology. *Curr. Opin. Pharmacol.* 10, 73–79.

Waldhoer, M., Fong, J., Jones, R. M., Lunzer, M. M., Sharma, S. K., Kostenis, E., Portoghese, P. S., and Whistler, J. L. (2005). A heterodimer-selective agonist shows in vivo relevance of G protein-coupled receptor dimers. *Proc. Natl. Acad. Sci. U.S.A.* 102, 9050–9055.

Wellman, P. J., Davis, K. W., and Nation, J. R. (2005). Augmentation of cocaine hyperactivity in rats by systemic ghrelin. *Regul. Pept.* 125, 151–154.

White, J. H., Wise, A., Main, M. J., Green, A., Fraser, N. J., Disney, G. H., Barnes, A. A., Emson, P., Foord, S. M., and Marshall, F. H. (1998). Heterodimerization is required for the formation of a functional GABA(B) receptor. *Nature* 396, 679–682.

Whorton, M. R., Bokoch, M. P., Rasmussen, S. G., Huang, B., Zare, R. N., Kobilka, B., and Sunahara, R. K. (2007). A monomeric G protein-coupled receptor isolated in a high-density lipoprotein particle efficiently activates its G protein. *Proc. Natl. Acad. Sci. U.S.A.* 104, 7682–7687.

Wilson, S. J., Roche, A. M., Kostetskaia, E., and Smyth, E. M. (2004). Dimerization of the human receptors for prostacyclin and thromboxane facilitates thromboxane receptor-mediated cAMP generation. *J. Biol. Chem.* 279, 53036–53047.

Wu, B., Chien, E. Y., Mol, C. D., Fenalti, G., Liu, W., Katritch, V., Abagyan, R., Brooun, A., Wells, P., Bi, F. C., Hamel, D. J., Kuhn, P., Handel, T. M., Cherezov, V., and Stevens, R. C. (2010). Structures of the CXCR4 chemokine GPCR with small-molecule and cyclic peptide antagonists. *Science.* 330, 1066–1071.

Xu, H., Staszewski, L., Tang, H., Adler, E., Zoller, M., and Li, X. (2004). Different functional roles of T1R subunits in the heteromeric taste receptors. *Proc. Natl. Acad. Sci. U.S.A.* 101, 14258–14263.

Yoshioka, K., Hosoda, R., Kuroda, Y., and Nakata, H. (2002). Hetero-oligomerization of adenosine A1 receptors with P2Y1 receptors in rat brains. *FEBS Lett.* 531, 299–303.

Zhang, F., Klebansky, B., Fine, R. M., Liu, H., Xu, H., Servant, G., Zoller, M., Tachdjian, C., and Li, X. (2010). Molecular mechanism of the sweet taste enhancers. *Proc. Natl. Acad. Sci. U.S.A.* 107, 4752–4757.

Zhang, F., Klebansky, B., Fine, R. M., Xu, H., Pronin, A., Liu, H., Tachdjian, C., and Li, X. (2008). Molecular mechanism for the umami taste synergism. *Proc. Natl. Acad. Sci. U.S.A.* 105, 20930–20934.

Zhu, W. Z., Chakir, K., Zhang, S., Yang, D., Lavoie, C., Bouvier, M., Hebert, T. E., Lakatta, E. G., Cheng, H., and Xiao, R. P. (2005). Heterodimerization of beta1- and beta2-adrenergic receptor subtypes optimizes beta-adrenergic modulation of cardiac contractility. *Circ. Res.* 97, 244–251.

Permissions

All chapters in this book were first published in TIN, by Frontiers; hereby published with permission under the Creative Commons Attribution License or equivalent. Every chapter published in this book has been scrutinized by our experts. Their significance has been extensively debated. The topics covered herein carry significant findings which will fuel the growth of the discipline. They may even be implemented as practical applications or may be referred to as a beginning point for another development.

The contributors of this book come from diverse backgrounds, making this book a truly international effort. This book will bring forth new frontiers with its revolutionizing research information and detailed analysis of the nascent developments around the world.

We would like to thank all the contributing authors for lending their expertise to make the book truly unique. They have played a crucial role in the development of this book. Without their invaluable contributions this book wouldn't have been possible. They have made vital efforts to compile up to date information on the varied aspects of this subject to make this book a valuable addition to the collection of many professionals and students.

This book was conceptualized with the vision of imparting up-to-date information and advanced data in this field. To ensure the same, a matchless editorial board was set up. Every individual on the board went through rigorous rounds of assessment to prove their worth. After which they invested a large part of their time researching and compiling the most relevant data for our readers.

The editorial board has been involved in producing this book since its inception. They have spent rigorous hours researching and exploring the diverse topics which have resulted in the successful publishing of this book. They have passed on their knowledge of decades through this book. To expedite this challenging task, the publisher supported the team at every step. A small team of assistant editors was also appointed to further simplify the editing procedure and attain best results for the readers.

Apart from the editorial board, the designing team has also invested a significant amount of their time in understanding the subject and creating the most relevant covers. They scrutinized every image to scout for the most suitable representation of the subject and create an appropriate cover for the book.

The publishing team has been an ardent support to the editorial, designing and production team. Their endless efforts to recruit the best for this project, has resulted in the accomplishment of this book. They are a veteran in the field of academics and their pool of knowledge is as vast as their experience in printing. Their expertise and guidance has proved useful at every step. Their uncompromising quality standards have made this book an exceptional effort. Their encouragement from time to time has been an inspiration for everyone.

The publisher and the editorial board hope that this book will prove to be a valuable piece of knowledge for researchers, students, practitioners and scholars across the globe.

List of Contributors

Stephanie Y. L. Ng, Leo T. O. Lee and Billy K. C. Chow
Endocrinology, School of Biological Sciences, The University of Hong Kong, Hong Kong, China

A. Couvineau, E. Ceraudo, Y.-V. Tan, P. Nicole and M. Laburthe
Faculté de Médecine Xavier Bichat, INSERM 773/ Centre de Recherche Biomédicale Bichat Beaujon (CRB3), Université Paris 7, Paris Cedex 18, France

Ingrid Langer
Institut de Recherche Interdisciplinaire en Biologie Humaine et Moléculaire, Faculté de Médecine, Université Libre de Bruxelles, Brussels, Belgium

Janna Blechman and Gil Levkowitz
Department of Molecular Cell Biology, Weizmann Institute of Science, Rehovot, Israel

Dora Reglodi and AndreaTamas
Department of Anatomy, Lendulet PACAP-Research Team of the University of Pécs and Hungarian Academy of Sciences, Pécs, Hungary

Miklos Koppan and Donat Szogyi
Department of Obstetrics and Gynaecology, University of Pécs, Pécs, Hungary

Laura Welke
Department of Anatomy, Ross University School of Medicine, Roseau, Commonwealth of Dominica

Meike Körner and Jean Claude Reubi
Division of Cell Biology and Experimental Research, Institute of Pathology, University of Berne, Berne, Switzerland

Emanuel Christ
Division of Endocrinology, Diabetology and Clinical Nutrition, University Hospital of Berne, Inselspital, Berne, Switzerland

Damian Wild
Division of Nuclear Medicine, Department of Radiology, University Basel Hospital, Basel, Switzerland

Mi Jin Moon, Sumi Park, Dong-Kyu Kim, Eun Bee Cho, Jong-Ik Hwang and Jae Young Seong
Graduate School of Medicine, Korea University, Seoul, Republic of Korea

Hubert Vaudry
INSERM U982, Laboratory of Neuronal and Neuroendocrine Differentiation and Communication, University of Rouen, Mont-Saint-Aignan, France

Véronique Gigoux and Daniel Fourmy
Université de Toulouse, Université Paul Sabatier, Toulouse, France

Arpád Dobolyi and Miklós Palkovits
Neuromorphological and Neuroendocrine Research Laboratory, Department of Anatomy, Histology and Embryology, Hungarian Academy of Sciences, Semmelweis University, Budapest, Hungary

Eugene Dimitrov and Ted B. Usdin
Section on Fundamental Neuroscience, National Institute of Mental Health, National Institute of Health, Bethesda, MD, USA

Jessica A. Krizo
Department of Biological Sciences, Kent State University, Kent, OH, USA

Eric M. Mintz
Department of Biological Sciences, Kent State University, Kent, OH, USA
School of Biomedical Sciences, Kent State University, Kent, OH, USA

Hsiao-Jou Cortina Chen, Jereme G. Spiers, Conrad Sernia and Nickolas A. Lavidis
School of Biomedical Sciences, The University of Queensland, Brisbane, QLD, Australia

Jereme G. Spiers, Hsiao-Jou Cortina Chen, Conrad Sernia and Nickolas A. Lavidis
School of Biomedical Sciences, The University of Queensland, Brisbane, QLD, Australia

Emily Alves and Femke T.A. Buisman-Pijlman
School of Medical Sciences, University of Adelaide, Adelaide, SA, Australia

Andrea Fielder
School of Midwifery, University of South Australia, Adelaide, SA, Australia

Nerelle Ghabriel
School of Midwifery, University of South Australia, Adelaide, SA, Australia
School of Psychology, University of South Australia, Adelaide, SA, Australia

Michael Sawyer
School of Paediatrics and Reproductive Health, University of Adelaide, Adelaide, SA, Australia
Research and Evaluation Unit, Women's and Children's Health Network, Adelaide, SA, Australia

Janet K. Bester-Meredith, Alexandria P. Fancher and Grace E. Mammarella
Department of Biology, Seattle Pacific University, Seattle, WA, USA

Jennifer Rainville
Department of Cell and Molecular Biology, Tulane University, New Orleans, LA, USA

Kevin Pollard
Neuroscience Program, Tulane University, New Orleans, LA, USA

NandiniVasudevan
Department of Cell and Molecular Biology, Tulane University, New Orleans, LA, USA
Neuroscience Program, Tulane University, New Orleans, LA, USA

Abimbola A. Akintola and Diana van Heemst
Department of Gerontology and Geriatrics, Leiden University Medical Center, Leiden, Netherlands

Jo E. Lewis
Queen's Medical Centre, School of Life Sciences, University of Nottingham Medical School, Nottingham, UK

John M. Brameld and Preeti H. Jethwa
Division of Nutritional Sciences, School of Biosciences, University of Nottingham, Loughborough, UK

Nicolette L. McGuire
Laboratory of Reproductive Neuroendocrinology, Department of Integrative Biology, University of California at Berkeley, Berkeley, CA, USA

George E. Bentley
Laboratory of Reproductive Neuroendocrinology, Department of Integrative Biology, University of California at Berkeley, Berkeley, CA, USA
Helen Wills Neuroscience Institute, University of California at Berkeley, Berkeley, CA, USA

Caroline Ménard
Neuroscience Division, Douglas Mental Health University Institute Research Center, Montreal, QC, Canada
Department of Psychiatry, McGill University, Montreal, QC, Canada
Laboratory of Neuroendocrinology of Aging, Centre Hospitalier de l'Université de Montréal Research Center, Montreal, QC, Canada
Department of Medicine, University of Montreal, Montreal, QC, Canada

Rémi Quirion
Neuroscience Division, Douglas Mental Health University Institute Research Center, Montreal, QC, Canada
Department of Psychiatry, McGill University, Montreal, QC, Canada

Sylvain Bouchard
Faculty of Medicine, University of Montreal, Montreal, QC, Canada

Guylaine Ferland
Hôpital du Sacré-Coeur de Montréal Research Center, Montreal, QC, Canada
Department of Nutrition, University of Montreal, Montreal, QC, Canada

Pierrette Gaudreau
Laboratory of Neuroendocrinology of Aging, Centre Hospitalier de l'Université de Montréal Research Center, Montreal, QC, Canada
Department of Medicine, University of Montreal, Montreal, QC, Canada

Md. Shahjahan, Takashi Kitahashi and Ishwar S. Parhar
Brain Research Institute, School of Medicine and Health Sciences, Monash University Malaysia, Petaling Jaya, Malaysia

Jean Luc Do Rego
INSERM, Mont-Saint-Aignan, France
European Institute for Peptide Research, IFRMP 23, Regional Platform for Cell Imaging, PRIMACEN, University of Rouen, Mont-Saint-Aignan, France
International Associated Laboratory Samuel de Champlain, Mont-Saint-Aignan, France

Jae Young Seong
Laboratory of G Protein-Coupled Receptors, Graduate School of Medicine, Korea University College of Medicine, Seoul, Korea

Van Luu-The
Research Center in Molecular Endocrinology, Oncology and Genetics, Laval University Hospital Center, Québec, QC, Canada

Delphine Burel, Jerôme Leprince, David Vaudry, Marie-Christine Tonon and Hubert Vaudry
INSERM, Mont-Saint-Aignan, France
European Institute for Peptide Research, IFRMP 23, Regional Platform for Cell Imaging, PRIMACEN, University of Rouen, Mont-Saint-Aignan, France
International Associated Laboratory Samuel de Champlain, Mont-Saint-Aignan, France
Laboratory of Neuronal and Neuroendocrine Differentiation and Communication, INSERM U982, University of Rouen, Mont-Saint-Aignan, France

Kazuyoshi Tsutsui
Laboratory of Integrative Brain Sciences, Department of Biology, Waseda University, Tokyo, Japan
Center for Medical Life Science of Waseda University, Tokyo, Japan

Georges Pelletier
Research Center in Molecular Endocrinology, Oncology and Genetics, Laval University Hospital Center, Québec, QC, Canada

Maud Kamal and Ralf Jockers
Department of Endocrinology, Metabolism and Cancer, INSERM U1016, Institut Cochin, Paris, France
CNRS UMR 8104, Paris, France
University Paris Descartes, Paris, France

Index

P

R

S

T

V

X

www.ingramcontent.com/pod-product-compliance
Lightning Source LLC
LaVergne TN
LVHW080926210926
848485LV00004B/740